The Department of Otolaryngology–Head and Neck Surgery at the University of Cincinnati evaluates and sees patients from around the United States and the world. All readers of this book worldwide are welcome to contact us for consultations or referrals, as you might need. Please use the following contact information (and mention that you are a reader):

to schedule consults/referrals for **Adult** ENT:

direct phone number: +1-513-475-8400
email: angie.keith@uchealth.com
website: www.uchealth.com/ent

to schedule consults/referrals for **Pediatric** ENT:

direct phone number: +1-513-636-4355
email: chmcent@cchmc.org
website: www.cincinnatichildrens.org/ent

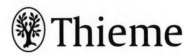

Otolaryngology Cases

The University of Cincinnati Clinical Portfolio

Second Edition

Myles L. Pensak, MD, FACS
H. B. Broidy Professor and Chairman
Department of Otolaryngology—Head and Neck Surgery
Professor of Neurologic Surgery
University of Cincinnati Academic Health Center
Cincinnati, Ohio

Catherine K. Hart, MD
Assistant Professor
Department of Otolaryngology—Head and Neck Surgery
University of Cincinnati Academic Health Center
Division of Pediatric Otolaryngology—Head and Neck Surgery
Cincinnati Children's Hospital Medical Center
Cincinnati, Ohio

Yash J. Patil, MD, FACS
Associate Professor
Department of Otolaryngology—Head and Neck Surgery
University of Cincinnati Academic Health Center
Cincinnati, Ohio

137 illustrations

Thieme
New York • Stuttgart • Delhi • Rio de Janeiro

Executive Editor: Timothy Y. Hiscock
Managing Editor: J. Owen Zurhellen IV
Editorial Assistant: Keith Palumbo
Director, Editorial Services: Mary Jo Casey
Production Editor: Torsten Scheihagen
International Production Director: Andreas Schabert
Editorial Director: Sue Hodgson
International Marketing Director: Fiona Henderson
International Sales Director: Louisa Turrell
Director of Institutional Sales: Adam Bernacki
Senior Vice President and Chief Operating Officer: Sarah Vanderbilt
President: Brian D. Scanlan
Printer: Replika Press Pvt. Ltd.

Library of Congress Cataloging-in-Publication Data

Names: Pensak, Myles L., editor. | Hart, Catherine K., editor. | Patil, Yash J., editor. | University of Cincinnati. Department of Otolaryngology and Maxillofacial Surgery.
Title: Otolaryngology cases : the University of Cincinnati clinical portfolio / [edited by] Myles L. Pensak, Catherine K. Hart, Yash J. Patil.
Description: Second edition. | New York : Thieme, [2018] | Includes bibliographical references and index.
Identifiers: LCCN 2016049909 (print) | LCCN 2016050231 (ebook) | ISBN 9781626234192 (soft cover : alk. paper) | ISBN 9781626234202 (eISBN) | ISBN 9781626234208
Subjects: | MESH: Otorhinolaryngologic Diseases | Otolaryngology | Diagnosis, Differential | Case Reports
Classification: LCC RF56 (print) | LCC RF56 (ebook) | NLM WV 150 | DDC 617.5/1–dc23
LC record available at https://lccn.loc.gov/2016049909

Thieme Publishers New York
333 Seventh Avenue, New York, NY 10001 USA
+1 800 782 3488, customerservice@thieme.com

Thieme Publishers Stuttgart
Rüdigerstrasse 14, 70469 Stuttgart, Germany
+49 [0]711 8931 421, customerservice@thieme.de

Thieme Publishers Delhi
A-12, Second Floor, Sector-2, Noida-201301
Uttar Pradesh, India
+91 120 45 566 00, customerservice@thieme.in

Thieme Publishers Rio de Janeiro, Thieme Publicações Ltda.
Edifício Rodolpho de Paoli, 25º andar
Av. Nilo Peçanha, 50 – Sala 2508
Rio de Janeiro 20020-906 Brasil
+55 21 3172-2297 / +55 21 3172-1896

Cover design: Thieme Publishing Group
Typesetting by DiTech Process Solutions

Printed in India by Replika Press Pvt. Ltd.   5 4 3 2 1

ISBN 978-1-62623-419-2

Also available as an e-book:
eISBN 978-1-62623-420-8

Important note: Medicine is an ever-changing science undergoing continual development. Research and clinical experience are continually expanding our knowledge, in particular our knowledge of proper treatment and drug therapy. Insofar as this book mentions any dosage or application, readers may rest assured that the authors, editors, and publishers have made every effort to ensure that such references are in accordance with **the state of knowledge at the time of production of the book.**

Nevertheless, this does not involve, imply, or express any guarantee or responsibility on the part of the publishers in respect to any dosage instructions and forms of applications stated in the book. **Every user is requested to examine carefully** the manufacturers' leaflets accompanying each drug and to check, if necessary in consultation with a physician or specialist, whether the dosage schedules mentioned therein or the contraindications stated by the manufacturers differ from the statements made in the present book. Such examination is particularly important with drugs that are either rarely used or have been newly released on the market. Every dosage schedule or every form of application used is entirely at the user's own risk and responsibility. The authors and publishers request every user to report to the publishers any discrepancies or inaccuracies noticed. If errors in this work are found after publication, errata will be posted at www.thieme.com on the product description page.

Some of the product names, patents, and registered designs referred to in this book are in fact registered trademarks or proprietary names even though specific reference to this fact is not always made in the text. Therefore, the appearance of a name without designation as proprietary is not to be construed as a representation by the publisher that it is in the public domain.

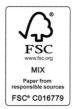

This second edition is dedicated to the caring support and professional staff whom we, the physicians of the Department of Otolaryngology–Head and Neck Surgery, are fortunate to work beside in the daily care of our patients at UC Health, Cincinnati Children's Hospital Medical Center, and the VA Medical Center.

Contents

XIV Trauma

XV Facial Plastic and Reconstructive Surgery

Foreword

I am quite honored to have been asked by Dr. Myles L. Pensak to write this Foreword for the second edition of his book, *Otolaryngology Cases: The University of Cincinnati Clinical Portfolio*. We have been blessed by the University of Cincinnati for educating several of our finest clinical faculty, three of whom have endowed professorships here at the University of North Carolina at Chapel Hill. Dr. William Shockley did his residency at the University of Cincinnati, Dr. Mark Weissler did his fellowship in Head and Neck Oncology there, and Dr. Amelia Drake did her Pediatric Otolaryngology fellowship at Cincinnati also. All three are fabulous teachers, outstanding clinicians, and wonderful investigators. Keeping that in mind, I reviewed the chapters for the second edition of this book and have found the style of each presentation to be outstanding. In every area of otolaryngology, a clinical pathology is presented in a patient-based scenario. The material is very easy for the reader to follow, and the differential diagnoses and management options are very current. Any reader can understand the rationale for therapy and the different modalities that are used in planning for diagnosis and management.

The bibliography at the end of each chapter allows the reader to probe further into the background information that would lead to management options for each clinical scenario. This is the kind of organized approach to patient care that one finds in the minds of the best clinicians in medicine. Dr. Pensak and his colleagues at the University of Cincinnati have done an outstanding job of conveying their expertise to the reader in a way that allows any clinician to understand the nuances of state-of-the-art diagnosis and therapy. There are many new chapters which reflect innovations in our specialty and offer the opportunity for the reader to become acquainted with the exciting new faculty at the University of Cincinnati. I feel that this book has an outstanding capacity to elevate the level of care in our field to that which would be available in one of the leading institutions in our country, the University of Cincinnati School of Medicine!

Harold C. Pillsbury III, MD
Chair, Department of Otolaryngology/Head and
Neck Surgery
University of North Carolina School of Medicine
Chapel Hill, North Carolina

Preface

The case study format has become popular as a teaching tool in a multiplicity of disciplines. Included among these are the familiar case studies in business, law, the social sciences and medicine. Despite an ever expanding universe of data in both basic and clinical science information, for the clinician the case study model remains a cornerstone of the pedagogic model. Moreover, the case study format encourages a disciplined approach to patient assessment and management options by establishing a uniform algorithm in obtaining and utilizing discreet points of data.

The first edition of this book had been published in 2010. This second edition includes new cases and updates on foundational chapters as well as over 20 new studies reflecting the changes in diagnostics and therapeutics that have become part of the clinical armamentarium of the contemporary otolaryngologist. As with our earlier edition, the faculty have carefully chosen illustrative examples of pathologic scenarios that are most likely to present to the general otolaryngologist. Updated illustrations and radiographic and pathologic studies accompany the text where visual illustration is felt to enhance the reader's understanding. Each chapter has a highlighted bibliography and associated test questions to ensure that salient parts emphasized in the case study are appreciated. The uniform format of the chapters is intended to optimize an appreciation for the efficient and cost effective management of our patients. The text is divided by subspecialty discipline to enhance the learning experience.

It is the hope of the authors that the text will provide a clearly articulated, well-organized state-of-the-art studies profile that will enable practitioners to optimize patient care. Readers are encouraged to visit the department's website www.ENT.uc.edu for further patient and professional information, as well as interdisciplinary links.

Myles L. Pensak, MD, FACS
Catherine K. Hart, MD
Yash J. Patil, MD, FACS

Acknowledgments

The authors extend their sincerest appreciation to Laura Hebert for her work on this book and her ongoing commitment to the tripartite mission of the Department of Otolaryngology–Head and Neck Surgery, University of Cincinnati Academic Health Center.

Contributors

Alessandro de Alarcon, MD
Director, Center for Pediatric Voice Disorders
Cincinnati Children's Hospital Medical Center
Department of Otolaryngology–Head and Neck
  Surgery
University of Cincinnati Academic Health Center
Cincinnati, Ohio

Douglas C. von Allmen, MD
Resident
Department of Otolaryngology–Head and Neck
  Surgery
University of Cincinnati Academic Health Center
Cincinnati, Ohio

John F. Barrord, MD
Assistant Professor
Department of Otolaryngology–Head and Neck
  Surgery
University of Cincinnati Academic Health Center
Cincinnati, Ohio

Hayley L. Born, MD
Resident Physician
Department of Otolaryngology–Head and Neck
  Surgery
University of Cincinnati Academic Health Center
Cincinnati, Ohio

Daniel I. Choo, MD
Professor and Director, Pediatric Otolaryngology
Department of Otolaryngology–Head and Neck
  Surgery
Cincinnati Children's Hospital Medical Center
University of Cincinnati Academic Health Center
Cincinnati, Ohio

Ryan M. Collar, MD, MBA
Assistant Professor
Department of Otolaryngology–Head and Neck
  Surgery
University of Cincinnati Academic Health Center
Cincinnati, Ohio

Robin T. Cotton, MD, FACS, FRCS(C)
Professor of Pediatrics and Otolaryngology–Head and
  Neck Surgery
University of Cincinnati Academic Health Center
Director, Aerodigestive Center
Division of Pediatric Otolaryngology–Head and Neck
  Surgery
Cincinnati Children's Hospital Medical Center
Cincinnati, Ohio

Ryan A. Crane, MD
Resident Physician
Department of Otolaryngology–Head and Neck
  Surgery
University of Cincinnati Academic Health Center
Cincinnati, Ohio

Michael A. DeMarcantonio, MD
Former Pediatric Fellow, Cincinnati Children's
  Hospital Medical Center
Department of Otolaryngology–Head and Neck
  Surgery
University of Cincinnati Academic Health Center
Cincinnati, Ohio
Staff Physician
Eisenhower Army Medical Center
Augusta, Georgia

Colin R. Edwards, MD
Resident
Department of Otolaryngology–Head and Neck
  Surgery
University of Cincinnati Academic Health Center
Cincinnati, Ohio

Brian D. Goico, MD
Former Chief Resident
Department of Otolaryngology–Head and Neck
  Surgery
University of Cincinnati Academic Health Center
Group Health TriHealth Physician Partners
Cincinnati, Ohio

Adam D. Goodale, MD
Resident
Department of Otolaryngology–Head and Neck
  Surgery
University of Cincinnati Academic Health Center
Cincinnati, Ohio

John H. Greinwald Jr., MD
Professor
Department of Otolaryngology–Head and Neck
  Surgery
University of Cincinnati Academic Health Center
Cincinnati Children's Hospital Medical Center
Cincinnati, Ohio

Thomas K. Hamilton, MD
Resident
Department of Otolaryngology–Head and Neck
  Surgery
University of Cincinnati Academic Health Center
Cincinnati, Ohio

Jeffrey J. Harmon, MD
Resident
Department of Otolaryngology–Head and Neck
  Surgery
University of Cincinnati Academic Health Center
Cincinnati, Ohio

Catherine K. Hart, MD
Assistant Professor
Department of Otolaryngology—Head and Neck
  Surgery
University of Cincinnati Academic Health Center
Division of Pediatric Otolaryngology—Head and Neck
  Surgery
Cincinnati Children's Hospital Medical Center
Cincinnati, Ohio

Christine H. Heubi, MD
Clinical Fellow
Division of Pediatric Otolaryngology–Head and Neck
  Surgery
Cincinnati Children's Hospital Medical Center
Cincinnati, Ohio

Brian L. Hendricks, MD
Resident
Department of Otolaryngology–Head and Neck
  Surgery
University of Cincinnati Academic Health Center
Cincinnati, Ohio

Brian Ho, MD
Clinical Surgical Senior Fellow
Cincinnati Children's Hospital Medical Center
University of Cincinnati Academic Health Center
Cincinnati, Ohio

David B. Hom, MD, FACS
Professor and Director, Division of Facial Plastic and
  Reconstructive Surgery
Department of Otolaryngology–Head and Neck
  Surgery
University of Cincinnati Academic Health Center
Cincinnati, Ohio

Rebecca J. Howell, MD
Assistant Professor of Laryngology
Department of Otolaryngology–Head and Neck
  Surgery
Associate Director, Voice, Swallowing, and Airway
  Center
University of Cincinnati Academic Health Center
Cincinnati, Ohio

Stacey L. Ishman, MD, MPH
Professor
Department of Otolaryngology–Head and Neck
  Surgery
University of Cincinnati Academic Health Center
Cincinnati Children's Hospital Medical Center
Cincinnati, Ohio

Niall D. Jefferson, MD, FRACS
Former Pediatric Fellow, Cincinnati Children's
  Hospital Medical Center
Department of Otolaryngology–Head and Neck
  Surgery
University of Cincinnati Academic Health Center
Cincinnati, Ohio
Conjoint Assistant Professor
John Hunter Hospital
Newcastle, New South Wales, Australia

Sid M. Khosla, MD
Associate Professor
Department of Otolaryngology–Head and Neck
  Surgery
University of Cincinnati Academic Health Center
Cincinnati, Ohio

Brittany A. Leader, MD
Resident
Department of Otolaryngology–Head and Neck
  Surgery
University of Cincinnati Academic Health Center
Cincinnati, Ohio

David R. Lee, MD
Resident
Department of Otolaryngology–Head and Neck
  Surgery
University of Cincinnati Academic Health Center
Cincinnati, Ohio

Jonathan R. Mark, MD
Assistant Professor
Department of Otolaryngology–Head and Neck
  Surgery
University of Cincinnati Academic Health Center
Cincinnati, Ohio

Amy M. Manning, MD
Resident
Department of Otolaryngology–Head and Neck
  Surgery
University of Cincinnati Academic Health Center
Cincinnati, Ohio

Charles M. Myer III, MD, FACS
Professor and Vice Chairman
Department of Otolaryngology–Head and Neck
  Surgery
University of Cincinnati Academic Health Center
Cincinnati Children's Hospital Medical Center
Cincinnati, Ohio

Charles M. Myer IV, MD
Assistant Professor
Department of Otolaryngology–Head and Neck
  Surgery
University of Cincinnati Academic Health Center
Division of Pediatric Otolaryngology–Head and Neck
  Surgery
Cincinnati Children's Hospital Medical Center
Cincinnati, Ohio

Patrick R. Owens, MD
Resident Physician
Department of Otolaryngology–Head and Neck
  Surgery
University of Cincinnati Academic Health Center
Cincinnati Children's Hospital Medical Center
Cincinnati, Ohio

Reena Dhanda Patil, MD, MBA
Assistant Professor
Veterans Affairs Site Director
Director of Medical Student Education
University of Cincinnati Academic Health Center
Cincinnati, Ohio

Yash J. Patil, MD, FACS
Associate Professor
Department of Otolaryngology–Head and Neck
  Surgery
University of Cincinnati Academic Health Center
Cincinnati, Ohio

Myles L. Pensak, MD, FACS
H. B. Broidy Professor and Chairman
Department of Otolaryngology–Head and Neck
  Surgery
Professor of Neurologic Surgery
University of Cincinnati Academic Health Center
Cincinnati, Ohio

Andrew J. Redmann, MD
Resident
Department of Otolaryngology–Head and Neck
  Surgery
University of Cincinnati Academic Health Center
Cincinnati, Ohio

Michael J. Rutter, MD
Professor
Department of Otolaryngology–Head and Neck
  Surgery
University of Cincinnati Academic Health Center
Cincinnati Children's Hospital Medical Center
Cincinnati, Ohio

Ravi N. Samy, MD, FACS
Chief, Division of Otology/Neurotology
Program Director, Neurotology Fellowship
Associate Professor
Department of Otolaryngology–Head and Neck
  Surgery
University of Cincinnati Academic Health Center
Cincinnati Children's Hospital Medical Center
Cincinnati, Ohio

Alfred M. Sassler, DO, FACS, FAAOA
Associate Professor
Department of Otolaryngology–Head and Neck
 Surgery
Director, ENT Allergy Program, Rhinology Division
University of Cincinnati Academic Health Center
Cincinnati, Ohio

Allen M. Seiden, MD
Professor
Department of Otolaryngology–Head and Neck
 Surgery
University of Cincinnati Academic Health Center
Cincinnati, Ohio

Tasneem A. Shikary, MD
Former Chief Resident
Department of Otolaryngology–Head and Neck
 Surgery
University of Cincinnati Academic Health Center
Group Health TriHealth Physician Partners
Cincinnati, Ohio

Sally R. Shott, MD
Professor
Department of Otolaryngology–Head and Neck
 Surgery
University of Cincinnati Academic Health Center
Cincinnati Children's Hospital Medical Center
Cincinnati, Ohio

David F. Smith, MD, PhD
Department of Otolaryngology–Head and Neck
 Surgery
University of Cincinnati Academic Health Center
Clinical Fellow, Sleep Medicine
Division of Pulmonary Medicine
Cincinnati Children's Hospital Medical Center
Cincinnati, Ohio

Shawn M. Stevens, MD
Fellow, Neurotology Otology and Skull Base Surgery
Department of Otolaryngology–Head and Neck
 Surgery
University of Cincinnati Academic Health Center
Cincinnati, Ohio

David L. Steward, MD, FACS
Professor and Director, Division of Head and Neck
 Surgery
Department of Otolaryngology–Head and Neck
 Surgery
University of Cincinnati Academic Health Center
Cincinnati, Ohio

Alice L. Tang, MD
Former Chief Resident
Department of Otolaryngology–Head and Neck
 Surgery
University of Cincinnati Academic Health Center
Cincinnati, Ohio
Head and Neck Oncology and Reconstructive Fellow
Vanderbilt University
Nashville, Tennessee

Kareem O. Tawfik, MD
Resident
Department of Otolaryngology–Head and Neck
 Surgery
University of Cincinnati Academic Health Center
Cincinnati, Ohio

Jamie L. Welshhans, MD
Resident
Department of Otolaryngology–Head and Neck
 Surgery
University of Cincinnati Academic Health Center
Cincinnati, Ohio

Nathan D. Wiebracht, MD
Resident
Department of Otolaryngology–Head and Neck
 Surgery
University of Cincinnati Academic Health Center
Cincinnati, Ohio

J. Paul Willging, MD
Professor
Department of Otolaryngology–Head and Neck
 Surgery
University of Cincinnati Academic Health Center
Director, Clinical Operations Division of Pediatric
 Otolaryngology
Cincinnati Children's Hospital Medical Center
Cincinnati, Ohio

Keith M. Wilson, MD, FACS
Associate Professor
Director, Head and Neck Oncologic Surgery
  Fellowship
Department of Otolaryngology–Head and Neck
  Surgery
University of Cincinnati Academic Health Center
Cincinnati, Ohio

Andre M. Wineland, MD, MSCI
Senior Clinical Fellow
Division of Pediatric Otolaryngology–Head and Neck
  Surgery
Cincinnati Children's Hospital Medical Center
Cincinnati, Ohio

Lee A. Zimmer, MD, PhD, FACS
Associate Professor and Director, Division of Rhinol-
  ogy and Anterior Skull Base Surgery
Department of Otolaryngology–Head and Neck
  Surgery
University of Cincinnati Academic Health Center
Cincinnati, Ohio

Part I
Pediatric Otology

I

1 Congenital Hearing Loss

Brian Ho and John H. Greinwald Jr.

1.1 History

A 20-month-old girl was referred for hearing evaluation after failing a newborn hearing screen at birth. The parents related a history of a full-term pregnancy and normal delivery, although complicated by maternal influenza at 6 months' gestation. The mother received promethazine hydrochloride (Phenergan, Wyeth, New Jersey), a histamine type 1 antagonist, during pregnancy for nausea. Family history included a cousin with Usher syndrome. The patient failed the newborn hearing screening with distortion product otoacoustic emissions (DPOAEs) absent for the 2- to 6-kHz range. Auditory brainstem response (ABR) testing via air and bone conduction was consistent with severe to profound bilateral sensorineural hearing loss (SNHL). Genetic testing was negative for *GJB2* (connexin 26) and Usher syndrome. She received sequential cochlear implants and is now rehabilitating her hearing and speech.

1.2 Differential Diagnosis—Key Points

About 6 in 1,000 children in the United States are born annually with mild to moderate hearing loss, and 1 in 1,000 are born with severe to profound SNHL. Fifty percent of hearing loss is due to environmental causes such as maternal infection (toxoplasmosis, rubella, cytomegalovirus [CMV]), prematurity, postnatal viral/bacterial infections (e.g., meningitis), or ototoxic drugs (e.g., antibiotics). The other 50% is due to genetic causes. Of the genetic hearing loss, 70% is nonsyndromic. The majority of nonsyndromic hearing loss is autosomal recessive (80%), with autosomal dominant (17%), X-linked (3%), and mitochondrial (< 1%) hearing losses making up the remainder of the group. Syndromic hearing loss makes up 30% of inherited hearing loss, meaning that these individuals have other phenotypic manifestations along with their hearing loss.

1.2.1 Autosomal Recessive (80%) Nonsyndromic Hearing Loss (70%)

Connexins

Mutations in the gap junction β-2 gene (*GJB2*) encoding the connexin 26 protein (Cx26) on the long arm of chromosome 13 (13q11) account for 50% of autosomal recessive nonsyndromic hearing loss (ARNSHL). The most common *GJB2* mutation is 35delG. Cx26 is expressed in the stria vascularis, spiral ligament, spiral limbus, and supporting cells of the cochlea, forming intercellular channels called *gap junctions*. Gap junctions allow potassium to be recycled from the endolymph to the stria vascularis to maintain the endolymphatic potential. Most *GJB2* mutations confer severe to profound hearing loss. A 342-kb deletion in the *GJB6* gene encoding the connexin 30 protein (Cx30) upstream from *GJB2* is responsible for 3% of heterozygotes (deaf individuals with a *GJB2* mutation on only one of two alleles) in the United States. Higher rates have been identified in Spanish populations (66%).

Enlarged Vestibular Aqueduct Syndrome

Patients with enlarged vestibular aqueduct syndrome (EVAS) have large vestibular aqueducts, hearing loss, and incomplete cochlear partitioning (Mondini's malformation) similar to that seen in Pendred's syndrome, without thyroid abnormalities. The hearing loss ranges from mild to profound, the audiogram is flat or downsloping, and the loss is sensorineural or mixed. SNHL can be progressive or sudden following head trauma. The *SLC26A4* mutation seen in Pendred's syndrome is identified in 25% of patients with EVAS. Interestingly, many patients with EVAS are found to be heterozygote for mutations in the SLC26A4 gene. This does not represent a dominant inheritance pattern, but a second, yet to be discovered, mutation is thought to be present.

Otoferlin

The *OTOF* gene encodes otoferlin, a membrane-anchored, calcium-binding protein that plays a role in the exocytosis of synaptic vesicles at the auditory inner hair cell ribbon synapse. It is associated with prelingual profound SNHL and inherited auditory neuropathy/auditory dyssynchrony (AN/AD), which is characterized by the presence of otoacoustic emissions (OAEs) and a cochlear microphonic on ABR (one early cochlear wave with no waves from the auditory pathway). Treatment

Table 1.1 Usher syndrome

Type	Common gene	% of patients	Hearing	Vestibular function	Visual	Clinical
1	MYO7A	40%	Congenital bilateral severe to profound SNHL	Abnormal	Early onset RP by age 10	Amplification ineffective Manual communication Late motor milestones
2	USH2A	60%	Moderate SNHL (sloping audiogram)	Normal	RP onset in second decade	Hearing aids effective Oral communication
3	USH3A	3%	Progressive SNHL	Variable or progressive	Variable onset of RP	Variable

Abbreviations: RP, retinitis pigmentosa; SNHL, sensorineural hearing loss

includes frequency modulation (FM) devices and hearing aids for mild to moderate hearing loss and cochlear implantation for severe SNHL.

1.2.2 Autosomal Dominant (20%) Nonsyndromic Hearing Loss (70%)

Connexins

Dominant mutations in the GJB2 and GJB6 genes have been reported but occur less frequently than recessive mutations.

WFS1 Gene

Mutations in the WFS1 gene confer SNHL affecting frequencies below 2000, Hz and worsening over time. Patients retain excellent understanding of speech, and many choose not to wear hearing aids.

COCH Gene

Mutations in the COCH gene are associated with high-frequency SNHL that presents in the second to fourth decade of life and progresses to profound SNHL by the fifth decade. Many experience recurrent bouts of vertigo similar to Meniere's disease.

1.2.3 Autosomal Recessive (80%) Syndromic Hearing Loss (30%)

Usher Syndrome

The incidence of Usher syndrome is 1 in 25,000, affecting 2 to 4% of the deaf population and 50% of the deaf and blind population. Individuals have SNHL, retinitis pigmentosa, and vestibular dysfunction. Three types of Usher syndrome are recognized (▶ Table 1.1). Electroretinography can identify photoreceptor abnormalities in children 2 years of age, which is earlier than can be done using funduscopic examination. Rehabilitation with hearing aids, cochlear implantation, and educational and vocational planning is essential.

Pendred's Syndrome

Pendred's syndrome accounts for 1 to 2% of profound congenital deafness. Mutations in the SLC26A4 (PDS) gene and pendrin protein affect iodine and chloride ion transport. The syndrome is characterized by severe to profound or progressive SNHL, cochlear abnormalities (Mondini's malformation, large vestibular aqueduct, malformed vestibular canals), vestibular dysfunction, and euthyroid goiter in early puberty or adulthood. Genetic testing is used to make the diagnosis because the perchlorate discharge test that was historically used is neither sensitive nor specific. Thyroid function tests should be obtained and exogenous thyroid hormone used rather than thyroid surgery.

Jervell and Lange-Nielsen Syndrome

Jervell and Lange-Nielsen syndrome accounts for 0.1% of profound deafness. It is characterized by severe to profound SNHL, QT-interval prolongation, large T waves, and torsades de pointes on electrocardiography (ECG), with ventricular arrhythmia, syncope, seizure, or sudden death in the second or third decade of life. There may be a family history of syncope, seizure, sudden infant death syndrome (SIDS), or sudden death, and first-degree relatives may have cardiac irregularities without SNHL. Mutations in *KVLQT1* and *KCNE1* that regulate potassium channels in the ear and heart have been identified in some families. Patients and family members should receive an ECG and be referred to cardiology for beta-blockade.

Biotinidase Deficiency

Biotin is a water-soluble B vitamin essential for gluconeogenesis, fatty acid synthesis, and amino acid catabolism. About 1 in 60,000 children are born without biotinidase and cannot recycle biotin. Failure to add biotin to the diet will result in irreversible SNHL, optic atrophy, seizures, hypertonia, developmental delay, ataxia, skin rash, alopecia, and conjunctivitis. Consider this disorder when a child presents with SNHL and ataxia.

Refsum's Disease

This rare disorder, caused by faulty phytanic acid metabolism, manifests as severe progressive SNHL and retinitis pigmentosa. Patients have a high serum concentration of phytanic acid and can be treated with dietary modification and plasmapharesise.

1.2.4 Autosomal Dominant Syndromic Hearing Loss (17%)

Waardenburg's Syndrome

Waardenburg syndrome accounts for 2% of profound deafness. Abnormalities in tissues of neural crest origin lead to SNHL (unilateral or bilateral), enlarged vestibular aqueduct, pigmentary changes such as a white forelock (varying age of first appearance), early graying of the hair, vitiligo, synophrys (eyebrows grow together), blue eyes or heterochromia iridis (different colored eyes), dystopia canthorum (lateral displacement of inner canthi), pinched nose, craniofacial abnormalities, neural tube defects, gastrointestinal dyskinesia,

and limb defects. Four types are recognized, the most common being type 1 (▶ Table 1.2).

CHARGE Syndrome

The CHARGE acronym stands for coloboma of the eye, heart anomaly, choanal atresia, retardation, and genitourinary and ear anomalies. The incidence is 0.1 to 1.2 per 10,000, and more than 75% of patients have mutations in the *CHD7* gene. A definite clinical diagnosis includes all four major characteristics: (1) coloboma of the iris, retina, choroid, or disc; (2) choanal atresia (bilateral or left-sided); (3) cranial nerve (CN) dysfunction (CNI, CNVII, CNVIII, CNIX, CNX); (4) characteristic ear (short, wide, asymmetric protruding pinna with little lobe, ossicular and Mondini's malformations, hypoplastic or absent semicircular canal). A probable diagnosis includes one major plus several minor characteristics, which include (1) developmental delay and hypotonia; (2) growth deficiency; (3) square face, prominent forehead and nasal bridge, and flat midface; (4) cleft lip, palate, or both; (5) cardiovascular malformations; (6) tracheoesophageal fistula; and (7) delayed puberty. Patients should be evaluated for respiratory distress, aspiration, swallowing, and hearing and also should be referred for neurologic, visual, cardiac, and urologic workup.

Branchio-oto-renal Syndrome (Melnick-Fraser Syndrome)

The incidence of branchio-oto-renal (BOR) syndrome is 1 in 40,000. *EYA1* gene mutations on chromosome 8q13 are identified in 40% of individuals with the BOR phenotype, which is inherited with high penetrance and variable expressivity. The clinical diagnosis is based on three major criteria, two major and two minor criteria, or one major criterion and an affected first degree relative (▶ Table 1.3). The combination of a hypoplastic cochlea, facial nerve deviated to the medial side of

Table 1.2 Waardenburg syndrome types

Type	Name	Common gene	Differentiating clinical feature(s)
1	Waardenburg syndrome	*PAX3*	Dystopia canthorum
2	Tietz syndrome	*MITF*	Dystopia canthorum absent
3	Klein-Waardenburg syndrome	*PAX3*	Features of type 1 plus upper limb defects
4	Shah-Wardenburg syndrome	*SOX10, EDNRB, EDN3*	Features of type 2 plus Hirschsprung's disease

Table 1.3 Branchio-oto-renal syndrome diagnostic criteria

Major	Minor
Hearing loss (conductive, sensorineural, mixed)	External ear
Prehelical pits	Middle ear
Branchial cleft cyst/fistula	Inner ear
Renal dysplasia/malformed calyces, aplasia, polycystic kidney	Tags

Table 1.4 Stickler syndrome

Type	Common Gene	Differentiating Clinical Feature(s)
1	COL2A1	Classic Stickler syndrome (see description in text)
2	COL11A1	More severe hearing loss and thick bundles throughout vitreous cavity of eye
3	COL11A2	No ocular abnormalities

the cochlea, funnel-shaped internal auditory canal, patulous eustachian tube, and kissing carotid arteries is pathognomonic for BOR.

Stickler Syndrome

The incidence of Stickler syndrome is 1 in 8,000; however, only 40% have SNHL. Stickler syndrome is a connective tissue disorder characterized by ocular findings (myopia, cataract, retinal detachment), hearing loss (high-frequency conductive loss or progressive SNHL), flat "scooped-out" midface, micrognathia, Pierre Robin sequence, spondyloepiphyseal dysplasia congenital, short stature, precocious arthritis, marfanoid habitus, and mitral valve prolapse. Evaluation of hearing, vision, the airway, and the heart is required. Contact sports should be avoided because of the risk of retinal detachment, and family members should be screened for visual or hearing impairment (▶ Table 1.4).

Neurofibromatosis Type 2

Mutations in the tumor suppressor gene schwannomin on chromosome 22q11 lead to neurofibromatosis type 2 (NF2). Diagnostic criteria include (1) bilateral acoustic neuromas or (2) unilateral acoustic neuroma or two of neurofibroma, meningioma, glioma, schwannoma, juvenile lenticular opacity, and a first-degree relative with NF2. Symptoms include unilateral hearing loss, tinnitus, imbalance, and vertigo in the second decade of life, with contralateral symptoms around 2 years later. Diagnosis requires magnetic resonance imaging (MRI) with gadolinium. Treatment includes observation, gamma knife, or surgery. Family members should receive genetic testing.

Treacher Collins Syndrome (Mandibulofacial Dysostosis)

Mutations in the TCOF1 gene and treacle protein lead to bilateral ear anomalies (microtia, aural atresia, conductive hearing loss, SNHL, vestibular dysfunction), downsloping palpebral fissures, coloboma of the outer lower eyelid, absent eyelashes, hypoplastic zygomatic arch, micrognathia, cleft palate, parotid hypoplasia, and normal intelligence. Evaluation of hearing and sleep apnea is required. In contrast, individuals with Goldenhar syndrome have unilateral facial anomalies and upper eyelid coloboma.

Apert-Crouzon Syndrome

The incidence of Apert syndrome is 1 in 65,000. FGFR2 mutations that result from increased paternal age lead to coronal suture craniosynostosis (prominent forehead, flat occiput), large fontanelles, mental retardation, hearing loss (fixed stapes footplate, wide cochlear aqueduct, absent internal auditory canal), downsloping palpebral fissures, proptosis, exposure keratitis, optic nerve anomalies, midface hypoplasia, downsloping corners of the mouth, narrow "byzantine" palate with cleft, dental anomalies, fused cervical vertebrae, tracheal anomalies, cardiac changes, genitourinary and gastrointestinal anomalies, and syndactyly of the hands and feet (digits 2, 3, and 4 joined in a middigital mass). Features of Crouzon syndrome are similar but without syndactyly. Evaluation of hearing, the airway, vision, and the heart is required.

Connexins

Keratoderma-ichthyosis-deafness (KID) syndrome, Vohwinkel syndrome (mutilating keratoderma), and palmoplantar hyperkeratosis are due to GJB2 mutations.

1.2.5 X-linked (3%) Hearing loss

Stapes Fixation with Perilymphatic Gusher

Mutations in *POU3F4* can lead to profound SNHL, mixed hearing loss, an enlarged internal auditory canal with a thin or absent lamina cribrosa (bony plate between the auditory canal and the cochlea), and stapes fixation with perilymphatic gusher during stapes surgery. Young males with a family history of X-linked hearing loss are most commonly affected; however, females can have mild expression of this gene.

Alport Syndrome

The incidence of Alport syndrome is 1 in 10,000. *COL4A5* mutations lead to high-frequency, progressive SNHL in the second decade, retinal flecks, lens protrusion, spherophakia, congenital cataract, and progressive glomerulonephritis. Symptoms are worse in males. Audiologic evaluation and early management of renal disease are essential.

Mohr-Tranebjaerg Syndrome (Deafness–Dystonia–Optic Atrophy Syndrome)

Mutations in *TIMM8A* cause progressive SNHL, dystonia, myopia, visual field reduction, cortical blindness, and mental deterioration.

Norrie Disease

Mutations in the *NDP* gene cause congenital rapidly progressive blindness, ocular degeneration, microphthalmia, progressive SNHL in the second decade, and progressive mental deterioration.

Otopalatodigital Syndrome

Mutations in the *FLNA* gene lead to otopalatodigital (OPD) syndrome type 1 (mild form) and OPD syndrome type 2 (severe form, death in first year). Features include conductive, sensorineural, or mixed hearing loss, cleft palate, oligohypodontia, short proximal thumbs, hypoplastic distal phalanges and great toe with large sandal gap, bowed limbs, joint restriction, prominent supraorbital ridges, downslanting palpebral fissures, hypertelorism, broad nasal bridge and tip, and normal intelligence.

Wildervanck Syndrome

Wildervanck syndrome affects women and its features are a combination of Klippel-Feil anomaly (SNHL or mixed hearing loss, facial asymmetry, fused cervical vertebrae, torticollis, renal and cardiovascular anomalies) and Duane syndrome (lateral rectus innervated by CNIII).

1.2.6 Mitochondrial (< 1%)

Mitochondrial proteins interact with chromosomal proteins to facilitate energy production. All mitochondrial inheritance comes from the maternal egg. Mitochondrial mutations are present in 1 to 2% of newborns, with the 12S rRNA *A1555G* mutation being the most commonly reported. This mutation is structurally similar to bacterial 16S rRNA, and aminoglycosides aimed at bacterial rRNA can erroneously attack mitochondrial rRNA, resulting in ototoxicity. Fifteen percent of people in the United States and most people in Mongolia with aminoglycoside ototoxicity have the *A1555G* mutation. Family members may have milder hearing loss without being exposed to ototoxic medications.

MELAS

MELAS stands for mitochondrial encephalopathy, lactic acidosis, and stroke. Hearing loss is also present.

MIDD

MIDD is maternally inherited diabetes and deafness.

Kearns-Sayre Syndrome

Kearns-Sayre syndrome comprises SNHL, ataxia, short stature, delayed puberty, ophthalmoplegia, and retinopathy.

MERRF

Myoclonic epilepsy with ragged red fibers (MERRF) includes SNHL, ataxia, epilepsy, and optic atrophy.

1.2.7 Chromosomal Hearing Loss

Down Syndrome

The incidence is 1 in 1,500 for mothers under age 30 and 1 in 50 for mothers over age 40. The most common cause is trisomy 21. The clinical diagnosis includes 4 of 10 features: (1) flat face, (2) slanted palpebral fissures, (3) anomalous auricles, (4) excess skin on the back of the neck, (5) hypotonia, (6) hyperflexible joints, (7) simian crease, (8) fifth finger midphalanx dysplasia, (9) pelvic dysplasia, and (10) poor startle reflex. Atlantoaxial instability is common, and a shoulder roll should not be used. Examination of hearing and the airway, heart, and pelvis is required.

Turner Syndrome

Females with Turner syndrome (monosomic X chromosome) have hearing loss (conductive, SNHL, mixed), webbed neck, short stature, and gonadal dysgenesis.

1.3 Test Interpretation

- Historically only children at risk underwent hearing evaluation. Risk factors include family history of SNHL, in utero infection (toxoplasmosis, rubella, CMV, herpes, syphilis), prematurity, syndromes, craniofacial anomalies, birth weight < 1,500 g, Apgar scores less than 3 at 5 minutes or less than 6 at 10 minutes, respiratory distress, mechanical ventilation longer than 10 days, hyperbilirubinemia requiring exchange transfusion, bacterial meningitis, ototoxic medication, head trauma, otitis media with effusion lasting 3 months, temporal bone fracture, neurodegenerative or demyelinating disease, or parental concern. Less than 50% of infants with hearing loss were detected, leading to implementation of the infant hearing screening program. Newborns at risk who pass the screen should be monitored for changes in hearing every 6 months for 3 years.
- Universal newborn screening has decreased the age of detection from 2.5 years to less than 4 months, resulting in decreased rates of speech and language delay. Automated OAEs (AOAEs) measure the outer cochlear hair cell response to acoustic stimuli presented through a probe in the external auditory canal. Transient evoked OAEs (TEOAEs) and DPOAEs assess frequency-specific function from 500 to 6000, Hz as long as there is no contamination by ambient noise, vernix, or middle ear pathology. Infants at risk for SNHL should undergo automated ABR (AABR) by presenting a click stimulus at 35 dB hearing loss to the auditory canal and recording from forehead surface electrodes. Screening AABR cannot differentiate the type or degree of hearing loss. This process has a sensitivity of 100%, specificity of 99.7%, referral rate of 2%, and positive predictive value of 83.3% (Hall et al2004). Infants who do not pass should have both ears retested within 1 month using AOAEs and AABR. Failure to pass retesting requires diagnostic OAEs and ABR by an audiologist to determine hearing thresholds. Click-evoked ABR tests the 1,000- to 4,000-Hz range, and tone burst ABR and auditory steady-state response (ASSR) testing provide frequency-specific information. The test battery should include air and bone conduction ABR, high-frequency tympanometry, OAEs, stapedial reflexes, tone burst ABR or ASSR or both, and behavioral audiometry. Reversing polarity during air conduction ABR ensures that the response is neural and not the cochlear microphonic. Amplification should be provided within 1 month, visual acuity assessed, and families offered genetic counseling.
- Children older than 5 months should undergo standard audiometric testing to establish the degree and nature of hearing loss for each ear.
- Syndromic children with SNHL should be tested for known associated features. A sequential diagnostic paradigm has been proposed for the workup of idiopathic ARNSHL for a more efficient and cost-effective approach (Preciado et al 2005, ▸ Fig. 1.1). This does not obviate the need for specific testing when dictated by clinical examination or imaging when planning surgical intervention for example, autoimmune inner ear disease, syphilis, CMV, toxoplasmosis.

1.4 Diagnosis

Bilateral SNHL

1.5 Medical Management

Hearing aids should be fitted as soon as the hearing loss is identified. Genetic counseling regarding the cause of the hearing loss, additional deficits, vocational planning, and the implications for siblings or future offspring should be offered. Appropriate referrals as part of an integrated team of practitioners should be made. These would include speech therapy and/or auditory verbal therapy, developmental pediatrics, social work, early intervention specialist or educational liaison, and audiologist.

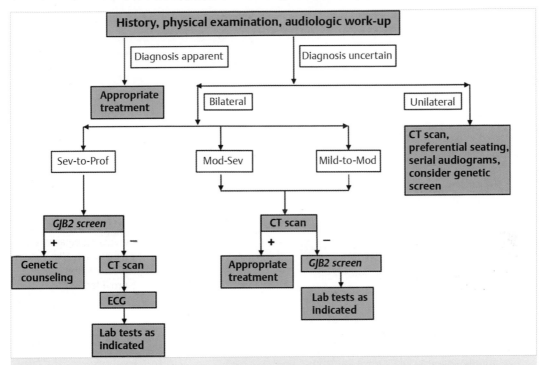

Fig. 1.1 Sequential diagnostic paradigm for the workup of idiopathic autosomal recessive nonsyndromic hearing loss. CT, computed tomography; ECG, electrocardiography; Mod, moderate; Prof, profound; Sev, severe. (From Preciado DA, Lawson L, Madden C, et al. Improved diagnostic effectiveness with a sequential diagnostic paradigm in idiopathic pediatric sensorineural hearing loss. Otol Neurotol 2005;26(4):610–661.)

1.6 Surgical Management

Indications for bone-anchored hearing aids include the following: (1) conductive or mixed hearing loss where conventional hearing aids cannot be used (e.g., anomaly of external or middle ear, chronic infection, unmanageable feedback), (2) unilateral conductive or mixed hearing loss, and (3) unilateral severe to profound SNHL. Indications for cochlear implantation include (1) bilateral severe to profound SNHL; (2) aided open-set sentence recognition (e.g., hearing in noise test [HINT]) score of 40% for Medicare, 60% for private payers; (3) when the patient does not benefit from amplification and aural rehabilitation; (4) implantable cochlea with nerve present; and (5) motivated patient and family.

1.7 Rehabilitation and Follow-up

Patients should have an audiologic reevaluation every 3 months during the first year and every 6 months thereafter. Hearing aids should be calibrated on a regular basis and new molds fitted when required. Periodic audiometric reevaluation is necessary to rule out fluctuation or progression of hearing loss. Speech-language therapy is imperative for the promotion of language and communication. Patients should see an otologist at least on an annual basis to reassess the accuracy of the initial diagnosis, inspect for diseases of the external and middle ear, and evaluate for progression of hearing loss and suitability of the patient's educational program, and as needed if changes are noted in hearing. Avoidance of ototoxic medications and of loud noise exposure by using hearing protection is essential. Children with cochlear implants require extensive rehabilitation involving specially trained audiologists, speech-language therapists, and auditory verbal therapists on a long-term basis to achieve maximal results. Parents must be made aware of this before implantation. With proper amplification, speech-language therapy, and educational programs, patients with congenital hearing loss can usually fully participate in social activities, school, and work.

1.8 Questions

1. Most nonsyndromic hearing loss is
   a) X-linked recessive.
   b) X-linked dominant.
   c) Autosomal recessive.
   d) Autosomal dominant.
   e) Mitochondrial.
2. Most autosomal recessive nonsyndromic hearing loss (ARNSHL) is due to
   a) Mutations in the *GJB6* gene.
   b) Mutations in the *EYA1* gene.
   c) Mutations that affect gap junctions in the stria vascularis.
   d) Mutations in the *WFS1* gene.
   e) Mitochondrial nonnuclear DNA.
3. Universal newborn hearing screening is based on the premise that
   a) The auditory brainstem response (ABR) measures action potentials from outer cochlear hair cells.
   b) Visual reinforcement audiometry is best used in children younger than 2 months.
   c) Outer hair cells in the cochlea emit signals spontaneously and following stimulation.
   d) Syndromic hearing loss is often difficult to diagnose in early childhood.
   e) Early intervention with a cochlear implant can help children with sensorineural hearing loss (SNHL) and a pure tone average of 50 dB or worse.

Answers: 1. c 2. a 3. c

Suggested Readings

Ballana E, Ventayol M, Rabionet R, Gasparini P, Estivill X. Connexins and deafness homepage. www.crg.es/deafness. Accessed Date: February 9, 2009

De Michele AM, Ruth RA. Newborn hearing screening. Medscape Reference; 2010. February 2008: http://emedicine.medscape.com/article/836646

Hall JW, III, Smith SD, Popelka GR. Newborn hearing screening with combined otoacoustic emissions and auditory brainstem responses. J Am Acad Audiol. 2004; 15(6):414–425

Isaacson B, Lee KH, Kutz JW, Roland PS, Sargent EW. Cochlear Implants, Indications. emedicine medscape com. July 2008: http://emedicine.medscape.com/article/857164-print

Johnson R, Greinwald J. Genetic hearing loss. In: Bailey BJ, Johnson JT, eds. Head & Neck Surgery—Otolaryngology. Lippincott Williams & Wilkins;Philadelphia, PA. 4th edition; 2006:Chapt 94

Preciado DA, Lawson L, Madden C, et al. Improved diagnostic effectiveness with a sequential diagnostic paradigm in idiopathic pediatric sensorineural hearing loss. Otol Neurotol. 2005; 26(4):610–615

Propst EJ, Blaser S, Gordon KA, Harrison RV, Papsin BC. Temporal bone findings on computed tomography imaging in branchio-oto-renal syndrome. Laryngoscope. 2005; 115(10):1855–1862

Smith RJ, Van Camp G. Deafness and hereditary hearing loss overview. GeneReviews. www.geneclinics.org/profiles/. January 2007 - July 2008

2 Single-Sided Deafness

Michael A. DeMarcantonio and Daniel I. Choo

2.1 History

A 6-year-old boy presented to the otolaryngology clinic with parental concerns of hearing loss. The patient's mother reported a normal pregnancy with negative screening for *toxoplasmosis, other agents, rubella, cytomegalovirus, and herpes simplex* (TORCH). The child passed his newborn hearing screening but had recently demonstrated difficulty hearing in noisy environments and had trouble paying attention at school. The patient had a history of recurrent acute otitis media with one set of tympanostomy tubes at 18 months of age. No audiogram was performed before or after surgery. The patient had no history of imbalance or vertigo.

The physical examination demonstrated myringosclerosis of the tympanic membranes without evidence of middle ear effusion. Weber lateralized to the left ear and Rinne was positive bilaterally. The remainder of the head and neck exam was normal. Neurologic exam showed normal cranial nerves, gait, and Romberg.

2.2 Differential Diagnosis—Key Points

Unilateral sensorineural hearing loss (SNHL) has an estimated prevalence of 3 to 5% in school-age children. The incidence of unilateral profound SNHL, also known as single-sided deafness (SSD), ranges from 0.1 to 3%. Historically, the effect of unilateral SNHL on speech-language development was undervalued. It has now become evident that unilateral SNHL is associated with an increase in grade failures, behavior problems, and need for educational assistance and speech therapy.

Possible etiologies of unilateral SNHL include congenital malformations, infections, ototoxic medications, and traumatic causes. Despite improvements in audiologic testing and imaging, 35 to 50% of children with unilateral SNHL continue to have an unknown etiology.

2.2.1 Congenital

Common congenital abnormalities include enlarged vestibular aqueduct (EVA), cochlear abnormalities, and cochlear nerve deficiency. EVA represents the most common inner ear malformation detected in patients with SNHL. While EVA most frequently occurs bilaterally, EVA can be unilateral in up to 40% of cases. EVA is frequently found in association with cochlear abnormalities ranging from mild asymmetry to classic Mondini's malformation. With the use of magnetic resonance imaging (MRI), congenital cochlear abnormalities are increasingly being identified in patients with SNHL. While malformations can be severe, including complete aplasia, common cavity, and Mondini's malformation, mild cochlear dysplasia represents the most common finding. Cochlear nerve deficiency is defined as an absent or hypoplastic cochlear nerve. Recent research has revealed that cochlear nerve deficiency is more common than previously appreciated, occurring in up to 26% of children with unilateral SNHL. Suspicion for cochlear nerve deficiency should be especially high in children identified with unilateral severe SNHL at birth.

2.2.2 Infectious Causes

Cytomegalovirus (CMV) is the most common intrauterine infection in the United States, causing up to 40% of all congenitally acquired hearing loss. Hearing loss is often detected at birth, but is also delayed in presentation in 33 to 50% of cases. SNHL may be unilateral in children with CMV and typically presents as a moderate to severe loss. Diagnosis of CMV is complicated by the fact that (pathologic) congenital CMV infection can only be confirmed in the newborn period. As a result, CMV may be the underlying pathology in an unquantifiable number of patients with unilateral SNHL. After birth, the mumps paramyxovirus may account for up to 2% of pediatric hearing loss cases. Typically hearing loss is unilateral and moderate to profound in severity. Bacterial meningitis results in hearing loss in 34% of children affected. While bilateral hearing loss appears more common, up to 40% of patients will present with unilateral hearing loss.

2.2.3 Environmental/Risk Factors

Children and parents should be questioned about common risk factors associated with hearing loss such as prematurity, hyperbilirubinemia, and noise exposure or exposure to ototoxic medications (aminoglycoside antibiotics, systemic chemotherapy, macrolides, and loop diuretics). A detailed trauma history should also be undertaken to rule out previous temporal bone fractures or closed head injuries. Lastly, causes of conductive hearing loss such as middle ear effusion, trauma, and ossicular malformations should be ruled out using clinical history, physical exam, and audiogram.

2.3 Test Interpretation

- An audiogram was performed at initial evaluation (▶ Fig. 2.1), demonstrating right-sided severe to profound SNHL and normal tympanograms bilaterally. An audiogram is essential to differentiate conductive hearing loss (CHL) from SNHL and assess the severity of hearing loss.

- A computed tomography (CT) scan was subsequently ordered (▶ Fig. 2.2), showing enlargement of the right vestibular aqueduct, with transverse dimensions at the operculum aperture measuring 1.8 mm (> 95th percentile), consistent with EVA. CT and MRI imaging can identify temporal bone abnormalities in up to 37% of children with previously unexplained SNHL. EVA is the most commonly identified abnormality, followed by anomalies of the cochlea and vestibule. Diagnosis of EVA was initially defined as a midpoint vestibular aqueduct width of greater than 1.5 mm. The vestibular aqueduct size on CT can quickly be compared with the width of the posterior semicircular canal as a rough estimate of enlargement. Recent research, using normative data, defines an enlarged vestibular aqueduct as having a midpoint and opercular width of ≥ 1.0 and 2.0 mm, respectively

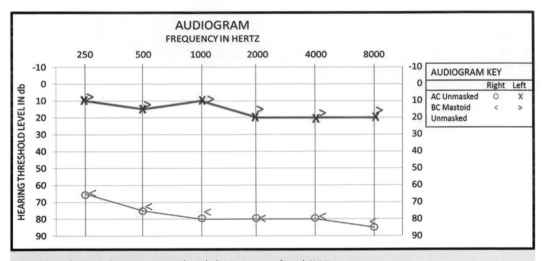

Fig. 2.1 Audiogram demonstrating right-sided severe to profound SNHL.

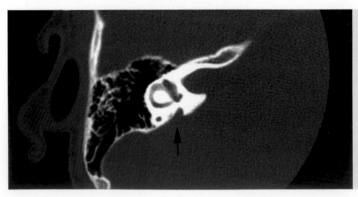

Fig. 2.2 CT of temporal bone showing right-sided EVA (arrow).

- Genetic testing should be considered in children with a diagnosis of SSD at birth and in patients with possible syndromic features.

While many congenital malformations, like EVA, can be detected on CT scan, MRI plays an essential role in SNHL diagnostic imaging. MRI should be considered in cases of congenital profound SNHL to evaluate for cochlear nerve deficiency, and in children with possible retrocochlear or intracranial pathology.

2.4 Diagnosis

SSD with EVA

2.5 Medical Management

Patients should be referred to audiology for hearing aid evaluation and assistance with school interventions. This patient was unlikely to benefit from a traditional hearing aid due to the severe to profound nature of the right-sided hearing loss and was counseled on the use of a contralateral routing of signal (CROS) hearing aid. A CROS hearing aid employs a microphone in the affected ear to detect sound and speech on the affected side, which are then routed to a receiver/speaker in the normal-hearing ear. CROS aids are now highly effective but do entail having an appliance in both the poorer-hearing ear and the normal-hearing ear.

Frequency modulation (FM) systems should be strongly considered in children with SSD. Particularly in a classroom setting, children with SSD often experience difficulty hearing in noise due to a poor signal-to-noise ratio. By implementing an FM system in classrooms, children with SSD (as well as all the other students in the classroom) receive a greatly enhanced signal (teacher/speaker)–to–noise (classroom noise) ratio, which allows them to "hear" better. While these devices have benefited recently from advances in technology, both CROS and FM systems remain limited by patient compliance. In children with unilateral EVA, parents should be counseled about the possible development of contralateral hearing loss and the risk of hearing loss progression following head trauma.

2.6 Surgical Management

The bone-anchored hearing aid (BAHA) is a good surgical option in patients with SSD, with a success rate of 96%. Children 5 years and older with profound unilateral hearing loss have been shown to have improvements in quality of life and perception in noise. However, BAHA has not been shown to improve sound localization in children with SSD. Recent refinements in surgical technique and device design have resulted in decreased surgical times, reduced complications, and abutment-free, magnet-based devices.

Cochlear implantation has been explored as a surgical treatment for SSD in adults. A recent systematic review identified 137 patients that underwent cochlear implantation for SSD. While some studies have shown improved sound localization and speech perception, no well-designed randomized studies have been performed to date. In children, only small cases series have been published with promising but limited results.

2.7 Rehabilitation and Follow-up

Patients with unilateral SNHL and SSD will require lifelong otolaryngology and audiology follow-up. Specifically, patients with EVA should undergo at least yearly audiogram to evaluate for progression of hearing loss and the development of contralateral hearing loss.

2.8 Questions

1. The following statements are true about enlarged vestibular aqueduct (EVA) except
   a) EVA is defined as an enlarged vestibular aqueduct having a midpoint and opercular width of ≥ 1.0 and 2.0 mm, respectively.
   b) EVA is the most common finding on imaging in unilateral sensorineural hearing loss (SNHL).
   c) EVA is frequently associated with common cavity deformity.
   d) Head trauma may result in progression of hearing loss.
2. Cytomegalovirus (CMV)
   a) Is an uncommon cause of congenital hearing loss.
   b) May result in delayed presentation of hearing loss.
   c) Always presents with bilateral hearing loss.
   d) Can be tested for in children as old as 3 years of age.
3. Unilateral hearing loss
   a) Remains of unknown etiology in 35 to 50% of children.

b) Occurs in 10% of school-age children.
c) Is most frequently a result of noise exposure and trauma in children.
d) Is rarely caused by cochlear nerve deficiency.

Answers: 1. c 2. b 3. a

Suggested Readings

Lieu JE, Tye-Murray N, Fu Q. Longitudinal study of children with unilateral hearing loss. Laryngoscope. 2012; 122(9):2088–2095

Kenna MA. Acquired Hearing Loss in Children. Otolaryngol Clin North Am. 2015; 48(6):933–953

Greinwald J, DeAlarcon A, Cohen A, et al. Significance of unilateral enlarged vestibular aqueduct. Laryngoscope. 2013; 123(6):1537–1546

Ghogomu N, Umansky A, Lieu JE. Epidemiology of unilateral sensorineural hearing loss with universal newborn hearing screening. Laryngoscope. 2014; 124(1):295–300

3 External Auditory Canal Atresia

Andre M. Wineland and Daniel I. Choo

3.1 History

A 5-year-old girl was referred from her pediatrician for evaluation of right-sided hearing loss. The family also expressed concerns on the overall appearance of the right ear. Other than the hearing loss and the shape of her right ear, she had no other complaints or significant medical history. She had met all of her developmental milestones and would soon start kindergarten. Her parents were concerned about teasing once she started school. They were seeking both a cosmetic and a functional solution. She had been wearing a soft-band bone-anchored hearing aid (BAHA) hearing aid since she was an infant.

On examination, the left ear was normal with an aerated middle ear space. The right pinna was uniformly small, but all subunits were present. A very short blind-ended pouch was the only rudiment of an external auditory canal (EAC). A repeat audiogram revealed normal hearing in the left ear and a maximum conductive hearing loss in the right ear. Balance function was normal. There was no facial asymmetry. The palate was intact and elevated symmetrically. She had a class I occlusal pattern without evidence of retrognathia or micrognathia.

3.2 Differential Diagnosis—Key Points

Ear malformations include incomplete development of the external ear (*microtia*), complete failure of external ear development (*anotia*), and failure to form the EAC (*aural atresia*). All three conditions represent an arrest in development with the external ear developing before the middle ear.

In 1926, Marx described three classes of microtia:
- *Class I*: Mild deformity. Smaller auricle (when compared to the other). All subunits of the auricle are accounted for.
- *Class II*: Auricle is one-half to two-thirds the size of the contralateral ear. Some, but not all, subunits are identifiable.
- *Class III*: Severely malformed auricle. Vestigial structure composed of rudimentary cartilage and fibrofatty tissue.

In 1957, Meurman expanded Marx's classification by describing a fourth group, *anotia*.

Aural atresia affects 1 to 17 per 10,000 births. Males are twice as likely to be affected as females. Unilateral atresia is three times more common than bilateral atresia, with the unilateral atresias occuring more commonly on the right. A craniofacial syndrome is identified in approximately 50% of the children with aural atresia. Common syndromes include Crouzon, Alpert, Pfeiffer, Klippel-Feil, branchio-oto-renal, 18q deletron syndrome, hemifacial microsomia, Treacher Collin, and Nager. Children with dysmorphisms should be referred for evaluation by a craniofacial team that includes clinicians from dentistry, plastic surgery, otolaryngology, speech-language pathology, audiology, clinical genetics, and ophthalmology. These children are also at risk of developmental anomalies of their cardiovascular and renal systems, and referrals to cardiology/urology/nephrology should be implemented as indicated by history and physical exam.

In 1992, Jahrsdoerfer et al developed a 10-point grading system to determine surgical candidacy based on key features from the computed tomography (CT) scan and appearance of the external ear. A score of 8 or above in experienced hands is associated with postoperative speech reception thresholds of less than 30 dB HL in 80% of cases. Traditionally, patients with a Jarhsdoerfer score of 6 or less were counseled against having atresia repair due to the low likelihood of success and higher risks of complications (e.g., facial nerve injury).

The following is a summary of this 10-point grading system:
- Stapes present = 2 points.
- Oval window open = 1 point.
- Middle ear space well developed = 1 point.
- Facial nerve identified in a normal position = 1 point.
- Malleus-incus complex present = 1 point.
- Mastoid pneumatization well developed = 1 point.
- Incus-stapes connection present = 1 point.
- Round window present = 1 point.
- External ear well formed = 1 point.

It is possible for a canal cholesteatoma (epithelial inclusion cyst) to develop in a stenotic EAC. Canal cholesteatomas may be suspected clinically when squamous debris is found in the ear canal remnant, and these are identified radiographically as widening of the EAC. These commonly occur in cases with minor aplasia with small EACs (< 4 mm). A canal cholesteatoma in the setting of aural atresia is a surgically managed disease.

3.3 Test Interpretation

An audiologic assessment is necessary in children affected by aural atresia. If bilateral atresia is present, a masking dilemma will exist that requires particularly skilled audiologic assessment and techniques to determine ear-specific hearing levels. As reflected in the case study, aural atresia is most commonly associated with a maximal conductive hearing loss in the affected ear. In cases of unilateral atresia, audiometric evaluation of the opposite ear is important in the rehabilitative planning and overall management of the child.

CT of the temporal bone is necessary for preoperative planning. ► Fig. 3.1 demonstrates the differences between well-developed temporal bones that are amenable to successful atresia repair and those temporal bones in which the middle ear and associated structures are poorly developed and typically lead to poor hearing outcomes. Although imaging studies may be obtained at any time before the surgical repair, it may be preferable to obtain scans closer to the surgical timeframe to avoid radiation exposure during infancy or early childhood periods and also to potentially avoid the need for repeat updated scans.

Surgical repair is partly dependent upon the type of reconstruction technique used for the microtia repair. Both techniques are discussed in further detail below. Briefly, in Nagata's technique, the children are often appropriate candidates when the child is 7 or 8 years of age. Measurement of the size of the head and the chest wall (i.e., rib size) often dictates when there is sufficient autologous tissue for grafting and reconstruction. In the Brent method, children can typically start slightly earlier (5 to 6 years of age).

3.4 Diagnosis

1. Class I 1 deformity of the right pinna
2. External auditory canal atresia

3.5 Medical Management

Adequate auditory stimulation should be provided to an infant as soon as reasonable. In cases of bilateral atresia, this can be accomplished with bone conduction hearing aids when the child is 4 to 6 months old. Whereas soft-band bone-anchored hearing aids (BAHAs) can be placed in the first couple months of life, implantable BAHAs are FDA approved at age 5 or older.

For candidates with poor Jahrsdoerfer scores, bone conduction hearing aids or BAHAs can provide serviceable hearing. It is ideal to provide binaural hearing in children for hearing in noisy

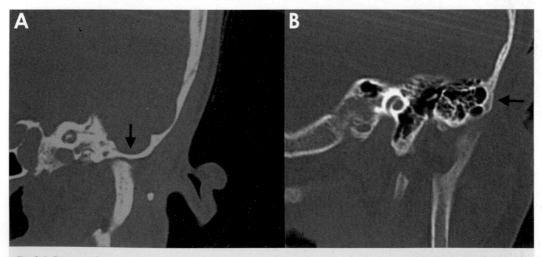

Fig. 3.1 Bone window, coronal CT images of the left ear from two different patients. (a) A poorly pneumatised temporal bone with a low-hanging tegmen (dura) as indicated by the arrow. Such anatomic challenges make successful atresia repair extremely unlikely. (b) In contrast, the arrow indicates a well-pneumatized temporal bone with sufficient space to create a widely patent ear canal and a mobile ossicular chain that would allow for excellent hearing outcomes.

environments and to provide directionality of sound for localization.

3.6 Surgical Management

Parental counseling for congenital aural atresia repair should be included properly by reviewing expectations, operative risks, and postoperative care. Common discussion points include (but are not limited to) long-term care of the ear/mastoid, potential risks of facial nerve injury, potential risk of inner ear damage, potential damage to the temporomandibular joint, and the potential need for revision surgery (canal restenosis, graft lateralization, and chronic otitis externa).

Once deemed a suitable candidate for aural atresia repair, surgery involves creating an auditory canal, removing the atretic plate, mobilizing or reconstructing the sound-conducting mechanism, creating a new external auditory meatus, and lining the newly created canal with a split-thickness skin graft. The canal is generally centered over the ossicular mass and bounded anteriorly by the temporomandibular joint, superiorly by the tegmen, and posteriorly by the mastoid air cell system (▶ Fig. 3.2). Entrance to the middle ear space

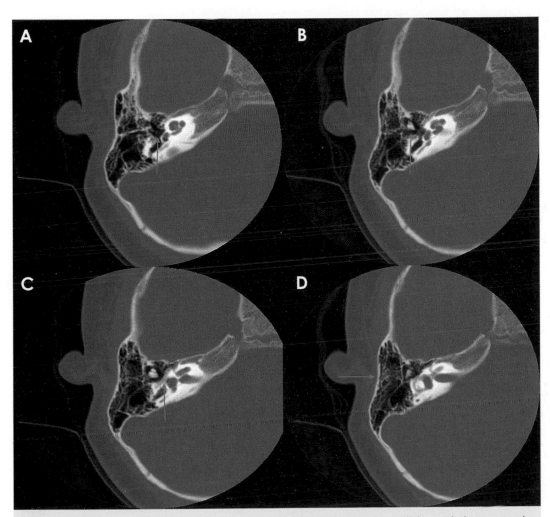

Fig. 3.2 Axial bone window CT images from a child with a right congenital aural atresia. All the panels demonstrate the robust aeration and development of the mastoid and middle ear cleft. **(a)** The arrow points toward the stapes that is critical for good hearing outcomes. **(b)** The arrow indicates the fused incus-malleus complex. **(c)** The arrow indicates the horizontal facial nerve. **(d)** The arrow highlights the general area in which creation of the ear canal would allow access to the ossicles for successful atresia repair.

occurs in the epitympanum to protect the ossicles and prevent inadvertent injury to the inner ear. Although facial nerve monitoring is routinely employed, vigilance for an aberrant facial nerve is mandatory.

A 30% revision rate is seen with long-term follow-up. The EAC has a tendency to restenosis over time. This may encroach on the tympanic membrane and interfere with hearing thresholds as well.

Microtia repair is classically performed before construction of the EAC, but this is not uniformly accepted. It is best to approach this issue of timing of each repair with the family and the surgeons performing each part of the procedure. There are two commonly described methods: Brent (1974) and Nagata (1985).

There are four stages of microtia repair according to Brent:
1. Fabrication of the auricular framework with contralateral costal cartilage.
2. Lobule transposition.
3. Framework elevation.
4. Tragus reconstruction.

There are two stages of microtia repair according to Nagata:
1. Fabrication of the auricular framework from ipsilateral costal cartilage, tragus reconstruction, and lobule transposition.
2. Framework elevation.

Alloplastic materials (silicone and Medpore) are also available to use in reconstruction. Although short-term results appear promising, long-term results are still lacking. Complete prosthetic auricles are also available, but usually reserved for failed reconstructions or based upon patient and family preference.

3.7 Rehabilitation and Follow-up

Continued aural rehabilitation is essential for all hearing-impaired children. Regular otologic examinations should be performed along with repeat audiologic testing. In addition, some patients may benefit from speech therapy.

3.8 Questions

1. True or false? The most common cause of hearing loss after aural atresia repair is ossicular refixation.
2. True or false? Magnetic resonance imaging (MRI) is the appropriate imaging modality to assess candidacy for aural atresia repair.
3. In the Jahrsdoerfer grading system, which counts as 2 points?
   a) Middle ear space.
   b) Pneumatization of the mastoid.
   c) Course of the facial nerve.
   d) Appearance of the external ear.
   e) Stapes.

Answers: 1. True 2. False 3. e

Suggested Readings

Brent B. Auricular repair with autogenous rib cartilage grafts: two decades of experience with 600 cases. Plast Reconstr Surg. 1992; 90(3):355–374, discussion 375–376

Brent B. The team approach to treating the microtia atresia patient. Otolaryngol Clin North Am. 2000; 33(6):1353–1365, viii

Brent B. Technical advances in ear reconstruction with autogenous rib cartilage grafts: personal experience with 1200 cases. Plast Reconstr Surg. 1999; 104(2):319–334, discussion 335–338

Calzolari F, Garani G, Sensi A, Martini A. Clinical and radiological evaluation in children with microtia. Br J Audiol. 1999; 33(5):303–312

Chang SO, Lee JH, Choi BY, Song JJ. Long term results of postoperative canal stenosis in congenital aural atresia surgery. Acta Otolaryngol Suppl. 2007; 558(558):15–21

De la Cruz A, Teufert KB. Congenital aural atresia surgery: long-term results. Otolaryngol Head Neck Surg. 2003; 129(1):121–127

Jahrsdoerfer RA, Yeakley JW, Aguilar EA, Cole RR, Gray LC. Grading system for the selection of patients with congenital aural atresia. Am J Otol. 1992; 13(1):6–12

Meurman Y. Congenital microtia and meatal atresia; observations and aspects of treatment. AMA Arch Otolaryngol. 1957; 66(4):443–463

Siegert R, Mattheis S, Kasic J. Fully implantable hearing aids in patients with congenital auricular atresia. Laryngoscope. 2007; 117 (2):336–340

Suutarla S, Rautio J, Ritvanen A, Ala-Mello S, Jero J, Klockars T. Microtia in Finland: comparison of characteristics in different populations. Int J Pediatr Otorhinolaryngol. 2007; 71(8):1211–1217

Teufert KB, De la Cruz A. Advances in congenital aural atresia surgery: effects on outcome. Otolaryngol Head Neck Surg. 2004; 131 (3):263–270

4 Otitis Media

Christine H. Heubi and Robin T. Cotton

4.1 History

A 7-month-old infant presented to the emergency department with a 1-week history of swelling behind his left ear that had increased in size over the past week. The family denied fever but did report symptoms of upper respiratory infection the week prior to the onset of ear swelling. He had not been seen by a primary care physician and had not been on any medications. Physical examination revealed an alert infant with a temperature of 37 °C. Auricular examination revealed proptosis of the left auricle with a large, fluctuant mass overlying the mastoid that was tender to palpation. Otoscopy revealed a bulging, erythematous left tympanic membrane. The right otoscopic exam also showed an erythematous tympanic membrane, but no postauricular tenderness. Facial nerve function appeared normal bilaterally. Numerous small lymph nodes were palpated in the posterior triangle of the neck. The remainder of the head and neck examination revealed no abnormality. A computed tomography (CT) scan of the temporal bone was ordered, as well as a complete blood count (CBC) with differential.

4.2 Differential Diagnosis—Key Points

Complications of otitis media can be classified according to extracranial and intracranial involvement (► Table 4.1). The differential diagnosis of extracranial complications of acute otitis media can be divided into two groups: intratemporal and extratemporal. Intracranial complications include sigmoid sinus thrombosis, brain or subdural abscess, otitic hydrocephalus, and meningitis. An accurate history, complete otolaryngologic and neurologic examination, and radiographic Imaging are needed to differentiate the various complications.

All cases of acute otitis media involve inflammation of the mastoid air cells. However, clinically significant acute mastoiditis is a clinical diagnosis based on the findings of suppurative otitis media, postauricular swelling with loss of postauricular crease, and protrusion of the auricle. Coalescent mastoiditis is a specific radiographic diagnosis based on CT and is differentiated from acute mastoiditis by radiographic evidence of loss of the bony septations.

Suppurative labyrinthitis occurs when bacterial invasion penetrates the otic capsule, usually via the round window or oval window. The classic presentation is rapid onset of vertigo, sensorineural hearing loss, nausea, and vomiting during an episode of acute otitis media. In the absence of associated meningitis, the cerebrospinal fluid pressure and analysis are normal. Suppurative acute petrositis occurs when there is extension of the middle ear infection into the petrous apex, resulting in symptoms of retro-orbital pain, persistent otorrhea, and sixth cranial nerve palsy. This symptom complex is known as the Gradenigo triad. Facial paralysis, usually unilateral, can occur during an episode of acute otitis media either secondary to direct inflammation through a bony dehiscence in the tympanic segment of the facial nerve or secondary to osteitis involving the bony fallopian canal.

Table 4.1 Complications of acute otitis media

I. Extracranial	II. Intracranial
A. Intratemporal	A. Extradural granulation tissue and/or abscess
1. Acute mastoiditis	
2. Coalescent mastoiditis	
3. Labyrinthitis	
4. Petrositis	
5. Facial nerve dysfunction	
6. Tympanic membrane perforation	
B. Extratemporal	B. Sigmoid sinus thrombosis
1. Subperiosteal abscess	
2. Bezold's abscess	
	C. Brain abscess
	D. Oticti hydrocephalus
	E. Meningitis
	F. Subdural abscess

Extratemporal complications occur when infection progresses to involve the cortical bone surrounding the mastoid air cells. Osteitis of the lateral cortex can result in the development of a subperiosteal abscess. The patient usually presents with more pronounced auricular protrusion, loss of the postauricular crease, and fluctuance over the mastoid. Osteitis of the medial or inferior mastoid cortex can result in the development of a deep neck space infection known as Bezold's abscess.

Acute mastoiditis can be accompanied by a significant amount of inflammation of the cartilaginous external auditory canal or granulation tissue, making visualization of the tympanic membrane difficult or impossible in the awake child. This can clinically mimic acute external otitis without middle ear or mastoid involvement. The physical examination can help differentiate the two entities. Manipulation of the external auditory canal by pulling on the tragus is extremely painful in acute external otitis, but not in mastoiditis. Occasionally, initial response to intravenous (IV) and ototopical treatments is needed to make an accurate diagnosis.

Intracranial complications of acute otitis media manifest with a broad range of signs and symptoms. Presentation can range from headache and lethargy to seizures and focal neurologic signs. Sigmoid sinus thrombosis classically presents with "picket fence" fevers, toxemia, septic embolization, and torticollis. However, further complications can occur with thrombus propagation, including jugular foramen syndrome, otitic hydrocephalus, coma, and even death.

Brain abscesses can be difficult to diagnose because the signs and symptoms are often subtle. Presentation depends on the stage of the abscess. The first stage, cerebritis, is accompanied by generalized symptoms of headache, malaise, fever, and drowsiness, followed by a quiescent or latent phase that can last for weeks. In the third phase, abscess formation occurs with focal neurologic signs. The final phase, termination, results in rupture of the abscess, leading to rapid deterioration and death.

Meningitis presents with classic findings of headache, fever, and neck rigidity. Kernig and Brudzinski signs are positive. Spread of infection to the meninges is by hematogenous dissemination, inner ear malformations (incomplete partitioning), or direct spread (middle fossa dehiscence, meningoencephalocele).

4.3 Test Interpretation

The CT scan (▶ Fig. 4.1) revealed a left coalescent mastoiditis and a large subperiosteal abscess with extensive dehiscence of the squamous portion of the temporal bone. There was a small intracranial, extradural component that was contiguous with the postauricular abscess. There was no sign of sigmoid sinus thrombosis. Opacification of the right middle ear space was also seen, with preservation of the mastoid trabeculae. The CBC showed a white blood cell count of 25.6 K/μL without a left shift.

CT is the appropriate modality to assess the mastoid and temporal bone. If intracranial involvement is suspected, contrast-enhanced magnetic resonance imaging (MRI) is a superior investigation. It is more sensitive for the detection of an early brain abscess, sigmoid sinus thrombosis, subdural abscess, and extradural granulation tissue. A white blood cell count can be used as a marker to monitor improvement with medical therapy. Blood cultures are necessary if sepsis is suspected.

4.4 Diagnosis

Left acute otomastoiditis with subperiosteal abscess

4.5 Medical Management

Empiric IV antimicrobial coverage should include coverage for the most common organisms that cause acute otitis media, including *Streptococcus pneumoniae, Haemophilus influenzae,* and *Moraxella catarrhalis.* Once culture results are obtained, coverage can be narrowed. Following surgical drainage, symptoms usually dissipate quickly, and oral antibiotic therapy can be instituted. Extensive disease or young age may merit consideration of a longer course of IV therapy. Ciprofloxacin-dexamethasone otic drops should be instilled after placement of tympanostomy tubes. This allows ototopical treatment of the infection and inflammation. Steroids can be administered to address inflammation associated with the facial nerve paralysis, if present.

4.6 Surgical Management

This patient was started on IV ceftriaxone and flagyl in the emergency room. He was taken to the operating room for bilateral myringotomy and

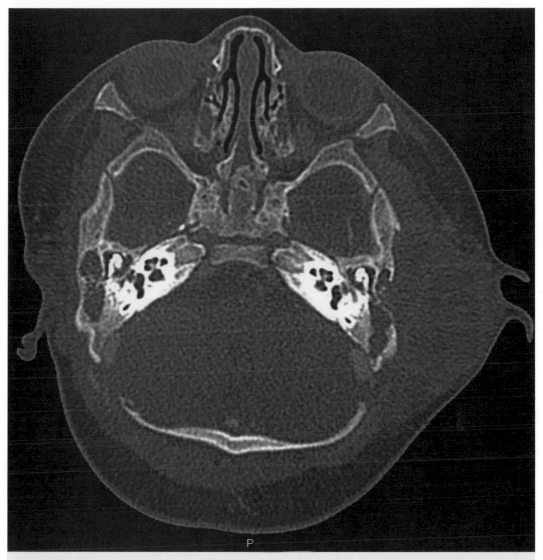

Fig. 4.1 Axial computed tomography scan of temporal bones: left mastoiditis with subperiosteal abscess.

tympanostomy tube placement, and treatment with ciprofloxacin-dexamethasone otic drops was initiated. Additionally, he underwent incision and drainage of the subperiosteal abscess, and a small Penrose drain was placed. Cultures taken at the time of surgery grew pan-sensitive *S. pneumoniae,* and his white blood cell count normalized. Flagyl was discontinued after the culture result was finalized. By postoperative day 7, scant serosanguineous drainage was seen emanating from the drain, and it was removed. Given the extensive destruction of the squamous portion of the temporal bone, which was felt to represent periosteomyelitis, the patient's

age, and the extent of the subperiosteal abscess, prolonged IV therapy with ceftriaxone was arranged for 4 weeks as an outpatient, and he continued on Ciprodex (Alcon) otic suspension for 14 days. He was discharged on postoperative day 7.

Cortical mastoidectomy with placement of a tympanostomy tube has historically been the preferred treatment for acute mastoiditis. More recently, the disease has been managed conservatively with IV antibiotics and myringotomy, often with tympanostomy tube placement for ototopical application of antibiotics. Whether to address the mastoid remains controversial. When an extracranial complication of acute otitis media and a coalescent mastoiditis is present, a cortical mastoidectomy is advised. When mastoid septa are intact, tympanostomy tube placement, medical treatment, and close observation constitute a reasonable initial approach. Any deterioration of the child warrants a mastoidectomy. In this particular patient, given the extensive destruction of the mastoid air cells, a cortical mastoidectomy was not needed.

4.7 Rehabilitation and Follow-up

The patient was seen in clinic 1 week after discharge, with a healed postauricular incision and a patent pressure-equalizing tube in place without evidence of infection. He continued on IV antibiotics for a total of 6 weeks, and a repeat CT scan obtained at 6 weeks showed resolution of the infection without any further destruction of the bone. At his last follow-up appointment 6 months after surgery, this child's pressure-equalizing tubes were intact bilaterally, his tympanic membranes were intact, and he had normal hearing per audiogram.

4.8 Questions

1. All of the following are complications of acute mastoiditis except
   a) Meningitis.
   b) Subperiosteal abscess.
   c) Cavernous sinus thrombosis.
   d) Brain abscess.

2. Gradenigo's triad, the symptom complex associated with petrositis, is characterized by all of the following except
   a) Cranial nerve VII palsy.
   b) Retro-orbital pain.
   c) Persistent otorrhea.
   d) Cranial nerve VI palsy.
3. Which of the following is not a common organism causing acute otitis media?
   a) Haemophilus influenzae.
   b) Moraxella catarrhalis.
   c) Streptococcus pneumoniae.
   d) Staphylococcus aureus.

Answers: 1. c 2. a 3. d

Suggested Readings

Bluestone CD, Klein JO. Intratemporal complications and sequelae of otitis media. In: Bluestone CD, Stool SE, Alper CU, et al, eds. Pediatric Otolaryngology. 4th ed. Philadelphia, PA: WB Saunders; 2003:687–763

Brown KD, Selesnick SH, Tang S. Complications of otitis media. In: Pensak ML, Choo DI, eds. Clinical Otology. 4th ed. New York, NY: Thieme; 2015:231–240

Budenz CL, El-Kashlan HK, Shelton C, Aygun N, Niparko JK. Complications of temporal bone infections. In: Flint PW, Haughey BH, Lund V, et al, eds. Cummings Otolaryngology. 6th ed. Philadelphia, PA: Elsevier Saunders; 2015:2156–2176

Chesney J, Black A, Choo D. What is the best practice for acute mastoiditis in children? Laryngoscope. 2014; 124(5):1057–1058

Harley EH, Sdralis T, Berkowitz RG. Acute mastoiditis in children: a 12-year retrospective study. Otolaryngol Head Neck Surg. 1997; 116(1):26–30

Rettig E, Tunkel DE. Contemporary concepts in management of acute otitis media in children. Otolaryngol Clin North Am. 2014; 47 (5):651–672

Part II

Adult Otology

5 Otitis Externa

David R. Lee and John H. Greinwald Jr

5.1 History

A 12-year-old boy presented with his mother with a 3-day history of worsening right ear pain, aural fullness, and an extremely tender right ear. His mother stated that they had recently spent the weekend at their lake house, and his symptoms hed worsened since that time. He had no significant past medical or surgical history but did report a muffled feeling and mild hearing loss in his right ear. He was taking a daily chewable multivitamin. On physical examination, he had extreme pain upon distraction of the pinna, erythema of the right external auditory canal (EAC), and mild otorrhea and crusting of the right ear.

5.2 Differential Diagnosis—Key Points

In the young, healthy population in the United States, acute inflammation of the external auditory meatus is most likely due to bacterial otitis externa. This is simply a cellulitis of the skin and soft tissue of the EAC. Fungal otitis externa, or otomycosis, is an uncommon cause of otitis externa but has some similar predisposing factors. Typically, otomycosis will present with severe itching but less pain than bacterial otitis externa. Malignant, or necrotizing, otitis externa is an infection that extends into the deeper soft tissues and bone adjacent to the EAC, and it can progress to include the skull base and cranial nerves. Patients who have diabetes mellitus or are immunocompromised are particularly at risk for both otomycosis and malignant otitis externa.

Bacterial otitis externa is an infectious process, most commonly caused by *Pseudomonas aeruginosa* and *Staphylococcus aureus*. Less commonly, it can be caused by *Proteus, Staphylococcus epidermidis,* diphtheroids, and *Escherichia coli.* Otomycosis is primarily caused by Conchicola albicans and Aspergillus species. Malignant otitis externa is most frequently caused by *P. aeruginosa* and infrequently is caused by *Aspergillus.*

Otitis externa can be caused by an underlying condition. Many dermatologic conditions can be the causative factor, including eczema, atopic dermatitis, and psoriasis. An infection of a hair follicle, or a furuncle, can be associated with an acute localized otitis externa. Rare causes of recurrent otitis externa include first branchial cleft anomalies and neoplasms and exostoses of the EAC.

5.3 Test Interpretation

A culture is not needed to confirm diagnosis in bacterial otitis externa and should only be obtained in infections that are refractory to treatment. In these refractory patients, a diagnosis of otomycosis can be confirmed by potassium hydroxide preparation identifying fungal elements or by a positive fungal culture.

Otoscopy will show an ear canal that is red and erythematous, and often discharge will be present. The tympanic membrane may be mildly inflamed but will be normally mobile on pneumatic otoscopy in otitis externa. Acute otitis media may present similarly to otitis externa, but the tympanic membrane will not be mobile on pneumatic otoscopy in otitis media with effusion. It may not be possible to visualize the tympanic membrane due to inflammation in otitis externa. Fungal otitis externa will reveal an erythematous EAC and fungal debris. In malignant otitis externa, granulation tissue can be seen on the floor of the EAC at the osteocartilaginous junction.

If malignant otitis externa is suspected, a biopsy must be taken to rule out carcinoma of the EAC. Further radiologic imaging is also helpful for malignant otitis externa. Specifically, high-resolution computed tomography (CT) imaging aids in depicting bony erosion. Magnetic resonance imaging (MRI) is not often utilized but may be considered if soft tissue extension is the predominant concern.

As this patient's presentation and physical exam was typical for uncomplicated bacterial otitis externa, a culture was not performed. Otoscopy revealed a moderately inflamed EAC with a normal-appearing tympanic membrane and a small amount of thin purulent discharge.

5.4 Diagnosis

Uncomplicated acute bacterial otitis externa

5.5 Medical Management

Simple otitis externa can successfully be treated using otic drop preparations that are antiseptic, acidifying, or antibiotic—or even any combination. Ofloxacin and ciprofloxacin are single-agent antibiotics with an excellent spectrum of coverage of the pathogens commonly found in otitis externa. Steroids can be added to preparations to help reduce canal edema and otalgia. Acetic acid, aluminum acetate, gentian violet, and alcohol are all acceptable antiseptic preparations. If the cellulitis extends past the EAC, systemic antibiotics are indicated. Pain management is a major goal in treating acute otitis externa, and pain is often best controlled using a nonsteroidal anti-inflammatory agent with or without an opioid.

Otomycosis can be treated by nonspecific antifungal agents such as thimerosal and gentian violet. Specific antifungals include clotrimazole and nystatin drops, and ketoconazole may also be utilized.

For malignant otitis externa, long-term parenteral antibiotics are the treatment of choice. Aminoglycosides like tobramycin and antipseudomonals like piperacillin, ticarcillin, or ceftazidime may be utilized. Outpatient ciprofloxacin or ofloxacin can be utilized, but only if the diagnosis was made early in the disease course and the patient can be closely followed. The underlying immunocompromised state or diabetes must be controlled in order to successfully treat malignant otitis externa.

For recurrent bouts of otitis externa due to water exposure, the use of earplugs during exposure and/or antibiotic or acidification drops after water exposure can be helpful.

5.6 Surgical Management

Initial surgical treatment of acute bacterial otitis media involves debris removal from the EAC with meticulous atraumatic débridement. If the canal is extremely stenotic from inflammation, a wick can be placed with the aid of a microscope in an effort to open the EAC and permit delivery of otic drops to the medial canal. If the diagnosis of malignant otitis externa is confirmed, surgical débridement may be necessary to remove all necrotic tissue. In severe cases of malignant otitis externa, an aggressive procedure such as circumferential petrosectomy may be required to control disease progression and preserve cranial nerve function.

5.7 Rehabilitation and Follow-up

There is no need to have regular follow-up in patients with uncomplicated acute otitis media. In recurrent episodes of otitis externa, patient education of environmental risk factors and precautions may be required.

5.8 Questions

1. A 37-year-old man with human immunodeficiency virus (HIV) presents with right-sided ear pain, fullness, and difficulty hearing that has progressively worsened over the past 3 days. On exam, there is significant edema of the external auditory canal (EAC), and the tympanic membrane is intact and mobile on insufflation. Remaining physical exam is noncontributory. What is the best initial course of treatment?
   a) Acetic acid and alcohol otic drops.
   b) Ofloxacin otic drops.
   c) Topical acetic acid/alcohol solution and oral ciprofloxacin.

2. A 49-year-old man with medical history significant for CAD, HTN, obesity, diabetes, and peripheral neuropathy presents with left-sided ear pain, drainage, difficulty hearing, and left-sided facial weakness that has worsened over the past several hours. On exam there is significant left periauricular adenopathy, thick purulent drainage from the left ear, and a small amount of granulation tissue adherent to the EAC, and the tympanic membrane is not visualized. Which of the following is the best course of action?
   a) Immediate transfer to local emergency department.
   b) Begin oral antipseudomonal antibiotics and follow up in 1 week.
   c) Admit and begin parenteral antibiotics.
   d) Admit, begin parenteral antibiotics, and biopsy area of granulation tissue.

3. Which of the following is the most commonly isolated organism in acute otitis externa?
   a) Staphylococcus aureus.
   b) Corynebacterium.
   c) Pseudomonas aeruginosa.
   d) Escherichia coli.

Answers: 1. c 2. d 2. c

Suggested Readings

Rosenfeld RM, et al. Clinical practice guideline: acute otitis externa. Otolaryngology. 2006; 134(4):4–23

Roland PS, Stroman DW. Microbiology of acute otitis externa. Laryngoscope. 2002; 112(7 Pt 1):1166–1177

6 Cholesteatoma

Tasneem A. Shikary and Myles L. Pensak

6.1 History

A 46-year-old man with a history of achondroplasia and recurrent right ear infections presented with progressive right-sided hearing loss, aural fullness, and refractory otorrhea that had worsened over the past year. More recently he developed dizziness with occasional vertiginous spells.

The patient reported recurrent ear infections as a child and multiple sets of pressure equalization tubes but denied any other pertinent otologic history. He also denied history of trauma and had no other significant comorbid conditions related to, or in addition to, his achondroplasia.

Otomicroscopic examination of the left ear revealed a normal external auditory canal with a mildly atelectatic and sclerotic tympanic membrane with clear middle ear space. Examination of the right ear demonstrated diffuse squamous debris with an opacified tympanic membrane and no visible landmarks. Using a 512 Hz tuning fork, Weber's test lateralized to the patient's left ear. Rinne's test was positive on the left but could not be detected on the right side. A fistula test was performed and left-beating nystagmus was noted. Gait's and Romberg's tests were normal and cranial nerve function was grossly intact.

6.2 Differential Diagnosis—Key Points

- A *cholesteatoma* is a lesion of the temporal bone consisting of keratinizing squamous epithelium lined by a fibrous matrix. Due to the inflammatory and enzymatic properties of the cholesteatoma matrix, as well as the expansile growth of the lesion caused by ongoing squamous deposition into the sac, cholesteatomas have a propensity for eroding important structures of the middle and inner ear. This process can be exacerbated by bacterial superinfections. Cholesteatoma may be localized to the epitympanum, or it may follow preformed pathways to invade the mastoid, middle ear, or petrous apex.
- Cholesteatoma may be acquired (most common), congenital, or iatrogenic in origin.
  a) *Primary acquired cholesteatoma* is thought to be due to long-standing negative middle ear pressure and retraction of the tympanic membrane resulting from chronic eustachian tube dysfunction. This typically is located in the posterior tympanum from the pars tensa or in the pars flaccida.
  b) *Secondary acquired cholesteatoma* is thought to result from the growth of squamous epithelium through a perforated tympanic membrane, or it can be iatrogenic as a result of implantation of squamous epithelium into the middle ear. The perforation may be infectious, traumatic, or iatrogenic in nature.
  c) *Congenital cholesteatoma* is thought to result from an embryonic rest of epithelial tissue that fails to involute during middle ear development and most commonly occurs in the anterior-superior quadrant with an intact tympanic membrane.
- There are four main theories for the pathogenesis for acquired cholesteatoma; (1) invagination of the tympanic membrane, i.e., retraction pocket cholesteatoma; (2) basal cell hyperplasia; (3) epithelial ingrowth through a perforation (migration theory); and (4) squamous metaplasia of middle ear epithelium. All of these theories are based on the notion that cholesteatoma develops from the outermost squamous layer of the tympanic membrane, with the foremost being the most universally accepted. However, the invagination theory does not explain what sustains growth of the cholesteatoma after the initial retraction occurs. The epitympanum, aditus, and antrum become blocked in the early phase of the disease and thus cannot be the driving force for further development of cholesteatoma. More recently the mucosal traction theory has been proposed to account for this gap. The mucosal traction theory describes three phases, the first phase is retraction, but this is only the inciting event. Retraction allows for mucosal contact between the tympanic membrane and the ossicles, which is a necessary precursor for phase 2, or migration that is driven by this mucosal contact. In the final phase keratin is produced that accumulates in the sac.
- The differential diagnosis of cholesteatoma includes chronic otitis media with or without suppuration, keratosis obturans, tuberculous otitis, osteoradionecrosis, squamous cell or basal cell carcinoma, foreign body reaction, granulomatous disease, and encephalocele.

6.3 Test Interpretation

A baseline audiogram should be obtained for all patients with cholesteatoma. An audiogram will typically show a conductive or possibly a mixed hearing loss. The patient in this case had a right mixed hearing loss with a sizable air–bone gap (▶ Fig. 6.1). In cases associated with dizziness, concern should be raised for an inner ear fistula or labyrinthine fistula that most commonly results from erosion of the lateral canal.

Imaging is not necessary to diagnose cholesteatoma but can aid significantly in pre-surgical planning given the propensity of these lesions to destroy orienting landmarks and/or expose critical anatomy. Imaging is recommended for all revision procedures in which cholesteatoma is suspected. Computed tomography (CT) of the temporal bone with 1-mm collimation and both axial and coronal reconstructions is the study of choice. ▶ Fig. 6.2 demonstrates the typical findings of a primary acquired cholesteatoma with a soft tissue mass in the epitympanum and bony erosion of the scutum, ossicles, and in this case of the labyrinth at the lateral semicircular canal. Magnetic resonance imaging (MRI) with diffusion weighted imaging is more sensitive and specific than CT for imaging of cholesteatoma, although this modality is not routinely used. On diffusion restricted MRI, cholesteatoma will appear as a hyperintense mass.

6.4 Diagnosis

Primary acquired cholesteatoma

6.5 Medical Management

The medical management of cholesteatoma includes in-office débridement and treatment of acute inflammatory changes. Dry ear precautions (e.g., with cotton ball and petroleum jelly) are mandatory. Ototopical antibiotics with steroids are used to reduce secondary infection and reduce granulation tissue formation. Systemic antibiotic therapy can also be used for concomitant infection. However, definitive treatment of cholesteatoma requires surgical intervention.

6.6 Surgical Management

The primary goal of therapy is to create a safe, dry ear. The options for management of cholesteatoma include canal wall up or canal wall down tympanomastoidectomy.

Factors that determine which surgical approach is warranted include extent of disease; presence of complications; mastoid pneumatization; patient factors such as comorbidities, age, and reliability; and the surgeon's technical ability. If patients have extensive disease, concern for poor follow-up, reduced mastoid pneumatization, and multiple comorbidities, then a canal wall down procedure should be strongly considered, as residual cholesteatoma is easily managed, although the mastoid bowl does need regular débridement. Canal wall up techniques maintain the normal position of the

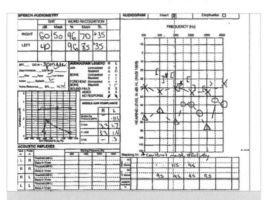

Fig. 6.1 An audiogram demonstrates profound right-sided deafness with left mixed hearing loss.

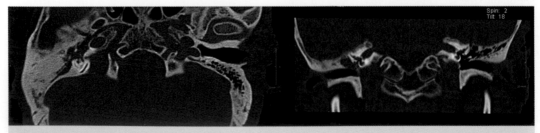

Fig. 6.2 Axial computed tomography scan cut that shows soft tissue mass in the epitympanic space with erosion of the tegmen and labyrinth.

tympanic membrane, but there are higher rates of recidivistic disease, which necessitates revision surgery. The most common site of residual or recurrent disease is the sinus tympani region, followed by the stapes footplate.

If a canal wall up technique is used, most surgeons utilize a combined postauricular transcanal and transmastoid exposure to completely extirpate cholesteatoma and a facial recess (posterior tympanotomy) approach as needed to access the mesotympanum. The canal wall down approach is the gold standard for treatment of cholesteatoma, particularly when an impending complication is present (e.g., cochlear fistula). The location of cholesteatoma, the extent of bone destruction, and the amount of mucosal inflammation will dictate whether reconstruction during the initial procedure is possible. Staging of the ear (also known as a second-look procedure) is often used to assess for recidivistic cholesteatoma and is typically performed 6 to 12 months after the initial procedure. At the time of the second look, an ossicular chain reconstruction can be performed.

In the current case, canal wall down tympanomastoidectomy was performed given the presence of a labyrinthine fistula, reduced mastoid pneumatization, and risk for recidivistic disease. Management of a labyrinthine fistula includes removing the matrix and repairing the defect with autologous tissue in cases of small fistula or leaving the matrix, exteriorizing the whole cavity, and then allowing it to re epithelialize.

6.7 Rehabilitation and Follow-up

A high index of suspicion is needed to assess for recurrence of disease over the life of the individual patient. If successful ossicular reconstruction is not achieved, consideration should be given to a bone-anchored hearing aid or referral for traditional hearing aid evaluation.

6.8 Questions

1. What is the most common site of recurrence for cholesteatoma?
   a) Sinus tympani and stapes footplate.
   b) Epitympanum.
   c) Mesotympanum.
   d) Facial recess.
2. What procedure is considered the gold standard for treatment of cholesteatoma?
   a) Mastoidectomy with facial recess.
   b) Canal wall up mastoidectomy.
   c) Canal wall down mastoidectomy.
   d) Tympanomastoidectomy.
3. What is the most common type of cholesteatoma?
   a) Congenital.
   b) Primary acquired.
   c) Secondary acquired.

Answers: 1. a 2. c 3. b

Suggested Readings

Glasscock ME III, Haynes DS, Storper IS, Bohrer PS. Surgery for chronic ear disease. In: Hughes G, Pensak M, eds. Clinical Otology. 3rd ed. New York, NY: Thieme; 2007

Persaud R, Hajioff D, Trinidade A, et al. Evidence-based review of aetiopathogenic theories of congenital and acquired cholesteatoma. J Laryngol Otol. 2007; 121(11):1013–1019

Smith JA, Danner CJ. Complications of chronic otitis media and cholesteatoma. Otolaryngol Clin North Am. 2006; 39(6):1237–1255

Collins WO, Choi SS. Otolaryngologic manifestations of achondroplasia. Arch Otolaryngol Head Neck Surg. 2007; 133(3):237–244

Jackler RK, Santa Maria PL, Varsak YK, Nguyen A, Blevins NH. A new theory on the pathogenesis of acquired cholesteatoma: Mucosal traction. Laryngoscope. 2015; 125 Suppl 4:S1–S14

Kuo CL. Etiopathogenesis of acquired cholesteatoma: prominent theories and recent advances in biomolecular research. Laryngoscope. 2015; 125(1):234–240

Copeland BJ, Buchman CA. Management of labyrinthine fistulae in chronic ear surgery. Am J Otolaryngol. 2003; 24(1):51–60

7 Otosclerosis

Brian D. Goico and Myles L. Pensak

7.1 History

A 54-year-old woman presented with a 10-year history of right-sided progressive hearing loss and tinnitus. She denied prior head trauma, chronic ear infections, aural fullness, vertigo, otalgia, or otorrhea. She was a lifelong nonsmoker and nondrinker. Her past medical history included hypertension and hyperlipidemia. Her physical examination demonstrated well-aerated middle ear spaces bilaterally without any masses or lesions appreciated. She had good tympanic membrane movement on pneumatic otoscopy. Her tuning fork Weber at 512 Hz lateralized to the right, and her Rinne was positive on the left and negative on the right at 512 Hz. She underwent an audiogram, which demonstrated a severe to profound mixed hearing loss in the right ear across all frequencies (► Fig. 7.1).

7.2 Differential Diagnosis—Key Points

- This patient demonstrated a significant unilateral mixed hearing loss across all frequencies with absent acoustic reflexes and a significant conductive component. There is a lengthy differential diagnosis for conductive or mixed hearing loss including effusion, cholesteatoma, tumors, tympanosclerosis, ossicular discontinuity, ossicular erosion, otosclerosis, osteogenesis imperfecta, superior semicircular canal dehiscence (SSCCD), tympanic membrane perforation, and Paget disease (osteitis deformans).
- History and physical examination are exceedingly important in determining the cause of conductive hearing loss. Otosclerosis is always in the top of the differential, especially in cases with no antedating otologic history of infection or

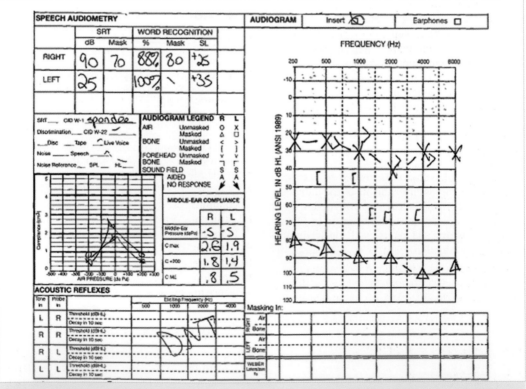

Fig. 7.1 Preoperative audiogram demonstrating a significant decrease in air conduction in the right ear. There is also a sensorineural loss due to cochlear otosclerosis.

trauma given that it is relatively common. More-over, not infrequently a positive family history is obtained. Otosclerosis is associated with hyper-vascularity of the cochlear promontory (Schwartz's sign) in about 10% of cases. SSCCD causes conductive hearing loss but is usually associated with vertiginous symptoms, especially with loud noises (Tullio's phenomenon) or pneu-matic otoscopy (Hennebert's sign). Autophony and pulsatile tinnitus are also frequent findings.

- Concomitant rhinosinusitis or upper respiratory infections may indicate effusions or eustachian tube dysfunction, both of which can be con-firmed on physical examination. Recurrent ear drainage and infections are associated with cho-lesteatoma and ossicular erosion. In this situa-tion, physical examination may reveal a chronic, nonhealing tympanic membrane perforation or deep retraction pocket and squamous debris.
- Previous head trauma may cause ossicular dis-continuity. Physical examination allows visual-ization of a tympanic membrane perforation or abnormal positioning of the ossicular chain. Finally, blue sclera, a history of frequent bone fractures, and concomitant neurologic findings are associated with osteogenesis imperfecta.
- Otosclerosis is histologically present in about 10% of the Caucasian population; however, only around 10% of those with histologic findings demonstrate symptoms (1% of this population cohort). It is less common in other ethnic groups and occurs more commonly in females, with a 2:1 ratio. In patients with clinical otosclerosis in one ear, 80% will histologically have contralateral involvement. The pathology is most commonly diagnosed in the fourth decade, and some data have shown it advances during pregnancy, although this has been refuted in other studies.
- Otosclerosis may manifest as conductive hearing loss, mixed hearing loss, or rarely, with only a sensorineural hearing loss (cochlear otosclero-sis). Most commonly, patients have a conductive or mixed loss with good word discrimination and absent acoustic reflexes. As with any type of hearing loss, it is frequently associated with tin-nitus. Although rare, vestibular symptoms may also be present.

7.3 Test Interpretation
7.3.1 Audiogram

The classic audiometric findings in otosclerosis include a significant conductive hearing loss that

progresses over time to a maximal conductive loss. Acoustic reflexes are absent. There is also a sensor-ineural hearing loss at 2,000 Hz (the resonant fre-quency of the ossicular chain) known as Carhart's notch. Sensorineural hearing loss may also be present, due to either cochlear otosclerosis or a concomitant loss such as in presbycusis.

7.3.2 Radiography

Radiographic studies are not essential for the diag-nosis of otosclerosis in a patient with a character-istic history and audiometric findings. However, a noncontrast high-resolution temporal bone com-puted tomography (CT) scan can be helpful at times. For example, this test may be helpful in the initial establishment of a diagnosis if an ossicular disruption, middle ear mass, SSCCD, or other cause of conductive loss is not ruled out on history and physical exam. Additionally, in patients with a mixed hearing loss, the CT scan may demonstrate cochlear involvement in otosclerosis by demon-strating a "halo sign" of demineralized bone around the otic capsule.

7.4 Diagnosis

Otosclerosis

7.5 Medical Management

All patients with a diagnosis of otosclerosis should be presented with the option of medical manage-ment, including fluoride supplementation and hearing amplification. Although fluoride has mini-mal evidence of clinical benefit in placebo-con-trolled studies, its historical use as an otosclerosis therapy and minimal side effect profile propagate its continued use. Hearing amplification by way of a hearing aid is a great alternative to surgery for patients with otosclerosis, eliminating the opera-tive risk of a stapedotomy or stapedectomy. Unfortunately, as hearing aids are not reimbursed by most insurance carriers, there is a financial con-sequence to this management plan.

7.6 Surgical Management

There are three surgical therapies that may be offered to patients with otosclerosis: bone-anch-ored hearing aid (BAHA), stapedotomy, or stape-dectomy. BAHA is an osseointegrated implant that allows direct transmission of sound through the skull to the cochlea, bypassing the fixed stapes. This therapy has been increasingly offered as an alternative option for patients with otosclerosis who cannot afford or tolerate hearing aids and want to avoid stapes surgery.

Stapedectomy or stapedotomy for treatment of the conductive hearing loss in otosclerosis is very effective; however, it also has potential operative risks that must be incorporated into an informed decision-making process with any otosclerosis patient considering elective surgery. The procedure entails removal of the stapes superstructure and creation of a hole in the stapes footplate (stapedotomy) or removal of the footplate (stapedectomy), with subsequent placement of a prosthesis between the vestibule and the lenticular process of the incus. One of the most feared risks is anacusis, which occurs in 1% of stapedectomy patients. Other risks include facial nerve injury, vertigo, dysgeusia, varying degrees of sensorineural hearing loss, tympanic membrane perforation, and perilymphatic fistula. Stapedectomy and stapedotomy should never be offered in an only hearing ear, an infected ear, or patients with X-linked stapes gusher syndrome. Substantial caution should be exercised in performing this procedure in patients with medical comorbidities, as in any elective procedure. In particular, patients on anticoagulation therapy who are unsafe to come off should strongly consider other treatment options. Even a small amount of bleeding will make the procedure more difficult and potentially increase the risk of complications. Additionally, this procedure should not be performed in patients who plan to scuba dive within 1 year of surgery or fly in nonpressurized airplane cabins.

This patient underwent a right transcanal tympanotomy and stapedotomy with an argon laser under general anesthesia (▶ Fig. 7.2). At her postoperative visit, she had a significant improvement in hearing and an audiogram demonstrated a closure of her right-sided air–bone gap to within 5 dB across all frequencies.

7.7 Rehabilitation and Follow-up

Postoperatively, patients need to avoid straining, strenuous activity, and nose blowing for several weeks. They should be instructed to keep their head elevated for several days postoperatively, and dry ear precautions should be implemented. Patients with bilateral otosclerosis should undergo at least 6 months to 1 year of observation between surgeries to ensure no delayed sensorineural hearing loss is noted.

7.8 Questions

1. Which of the following causes of conductive hearing loss is associated with dizziness on pneumatic otoscopy?
   a) Otosclerosis.
   b) Superior semicircular canal dehiscence (SSCCD).
   c) Glomus tympanicum.
   d) Osteogenesis imperfecta.
2. What does a "halo sign" on a temporal bone computed tomography (CT) scan indicate?
   a) Stapes fixation.
   b) SSCCD.
   c) Glomus tympanicum.
   d) Cochlear otosclerosis.
3. Which of the following is not an absolute contraindication to stapedectomy?

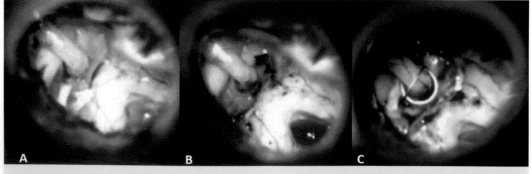

Fig. 7.2 (a) View of middle ear space demonstrating normal incudostapedial joint. (b) Stapes superstructure removed, demonstrating thickened footplate beneath. (c). Robinson's bucket handle prosthesis in position over fascia graft that is placed over stapedotomy.

a) Only hearing ear.
b) X-linked stapes gusher.
c) Mixed hearing loss.
d) Active acute otitis media.

Answers: 1. b 2. d 3. c

Suggested Readings

Fritsch MH, Naumann IC. Phylogeny of the stapes prosthesis. Otol Neurotol. 2008; 29(3):407–415

Hentschel MA, Huizinga P, van der Velden DL, et al. Limited evidence for the effect of sodium fluoride on deterioration of hearing loss in patients with otosclerosis: a systematic review of the literature. Otol Neurotol. 2014; 35(6):1052–1057

Lempert J. Improvement of hearing in cases of otosclerosis a new one stage surgical technic. Arch Otolaryngol. 1938; 28(1):42–97

Lippy WH, Berenholz LP. Pearls on otosclerosis and stapedectomy. Ear Nose Throat J. 2008; 87(6):326–328

Merkus P, van Loon MC, Smit CF, Smits C, de Cock AF, Hensen EF. Decision making in advanced otosclerosis: an evidence-based strategy. Laryngoscope. 2011; 121(9):1935–1941

Schrauwen I, Van Camp G. The etiology of otosclerosis: a combination of genes and environment. Laryngoscope. 2010; 120(6):1195–1202

8 Sudden Sensorineural Hearing Loss

Niall D. Jefferson and John H. Greinwald Jr.

8.1 History

A 68-year-old woman presented with new, rapid onset hearing loss in the right ear associated with some imbalance, which has since resolved. Her hearing had previously been normal. She had no recent viral symptoms. She had a history of non–insulin dependent diabetes mellitus and smoked half a pack of cigarettes per day. She denied headache, vertigo, or visual changes. There had been no head trauma.

Physical examination of both ears revealed normal external auditory canals and intact tympanic membranes bilaterally. The Rinne was equivocal on the right and the Weber lateralized to the left ear. The remainder of the cranial nerve examination was normal. The cerebellar examination was normal and Romberg's test was unremarkable.

8.2 Differential Diagnosis—Key Points

Sudden sensorineural hearing loss (SSNHL) is the term used to describe an abrupt onset of hearing loss of at least 30 dB in three contiguous frequencies on a standard audiogram within 3 days or less. SSNHL is typically variable in severity and is usually unilateral, although bilateral involvement up to 4% has been reported. A cause for SSNHL is identified in only 10 to 15% of patients at the time of presentation. A large number of theories regarding the cause of this condition have been proposed, although the ultimate etiology often remains unknown. The clinical history and physical examination can help narrow the potential diagnoses. Given that the list of possible causes is plentiful, it can be helpful to categorize the potential causes into traumatic, infectious, inflammatory, vascular, neoplastic, toxic, and idiopathic. Importantly, the nonidiopathic causes should be identified early and management instituted, the most pressing being stroke, malignancy, and vestibular schwannoma.

- *Infectious:* Many infectious processes can affect the inner ear. Viral infections are the most commonly implicated, although the evidence remains circumstantial. Noncontrolled studies report a recent viral illness in 17 to 33% of patients presenting with SSNHL; this becomes less compelling when considering that 25% of patients without hearing loss visiting an otolaryngologist report a viral-like illness in the preceding month. Bacterial and even fungal infections have been implicated. Despite the lack of solid evidence, infection (especially viral) remains the most likely culprit in many cases of SSNHL.
- *Traumatic:* Trauma to the inner ear, whether physical, acoustic, or barotrauma, can cause sudden deafness secondary to a perilymphatic fistula or cochlear membrane breaks.
- *Immune-mediated inner ear disease:* A number of recognized autoimmune conditions including Cogan's syndrome and systemic lupus erythematosus have been documented as causing hearing loss. The evidence supporting an autoimmune cause for SSNHL has been growing over time. With improving markers for inner ear autoimmunity, it is possible that a greater link will be elucidated as a cause for SSNHL.
- *Vascular:* The cochlea has an end-organ blood supply with no collateral vasculature and therefore is at risk of vascular compromise. This can occur as a result of thrombosis, embolus, or vasospasm. Other possible mechanisms include atherosclerosis, hypotension, hematologic diseases such as leukemia, sickle cell anemia, macroglobulinemia, and polycythemia. SSNHL can be more common and more severe in patients with diabetes.
- *Neoplastic:* Between 2.7 and 10% of individuals presenting with SSNHL have retrocochlear pathology. The most common of these is a vestibular schwannoma (VS). Ten percent to 20% of patients with a VS will report a sudden decrease in their hearing at some point in their history.
- *Miscellaneous:* Iron deficiency anemia has been identified as a risk factor for SSNHL. A study of 4,000 individuals with SSNHL and 12,000 controls reported that 4.3% of the hearing loss group had iron deficiency anemia compared with 3% of the control group. The association between anemia and hearing loss appeared greatest in patients aged 44 years and younger.

8.3 Test Interpretation

SSNHL has a reported incidence of between 5 and 160 cases per 100,000 members of the population.

Associated with this are a multitude of medical visits to emergency departments, audiologists, primary care providers, and otolaryngologists. As outlined above, despite a comprehensive history and physical examination the etiology remains unknown in the majority of cases. This leads to extensive testing and a significant associated cost to the health care system. The clinical practice guidelines on SSNHL released by the American Academy of Otolaryngology–Head and Neck Surgery (AAO-HNS) in 2012 made recommendations in relation to testing and are outlined in ▶ Table 8.1.

Conductive hearing loss and SSNHL have significantly different management paradigms; therefore, determining the nature of the hearing loss through the history, physical examination, tuning fork exam, and audiometry is essential. Associated with the history and physical examination will be identifying whether there is a definable underlying condition such as Meniere's disease, an autoimmune or metabolic condition that, if identified, should be managed in accordance with best practice for that condition.

Computed tomography (CT) scanning is not recommended in most cases of SSNHL because it carries an associated radiation exposure and cost and offers little to the management of this condition. Exceptions to this are cases of trauma, chronic ear disease, or focal neurologic findings.

As indicated above, accurate audiometric evaluation confirms the diagnosis of SSNHL and allows for monitoring for improvement during follow-up.

While specific blood tests may be warranted in selected cases such as testing for Lyme disease in endemic areas, shotgun testing without consideration of patient or geographic risk factors is discouraged. The associated cost of extensive testing and the potential harm related to false negative or false positive results can be significant.

Retrocochlear pathology, with VS being the most common, is an important consideration in the patient that presents with SSNHL. Prevalence rates of cerebellopontine angle (CPA) tumors identified in SSNHL patients have been reported between 2.7 and 10.2% on magnetic resonance imaging (MRI). Symptoms associated with CPA tumors include tinnitus in the affected ear, otalgia, and paresthesia; however, these symptoms are rare enough in practice that their absence cannot be relied upon to exclude a retrocochlear lesion. While there are no randomized trials examining investigation versus no investigation for VS, the cost of screening compares favorably to the cost of treating larger tumors as well as the associated poorer hearing outcomes with a larger lesion.

In this case, the pure tone audiogram revealed a severe to profound SSNHL in the right ear, worse in the high frequencies. An MRI scan performed was normal with no evidence of retrocochlear pathology.

8.4 Diagnosis

Idiopathic unilateral, right-sided SSNHL

8.5 Medical Management

A number of therapeutic strategies have been proposed in the management of SSNHL, including the use of vasodilators, antiviral agents, thrombolytics, antioxidants, hemodilution, and hyperbaric oxygen. The most accepted treatment has been steroids, administered systemically or intratympanically, either alone or in combination.

Table 8.1 Summary of SSNHL American Academy of Otolaryngology–Head and Neck Surgery 2012 clinical practice guidelines

Evidence-based statement	Statement strength
Exclusion of conductive hearing loss	Strong recommendation
Modifying factors	Recommendation
Computed tomography	Strong recommendation against
Audiometric confirmation of idiopathic SSNHL	Recommendation
Laboratory testing	Strong recommendation against
Retrocochlear pathology	Recommendation
Abbreviations: SSNHL, sudden sensorineural hearing loss.	

The first evidence supporting the use of steroids was by Wilson et al in 1980. Since then a number of randomized, pseudorandomized, and non-randomized trials have been performed examining the benefit of steroids in the management of this condition. The AAO-HNS clinical practice guidelines from 2012 refrained from making strong recommendations for or against the use of steroids given the nature of the available evidence. Crane et al in January of 2015 released a meta-analysis of randomized trials relating to the use of steroids for SSNHL. They found that the available evidence does not support the use of systemic steroids, as steroids provided no benefit compared to placebo. In addition there was an absence of treatment effect of intratympanic over systemic steroids. There may be benefit for intratympanic steroids in salvage cases. However, as the authors point out, this finding must be interpreted with caution, as any treatment failure could be considered a salvage case.

Overall, the available evidence indicates that the mode of administration of steroids for SSNHL does not seem to significantly affect the outcome. Steroids do not seem to have a treatment effect as a primary treatment for SSNHL. Finally, while the available evidence seems to suggest a role for intratympanic steroids as a salvage treatment, as outlined above, this should be accepted with caution and the clinician should reconsider the use of steroids in the setting of SSNHL as either primary or salvage treatment.

8.6 Surgical Management

There is no role for surgery in the acute management of true idiopathic SSNHL. There is a role for surgery in the repair of perilymphatic fluid leak in cases of SSNHL associated with a positive fistula test or a history of recent trauma or barotrauma or in cases of SSNHL associated with a CPA tumor. In some cases, patients may meet the indications for cochlear implantation, which is discussed in Chapter 11.

8.7 Rehabilitation and Follow-up

Fortunately the rates of spontaneous recovery for SSNHL are generally good, ranging from 47 to 63%. Negative prognostic indicators include age younger than 15 years or greater than 65 years, an elevated erythrocyte sedimentation rate (ESR) (> 25), vertigo or vestibular changes on electronystagmography, hearing loss in the opposite ear, or a severe hearing loss at the initial evaluation.

Clinicians should educate patients about the natural history of the condition and about risks and benefits of current treatment options and their limitations given the current evidence.

Follow-up audiometry should be performed within 6 months of diagnosis to assess for other etiologies in patients who have progression of their hearing loss and to identify those patients who may benefit from rehabilitation. If treatment is initiated, earlier audiometric testing may be indicated to assess response to the intervention.

Patients with an incomplete recovery should be counseled about the possible benefits of hearing assistive technology, amplification, and possible implantation, as well as other supportive measures.

This patient was monitored with serial audiograms, which demonstrated progressive improvement in her hearing thresholds to the point that a hearing aid in the right ear was sufficient.

8.8 Questions

1. Standard evaluation of sudden sensorineural hearing loss (SSNHL) should include all of the following except
   a) Complete history and physical examination.
   b) Audiogram.
   c) Computed tomography (CT) scan of the head.
   d) Magnetic resonance imaging (MRI) of the brain.
2. Management options for cases of SSNHL include
   a) Education about the natural history.
   b) Serial audiometry.
   c) Trial of hearing assistive technology.
   d) Possible implantation.
   e) All of the above.
3. SSNHL is defined as
   a) Abrupt hearing loss of at least 30 dB in three contiguous frequencies within 3 days or less.
   b) Abrupt hearing loss of at least 30 dB in two contiguous frequencies within 3 days or less.
   c) Abrupt hearing loss of at least 20 dB in three contiguous frequencies within 3 days or less.
   d) Abrupt hearing loss of at least 20 dB in two contiguous frequencies within 3 days or less.

Answers: 1. c 2. e 3. a

Suggested Readings

Byl FM, Jr. Sudden hearing loss: eight years' experience and suggested prognostic table. Laryngoscope. 1984; 94(5 Pt 1):647–661

Conlin AE, Parnes LS. Treatment of sudden sensorineural hearing loss: I. A systematic review. Arch Otolaryngol Head Neck Surg. 2007; 133(6):573–581

Crane RA, Camilon M, Nguyen S, Meyer TA. Steroids for treatment of sudden sensorineural hearing loss: a meta-analysis of randomized controlled trials. Laryngoscope. 2015; 125(1):209–217

Stachler RJ, Chandrasekhar SS, Archer SM, et al. American Academy of Otolaryngology-Head and Neck Surgery. Clinical practice guideline: sudden hearing loss. Otolaryngol Head Neck Surg. 2012; 146 (3) Suppl:S1–S35

9 Labyrinthine Fistula

Shawn M. Stevens and Ravi N. Samy

9.1 History

A 40-year-old female woman presented to your office with complaints of sudden hearing loss, fluctuating dizziness, and aural fullness. The hearing loss and dizziness had come on suddenly approximately 6 weeks ago. She stated her hearing was initially "muffled" on the left but had progressed over the last week to the point that she could not hear anything from that ear. She also noted disequilibrium as well as true vertigo spells lasting seconds when she bent over or lifted heavy objects. She did note intermittent purulent drainage from the left ear since her symptoms began.

She had a long history of chronic ear disease and had undergone two prior tympanoplasties for cholesteatoma on the left. Both of these had been performed by an otolaryngologist in a different state. She reported the latter surgery had been performed roughly 4 years ago and entailed a canal wall down approach. She was aware of few other details regarding this procedure, and operative notes were not available for either procedure. Aside from mild intermittent asthma, her remaining history was unremarkable. She had quit smoking roughly 15 years ago.

On exam, you noted a well-appearing woman in no distress. The patient's head and neck exam was largely unremarkable. Her cranial nerve exam was normal with symmetric facial function and intact sensation. You did note crusted drainage emanating from the left external auditory canal. The auricle appeared normal without evidence of external infection. There was no pain with manipulation of the pinna or tenderness to palpation over the temporal fossa, mastoid, or upper neck. Weber's test performed with a 512-Hz fork lateralized to the right. Rinne's test was positive on the right but could not be detected on the left (she heard it on the right when the tuning fork was placed on bone). The patient had a subtle spontaneous right-beating nystagmus that was more pronounced under Frenzel goggles. A Dix-Hallpike test was negative.

Otomicroscopic exam was normal on the right side aside from mild retraction of the tympanic membrane and mild myringosclerosis. Extensive mucopurulent debris was noted on the left to be filling her external canal. This was removed with a no. 3 suction and revealed a thickened tympanic membrane with a large central perforation filled with granulation tissue. Squamous debris was noted within the middle ear space. A fistula test performed with a pneumatic otoscope was positive on the left under both positive and negative pressure (Hennebert's sign).

9.2 Differential Diagnosis—Key Points

At this point in the patient's history, given her presentation with sudden hearing loss and fluctuating dizziness, there would be significant concern for development of a labyrinthine fistula. The addition of active middle ear disease (possibly recidivistic cholesteatoma) and a positive fistula test further support this notion.

- Labyrinthine fistulas may develop through any abnormal breach in the dense otic capsule bone that connects the fluid-filled spaces of the membranous labyrinth to the surrounding anatomy of the middle ear, mastoid cavity, or middle fossa. The oval and round windows represent the only natural "weak" points in the continuity of the otic capsule.
- Labyrinthine fistulas may occur via a number of mechanisms. These include temporal bone fracture, barotrauma, and iatrogenic injury. They may also arise spontaneously, in the setting of chronic ear disease, and in the form of superior semicircular canal dehiscence. Although each of these mechanisms is highly unique, the resulting clinical manifestations can be remarkably similar.
- A communication between the endolymphatic and perilymphatic spaces of the labyrinth or passage of perilymph from the labyrinth into the middle ear or mastoid can lead to hearing loss and/or vestibular disturbances.
- Perhaps the most well described instance of labyrinthine fistula is as a complication following stapes surgery. In such cases, the stapes prosthesis can become displaced, partially dislodged, or subluxed, resulting in leakage of perilymph from the footplate fenestra. Patients will present with imbalance, hearing loss, and possibly vertigo related to straining, positioning, or loud sounds. Management entails middle ear exploration with revision of the prosthesis or patching of the fenestra.

- Superior semicircular canal dehiscence has received the most in-depth scientific investigation out of the various etiologies of labyrinthine fistula. This entity has a somewhat unique presentation and management strategy, and for this reason it is covered in chapter 19.
- Traumatic fistulas (e.g., after motor vehicle accident) can be more ambiguous in presentation and may be masked by concomitant injuries, diminished mental status, or intentional sedation for ventilator management. Temporal bone fractures may extend to involve the otic capsule or cause traumatic disruption of the ossicular chain. Sensorineural hearing loss related to traumatic inner ear fistulas is typically irreversible. In select cases, middle ear exploration may be considered in patients suffering from vertigo or fluctuating hearing loss.
- Spontaneous perilymph fistula (PLF) remains one of the most controversial topics in otolaryngology. This is mainly due to a lack of a gold standard test that is sensitive and specific for such a diagnosis. Established indications for surgery remain unclear, and the pathogenesis of spontaneous PLF is not well understood. Patients will typically present with fluctuating sensorineural hearing loss, dizziness/vertigo, tinnitus, and aural fullness. Fistula tests performed with pneumatic otoscopy may elicit evoked nystagmus (Hennebert's sign). Surgery, when indicated, entails middle ear exploration focusing on the annular ring of the oval window and the round window niche where spontaneous PLF is thought to arise. If a fistula is detected, the windows are bolstered with fascia. In appropriately selected cases, vestibular complaints may improve in roughly two-thirds of patients. Hearing loss, however, will remain unchanged or worsen in 70 to 90% of patients as reported in the largest series on the topic.
- Chronic otitis media, typically in association with cholesteatoma, can result in erosion of otic capsule bone. The reported rate of labyrinthine fistula in chronic ear disease varies from 2 to 12%. It is most often reported during revision surgery, especially following a canal wall down mastoidectomy. Patients will typically present in a manner similar to poststapedectomy perilymph fistula: fluctuating vertigo, hearing loss, and spontaneous nystagmus. Fistula tests are typically positive, but they may be negative in some cases due to cholesteatoma or diseased mucosa limiting pressure compliance changes or obstructing the fistula site.

- The most common locations for a labyrinthine fistula to arise in the setting of chronic ear disease are (in decreasing order of frequency) the lateral semicircular canal, the oval window, and the promontory.

9.3 Test Interpretation

Further testing in this scenario was warranted because of the patient's constellation of symptoms. The concerning factor here was the patient's sudden and severe degree of hearing loss. This patient was immediately placed on high-dose oral steroids with a proton pump inhibitor. Tests to be considered in this case would include

- *Audiogram:* Audiologic testing demonstrated normal hearing on the right side, with a speech reception threshold at 10 dB and a speech discrimination score of 100%. On the left side, a profound sensorineural hearing loss was noted at all frequencies. Speech testing could not be conducted on the left. Immittance testing was notable for a type B, high-volume tympanogram on the left and a type As curve of the right (▶ Fig. 9.1).
- *Electronystagmography-videonystagmography:* These tests demonstrated spontaneous right-beating nystagmus. A significant left-sided vestibulopathy was noted on caloric testing. A positive fistula test was again established on the left.
- *Vestibular evoked myogenic potentials (VEMPs):* These would be useful in cases of suspected superior semicircular canal dehiscence but would not have added much useful information in this patient's presentation.
- *Radiography:* A high-resolution computed tomography (CT) scan of the temporal bones with 0.67-mm collimations and coronal reconstructions would be the most useful test. American Academy of Otolaryngology–Head and Neck Surgery (AAO-HNS) guidelines do recommend such CT imaging in all cases of chronic ear disease where cholesteatoma is suspected and revision surgery is under consideration. In this case, close inspection should be made of the otic capsule structures at risk for fistulas, including the lateral semicircular canal, round/oval windows, and bony promontory. CT imaging should also be inspected for evidence of recurrent cholesteatoma, high-riding jugular bulb, tegmen dehiscences, and/or a thin or dehiscent fallopian canal. The addition of Stenver and Pöschl views would be helpful in assessing for superior canal

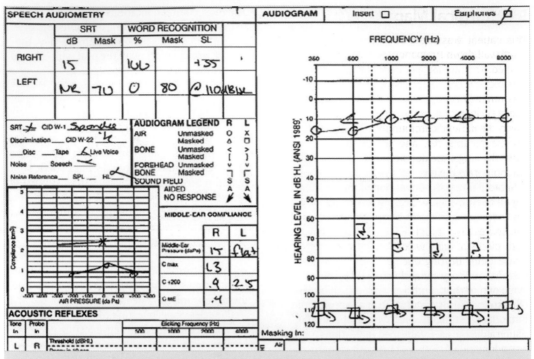

Fig. 9.1 Audiogram from a patient with suspected left labyrinthine fistula related to cholesteatoma. An asymmetric, profound left sensorineural hearing loss is demonstrated. Speech audiometry testing was not perceived by the patient on the left.

dehiscence, if this is under consideration. CT, in this case, revealed a labyrinthine fistula with erosion of the otic capsule at the promontory and a soft tissue communication between the middle and inner ears (▶ Fig. 9.1). Soft tissue densities within the middle ear were suggestive of diseased mucosa or cholesteatoma.

9.4 Diagnosis

- Labyrinthine fistula (via the bony promontory) related to cholesteatoma/chronic ear disease
- Profound sensorineural hearing loss secondary to inner ear fistula

9.5 Medical Management

The patient was immediately treated with high-dose oral steroids and supportive care, both of which were initiated during her work-up. Unfortunately, her hearing failed to improve although her dizziness and vertigo did get better during the preoperative period. Serial aural toilet was conducted in the clinic, and strict dry ear precautions were

observed. Medicated drops were used in the left ear with resolution of her drainage and granulation tissue. Although the definitive treatment for this disease is surgical, medical optimization can reduce technical difficulties encountered during revision chronic ear surgery and potentially reduce the rate of postoperative morbidity.

In cases of known or suspected labyrinthine fistulas, systemic steroids have been shown to have some efficacy in prevention of further deterioration of sensorineural hearing. There is debate in the literature concerning the appropriate time to intervene surgically for a labyrinthine fistula. This timing is highly dependent on the causative mechanism, the patient's overall health, and the preoperative hearing status. Efforts should be made, when possible, to save as much hearing and vestibular function as possible via expedited surgical intervention. Once severe to profound hearing loss has ensued, however, this tends to be irreversible. In the present case, it was felt that the benefits of medically reducing middle ear inflammatory disease outweighed the risks of an immediate surgical intervention.

9.6 Surgical Management

This patient was taken to the operating room. A canal wall down tympanomastoidectomy was performed. The labyrinthine fistula was identified, as was recidivistic cholesteatoma. All diseased tissue was removed from this area, and the promontory dehiscence was plugged with temporalis fascia. Given the patient's profound hearing loss, multiple disease recurrences, and desire to avoid future bowl cleanings, the decision was made to close off and obliterate the ear.

Subtotal petrosectomy was conducted, removing all remaining air cell tracts. All epithelial surfaces were removed from the mastoid and middle ear spaces. The eustachian tube was obliterated with pieces of bone wax mixed with oxidized cellulose (after drilling out the protympanum). The external auditory canal skin was then everted and oversewn with an imbricating stitch. A musculoperiosteal flap was then rotated inward to reinforce the external auditory canal closure. To obliterate the resulting middle ear/mastoid cavity, an abdominal fat graft was harvested from the left lower quadrant. The wound was then closed in layers.

9.7 Rehabilitation and Follow-up

As anticipated, the patient did not recover hearing in the diseased ear. Her dizziness and vertigo did resolve following surgery. She has not had any significant postoperative complications. Following middle ear/mastoid obliteration, especially in cases such as this associated with cholesteatoma, patients should be followed clinically. Magnetic resonance imaging (MRI) with diffusion weighted imaging may be considered, as this carries good sensitivity and specificity for recidivistic disease. The patient has several options for hearing rehabilitation in the future. These would include contralateral routing of signal (CROS) hearing aid and osseointegrated hearing aid. Cochlear implantation for single-sided deafness is currently under investigation, but outcomes data are limited.

9.8 Questions

1. True or false? All suspected labyrinthine fistulas must be explored urgently.
2. Which of the following would not be an expected location for a labyrinthine fistula in a patient with chronic ear disease and recurrent cholesteatoma?
   a) Protympanum.
   b) Oval window.
   c) Cochlear promontory.
   d) Lateral semicircular canal.
3. The surgical management of spontaneous perilymph fistula is a controversial topic in otolaryngology. One of the primary problems underlying this is
   a) Poor hearing outcomes following surgical intervention.
   b) A relatively high rate of iatrogenic facial nerve injury during middle ear exploration.
   c) The procedure is technically challenging.
   d) There is no gold standard diagnostic test for this disorder.

Answers: 1. False 2. a 3. d

Suggested Readings

Albera R, Canale A, Lacilla M, Cavalot AL, Ferrero V. Delayed vertigo after stapes surgery. Laryngoscope. 2004; 114(5):860–862

Hornibrook J. Perilymph fistula: fifty years of controversy. ISRN Otolaryngol. 2012; 2012(12):281248

Maitland CG. Perilymphatic fistula. Curr Neurol Neurosci Rep. 2001; 1(5):486–491

Minor LB. Labyrinthine fistulae: pathobiology and management. Curr Opin Otolaryngol Head Neck Surg. 2003; 11(5):340–346

Sim RJ, Jardine AH, Beckenham EJ. Long-term outcome of children undergoing surgery for suspected perilymph fistula. J Laryngol Otol. 2009; 123(3):298–302

10 Meniere's Disease

Patrick R. Owens and Myles L. Pensak

10.1 History

A 63-year-old female woman presented with a chief complaint of vertigo and right-sided hearing loss present for the past 6 years. The episodes lasted for several hours, were associated with nausea and vomiting, and had been more frequent over the past 6 months. She reported a fluctuating hearing loss accompanied by aural fullness and tinnitus on the right. She had no history of ear surgery or family history of ear disease. She had no history of noise exposure, ototoxic medications, head trauma, or allergies. Physical examination revealed a Weber at 512 Hz that lateralized to the left, and her Rinne at 512 Hz was positive bilaterally. Otomicroscopic examination revealed normal tympanic membranes without effusion, and a negative fistula test was obtained. The remainder of her head and neck and neuro-otologic examinations were normal.

10.2 Differential Diagnosis—Key Points

- Meniere's disease is characterized by episodic vertigo, fluctuating sensorineural hearing loss, tinnitus, and aural fullness. Attacks generally last 20 minutes to hours. There is variability in the symptoms and progression of the disease. It primarily affects white individuals with a peak incidence between 40 and 60 years. Meniere's disease can rarely occur in children. While the pathobiology and clinical presentation is similar, Meniere's syndrome has a defined etiology, while Meniere's disease, by definition, is idiopathic.
- The differential diagnosis includes perilymphatic fistula, dizziness associated with otitis media, benign positional vertigo of childhood, tumors of the skull base (e.g., meningiomas and acoustic neuromas), and autoimmune inner ear disease. An autoimmune inner ear disease work-up must be considered in patients with bilateral Meniere's disease. Migraine-associated vestibulopathy (MAV) should also be considered in the differential.
- The pathogenesis stems from endolymphatic hydrops, most likely from overproduction or insufficient absorption through the endolymphatic sac, from either an anatomic or functional standpoint. One theory involves microruptures of the membranous labyrinth with leakage of potassium-rich endolymph into the perilymphatic space. Autoimmune, viral, or ischemic factors may also contribute.
- Allergy can play a role in Meniere's exacerbations. It is theorized that antigenic exposure leads to fluid changes in the endolymphatic sac, ion disturbances, and vestibulocochlear neurotoxicity. Accumulation of immune complexes may affect the sac's filtering ability. Endolymphatic hydrops results in saccular distention, which causes the sac to abut the stapes footplate with a resultant positive Hennebert's sign or Tullio's phenomenon. As a result of this phenomenon, stapes procedures are contraindicated in active Meniere's disease.
- Meniere's disease is the idiopathic presentation of the syndrome of sensorineural hearing loss, tinnitus, vertigo, and aural fullness. Clinically, vertiginous attacks generally last 20 minutes to hours. Recurrent vestibulopathy and atypical Meniere's disease may be confounding diagnoses. A rare presentation is the drop attacks of Tumarkin, characterized by sudden falls secondary to spatial disorientation but without loss of consciousness. Lermoyez's syndrome is characterized by improving hearing status and reduced tinnitus with the onset of vertigo. Horizontal nystagmus is present during acute attacks. Hearing loss is typically low frequency and fluctuating in the early period but can progress to a moderate sensorineural hearing loss in all frequencies.

10.3 Test Interpretation

Standard testing consists of an audiogram with a typical flat or low-frequency hearing loss (▶ Fig. 10.1). Electronystagmography for evaluation of vestibular function and electrocochleography (ECochG) can also be considered. ECochG may demonstrate increased SP:AP ratios, with 0.4 being the upper limit of normal. Magnetic resonance imaging (MRI) with gadolinium is necessary to rule out other pathologic conditions that can mimic Meniere's disease, including retrocochlear pathologies such as acoustic neuromas.

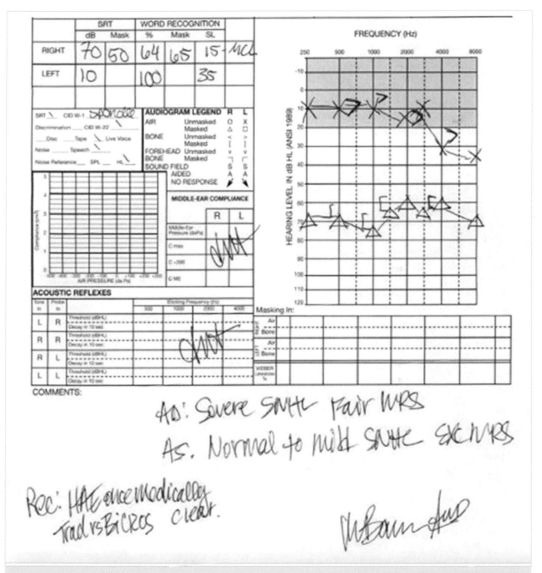

Fig. 10.1 Asymmetric sensorineural hearing loss on the right ear with fair word recognition score. Low-frequency sensorineural hearing loss is common in patients with Meniere's disease.

10.4 Diagnosis

Right-sided Meniere's disease

10.5 Medical Management

Medical treatment consists of lifestyle changes; salt restriction with a 2-g sodium diet and diuretics are used to reduce endolymph accumulation (hydrops). Additionally, patients are often advised to stop smoking and to limit alcohol and caffeine consumption, although there is very limited evidence that this impacts endolymphatic hydrops. Stress reduction is also important. Any allergy symptoms that are related to episodes should be addressed and managed. This has been shown to increase quality of life and improve symptomatology in patients. Symptomatic treatment for acute episodes includes sedatives or antiemetics. Disequilibrium may persist between vertigo attacks. Vestibular rehabilitation is of benefit to minimize disequilibrium and risk of falls. Intratympanic steroids can be used as a nonablative office procedure for their anti-inflammatory, immunosuppressive, and possible antioxidant effects. There is increasing empiric evidence to suggest temporary efficacy for this therapy. However, double-blind studies are currently not reported. There may be a role for positive pressure application to the middle ear as a means for redistributing inner ear fluids. Use of the Meniett device may provide benefit for vertigo reduction in select patients.

10.6 Surgical Management

For about 10 to 25% of patients, medical therapy fails and surgical therapy is required. Despite ablative procedures, central adaptation is still needed. Hearing conservation procedures should be attempted before hearing ablative procedures in patients with functional hearing and include endolymphatic sac decompression with or without mastoid shunt placement. There remains debate regarding the efficacy of these procedures since a meta-analysis showed insufficient evidence compared to placebo. However, it has been the experience of the University of Cincinnati faculty that carefully selected patients with vertigo experience a significantly improved quality of life with shunting. Vestibular neurectomy (via retrosigmoid or middle cranial fossa routes) is also an excellent option for severe vertigo for disabled patients. Additional ablative treatments would include intratympanic gentamicin (aminoglycoside therapy), which can reduce vestibular attacks with greater success than shunting but less effectively than vestibular neurectomy. Intratympanic gentamicin has a greater than 5 to 15% chance of increased hearing loss with tinnitus. Surgical ablation procedures with a labyrinthectomy are reserved for those patients with a nonserviceable hearing ear.

10.7 Rehabilitation and Follow-up

Meniere's disease affects an individual's quality of life because of changes in the cochleovestibular system. The patient will need long-term follow-up to assess for progression of symptoms, along with serial audiograms to monitor hearing. Patients can also develop symptoms in the contralateral ear with a reported frequency of 25 to 40%. Because of the potential for bilateral involvement, very careful consideration must be given before recommending an irreversible ablative procedure for the symptomatic side. Tinnitus and hearing loss can often be successfully managed with use of a hearing aid.

10.8 Questions

1. The following are treatments for Meniere's disease that are considered ablative except
   a) Labyrinthectomy.
   b) Vestibular neurectomy.
   c) Endolymphatic sac decompression.
   d) Intratympanic gentamicin injection.
2. The most common pattern of hearing loss associated with Meniere's disease is
   a) High-frequency picket fence sensorineural hearing loss.
   b) Mixed conductive and sensorineural hearing loss.
   c) High-frequency sensorineural hearing loss.
   d) Low-frequency sensorineural hearing loss.
3. Meniere's syndrome has been associated with all the following except
   a) Otosclerosis.
   b) Autoimmune inner ear disease.
   c) Syphilis.
   d) Lyme disease.

Answers: 1. c 2. d 3. a

Suggested Readings

Schuknecht HF. Meniere's disease: a correlation of symptomatology and pathology. Laryngoscope. 1963; 73:651–665

Boleas-Aguirre MS, Lin FR, Della Santina CC, Minor LB, Carey JP. Longitudinal results with intratympanic dexamethasone in the treatment of Ménière's disease. Otol Neurotol. 2008; 29(1):33–38

Gates GA, Verrall A, Green JD, Jr, Tucci DL, Telian SA. Meniett clinical trial: long-term follow-up. Arch Otolaryngol Head Neck Surg. 2006; 132(12):1311–1316

Glasscock ME, III, Gulya AJ, Pensak ML, Black JN, Jr. Medical and surgical management of Meniere's disease. Am J Otol. 1984; 5(6):536–542

Brinson GM, Chen DA, Arriaga MA. Endolymphatic mastoid shunt versus endolymphatic sac decompression for Ménière's disease. Otolaryngol Head Neck Surg. 2007; 136(3):415–421

Lee L, Pensak ML. Contemporary role of endolymphatic mastoid shunt surgery in the era of transtympanic perfusion strategies. Ann Otol Rhinol Laryngol. 2008; 117(12):871–875

Pullens B, Giard JL, Verschuur HP, van Benthem PP. Surgery for Ménière's disease. Cochrane Database Syst Rev. 2010(1):CD005395

Bodmer D, Morong S, Stewart C, Alexander A, Chen JM, Nedzelski JM. Long-term vertigo control in patients after intratympanic gentamicin instillation for Ménière's disease. Otol Neurotol. 2007; 28(8):1140–1144

De La Cruz A, Borne Teufert K, Berliner KI. Transmastoid labyrinthectomy versus translabyrinthine vestibular nerve section: does cutting the vestibular nerve make a difference in outcome? Otol Neurotol. 2007; 28(6):801–808

Derebery MJ. Allergic management of Meniere's disease: an outcome study. Otolaryngol Head Neck Surg. 2000; 122(2):174–182

11 Cochlear Implant

Kareem O. Tawfik and Ravi N. Samy

11.1 History

A 79-year-old woman presented with a history of subjective, slowly progressive bilateral hearing loss over approximately 20 years. She wore conventional hearing aids, but over time their benefit had waned considerably. She complained of difficulty understanding speech in noisy environments and reported constant, bilateral nonpulsatile tinnitus. She denied a history of ear infections, ear surgery, head trauma, otorrhea, otalgia, aural fullness, dizziness, or visual problems. A focused head and neck examination revealed no abnormalities, and otomicroscopic examination was normal. The patient could not hear the Weber tuning fork examination; Rinne was positive bilaterally.

11.2 Differential Diagnosis—Key Points

- This physical examination was consistent with bilateral sensorineural hearing loss, which in this patient might be secondary to presbycusis. Audiometric testing was needed to define the nature and extent of hearing loss.
- The differential diagnosis of bilateral sensorineural hearing loss is lengthy and includes a variety of conditions: (1) hearing loss associated with systemic manifestations (infectious, immunologic, metabolic), (2) syndromic and nonsyndromic congenital hearing loss, (3) ototoxicity, (4) autoimmune inner ear disease (AIED), (5) idiopathic hearing loss, or (6) age-related hearing loss (i.e., presbycusis).
- A thorough history, physical examination, and audiometric and imaging studies are useful in identifying a specific cause. Serologic testing can be useful for AIED testing, as well as for hearing loss due to less common etiologies (such as syphilis). Although the precise cause for deafness cannot always be determined, it is helpful to classify patients into three categories: (1) postlingually deafened (deaf at or after 5 years of age), (2) congenitally deafened children (prelingual deafness), and (3) congenitally deafened adolescents and adults. In general, cochlear implantation results in favorable outcomes in patients with postlingual deafness compared to those with prelingual deafness. Similarly, patients with a short duration of antecedent deafness tend to have improved outcomes compared to those with long-standing hearing loss.
- Anatomic conditions that preclude successful cochlear implantation may be congenital or acquired. *Michel's aplasia* (cochlear agenesis) and *small internal auditory canal syndrome*, in which the cochlear nerve may be congenitally deficient or absent (also known as *cochlear hypoplasia* or *aplasia*, respectively), are examples of congenital anomalies precluding cochlear implantation. Acquired conditions hindering or precluding implantation include cochlear ossification (e.g., labyrinthitis ossificans after bacterial meningitis), cochlear trauma (e.g., temporal bone fractures), or cochlear nerve trauma (e.g., disruption of the cochlear nerve or sacrifice of the internal auditory artery during resection of a vestibular schwannoma).

11.3 Test Interpretation

For this patient, audiometric testing showed bilateral severe to profound sensorineural hearing loss, speech reception thresholds of 80 dB AD and 75 dbdB AS, and word recognition scores of 4% AD and 12% AS. Consonant-nucleus-consonant (CNC) test (an open-set word recognition test composed of a list of monosyllabic words administered in quiet) and AzBio test (an open-set sentence recognition test administered in quiet) scores in bilateral aided conditions were both 0%. Tympanometry revealed type A tympanograms, and acoustic reflexes were absent bilaterally. High-resolution computed tomography (CT) imaging of the temporal bones revealed normal pneumatization of the temporal bones and normal inner ear anatomy. The internal auditory canals were not widened.

11.4 Diagnosis

Bilateral profound sensorineural hearing loss due to presbycusis

11.5 Medical Management

Patients with mild to moderate sensorineural hearing loss often respond well to conventional amplification with hearing aids. Accordingly, criteria for cochlear implant candidacy (see below) require that hearing aids be attempted before implantation. When cochlear implantation is being considered, it is important that otitis externa or otitis media be absent. One should never implant an actively infected ear due to the risk of bacterial colonization of the implant and the potential for bacterial spread to the intracranial cavity. It is thought that the electrode array may serve as a conduit for bacterial spread to the inner ear. From the cochlea, bacteria may reach the intracranial cavity by way of the cochlear aqueduct or the auditory nerve.

11.6 Surgical Management

Cochlear implantation has been clinically approved by the U.S. Food and Drug Administration (FDA) for both prelingually and postlingually deafened children and adults. In addition to the FDA, insurance companies and the Centers for Medicare and Medicaid Services have established candidacy criteria for implantation. In general, adult candidacy includes patients who are 18 years or older with moderate to profound hearing loss with minimal benefit from hearing aids and no medical contraindications. Criteria for speech perception testing vary between manufacturers; patients must generally have scores ≤ 60% in best aided conditions. Prelingually deafened children may be as young as 12 months of age and exhibit profound hearing loss and limited benefit from hearing amplification while undergoing an early intervention program. Older children able to participate in open-set speech recognition testing should have scores ≤ 30%. Children younger than 12 months are candidates for cochlear implantation if at risk for labyrinthitis ossificans (e.g., following trauma or meningitis).

Preoperative assessment includes a thorough history and physical examination, auditory testing, radiologic evaluation, and psychosocial and educational assessment. Generally, auditory testing includes pure tone and speech reception thresholds, speech discrimination, and specialized audiologic testing for potential cochlear implant candidates (e.g., the hearing in noise test [HINT], as well as CNC and AzBio). Radiologic evaluation includes a CT scan or magnetic resonance imaging (MRI) of the temporal bone to determine mastoid pneumatization, inner ear patency, and potential ear anomalies. Whereas MRI is superior for assessment of retrocochlear pathology (e.g., cochlear nerve deficiency, vestibular schwannoma) or

central nervous system pathology (demyelinating disease, stroke), CT is superior to MRI for delineating temporal bone anatomy. Preoperative evaluation also includes assessment of the patient's family support and motivation for success. For children and adults, it is important to formalize a multidisciplinary education plan before surgery.

A cochlear implant device consists of an external portion (sound processor) and an implanted portion (internal receiver/stimulator). The sound processor contains a microphone and a magnet with associated radiofrequency coil that connects to the implanted portion and stimulates the active electrode. The electrode is placed through the cochleostomy into the scala tympani of the cochlea. The commercially available implants in the United States are the Advanced Bionics (Sylmar, CA), Med-El (Innsbruck, Austria), and Cochlear Nucleus (Sydney, Australia) implant systems.

The most common method of implantation involves a postauricular mastoidectomy with facial recess to gain access to the round window. A well is prepared in the squamous temporal bone for placement of the receiver/stimulator. A cochleostomy is created anterior/inferior and separate from the round window (a cochleostomy approach) but may also be situated in continuity with the round window at its anteroinferior margin (an extended round window approach); alternatively, the electrode may be inserted through the round window itself (a round window approach). In all approaches, the electrode is inserted into the scala tympani of the cochlea. Careful insertion of the active electrode is performed.

In the past decade, refinements in surgical technique have focused on hearing preservation. Ideally, cochlear implantation is accomplished by atraumatic insertion of the electrode array in the scala tympani. Traumatic insertions, most notably involving trans-scalar insertion (wherein the electrode array passes from the scala tympani to the scala vestibuli), have been associated with worse implant performance. Preservation of functional residual hearing allows implant recipients to perceive low-frequency acoustic stimulation while benefiting from improved speech understanding, particularly in the high frequencies, by electric stimulation. This combined-modality hearing mechanism is also known as electroacoustic stimulation and may be particularly advantageous to hearing in noisy environments. "Soft surgery" describes a combination of techniques designed to minimize cochlear trauma during implantation. These include minimizing the size of the cochleostomy as much as possible, situating the cochleostomy in such a way as to facilitate insertion into the scala tympani, preserving an intact ossicular chain, and avoiding aspiration of the cochlear perilymph. Some studies suggest round window insertions may cause less trauma than cochleostomy insertions.

Meticulous attention to detail in wound closure and avoidance of infection are important, as wound healing problems are the most common complications. Additional complications of cochlear implantation include bleeding, infection, facial nerve injury, dizziness, taste changes, tinnitus, cerebrospinal fluid leaks, meningitis, and false insertion of the electrode into the hypotympanic cells. Late complications can include device failure, infection, migration, and extrusion, which may require device removal. It is recommended that pneumococcal vaccination (Pneumovax and Prevnar 13) be given to all cochlear implant recipients to reduce the risk of meningitis.

11.7 Rehabilitation and Follow-up

After cochlear implantation, around 2 to 4 weeks of healing time is allowed before activating the device. When activation occurs, computer software programs are used to identify appropriate settings for the patient (also known as *mapping*). These settings are adjusted to create a map that customizes the device to the patient's specific hearing needs. Close follow-up with the audiologist is needed throughout the first year to achieve this customization. Aural rehabilitation and educational programs are crucial to successful implantation in both children and adults.

Hearing outcomes depend on many factors, including the etiology of deafness (prelingual or postlingual), duration of deafness, age at implantation (for children), mode of communication, socioeconomic status, motivation, family support, and others.

11.8 Questions

1. Into what portion of the cochlea should the active electrode be inserted?
   a) Scala media.
   b) Scala vestibuli.
   c) Scala tympani.
   d) Stria vascularis.
2. What is the most common complication of cochlear implant surgery?
   a) Poor wound healing.
   b) Facial nerve injury.
   c) Dysgeusia.
   d) Cerebrospinal fluid leak.
3. Meningitis can cause what condition that may preclude cochlear implantation?
   a) Sensorineural hearing loss.
   b) Hydrocephalus.
   c) Labyrinthitis ossificans.
   d) Endolymphatic hydrops.

Answers: 1. c 2. a 3. c

Suggested Readings

Adunka OF, Buchman CA. Cochlear Implants and Other Implantable Auditory Prostheses. In: Bailey BJ, Johnson JT, eds. Head & Neck Surgery—Otolaryngology. Vol 2. 5th ed. Philadelphia, PA: Lippincott Williams & Wilkins; 2014:2624–2653

Adunka O, Unkelbach MH, Mack M, Hambek M, Gstoettner W, Kiefer J. Cochlear implantation via the round window membrane minimizes trauma to cochlear structures: a histologically controlled insertion study. Acta Otolaryngol. 2004; 124(7):807–812

Roland JT, Jr, Gantz BJ, Waltzman SB, Parkinson AJ, Multicenter Clinical Trial Group. United States multicenter clinical trial of the cochlear nucleus hybrid implant system. Laryngoscope. 2016; 126 (1):175–81

Roland PS, Wright CG. Surgical aspects of cochlear implantation: mechanisms of insertional trauma. Adv Otorhinolaryngol. 2006; 64:11–30

Skarzynski H, Lorens A, Piotrowska A, Anderson I. Preservation of low frequency hearing in partial deafness cochlear implantation (PDCI) using the round window surgical approach. Acta Otolaryngol. 2007; 127(1):41–48

Wanna GB, Noble JH, Carlson ML. Impact of electrode design and surgical approach on scalar location and cochlear implant outcomes. Laryngoscope. 2014; 124 Suppl 6:S1–S7

12 Benign Paroxysmal Positional Vertigo

Adam D. Goodale and Myles L. Pensak

12.1 History

A 58-year-old woman presented to the clinic for evaluation of dizziness. She had experienced several episodes of the room spinning, particularly when lying down in bed at night, for the past several weeks. These episodes lasted for several minutes and were associated with nausea. She reported the dizziness happened only when she rolled to the right, but never when rolling to the left. There was no associated hearing loss, tinnitus, or aural fullness. She denied falls or balance issues. She did report a previous history of vestibular neuritis several years ago, but had not had any vertigo since then.

On physical exam, her ear canals were patent with normal-appearing tympanic membranes. She had no vertigo with pneumatic otoscopy. No spontaneous nystagmus was noted. Her Romberg and Fukuda tests were normal. When her head was rotated to the right and she was laid flat with her head extended over the table, she experienced vertigo with an upbeating, rotary nystagmus observed, which lasted for approximately 30 seconds.

12.2 Differential Diagnosis—Key Points

- Benign paroxysmal positional vertigo (BPPV) is the most common peripheral vestibular disorder, accounting for approximately 40% of all vestibular complaints. It is thought to be caused by either canalolithiasis, when there is free-floating debris within the semicircular canals, or cupulolithiasis, when otoconia debris is lodged in the cupula of the semicircular canals, resulting in asymmetric vestibular nerve activity and the sensation of vertigo.
- Patients with BPPV classically complain of brief episodes of vertigo with certain head maneuvers, most commonly rolling over in bed. Episodes have a 5- to 10-second latency period and last 30 to 60 seconds. BPPV is most commonly idiopathic in origin but can be seen following head trauma, vestibular neuritis, or stapes surgery.
- In patients with BPPV, the posterior semicircular canal is the affected canal in 90% of cases and the horizontal canal in 10% of cases. The superior canal is rarely involved due to gravity.

- Peripheral vertigo is typically characterized by the duration of vertigo as well as associated symptoms. Brief episodes of vertigo, lasting less than 60 seconds, are most commonly due to BPPV or superior semicircular canal dehiscence (SSCCD). Patients with SSCCD have vertigo elicited by loud sounds or changes in middle ear or intracranial pressure. They also commonly have conductive hearing loss and autophony.
- Episodic vertigo lasting for minutes to hours is commonly experienced with both Meniere's disease and perilymph fistula. Patients with Meniere's disease classically experience low-frequency sensorineural hearing loss, aural fullness, and tinnitus associated with their vertigo. Perilymph fistulas are often the result of head trauma or barotrauma, but they may result from chronic ear disease. These patients often have fluctuating or progressive hearing loss and vertigo immediately following a traumatic event.
- Vertigo lasting longer than 24 hours is commonly due to vestibular neuritis, labyrinthitis, or immune-mediated inner ear disease (IMIED). Vestibular neuritis manifests as acute onset vertigo with associated nausea and vomiting. Labyrinthitis has a similar presentation, but patients will more commonly experience concomitant hearing loss. Both of these clinical entities are thought to be caused by reactivation of latent herpes zoster virus in the vestibular ganglion. IMIED is often a primary inner ear process with only 15 to 30% of patients having an associated systemic autoimmune condition. These patients usually have fluctuating or progressive sensorineural hearing loss that may have associated vertigo. Symptoms may improve with high-dose steroids.
- Other causes of peripheral vestibular disorders to consider include migraine-associated vertigo; vestibular schwannoma; medication toxicity, particularly from aminoglycosides and chemotherapy; and chronic unilateral vestibular hypofunction.

12.3 Test Interpretation

Observing for nystagmus during the Dix-Hallpike maneuver is the key to diagnosing BPPV. During this maneuver, the posterior canal on the tested side is brought into a vertical plane that will cause loose otoconia to move in an excitatory direction with lying down. A positive test will show a latency of 5 to 10 seconds with vertigo lasting between 30 and 60 seconds associated with a rotary nystagmus toward the downward side. The nystagmus should fatigue with repeat testing. When the horizontal canal is the affected canal, the Dix-Hallpike maneuver will elicit a horizontal nystagmus, rather than rotary, toward the affected ear.

Patients should have an audiogram performed at the time of presentation to evaluate for inner ear disorders. In the initial setting, vestibular testing has little value in managing patients with BPPV; however, if symptoms persist, vestibular testing should be performed.

12.4 Diagnosis

Benign paroxysmal positional vertigo

12.5 Medical Management

Patients found to have BPPV should be educated on the nature and mechanism of their illness. In the majority of cases, symptoms related to BPPV are self-limited and resolve over weeks to months. There are various repositioning maneuvers, including Epley's repositioning procedure and Semont's maneuver, that should be tried if symptoms last more than 1 to 2 weeks. These maneuvers attempt to move the free-floating particles from the posterior canal into the vestibule. Approximately 90% of patients have resolution of their symptoms after one or two repositioning treatments. After repositioning, patients are instructed to avoid lying flat or bending over for 24 to 48 hours. When the horizontal canal is involved, patients should be treated with a "log rolling" maneuver for canalith repositioning. Vestibular suppressants have no benefit and should be avoided when treating BPPV; however, antiemetics can be useful.

12.6 Surgical Management

Surgical treatment for BPPV is reserved for patients with persistent and disabling symptoms lasting longer than 1 year. These patients should have failed repositioning maneuvers, medical treatment, and physical therapy. The two main surgical procedures used to treat BPPV are singular neurectomy and posterior semicircular canal occlusion.

Singular neurectomy involves a transcanal approach to identify and transect the singular nerve, which provides afferent neural input from the posterior semicircular canal. This procedure is technically challenging due to the variable location of the singular nerve, difficulty identifying the nerve when drilling, and complicated exposure around the round window niche. This procedure has fallen out of favor due to its difficulty and high rate of sensorineural hearing loss, which has been reported to be as high as 40%.

Posterior semicircular canal occlusion utilizes a transmastoid approach to expose the posterior semicircular canal. The canal is carefully opened, perilymph is wicked away, and the canal is filled with a fascial plug and bone dust to eliminate endolymph flow. This procedure is effective at eliminating vertigo with a relatively low incidence of sensorineural hearing loss of 5%. This is the preferred surgical procedure, given its technical simplicity and better hearing outcomes.

12.7 Rehabilitation and Follow-up

Most patients with BPPV will have resolution of symptoms with either observation or canalith repositioning procedures. Patients should be reassessed 1 month after treatment to ensure resolution of symptoms. Patients with persistent symptoms should be counseled on the risk of falls and referred to physical therapy for further treatment. Additionally, other causes of vertigo should be considered for patients with persistent BPPV.

12.8 Questions

1. The singular nerve, which receives afferent input from the posterior semicircular canal, arises from what nerve?
   a) Superior vestibular nerve.
   b) Cochlear nerve.
   c) Facial nerve.
   d) Inferior vestibular nerve.
2. A construction worker presents to the clinic after being in near proximity to an explosion at work. He reports episodic vertigo and fluctuating hearing loss for the past day. On examination of the left ear, the ear canal and tympanic membrane appear normal. However, on pneumatic otoscopy, the patient experiences a brief

episode of vertigo. The remainder of his head and neck exam is normal, as well as his audiogram. What is the recommended treatment at this time?

a) Middle ear exploration.

b) Bed rest.

c) High-dose corticosteroids.

d) Epley's maneuver.

3. Which of the following findings is consistent with central vestibular pathology?

a) Nystagmus is horizontal, rotary in nature.

b) Nystagmus is enhanced with visual fixation.

c) Nystagmus is suppressed with visual fixation

d) Lack of associated neurologic symptoms.

Answers 1. d 2. b 3. b

Suggested Readings

Bhattacharyya N, Baugh RF, Orvidas L, et al. American Academy of Otolaryngology, Head and Neck Surgery Foundation. Clinical practice guideline: benign paroxysmal positional vertigo. Otolaryngol Head Neck Surg. 2008; 139(5) Suppl 4:S47–S81

Leveque M, Labrousse M, Seidermann L, Chays A. Surgical therapy in intractable benign paroxysmal positional vertigo. Otolaryngol Head Neck Surg. 2007; 136(5):693–698

Parnes LS, McClure JA. Posterior semicircular canal occlusion for intractable benign paroxysmal positional vertigo. Ann Otol Rhinol Laryngol. 1990; 99(5 Pt 1):330–334

13 Vestibular Migraine

Andre M. Wineland and John H. Greinwald Jr.

13.1 History

A 32-year-old woman was referred by her primary care physician for evaluation of headaches and dizziness. She described a history of migraines but more recently had experienced seven distinct spontaneous vertigo episodes that impaired daily activities and lasted between 5 minutes and 72 hours. Exacerbating factors included stress, lack of sleep, menstruation, and certain foods. She had tried over-the-counter remedies but had never seen a physician for medical treatment until recently. She was otherwise in good health.

On physical examination she was afebrile with normal vital signs. She was in no distress. Cranial nerve exam was normal. There was no spontaneous nystagmus. Vestibular exam was normal. Otologic exam was unremarkable. The head and neck exam was also unremarkable. An audiogram demonstrated normal hearing.

13.2 Differential Diagnosis—Key Points

Vertigo is the illusion of movement of the person in relation to the surrounding environment. Vertigo can be seen in a number of conditions:

- Benign paroxysmal positional vertigo (BPPV) is associated with vertigo and head movement and is due to cupulolithiasis and/or canalithiasis in the posterior semicircular canal. Vertigo is self-limited and the majority of times can be treated with repositioning techniques.
- Vestibular neuronitis is characterized by severe vertigo, nausea, and vomiting due to viral inflammation of the vestibular nerve. Symptoms improve over the course of days to weeks. Hearing is preserved.
- Meniere's disease is characterized by severe episodes of vertigo often associated with fluctuation in hearing, aural fullness, and tinnitus. Symptoms improve over hours to days. Low-salt diet and diuretics are common first-line treatments.
- Oval and round window perilymph fistulas are seen most commonly in a posttraumatic setting. Patients present with sensorineural hearing loss and severe vertigo. Vertigo can be elicited with coughing/straining.
- Superior semicircular canal dehiscence syndrome is characterized by vertigo induced by sound and/or pressure.
- Acute or chronic otitis media can manifest with vertigo.
- Intracranial tumors (e.g., acoustic neuroma, meningioma, cholesterol granuloma, paraganglioma, arachnoid cyst, metastatic tumor) can present with vertigo.
- Autoimmune inner ear disease can present with fluctuant or progressive unilateral or bilateral sensorineural hearing loss that can be associated with vertigo.
- Labyrinthitis can present with sensorineural hearing loss and vertigo.
- While medications are often associated with vertigo, true vertiginous symptoms are rarely elicited.
- Mal de debarquement syndrome is not a true vertigo but rather the persistent rocking sensation commonly described after disembarking from a long boat excursion.
- Transient ischemic attacks result in temporary loss of blood flow resulting in neurologic dysfunction. Sudden onset of symptoms in the elderly with lack of preceding history warrants further vascular evaluation.
- Anxiety and depression are often comorbid conditions with chronic otologic processes. Over 50% of patients with vestibular migraine have comorbid psychiatric disorders.
- Migraine-associated vertigo can be diagnosed in patients with episodic vertigo, lightheadedness, and disequilibrium associated with migraine headaches.

According to the International Headache Society (IHS), migraines are separated into those with aura and those without aura.

13.2.1 Migraine without Aura

Untreated headache lasts 4 to 72 hours in adults and 2 to 48 hours if < 15 years old. The patient must experience either (1) nausea and/or vomiting or (2) phonophobia/photophobia. The headache must also have at least two of the following findings:
- Unilateral.
- Pulsatile quality.

- Severe enough to inhibit daily activities.
- Aggravated by physical activity.

13.2.2 Migraine with Aura

Aura is defined by at least two attacks:
- Reversible central nervous system dysfunction (e.g., vision, hearing, vertigo, ataxia, level of consciousness, paresthesia, paresis).
- Gradual onset of symptoms that typically subside in < 1 hour.
- Headache occurring before, during, or after the aura.

Vestibular migraine (VM) can be divided into definite and probable versions (▸ Table 13.1, ▸ Table 13.2). Symptoms must affect daily activities to be considered. The duration of episodes varies from minutes to hours to days, but would be rare for symptoms to exceed 72 hours. Phonophobia are often visual auras associated with vestibular migraines. Lastly, vestibular migraine is a diagnosis of exclusion and a specific age or range is not a requirement.

Neuropathophysiology

The "spreading wave of depression" was described by Cutrer and Baloh in 1992 and is the most commonly accepted theory regarding the pathophysiology of vestibular migraine. The inciting stimulus creates a transient wave that suppresses neuronal activity, resulting in large shifts of potassium (K+) and calcium (Ca++) resulting in decreased blood flow. Vertigo is believed to occur from the release of neuropeptides (e.g., neurokinin A, calcitonin gene-related peptide, neuropeptide substance P). Calcium channel blockers, beta-blockers, and tricyclic antidepressants are thought to block the release of these neuropeptides and are often included in the medical management.

An alternative theory includes temporary ischemia from vasospasm of the internal auditory artery. There continues to be active research into the area extending to functional neuroimaging, which will not be discussed in this chapter.

13.3 Test Interpretation

As with many vertiginous work-ups, the history is more helpful than physical exam findings, as many times the neuro-otologic exam is normal.

Vestibular tests are not specific enough to be included as diagnostic criteria for vestibular migraine. However, they can be useful when excluding other disease processes (e.g., Meniere's disease, perilymphatic fistula, dehiscent semicircular canal). Oculomotor and vestibulo-ocular reflex, video electronystagmography, calorics, rotational chair, audiogram, auditory brainstem response test, computerized dynamic posturography, and vestibular evoked myogenic potentials are common vestibular tests that may be incorporated in further evaluating a vertiginous patient.

13.4 Diagnosis

Vestibular migraine

Table 13.1 Diagnostic criteria for vestibular migraine

a) At least five episodes with vestibular symptoms of moderate or severe intensity, lasting 5 minutes to 72 hours

b) Current or previous history of migraine with or without aura

c) One or more migraine features with at least 50% of vestibular episodes:
  - headache with at least one of the following characteristics:
  - unilateral, pulsating, moderate/severe pain intensity, aggravation by routine activity
  - photophobia/phonophobia
  - visual aura

d) Not better accounted for by another vestibular or headache diagnosis

Table 13.2 Probable VMC

a) At least five episodes with vestibular symptoms of moderate or severe intensity, lasting 5 minutes to 72 hours

b) Only one of the vestibular migraine criteria is fulfilled (migraine history or migraine features during episode)

c) Not better explained by another vestibular or headache diagnosis

13.5 Medical Management

Optimal management for vestibular migraine involves a combination of medications, vestibular rehabilitation, and lifestyle modifications (sleep hygiene, restricted diet). The wide variety of medications commonly used to treat vestibular migraines reflects the potential difficulty in optimal management. Commonly used medications include beta-blockers, antidepressants, calcium channel blockers, anticonvulsants, nonsteroidal anti-inflammatory drugs (NSAIDs), and triptans. Starting medical therapy has been shown to increase compliance with vestibular rehabilitation. A food diary will often identify offending agents, such as monosodium glutamate (MSG), alcohol, aged cheese, chocolate, and aspartame. A food elimination diet for 1 month will help identify potential triggers.

13.6 Surgical Management

There are no widely accepted surgical options for managing vestibular migraines.

13.7 Rehabilitation and Follow-up

Vestibular rehabilitation therapy (VRT) has been shown to improve the dizziness handicap, activities-specific balance confidence, dynamic gait, and computerized dynamic posturography measures in patients who suffer from vestibular migraine. VRT is an exercise-based program aimed at promoting compensation for a damaged vestibular system. VRT is tailored toward the patient's specific vestibular issue(s), and a custom approach is created for them. Well-trained providers and willing patients are paramount to obtain maximal benefit from VRT.

13.8 Questions

1. True or false? During the work-up of vestibular migraine, the patient's history is more helpful than ancillary testing.
2. Provoking factors of vestibular migraine include which of the following?
   a) Hypoglycemia.
   b) Stress.
   c) Poor sleep.
   d) Caffeinated beverages.
   e) Monosodium glutamate.
   f) All of the above can provoke a vestibular migraine.
3. Treatments for vestibular migraine include which of the following?
   a) Food elimination diet.
   b) Amlodipine.
   c) Topiramate.
   d) Diclofenac.
   e) All of the above can be used to treat vestibular migraine.

Answers: 1. True 2. f 3. e

Suggested Readings

Bisdorff A, Von Brevern M, Lempert T, Newman-Toker DE. Classification of vestibular symptoms: towards an international classification of vestibular disorders. J Vestib Res. 2009; 19(1–2):1–13

Dieterich M, Obermann M, Celebisoy N. Vestibular migraine: the most frequent entity of episodic vertigo. J Neurol. 2016; 263 Suppl 1:S82–S89

Gottshall KR, Moore RJ, Hoffer ME. Vestibular rehabilitation for migraine-associated dizziness. Int Tinnitus J. 2005; 11(1):81–84

Headache Classification Subcommittee of the International Headache, Society. The International Classification of Headache Disorders: 2nd edition. Cephalalgia. 2004; 24(suppl 1):9–160

Lempert T, Neuhauser H, Daroff RB. Vertigo as a symptom of migraine. Ann N Y Acad Sci. 2009; 1164:242–251

Lempert T, Olesen J, Furman J, et al. Vestibular migraine: diagnostic criteria. J Vestib Res. 2012; 22(4):167–172

Neuhauser H, Leopold M, von Brevern M, Arnold G, Lempert T. The interrelations of migraine, vertigo, and migrainous vertigo. Neurology. 2001; 56(4):436–441

Shepard NT, Telian SA. Programmatic vestibular rehabilitation. Otolaryngol Head Neck Surg. 1995; 112(1):173–182

14 Tinnitus

Brian L. Hendricks and Ravi N. Samy

14.1 History

A 33-year-old white woman presented for evaluation of constant left-sided pulsatile tinnitus, which she had noticed over the last 6 months. She felt that it had been getting worse. She also reported occasional left-sided otalgia and headaches. She denied vertigo, aural fullness, hearing loss, or otorrhea. Her otologic history was significant for a history of left-sided auricular trauma during her childhood, but it was negative for any prior otologic surgery. She denied any significant history of otitis media. She had worked in a loud factory since the age of 18 and reported that she seldom wore hearing protection. Her family history was significant for her father dying of a ruptured intracranial aneurysm.

On neuro-otologic examination, Weber's examination was midline, Rinne's examination was positive bilaterally, examination of the pinnae was normal, and microscopic examination revealed normal tympanic membranes and mobility bilaterally. Compression of the ipsilateral jugular vein and provocative head movement failed to abate the patient's tinnitus. Auscultation with Toynbee's tube failed to demonstrate audible pulsatile tinnitus. Examination of the cranial nerves (CNs) revealed normal function of CNII through CNXII.

Audiometric testing revealed normal hearing acuity and normal tympanometry. Outside high-resolution computed tomography (CT) of the temporal bone showed no intratemporal tumors, but the skull base appeared thin. A carotid artery duplex study demonstrated mild irregularities of bilateral carotid systems without any hemodynamically significant stenosis.

14.2 Differential Diagnosis—Key Points

- Tinnitus is a symptom that has a wide variety of potential etiologies both within and beyond the field of otolaryngology. As such, it is important to have a routine diagnostic approach or algorithm in order to narrow down the range of possibilities. All evaluations should begin with a detailed history, complete head and neck examination, and audiogram. During this early portion of the work-up, several distinctions are key to make prior to moving forward. These include differentiating pulsatile versus nonpulsatile, subjective versus objective, and acute versus paroxysmal versus chronic, as well as any associated symptoms such as hearing loss, vertigo, headache, and autophony. Patients should also be asked about any history of head trauma.

a) Pulsatile tinnitus generally suggests a vascular etiology, though only approximately 70% of patients with pulsatile tinnitus have a distinctly identifiable cause. Patients with an audible neck bruit and/or history of significant atherosclerotic disease can be further evaluated with carotid Doppler imaging or CT angiography (CTA) of the neck. Patients whose symptoms abate with compression of the ipsilateral jugular vein may warrant CT venogram to evaluate the sigmoid and transverse sinuses. Those with autophony and/or a conductive hearing loss should be evaluated for patulous eustachian tube, as well as undergo noncontrast CT imaging to evaluate for superior semicircular canal dehiscence. Masses visible on otologic examination should be further characterized with CT and perhaps magnetic resonance imaging (MRI) with contrast. Those patients without any relevant findings with the above work-up should be considered for MRI/magnetic resonance angiography (MRA) imaging to evaluate for arteriovenous anomalies or other intracranial etiologies. MRI may be considered in obese patients with no other suggestive findings to rule out idiopathic intracranial hypertension.

b) Nonpulsatile tinnitus is much more common than pulsatile tinnitus, and it has an even wider array of possible etiologies. Patients with any form of hearing loss may experience chronic tinnitus, but those patients with acute hearing loss and tinnitus should be treated appropriately for sudden sensorineural hearing loss. Other potential etiologies of nonpulsatile tinnitus include prior neurologic or otologic trauma, Meniere's disease, superior semicircular canal dehiscence, vestibular schwannoma, idiopathic intracranial hypertension, Chiari's malformation, ototoxic medication usage, and perilymphatic fistula; however, the history should help narrow the above differential diagnosis. Patients with unilateral tinnitus and an asymmetric hearing loss should have MRI with gadolinium to evaluate for possible vestibular schwannoma. Patients experiencing paroxysmal tinnitus may ultimately require an MRI with contrast to evaluate for intracranial pathology.

c) Objective tinnitus that can be confirmed with direct auscultation of the neck or periauricular region can suggest carotid atherosclerosis or dural arteriovenous malformation. Objective findings on auscultation of the external auditory canal would indicate possible myoclonus of the palate or middle ear (but this tends to be a rapid, rhythmic tinnitus rather than a pulsatile tinnitus).

- Vascular anomalies of the middle ear: Vascular anomalies in the middle ear often present with pulsatile tinnitus. An aberrant or laterally displaced petrous carotid artery, a dehiscent or high-riding jugular bulb, a persistent stapedial artery, and an intratympanic carotid aneurysm represent the most common types of vascular anomalies.

To diagnose an aberrant carotid artery, high-resolution CT reveals the petrous carotid artery entering the middle ear through an enlarged inferior tympanic canaliculus, an enhancing hypotympanic "mass," and the carotid foramen and vertical segment of the petrous internal carotid artery are absent. Accurate radiographic diagnosis is imperative because this "mass" should never be biopsied. A persistent stapedial artery is usually noted with an enlarged anterior tympanic segment of the fallopian canal and an absent foramen spinosum on high-resolution CT scan. This entity may be associated with an aberrant petrous carotid artery.

A high riding jugular bulb is the most common vascular anomaly of the middle ear and is easily seen on CT scan of the temporal bone. It is defined as a jugular bulb extending above the inferior tympanic annulus. On otoscopic examination, this is seen as a blue-hued mass protruding from the hypotympanum. High-resolution CT scan reveals a focal absence of the sigmoid plate, and the jugular bulb appears to enter the middle ear as a mass. Accurate radiographic diagnosis is also imperative because this "lesion" should never be biopsied.

- Idiopathic intracranial hypertension: (IIH): IIH (or *pseudotumor cerebri* or *benign intracranial hypertension*) often presents with retro-ocular and pulsatile headache, pulsatile tinnitus, papilledema, and elevated intracranial pressure. This process is most prevalent in obese women of childbearing age. If left untreated, IIH may progress to permanent visual field deficits and blindness. The associated pulsatile tinnitus is thought to derive from turbulent venous flow in the transverse and sigmoid sinuses. Diagnosis is confirmed with elevated cerebrospinal fluid pressure (demonstrated with lumbar puncture) and radiographic imaging. The increased intracranial pressure of IIH may contribute to a venous pathology of sigmoid sinus diverticulum, which can be surgically corrected.

- Venous etiology: Venous hum tinnitus can be demonstrated in patients with a tortuous sigmoid sinus or a previous history of sigmoid sinus thrombosis and subsequent recanalization. Diagnosis is confirmed with elimination of the tinnitus with gentle jugular vein compression or by turning the patient's head to the contralateral side.

- Palatal myoclonus: Palatal myoclonus is caused by contraction of tensor palatini, levator veli palatini, tensor tympani, salpingopharyngeus, or superior constrictor muscles. It is described as a clicking sound that is rapid (up to 60 to 200 beats per minute), repetitive, and intermittent. The tinnitus does not dissipate while the patient is asleep. The muscle spasms may be seen either transorally or transnasally. Because of the rapidity of the clicking, this entity does not typically have a "heartbeat" or pulsatile nature.

- Jugulotympanic paraganglioma: These represent a common cause of pulsatile tinnitus. Glomus bodies are neural crest derivatives that reside along the course of Jacobson's and Arnold's nerves and in the region of the jugular bulb. Paragangliomas are thought to arise from these glomus bodies and migrate in close association with sympathetic ganglia. These highly vascular masses belong to the diffuse neuroendocrine system and are composed of chief cells and oxyphil cells. Paragangliomas usually grow slowly and may be present for several years before causing symptoms.

In addition to pulsatile tinnitus, associated symptoms are usually based on location and nearby involved anatomic structures. Involvement of the middle ear can lead to conductive hearing loss, aural bleeding, and Brown's sign (blanching of the lesion with positive pressure). Symptoms suggestive of tumor extension into associated structures include vertigo, sensorineural hearing loss, otalgia, and lower cranial neuropathy (CNIX–CNXII).

• Dural arteriovenous malformation (AVM): Dural AVM, or dural arteriovenous fistula, is one of the most common anomalies identified in patients with pulsatile tinnitus. In these vascular anomalies, an arteriovenous shunt is contained within the leaflets of the dura mater. The arterial supply is exclusively supplied by branches of the carotid or vertebral arteries before they penetrate the dura mater. A dural AVM may represent a true fistula, which is defined as a single or multiple dilated arterioles that connect directly to a vein without a nidus, and they are high pressure and high flow. Most commonly, these are found adjacent to a dural venous sinus, with a slight left-sided predominance. The junction of the transverse and sigmoid sinuses is the most common location.

Table 14.1 Clinical symptoms reported in 27 cases of dural arteriovenous malformations

Symptom	n (%)
Pulsatile tinnitus	25 (92%)
Occipital bruit	24 (89%)
Headache	11 (41%)
Visual impairment	9 (33%)
Papilledema	7 (26%)

Source: From Sundt TM Jr, Piepgras DG. The surgical approachapproach to arteriovenous malformations of the lateral and sigmoidsigmoid dural sinuses. J Neurosurg 1983;59:32–39.

Evidence suggests that dural AVMs of the transverse–sigmoid junction are acquired, not congenital, lesions that result from collateral revascularization after a previous thrombosis of the involved dural venous sinus. This is most commonly seen from sigmoid sinus thrombosis secondary to infection or trauma. In most cases, the occipital artery is the dominant arterial feeding vessel (▶ Table 14.1).

Depending on the direction of flow, these lesions may be life threatening, and complete evaluation for pulsatile tinnitus is warranted. Physical examination may reveal a loud bruit that may be auscultated over the mastoid or occiput. Dural AVMs are most commonly diagnosed via a combination of contrast-enhanced MRI and time-of-flight MRA or CT angiography.

14.3 Test Interpretation

Investigating the cause of pulsatile tinnitus is necessary because potentially life-threatening pathology may be present. Pure tone audiometry and speech audiometry are necessary tests, and tympanometry may objectively demonstrate pulsations. Pulsatile tinnitus is frequently associated with a low-frequency hearing loss, which is thought to be artifact. Otic capsule and temporal bone invasion by a paraganglioma will likely lead to a sensorineural hearing loss. If paraganglioma is suspected, evaluation of catecholamine secretion is imperative.

Auscultation: Auscultation of the upper neck and postauricular region can assist in the diagnosis of carotid atherosclerosis and dural AVMs. Toynbee's auscultation tube can be inserted into the external auditory canal in order to listen for myoclonus of the stapedius, tensor tympani, or muscles of the palate.

Blood tests: Hemoglobin level and thyroid function studies can be ordered to evaluate for potential anemia or hyperthyroidism that may result in a hyperdynamic cardiac state.

Radiographic evaluation: Carotid ultrasonography can be useful when the suspicion for atherosclerosis is high. High-resolution CT scan of the temporal bone demonstrates bony anatomy of the cranial base foramina (otosclerosis and superior canal dehiscence have also been rarely reported to cause pulsatile tinnitus). CTA will delineate vascular anomalies of the middle ear and cranial base. MRI, with and without gadolinium, and MRA are useful together to identify paragangliomas and dural AVMs.

Four-vessel angiography: This study is useful in delineating dural AVMs and for definitive or preoperative embolization of these lesions or paraganglioma (▶ Fig. 14.1).

14.4 Diagnosis

Dural AVM

14.5 Medical Management

Dural AVMs may be observed if they are small and the patient's symptoms are amenable. Therapy for dural AVMs is usually endovascular embolization with or without microneurosurgical resection, but stereotactic radiosurgery has been described as a viable treatment in patients with benign AVM that has failed other treatments. Radiosurgery is contraindicated in large dural AVMs or in those at risk of hemorrhage.

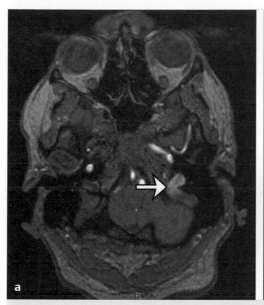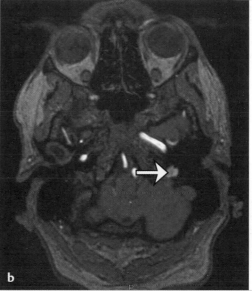

Fig. 14.1 (a,b) Axial T1-weighted postcontrast magnetic resonance images demonstrate a high-flow left dural arteriovenous fistula at the level of the distal sigmoid sinus–jugular bulb region, with arterial supply from transosseous arterial vessels in the region of the left jugular tubercle and occipital condyle. Note the high-contrast uptake in the left jugular bulb and sigmoid sinus junction compared with the right side.

14.6 Surgical Management

Indications for treatment of a dural AVM include neurologic dysfunction, bleeding from the lesion, or intractable symptoms. Referral to neurosurgical colleagues is warranted for evaluation for possible treatment or expectant management. Endovascular embolization may be performed via transarterial or transvenous access. Preoperative embolization usually facilitates surgical intervention because blood loss can be rapid and extensive.

14.7 Rehabilitation and Follow-up

Patients with dural AVM will need to be followed if expectant management is chosen, as these lesions put the patient at risk for life-threatening hemorrhage. In addition, serial imaging will be required of patients who undergo treatment in order to assess for recurrence or need for further interventions.

14.8 Questions

1. Which of the following is not a common treatment option for a dural arteriovenous malformation (AVM)?
   a) Endovascular embolization.
   b) Injection sclerotherapy.
   c) Surgical excision.
   d) Gamma Knife radiosurgery (Elekta AB, Stockholm, Sweden)
2. Which of the following is best suited to characterize a suspected glomus tumor (paraganglioma)?
   a) Computed tomography (CT) with contrast.
   b) MRI
   c) Magnetic resonance imaging (MRI). Neck ultrasound.
   d) Both CT and MRI.
3. All of the following are a potential cause of nonvascular pulsatile tinnitus except
   a) Idiopathic intracranial hypertension (IIH).
   b) Semicircular canal dehiscence.
   c) Myoclonus.
   d) Patulous eustachian tube.
   e) Otosclerosis.

Answers: 1. b 2. b 3. c

Suggested Readings

Cosetti MK, Roehm PC. Tinnitus and hyperacusis. In: Johnson JT, Rosen CA, eds. Bailey's Head and Neck Surgery: Otolaryngology. 5th ed. Philadelphia, PA: Lippincott Williams & Wilkins; 2014: 2597–2614

Langguth B, Biesinger E, Del Bo L, et al. Algorithm for the diagnostic and therapeutic management of tinnitus. In: Moller AR, Langguth B, eds. Textbook of Tinnitus. New York, NY: Springer; 2011: 381–385
Mattox DE, Hudgins P. Algorithm for evaluation of pulsatile tinnitus. Acta Otolaryngol. 2008; 128(4):427–431
Otto KJ, Hudgins PA, Abdelkafy W, Mattox DE. Sigmoid sinus diverticulum: a new surgical approach to the correction of pulsatile tinnitus. Otol Neurotol. 2007; 28(1):48–53

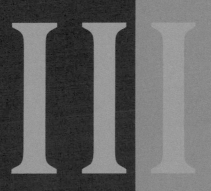

Part III

Neurotology and Skull Base

III

15 Acoustic Neuroma

Shawn M. Stevens and Ravi N. Samy

15.1 History

A 21-year-old woman presented to the emergency room after the sudden onset of a severe occipital headache that woke her from sleep. This had progressively worsened despite treatment with over-the-counter analgesics. She also experienced severe nausea and had an episode of violent projectile vomiting. The vomiting was of greatest concern to her and prompted her to seek definitive evaluation. She had also noted fluctuating hearing loss on the left for the past 2 years but had not pursued evaluation for this. She denied visual blurring, diplopia, facial weakness or numbness, dysphagia, dysphonia, or vertigo. She had felt imbalanced recently but had not noted ataxia or difficulty completing her normal tasks. Her past medical history was unremarkable. She had one uneventful pregnancy during the past year resulting in spontaneous vaginal delivery of a healthy newborn. Family history was negative.

Examination revealed a well-developed, well-nourished woman in no acute distress. The patient had normal vital signs, and her body mass index was measured at 26 kg/m^2. Her pupils were equally reactive to light and accommodation. Visual acuity was intact to finger counting. Both external auditory canals (EACs) and tympanic membranes were normal. The patient noted tingling of the left EAC with notable finding of numbness of the posterior-inferior quadrant on exam. Close inspection demonstrated a bidirectional nystagmus with a right-predominant fast phase. Facial nerve function was a House-Brackmann I/VI bilaterally. The remaining cranial nerve (CN) and neurologic examinations were normal. Tuning fork testing at 512 Hz revealed a Weber lateralizing to the right side with bilaterally positive Rinne's tests.

15.2 Differential Diagnosis—Key Points

- The differential diagnosis of severe headache with vomiting in a young female is broad but should raise concerns for an intracranial tumor or other disease process. The concomitant findings of bidirectional nystagmus, asymmetric subjective hearing loss, and conchal hypesthesia would further raise concern for a tumor. Differential diagnoses would include a benign cerebellopontine angle (CPA) lesion (acoustic neuroma, meningioma, facial neuroma), a benign or malignant tumor of the brainstem/central nervous system (glioma, glioblastoma, astrocytoma, ependymoma, and medulloblastoma), vascular lesion (arteriovenous malformation or other posterior fossa vascular anomaly), diseases causing elevated intracranial pressure (idiopathic intracranial hypertension, hydrocephalus), cerebrovascular accident, migraine-associated vertigo, or an episode of labyrinthitis. Given the patient's age and recent gravida status, pregnancy should be ruled out.

- The majority of CPA tumors are slow growing and are typically found incidentally or in relation to sudden or asymmetric sensorineural hearing loss. CPA and other intracranial tumors in young people and females of childbearing age have been known to present differently than in older patients. Tumor growth can be rapid and may result in large lesions at the time of presentation. These may exert significant mass effect on the brainstem and can be associated with development of hydrocephalus in up to one-third of cases. Presenting symptoms such as headache and severe nausea/vomiting would not be uncommon for a tumor in this patient demographic.

- A bidirectional nystagmus with a predominant fast phase away from the ear with reported hearing loss could be consistent with Bruns's nystagmus. This rare finding occurs most frequently in association with large CPA tumors > 3 cm and may help narrow the differential diagnosis. On close inspection, the examiner would note a slow-beating, large-amplitude nystagmus when looking toward the affected ear and a fast-beating, small-amplitude nystagmus when looking toward the opposite ear (also known as jerk nystagmus).

- The finding of left EAC paresthesias would also raise concerns for a large CPA tumor or brainstem lesion. Known as Hitselberger's sign, paresthesia and/or hypoesthesia of the posterior EAC can be caused by tumor compression of CNIX and CNX and resulting dysfunction of the distal auricular sensory branch (Arnold's nerve).

- Immediate investigative studies for this patient and presentation should include contrasted magnetic resonance imaging (MRI) of the brain and brainstem, basic laboratory testing, urine human chorionic gonadotropin (HCG) and toxicology screens, and audiometric testing if feasible. If MRI cannot be obtained in a time-sensitive fashion, computed tomography (CT) imaging is indicated to assess for life-threatening issues.
- Audiometric findings suggestive of a CPA lesion would include prolonged or disproportionate interwave latencies on auditory brainstem response, absent ipsilateral acoustic reflexes, rollover (paradoxical worsening of word recognition scores with louder presentations), and disproportionately low speech scores in comparison to pure tone thresholds.

15.3 Test Interpretation

Gadolinium-enhanced MRI scanning was undertaken and revealed a large, enhancing left CPA mass with extension into the internal auditory canal (IAC) and significant mass effect on the brainstem and adjacent cerebellum (▶ Fig. 15.1). This was hypointense on T2-weighted imaging. The lesion measured 4.8 × 4.4 cm in greatest

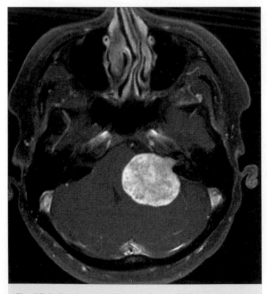

Fig. 15.1 Preoperative T1-weighted, gadolinium-enhanced, axial MRI image depicting a large enhancing mass in the left cerebellopontine angle. The tumor is exerting significant mass effect on the brainstem with midline shift. There is heterogeneous signal intensity within the tumor suggestive of cystic components.

dimensions and was heterogeneous with cystic components. There was a mild communicating hydrocephalus.

Laboratory panels, urinalysis, and urine toxicology showed no significant abnormalities. A urine HCG test was negative. The patient was able to transfer to clinic for performance of an audiogram. This demonstrated a moderate severe sloping to profound sensorineural hearing loss in the left ear with normal hearing on the right. Acoustic reflexes were absent on the left. Speech discrimination was 20% at 70 dB on the left.

15.4 Diagnosis

Acoustic neuroma (vestibular schwannoma)

15.5 Medical Management

Management options for unilateral, sporadic acoustic neuroma, a benign tumor of the vestibular nerves, would generally include observation with serial imaging, radiation therapy, and surgical resection. Management options in younger patients and those with large tumors generally involve surgery.

When counseling patients with an acoustic neuroma, important considerations include the patient's age, overall health status, significant comorbidities, and residual hearing level, and the initial tumor size on presentation. For smaller tumors, the patient should be educated that the tumor is benign; for this reason, patient desires should be heavily weighted in treatment discussions. Observation with serial MRI is a viable option because a large proportion (40–60%) of tumors will remain stable in size over a 3- to 5-year period. Patients in whom MRI is contraindicated should be observed with contrasted CT. In cases of large tumors (> 2–2.5 cm), rapidly growing tumors, brainstem compression, and/or hydrocephalus, surgery is the standard of care.

Medical management options for acoustic neuromas are currently limited in scope and efficacy. For sporadic tumors, which represent the majority of cases, one retrospective clinical study has suggested that use of aspirin may slow or halt the growth of some tumors. A translational study investigating these findings was able to demonstrate that COX-2 serves as a growth modulator in vestibular schwannomas. Prospective studies exploring the clinical outcomes of aspirin and nonsteroidal anti-inflammatory drug (NSAID) use for acoustic neuromas do not currently exist. For patients with germline mutations leading to acoustic neuroma formation and rapid progression (neurofibromatosis type 2), [NF2]), limited benefit has been derived from use of monoclonal antibodies, mTOR inhibitors, and tyrosine kinase receptor antagonists. Medications currently under phase II investigation include everolimus, lapatinib, erlotinib, and rapamycin. Given the different pathobiology underlying NF2, these benefits have not been realized in patients with sporadic tumors.

Stereotactic radiosurgery (< 5 fractions of radiation therapy) is aimed at halting growth of the tumor and should not be considered as a curative option. It is well suited to treatment of smaller tumors (< 1.5–2.0 cm), older patients, and those unable to tolerate surgery. Patients should be adequately counseled with respect to the risks and benefits of this treatment in contrast to surgery, and consultation with a neurotologist and/or neurosurgeon and a radiation oncologist is recommended.

Radiosurgery carries risk for development of hearing loss, vertigo, facial nerve dysfunction, delayed tumor growth, and in rare cases, radiation-induced malignant transformation. In events of radiation failure for tumor control, this modality may increase the technical difficulty and risk level associated with salvage surgical interventions in the future. If the presenting tumor is large or has cystic components or there is evidence of brainstem compression, radiotherapy is generally not recommended. Although debate exists, it is generally not recommended that younger patients (< 50–55 years old) receive radiosurgery given the risks for recurrent tumor growth and malignant transformation during the patients' long remaining life spans.

15.6 Surgical Management

Surgery is the only curative option for acoustic neuromas and other CPA tumors. Classically, three approaches have been described and include retrosigmoid, translabyrinthine, and middle fossa routes. The translabyrinthine approach is the most commonly used approach for resection of CPA tumors among neurotologists and is generally selected for patients with poor preoperative hearing and all tumor sizes. The retrosigmoid approach is also well suited for tumors of all sizes (particularly those situated within the CPA); neurosurgeons tend to favor this approach for large tumors

with significant brainstem compression. This approach is of limited use for smaller tumors located in the lateral aspect (fundus) of the IAC. The middle fossa approach is typically reserved for tumors of the IAC but can also be used for hearing preservation in tumors extending beyond the porus acusticus.

Both the retrosigmoid and middle fossa approaches allow for hearing preservation in patients with serviceable hearing and are associated with good outcomes (▶ Table 15.1). The translabyrinthine approach will result in loss of any residual hearing, should it exist. The surgical approach should be chosen on a case by case basis and selected in conjunction with patient preferences and presenting features. The patient in this procedure underwent a retrosigmoid approach given the size of her tumor at presentation and the degree of brainstem compression. In this case, near-total resection of the tumor was achieved, leaving a thin rind of tumor capsule on the facial nerve traversing the CPA (to preserve anatomic continuity and reduce the risk of postoperative complete facial palsy). This is a common and accepted approach to large tumors in which the facial nerve may be thinly splayed across the bulk of the tumor.

15.7 Rehabilitation and Follow-up

The patient awoke with a partial facial nerve palsy and could not fully close her eye with maximal effort (House-Brackmann IV/VI). Strict eye care with artificial tears, lubrication, and a moisture chamber was utilized to prevent exposure keratitis of the cornea. Temporary measures to facilitate eye closure include gold weight placement in the upper eyelid while waiting for future return of

Table 15.1 American Academy of Otolaryngology- Head and Neck Surgery hearing preservation reporting guidelines

Class	PTA (dB HL)	WRS (%)
A	≤ 30	≥ 70
B	> 30 - 50	≥ 50
C	> 50	≥ 50
D	Any level	< 50

Abbreviations: PTA, pure tone average; WRS, word recognition score; dB, decibel; HL, hearing level.

function, which may be anticipated in this case if improvement in eye closure does not occur rapidly or if there is any concern about eye protection or corneal hypesthesia. The remnant tumor capsule left on the splayed facial nerve will continue to be monitored with serial MRI starting 12 months from surgery. The patient was enrolled in vestibular rehabilitation therapy and encouraged to maintain high activity levels in order to expedite central compensation for her postsurgical vestibulopathy.

15.8 Questions

1. What surgical approach would not be suitable for resection of an acoustic neuroma that is 4 cm in greatest dimension with evidence of brainstem compression?
   a) Middle fossa approach.
   b) Retrosigmoid approach.
   c) Translabyrinthine approach.
2. Which of the following surgical approaches cannot be used for hearing preservation in acoustic neuromas?
   a) Retrosigmoid approach.
   b) Middle fossa approach.
   c) Translabyrinthine approach.
3. With respect to the American Academy of Otolaryngology–Head and Neck Surgery guidelines on hearing preservation, which preoperative hearing class would be considered to constitute serviceable hearing?

a) Class B (pure tone average [PTA] 35/word recognition score [WRS ≥] ≥ 60).
b) Class D (PTA 90/WRS 8).
c) Class A (PTA 65/WRS 24).
d) Class C (PTA 55/WRS 45).

Answers: 1. a 2. c 3. a

Suggested Readings

Battaglia A, Mastrodimos B, Cueva R. Comparison of growth patterns of acoustic neuromas with and without radiosurgery. Otol Neurotol. 2006; 27(5):705–712

Bennett M, Haynes DS. Surgical approaches and complications in the removal of vestibular schwannomas. Otolaryngol Clin North Am. 2007; 40(3):589–609, ix–x

Dilwali S, Kao SY, Fujita T, Landegger LD, Stankovic KM. Nonsteroidal anti-inflammatory medications are cytostatic against human vestibular schwannomas. Transl Res. 2015; 166(1):1–11

Doherty JK, Friedman RA. Controversies in building a management algorithm for vestibular schwannomas. Curr Opin Otolaryngol Head Neck Surg. 2006; 14(5):305–313

Peng KA, Wilkinson EP. Optimal outcomes for hearing preservation in the management of small vestibular schwannomas. J Laryngol Otol. 2016; 130(7):606–610

Peng KA, Wilkinson EP. Optimal outcomes for hearing preservation in the management of small vestibular schwannomas. J Laryngol Otol. 2016; 20:1–5

Shah KJ, Chamoun RB. Large Vestibular Schwannomas Presenting during Pregnancy: Management Strategies. J Neurol Surg B Skull Base. 2014; 75(3):214–220

Staecker H, Nadol JB, Jr, Ojeman R, Ronner S, McKenna MJ. Hearing preservation in acoustic neuroma surgery: middle fossa versus retrosigmoid approach. Am J Otol. 2000; 21(3):399–404

16 Glomus Jugulare

Shawn M. Stevens and Ravi N. Samy

16.1 History

A 68-year-old African-American woman presented with a chief complaint of pulse synchronous tinnitus in the left ear. This had progressively worsened over the past few years. She also noted some muffling of her hearing and aural fullness, both on the left. During the history, she expressed concern that some foods and drinks would "get stuck" when swallowing and that she would occasionally choke on liquids. She noted her voice had been deep and hoarse for years, but she attributed this to being a heavy smoker. She denied headaches, dizziness, or other neurologic deficits.

Her medical history was significant for well-controlled diabetes mellitus type 2, severe chronic obstructive pulmonary disorder (COPD) requiring daily nebulizer use, and coronary artery disease with stent placement 2 years ago. She had previously taken warfarin following this procedure but had stopped it at the discretion of her cardiologist. She had never had issues with high blood pressure or flushing. She had no other pertinent surgical or otologic history, and the remainder of her medical history was unremarkable. There was no known family history of skull base or intracranial tumors.

Physical examination of the pinnae and external auditory canals bilaterally was unremarkable. Otomicroscopic examination was normal on the right. On the left, however, there was a violaceous mass medial to an intact tympanic membrane causing it to bulge outward slightly. Pneumatic otoscopy revealed blanching of the mass. Tuning fork testing at 512 Hz revealed Weber's test that lateralized to the left ear with a negative Rinne on that side. Her cranial nerve exam was unremarkable with the exception of a hypomobile left true vocal fold on flexible nasopharyngoscopic exam. There were no neck masses, and her remaining exam was unremarkable.

16.2 Differential Diagnosis—Key Points

- Tinnitus, this patient's chief complaint, can generally be categorized as either subjective or objective. Pulse synchronous tinnitus typically falls into the latter category. The differential diagnosis for this is more broadly reviewed in chapter 14 but would include dural arteriovenous malformation, jugulotympanic paraganglioma (glomus tumor), other temporal bone tumors, vascular anomaly of the middle ear (e.g., aberrant carotid artery), sigmoid sinus dehiscence/diverticulum, encephalocele, idiopathic intracranial hypertension, stapedius muscle spasm, patulous eustachian tube, and myopalatal clonus.
- Jugulotympanic paragangliomas may arise from Arnold's nerve (branches of IX and X) or Jacobson's nerve (branch of IX). This occurs within the jugular bulb and/or the tympanic cleft. Though slow growing, these tumors are generally benign and arise from rests of neuroendocrine cells associated with parts of the peripheral nervous system. Carotid body tumors, glomus vagale tumors, and pheochromocytomas are examples of extratympanic paragangliomas. Jugulotympanic paragangliomas arise either within the jugular bulb or in association with Arnold's (branches of IX and X) and/or Jacobsen's (branch of IX) nerves. Though slow growing, these tumors can be locally aggressive and quite extensive by the time they become symptomatic. The most common findings are a violaceous middle ear mass, pulsatile tinnitus, and hearing loss (conductive, mixed, or sensorineural). Headaches and dizziness are also common findings. Blanching with pneumatic otoscopy (Brown's sign) is suggestive but not pathognomonic. The pulsatile tinnitus reflects the vascular nature of the tumor and is due to turbulent blood flow.
- Glomus jugulare tumors are often associated with variable levels of dysfunction of cranial nerves IX through XI, which are disrupted as they course through the jugular foramen. Nerves VII, VIII, and XII can also be affected by large tumors. For this reason, a thorough history and exam including assessment of vocal cord function is of great importance in future treatment planning. If a glomus tumor is suspected, patients should also be screened for tumors that secrete catecholamines (poorly controlled hypertension, flushing) and for bilateral disease, which has been reported in 4 to 8% of cases. Glomus tumors are most commonly sporadic, but hereditary paraganglioma syndromes have been described and are associated with a series of germline mutations to succinate dehydrogenase. These patients typically are younger at

presentation (< 40 years), may have prior history of pheochromocytoma, and are more likely to have malignant variants (capable of distant metastases).

- Vascular anomalies of the middle ear most often manifest with pulsatile tinnitus. These anomalies include high-riding jugular bulb, aberrant internal carotid artery, and petrous carotid artery aneurysms. These anomalies are readily identified using high-resolution computed tomography (CT) scans of the temporal bone. A high-riding jugular bulb (which occurs in 6% of patients) is the most common finding and occurs when the jugular bulb extends superior to the inferior tympanic annulus.
- The differential diagnosis for temporal bone tumors, particularly those of the jugular foramen and posterior fossa, would include schwannomas, meningiomas, chordomas, chondrosarcomas, endolymphatic sac tumors, and other sarcomas.

16.3 Test Interpretation

An assessment should begin with a complete audiometric evaluation that includes pure tone thresholds, speech reception threshold and discrimination, tympanometry, and acoustic reflexes. Typically, the audiogram will show conductive or mixed hearing loss when vascular anomalies or tumors of the middle ear are present. Sensorineural hearing loss can be present if there is extension into the otic capsule, temporal bone, or internal auditory canal.

Both high-resolution CT of the temporal bones and magnetic resonance imaging (MRI) with gadolinium should be obtained unless a direct contraindication exists. CT imaging will provide excellent detail of the temporal bone anatomy and be useful in identification of bony dehiscences, sigmoid diverticula, and high-riding jugular bulb. It may also be suggestive of jugulotympanic paragangliomas and other posterior fossa tumors. Glomus tympanicum tumors typically present as a soft tissue density within the middle ear cleft. Glomus jugulare tumors can be extensive and typically are associated with bony erosion and loss of clear foraminal margins. Jugular foramen schwannomas and meningiomas may be associated with bony remodeling but do not erode bone as glomus tumors often do.

Multiplanar MRI is especially critical for diagnosis of glomus jugulare tumors. T1-weighted images will have intermediate signal intensity, whereas T2 imaging has high signal intensity. Flow voids are present in both (salt and pepper pattern), and the tumor will strongly enhance with contrast. Axial and coronal formats should be assessed for the degree of bony and intracranial extension. Tumors should also be tracked inferiorly, as glomus jugulares have been known to extend into the upper neck. There are two major classification schemes to describe tumor extent, which are outlined in ▶ Table 16.1. MRI is also helpful for determining

Table 16.1 Classification schemes for paragangliomas

Glasscock-Jackson staging system for jugular paraganglioma tumors	
Grade	Definition
I	A small tumor involving the jugular bulb, middle ear, and mastoid
II	A tumor extending under the internal auditory canal; +/– intracranial extension
III	A tumor extending into the petrous apex; +/– intracranial extension
IV	A tumor extending to the clivus or infratemporal fossa; +/– intracranial extension
Fisch staging system for jugulotympanic paraganglioma tumors	
Class	Definition
A	Tumors limited to the middle ear space
B	Tumors limited to the middle ear or mastoid without involvement of the infralabyrinthine space of the temporal bone
C	Tumors involving infralabyrinthine and apical spaces of the temporal bone, with extension into the apex
D1	Tumors with intracranial extension < 2 cm in diameter
D2	Tumors with intracranial extension > 2 cm in diameter

the presence of synchronous paragangliomas of the head and neck (e.g., contralateral carotid body tumor).

Carotid and vertebral angiography (four-vessel angiography) is typically not needed for diagnostic purposes for glomus tumors. However, angiography with preoperative embolization is performed before the surgical extirpation of a glomus jugulare tumor to reduce the amount of intraoperative blood loss and the subsequent transfusion of blood products. Angiography can also serve a diagnostic role in cases where a jugular foramen schwannoma or meningioma must be ruled out (much less vascular tumors).

Laboratory evaluation must include urine and serum catecholamines because around 4% of paragangliomas are hormonally active. It should be noted that if screening reveals excess catecholamines, adrenal imaging (octreotide scan) is important to rule out a concomitant pheochromocytoma. In addition, endocrinology consultation is obtained and α-blockade antihypertensive agents are prescribed. This patient's CT scan revealed a rather large mass arising from the jugular foramen with evidence of bony erosion and intracranial and cervical extensions (▶ Fig. 16.1). MRI revealed an enhancing left jugular foramen mass with flow voids and extension into the neck (▶ Fig. 16.2).

16.4 Diagnosis

Glomus jugulare

16.5 Medical Management

Treatment options for glomus jugulare tumors include fractionated radiation therapy (RT), stereotactic radiosurgery (SRS), microsurgical resection, and observation. Observation is typically reserved for asymptomatic patients with a limited life expectancy (the old and the infirm). During treatment planning, factors such as patient age, general health, medical comorbidities, tumor size, involvement of critical structures, and the patient's wishes dramatically affect treatment decisions. Preexisting cranial neuropathies also play a key role in decision making.

Radiation (either RT or SRS) currently constitutes the mainstay of treatment for growing glomus jugulare tumors at most centers. This especially holds true for older patients and those with multiple significant comorbid conditions in whom iatrogenic injury to lower cranial nerves would be poorly tolerated. Tumor control rates are comparable to surgery (typically ~ 90%), but neither RT nor SRS is curative. The durability of tumor control remains under investigation, and delayed growth has been documented in 10 to 20% of cases

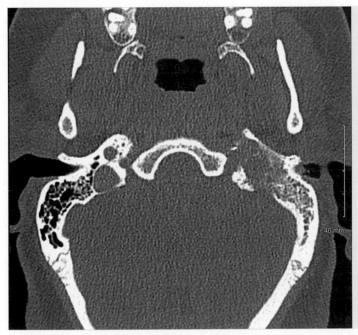

Fig. 16.1 Axial computed tomography scan of temporal bone demonstrating jugular foramen erosion on the left by a glomus jugulare tumor.

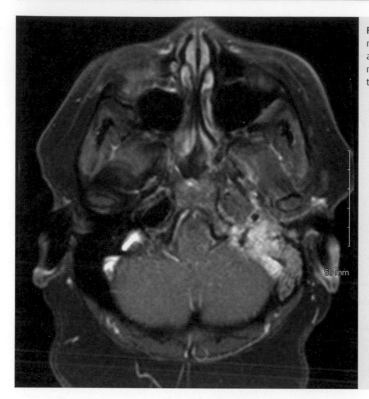

Fig. 16.2 Axial T1-weighted, gadolinium-enhanced MRI image revealing an enhancing left jugular foramen mass with intracranial extension. Notice flow void patterns in the mass.

as far out as 10 to 15 years from treatment. With current shielding techniques and fractionation regimens, side effects and collateral damage are typically minimal and well tolerated.

16.6 Surgical Management

Surgical management is the only curative treatment option for glomus jugulare. In young, healthy patients with large tumors and preexisting cranial neuropathies (i.e., little risk of iatrogenic cranial nerve injury), surgery should be considered a primary treatment modality. For patients with large tumors (Fisch C/D, Glasscock-Jackson III/IV, see ▶ Table 16.1) and normal cranial nerves, the algorithm is less clear. There is evidence these patients may respond favorably to subtotal tumor resection followed by close observation and use of SRS for regrowth. The extent of the tumor is vitally important and dictates the best surgical approach for each individual. All surgical approaches are based on having adequate control of vital structures in close approximation to the tumor, such as the lower cranial nerves and the internal carotid artery and internal jugular vein.

The facial nerve lies in close proximity to the jugular bulb. This necessitates either the fallopian bridge technique (working around a suspended, immobilized mastoid segment of the facial nerve) or facial nerve mobilization techniques for adequate access. The carotid artery must be controlled proximally in the neck. In larger tumors, an infratemporal fossa approach is necessary to control the petrous carotid artery. Cranial nerves IX, X, XI, and XII must be assessed during the tumor resection as well. If they are uninvolved, it might be possible to spare their function. In addition to these critical structures, preoperative assessment of intracranial involvement is important; cerebrospinal fluid (CSF) leaks and posterior fossa hemorrhage can occur, though rarely.

16.7 Rehabilitation and Follow-up

Following surgery, cranial nerve deficits are the most common morbidities and can be especially devastating in elderly and infirm patients. In patients with a normal cranial nerve exam at presentation, the rate of iatrogenic neuropathy following surgery ranges from 18 to 39%. Cranial nerve VII may be weak postoperatively if mobilized. Postoperative attention to eye protection is critical so that ocular morbidities can be avoided. Injury to the lower cranial nerves will affect speech and swallowing to varying degrees. Rehabilitation with speech therapy is critical in achieving adequate speech and swallowing and can be assisted by vocal cord medialization. Auditory rehabilitation with hearing aids or osseointegrated bone conduction implants may be considered in appropriate candidates. For patients treated via RT, SRS, or observation, surveillance for tumor growth is indicated with serial MRI scan performed at yearly intervals. Octreotide scanning can also be performed to monitor for recurrence.

In the presented case, the patient elected to undergo SRS. She was referred to speech-language pathology for swallowing rehabilitation. Surveillance imaging has demonstrated no growth to date. She had no adverse effects from her radiation and has not developed any new symptoms or cranial nerve deficits. She utilizes a traditional hearing aid on the side of the tumor.

16.8 Questions

1. In a 50-year-old, healthy man with a large glomus jugulare tumor and multiple preexisting cranial neuropathies, what is the treatment modality of choice to achieve cure?
   a) Surgical resection.
   b) Stereotactic radiosurgery.
   c) Hypo fractionated radiation.
   d) Definitive embolization.
2. A 95-year-old woman in reasonably good health with an intermediate-size glomus jugulare tumor would be considered for what treatment option that other patients might not?
   a) Surgical resection.

b) Hypo fractionated radiation.
c) Observation with serial imaging.
d) Octreotide suppression therapy.
3. Germline mutations to what are strongly associated with hereditary paraganglioma syndromes?
   a) Chromosome 17p.
   b) Succinate dehydrogenase.
   c) Thymidylate synthase.
   d) PAX3.

Answers: 1. a 2. c 3. b

Suggested Readings

Brackmann DE, Arriaga MA. Surgery for glomus and jugular foramen tumors. In: Brackmann DE, Shelton C, Arriaga MA, eds. Otologic Surgery. Philadelphia, PA: WB Saunders Co; 2001:478–492

Foote RL, Pollock BE, Gorman DA, et al. Glomus jugulare tumor: tumor control and complications after stereotactic radiosurgery. Head Neck. 2002; 24(4):332–338, discussion 338–339

Gilbo P, Morris CG, Amdur RJ, et al. Radiotherapy for benign head and neck paragangliomas: a 45-year experience. Cancer. 2014; 120 (23):3738–3743

Kaylie DM, O'Malley M, Aulino JM, Jackson CG. Neurotologic surgery for glomus tumors. Otolaryngol Clin North Am. 2007; 40 (3):625–649, x

Ramina R, Maniglia JJ, Fernandes YB, Paschoal JR, Pfeilsticker LN, Coelho Neto M. Tumors of the jugular foramen: diagnosis and management. Neurosurgery. 2005; 57(1) Suppl:59–68, discussion 59–68

Thomas AJ, Wiggins RH, III, Gurgel RK. Nonparaganglioma jugular foramen tumors. Otolaryngol Clin North Am. 2015; 48(2):343–359

Wanna GB, Sweeney AD, Carlson ML, et al. Subtotal resection for management of large jugular paragangliomas with functional lower cranial nerves. Otolaryngol Head Neck Surg. 2014; 151 (6):991–995

17 Petroclival Meningioma

Shawn M. Stevens and Myles L. Pensak

17.1 History

A 51-year-old woman was referred to your office with a 6-month history of left hemicranial headache, imbalance, and left facial tingling. The dysesthesias in her left face were described as intermittent but not painful. She denied diplopia, visual blurring, hearing loss, aural fullness, and nausea/vomiting. There were no other cranial neuropathies or gross motor or sensory deficits. There was no prior history of head trauma or recent infections. The remainder of her medical history was unremarkable.

Her examination revealed a well-appearing, slightly anxious woman in no distress. On gross neurologic examination she had notable unsteadiness with positive Fukuda's step test to the left. Her Rhomberg was also unstable, with a left sway that worsened when she closed her eyes. Her gait was normal, and she was able to perform rapid alternating, rotary, and translational movements with her bilateral upper and lower extremities. Gross motor and sensory function was intact.

On head and neck exam, there was no evidence of masses or lesions in the neck. There was no spontaneous or positional nystagmus noted either during primary inspection or with use of Frenzel's goggles. The cranial nerve (CN) examination revealed reduced sensation in the V1 and V2 distribution on the left side but was otherwise normal. Her corneal reflex on the left was notably diminished compared to the right. Extraocular movements were intact and symmetric, as was her pupillary exam. Otomicroscopic exam revealed normal external auditory canals and tympanic membranes bilaterally. Fistula tests were negative. Weber's test with a 512-Hz fork was detected in the midline. Rinne's test was positive bilaterally.

17.2 Differential Diagnosis—Key Points

Given the age of this female patient and her presenting symptomatology, the top diagnoses on the differential would include migraine and migraine-associated vertigo. While these diagnoses can rarely be associated with facial hypoesthesias (presenting as auras), unilateral trigeminal symptoms associated with ipsilateral hemicranial headaches raise some suspicion for an intracranial tumor or lesion. Given her imbalance, this could possibly involve the petrous apex, posterior fossa, cerebellopontine angle (CPA), or brainstem. Diagnoses of stroke, trigeminal neuralgia, and meningitis should also be entertained, although the presentation in this patient would be atypical for these.

- Petrous apex lesions on the differential include cholesterol granuloma and epidermoid tumor. These are known to manifest with any combination of symptoms, the most common being hearing loss, tinnitus, vestibular dysfunction, aural fullness, vision changes, and headache. Cranial neuropathies may also be seen in nerves V, VI, VII, and VIII. A patient with petrous apicitis would typically present with a history of acute otitis/mastoiditis in combination with retrobulbar pain, diplopia, and otorrhea (Gradenigo's triad).

- CPA lesions would include acoustic neuromas, meningiomas, and rarely, facial nerve neuromas. These lesions more commonly present with hearing loss, dizziness/imbalance, and sometimes facial twitching. Other cranial neuropathies can develop, although an isolated trigeminal hypoesthesia would be rare.

- Tumors can rarely arise along various aspects of the posterior fossa. This territory extends from the clivus and Meckel's cave anteriorly to the sigmoid sinus posteriorly. Tumors in this region could include chordomas, chondromas, various sarcomas, malignant metastases from distant sites, glomus tumors, trigeminal neuromas, schwannomas, petroclival (PC) meningiomas, and endolymphatic sac tumors.

- Roughly 20% of intracranial masses are meningiomas. Of these, only 10% are located in the posterior fossa. PC meningiomas represent a particularly rare subclass and constitute a mere 2% of all intracranial meningiomas. These benign but locally aggressive tumors arise from dural attachments to the PC synchondrosis, typically near the upper two-thirds of the clivus. They can grow to considerable size and present with highly variable rates of growth and degrees of invasiveness. Some tumors have been known to involve multiple key structures including the internal auditory canal (IAC), Meckel's cave, cavernous sinus, jugular foramen, orbit, and brainstem.

- Metastatic neoplasms should be in the differential diagnosis for older patients, with the petrous apex being the most common site for metastasis within the temporal bone. Breast, lung, prostate, melanoma, and malignant neoplasms of the kidney are the most common to metastasize to the temporal bone.
- Arachnoid cysts may arise in the posterior fossa and represent benign structures filled with cerebrospinal fluid. (CSF). The cysts may very rarely lead to erosion of the petrous apex and cause compression of the cranial nerves, brainstem, or cerebellum.

17.3 Test Interpretation

The initial evaluation of this patient would include a baseline audiogram, videonystagmography (VNG), and acoustic reflexes. Absence of the latter would be suggestive of a CPA tumor such as an acoustic neuroma. VNG testing would help differentiate a peripheral versus central etiology of the patient's imbalance.

Unless contraindicated, the key study in this case would be multiplanar, gadolinium-enhanced magnetic resonance imaging (MRI) with IAC protocol. High-resolution computed tomography (CT) of the temporal bone would serve as an adjunct to MRI and be useful for assessing local bone invasion versus expansion if a tumor were detected. CT can also detect microcalcifications, which are suggestive of some tumors such as a meningioma.

In this case, the patient's audiogram was normal and acoustic reflexes were intact. VNG demonstrated findings suggestive of a central pathology. Caloric and rotary chair testing were both normal. MRI demonstrated a mass in the region of the left PC synchondrosis that was hyperintense on T1-weighted imaging and enhanced with gadolinium. A dural tail was noted. There was mild to moderate mass effect on the brainstem with midline shift (▶ Fig. 17.1). The tumor extended from the IAC to the clivus and appeared to be confined to the posterior fossa (inferior to the tentorium). There was no involvement of Meckel's cave. CT was negative for bone erosion but did demonstrate microcalcifications within the tumor.

17.4 Diagnosis

Petroclival (PC) meningioma

17.5 Medical Management

PC meningiomas are rare tumors that arise in a relatively inaccessible anatomic region. Given this, much debate still exists over the most effective management strategy. In general, patients may be presented with three options: observation, stereotactic radiosurgery (SRS), and microsurgical

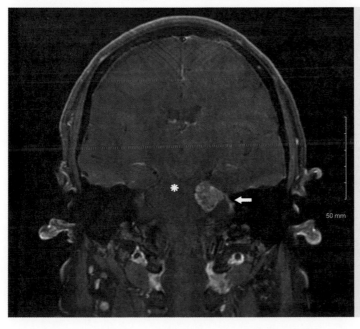

Fig. 17.1 Petroclival meningioma shown on a coronal, gadolinium-enhanced, T1-weighted image. The arrow indicates a dural tail. Mass effect from the tumor with midline shift of the brainstem is noted (asterisk).

resection. Selection of any one of these strategies must take into acount the patient's age, personal preferences, medical condition, and presenting symptoms (especially cranial neuropathies), and both the location and size of the tumor.

In cases of small tumors, observation is a reasonable option. This is especially the case in asymptomatic, elderly, and/or infirm patients given the high rate of morbidity associated with surgery. Close follow-up is necessary, however, as up to 75% of these tumors will exhibit growth at some point. It has also been shown that 50% of asymptomatic patients will go on to develop at least one CN deficit and that 20% of patients who presented with one CN deficit will develop an additional deficit in another cranial nerve.

Radiation therapy may be used as a primary intervention or as adjuvant therapy following subtotal surgical resection. Although not curative, good to excellent tumor control rates have been described. In the modern era, SRS has almost fully replaced conventional fractionated radiation. Progression-free survival rates following treatment have been quoted as high as 97%, 93%, 87%, 84%, and 80% at 3, 5, 8, 10, and 12 years, respectively. Patients should be made aware, however, that up to 10% of tumors have been shown to grow immediately following SRS and that rare cases of malignant transformation have been described. Additionally, up to 10% of patients will develop a new cranial neuropathy following SRS even in cases of quiescent tumor growth.

17.6 Surgical Management

The indications for surgical management include documented tumor growth and/or the development of neurologic deficits. In cases where surgery is indicated, multiple approaches are available to the surgeon. Factors considered during selection of a surgical approach include the tumor size and its location relative to the IAC, tentorium (superior, inferior, or combined), cavernous sinus, orbit, petrous carotid, and brainstem. The patient's age, preoperative hearing, and existing cranial nerve deficits should be considered in the surgical strategy. Given the high rates of morbidity that have been associated with gross total resection, most surgeons now advocate for subtotal resections followed by adjuvant use of SRS to preserve quality of life. Ten-year progression-free survival rates using this approach are roughly 80%.

Three primary surgical approaches (along with a large number of variants) have been described for resection of a PC meningioma: orbitozygomatic, transpetrosal (anterior, posterior, and combined), and retrosigmoid approaches. The orbitozygomatic approach is indicated for large lesions in the suprasellar, parasellar, and retrosellar areas, as well as for lesions extending into the cavernous sinus and the orbit. The transpetrosal approach has three key variants. The use of these is dependent on the tumor location, existing cranial nerve deficits, and the patient's hearing.

The anterior petrosal approach (Kawase's approach) is best suited for patients with intact hearing and PC meningiomas located medial to the IAC and without extensive involvement of the posterior fossa. The posterior transpetrosal approach itself has three variants, which themselves are extensions of a mastoidectomy: retrolabyrinthine, translabyrinthine, and transcochlear/transotic. Selection of the latter two provides the most direct route to the posterior fossa but is only an option in patients who have significant hearing loss.

Finally, the retrosigmoid approach has been used for lesions with significant mass in the posterior fossa and involving the cerebellopontine angle. A modification of this, the retrosigmoid intradural suprameatal approach, includes a retrosigmoid craniotomy and intradural drilling of the bone located above and anterior to the IAC. This allows access to lesions extending as far anterior as the clivus.

In this case the patient underwent gross total excision of her PC meningioma using a retrosigmoid approach. She recovered well from the procedure and had no neurotologic complications. Her postural stability has significantly improved following the procedure through vigorous vestibular rehabilitation. Her headache has improved to a lesser degree. Her facial hypoesthesia was initially worse but is gradually improving back to her preoperative baseline. Studies have shown such a preoperative deficit will be permanent in many cases.

17.7 Rehabilitation and Follow-up

Following surgical interventions, the incidence of new and permanent cranial nerve palsy ranges from 20 to 76%. Depending on the neurologic impairment of the patient resulting from the disease or treatment, audiologic, facial nerve, vestibular, or ophthalmologic rehabilitation may be necessary. Studies have shown that CNV and CNVIII were most likely to improve following surgery. CNVI, conversely, is the most likely to be permanently injured. The facial nerve is also at risk for injury. Other major complications following surgery may include CSF leaks, hydrocephalus, brainstem infarctions, meningitis, and cerebral edema (temporal lobe retraction or damage to vein of Labbé). Patients receiving both gross total and subtotal resection should be followed with MRI in surveillance for recurrence or regrowth.

17.8 Questions

1. A patient being observed with a small, asymptomatic petroclival (PC) meningioma could be expected to experience all of the following except
   a) Development of a new cranial nerve (CN) palsy.
   b) Tumor growth.
   c) Cerebrospinal fluid (CSF) leak.
   d) Tumor quiescence.
2. Which of the following would not be part of the differential diagnosis for a posterior fossa tumor?
   a) PC meningioma.
   b) Endolymphatic sac tumor.
   c) Chondrosarcoma.
   d) Cholesterol granuloma.

3. Following PC meningioma removal using a retrosigmoid approach, which preoperative CN deficit would be most likely to improve?
   a) CNV.
   b) CNII.
   c) CNVII.
   d) CNVI.

Answers: 1. c 2. d 3. a

Suggested Readings

Abdel Aziz KM, Sanan A, van Loveren HR, Tew JM, Jr, Keller JT, Pensak ML. Petroclival meningiomas: predictive parameters for transpetrosal approaches. Neurosurgery. 2000; 47(1):139–150, discussion 150–152

Hunter JB, Weaver KD, Thompson RC, Wanna GB. Petroclival meningiomas. Otolaryngol Clin North Am. 2015; 48(3):477–490

Isaacson B, Kutz JW, Roland PS. Lesions of the petrous apex: diagnosis and management. Otolaryngol Clin North Am. 2007; 40(3):479–519, viii

Pensak ML, Van Loveren H, Tew JM, Jr, Keith RW. Transpetrosal access to meningiomas juxtaposing the temporal bone. Laryngoscope. 1994; 104(7):814–820

Starke R, Kano H, Ding D, et al. Stereotactic radiosurgery of petroclival meningiomas: a multicenter study. J Neurooncol. 2014; 119(1):169–176

Xu F, Karampelas I, Megerian CA, Selman WR, Bambakidis NC. Petroclival meningiomas: an update on surgical approaches, decision making, and treatment results. Neurosurg Focus. 2013; 35(6):E11

18 Temporal Bone Fracture

Douglas C. von Allmen and Myles L. Pensak

18.1 History

A 48-year-old man was found by his significant other at the base of scaffolding following a presumed fall from 20 feet. Emergency medical services were alerted and the patient was intubated at the scene. Upon arrival at the emergency department he was noted to have a Glasgow Coma Scale (GCS) of 1T5. Physical exam revealed patent external auditory canals, without bloody discharge. Further examination of the right ear demonstrated hemotympanum. Palpation of the mastoid area and head did not reveal any bony abnormalities or step-offs. Pupils were 3 mm, round, and sluggishly reactive to light stimulus. No facial asymmetry was noted; however, due to the patient's mental status, facial nerve exam and tuning fork exam could not be performed at the time of initial examination.

18.2 Differential Diagnosis—Key Points

- Temporal bone fractures are traditionally characterized as longitudinal (80%), transverse (20%), or mixed based on the orientation of the fracture with relationship to the petrous portion of the temporal bone (longitudinal fractures in the coronal plane, transverse fractures perpendicular to the petrous ridge). Longitudinal fractures are thought to result from a lateral blow to the parietal or temporal bone, while transverse fractures are thought to result from a blow to the occiput or frontal bone. The alternative classification of otic capsule involving versus otic capsule sparing may represent a more practical classification with regard to clinical presentation and risk of sequelae such as profound hearing loss, cerebrospinal fluid (CSF) leak, and facial nerve injury. Otic capsule–involving fractures, compared to otic capsule–sparing fractures, are 5 times more likely to have facial nerve injury, 8 times more likely to have CSF leak, and 25 times more likely to have sensorineural hearing loss (SNHL).
- Bilateral otologic examination should consist of careful exam of the external auditory canal (EAC) for lacerations and persistent clear or serosanguinous drainage suggestive of CSF

drainage. EAC laceration may require wick placement to prevent canal stenosis. Weber's and Rinne's tuning fork exams allow for the identification of conductive versus sensorineural hearing loss. Conductive loss commonly occurs due to blood in the mastoid and may also represent damage or disarticulation of the ossicles. SNHL may represent an otic capsule–involving fracture but can also be indicative of long-standing prior hearing loss or acute SNHL unrelated to the fracture.

- A full neurologic exam in addition to the ear exam and tuning fork exam is important to obtain to identify the presence of other injuries. Temporal bone fractures, due to the high degree of force involved, are commonly associated with other fractures and brain and vascular injuries. For example, the patient in the scenario above sustained a small-segment carotid dissection. Subdural and epidural hematomas are also common in these patients, and as a result, cooperation with other treatment teams such as neurosurgery and trauma surgery is important to establish priorities of care. Facial nerve examination, although oftentimes difficult to obtain in patients with other head injuries, is important for early identification of facial nerve paralysis.
- An eye exam is important to identify nystagmus to aide in the diagnosis of associated vestibulopathy. Benign paroxysmal positional vertigo is common after head trauma. However, in the acute setting during initial evaluation, nystagmus may suggest labyrinthine injury, otic capsule involvement, or perilymph fistula.

18.3 Test Interpretation

- In the setting of profound right-sided SNHL, as seen in the patient in the above example, Weber's test lateralizes to the left and Rinne's test will be positive on the right.
- Pure tone audiogram reveals profound SNHL on the right.
- Obtaining a computed tomography (CT) scan of the temporal bones is important to determine the anatomic involvement of the fracture line with the focus on otic capsule and facial nerve involvement. A recent study demonstrated nearly 50% of otic capsule–involving fractures

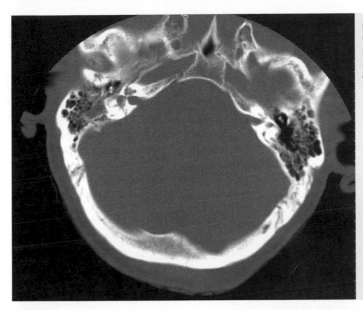

Fig. 18.1 Noncontrast axial CT scan of temporal bone demonstrating right-sided temporal bone fracture with involvement of the cochlea and vestibule.

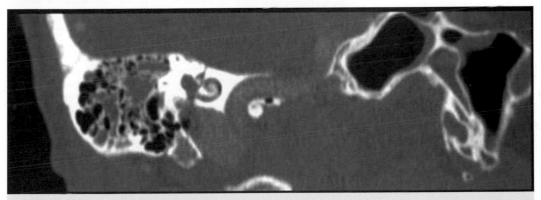

Fig. 18.2 Noncontrast coronal CT scan of temporal bone with cochlear involvement and associated jugular bulb hematoma.

have pneumolabyrinth, which can aid in identification of otic capsule involvement. CT scan from the patient above showed a right-sided temporal bone fracture with otic capsule involvement (▶ Fig. 18.1 and, ▶ Fig. 18.2).

18.4 Diagnosis

Right otic capsule–involving temporal bone fracture

18.5 Medical Management

Temporal bone fractures are generally treated conservatively unless neurologic complications are present that require urgent surgical intervention. Hemotympanum causing conductive hearing loss generally will resolve over the course of several weeks. A repeat audiogram to confirm the degree of hearing loss should be scheduled after resolution of the hemotympanum to avoid confounding results. Long-term or permanent hearing loss may be addressed with nonsurgical methods such as hearing aids.

Immediate onset facial nerve paralysis with loss of stimulation via maximal stimulation test (MST) or 90% degeneration on electroneuronography (ENoG) within 14 days requires facial nerve exploration. Delayed onset paralysis or persistent nerve stimulability should be treated with high-dose systemic corticosteroids and observed.

Antibiotic use in temporal bone fracture is limited. CSF fistulas occur in 17% of temporal bone fractures. No studies thus far have demonstrated a statistically significant benefit to prophylactic antibiotics with regard to the prevention of meningitis in the temporal bone fracture population. Due to the relatively low risk of meningitis in the acute setting and high rate of spontaneous closure within 1 week (55–85%), they may be managed conservatively with head elevation, stool softeners, bed rest, and lumbar drain.

Future otologic examination to evaluate for potential cholesteatoma formation should be performed due to the multiple mechanisms for epithelial entrapment. These mechanisms include entrapment of epithelium in the fracture line, ingrowth through persistent unhealed fracture line, ingrowth through a persistent tympanic membrane perforation, and trapping of epithelium medial to a canal stenosis.

Vestibulopathy associated with head trauma is common and should be treated with vestibular suppression medications such as meclizine and diazepam in addition to vestibular rehabilitation. Benign paroxysmal positional vertigo may present at the onset of injury or may be delayed in presentation and should be treated with Epply's maneuver once out of the acute injury setting to avoid aggravation of possible neurologic complications such as CSF leak.

18.6 Surgical Management

Early surgical management is indicated following facial nerve paralysis with evidence of wallerian degeneration as diagnosed with MST or ENoG. Facial nerve exploration can be performed by identifying the facial nerve and tracing its course to identify the area of injury. Injury distal to the geniculate ganglion can be addressed via a transmastoid approach, while proximal lesions are more easily addressed with a middle cranial fossa approach. Otic capsule–disrupting fractures with complete SNHL can be managed with obliteration of the middle ear and eustachian tube, while otic capsule–sparing temporal bone fractures with persistent CSF leak may require a middle cranial fossa approach to repair the leak site. If no facial nerve transection is identified, decompression along the entire length of the nerve should be performed. Transection of the facial nerve is managed with a greater auricular cable graft or direct anastomosis.

Surgical intervention for hearing loss may be performed after the acute injury has resolved. A patient with profound SNHL associated with otic capsule damage may be eligible for a cochlear implant. Patients with persistent conductive loss following resolution of hemotympanum may require tympanoplasty with possible ossicular chain reconstruction. Additionally, surgical management of CSF leak may be necessary if unresponsive to conservative measures. Surgical planning for repair, much like facial nerve repair, is based on otic capsule involvement to determine whether a hearing-preserving approach is necessary.

18.7 Rehabilitation and Follow-up

Long-term management following temporal bone fracture includes management of hearing loss, vestibulopathy, and sequelae related to traumatic brain injury (TBI) or vascular injuries sustained from the head trauma. Audiogram following the acute injury period is essential to evaluate the degree of hearing loss and direct further management.

18.8 Questions

1. A 37-year-old patient with a left-sided otic capsule–involving temporal bone fracture presents with left-sided House-Brackmann VI/VI. Which of the following is the next best test?
   a) Computed tomography angiography (CTA).
   b) Electroneuronography (ENoG).
   c) Audiogram.
   d) Magnetic resonance imaging (MRI).
2. Persistent clear otorrhea is found on exam 24 hours following temporal bone fracture and tests positive for beta-2 transferrin. What is the next best step in management?
   a) Surgical repair of cerebrospinal fluid (CSF) leak.
   b) Antibiotics.
   c) Bed rest, stool softeners, and precautions against Valsalva maneuvers.
   d) Lumbar drain.
3. Which of the following approaches should be taken for a facial nerve exploration and repair in an otic capsule–involving right temporal bone fracture with anacusis?
   a) Middle cranial fossa.
   b) Combined transmastoid and middle cranial fossa.
   c) Transmastoid/supralabyrinth.
   d) Translabyrinth.

Answers: 1. b 2. c 3. d

Suggested Readings

Little SC, Kesser BW. Radiographic classification of temporal bone fractures: clinical predictability using a new system. Arch Otolaryngol Head Neck Surg. 2006; 132(12):1300–1304

Johnson J. Bailey's Head and Neck Surgery: Otolaryngology. Lippincott Williams & Wilkins; 2013

Choi HG, Lee HJ, Lee JS, et al. The Rates and Clinical Characteristics of Pneumolabyrinth in Temporal Bone Fracture. Otol Neurotol. 2015; 36(6):1048–1053

Patel A, Groppo E. Management of temporal bone trauma. Craniomaxillofac Trauma Reconstr. 2010; 3(2):105–113

19 Superior Canal Dehiscence

Kareem O. Tawfik and Ravi N. Samy

19.1 History

A 42-year-old man presented with a 2-year history of chronic imbalance. Symptoms occurred daily and were exacerbated by loud noises and nose blowing. He had suffered multiple falls in the past and reported pulsatile tinnitus. He denied a history of hearing loss, ear infections, ear surgery, head trauma, otorrhea, otalgia, aural fullness, dizziness, or visual problems. Physical examination revealed a normal head and neck examination, including otomicroscopic examination of the ear canals and tympanic membranes. Weber's tuning fork examination at 512 Hz lateralized to the right ear, and Rinne's test was normal in both ears. Bilaterally, Hennebert's test elicited mild subjective dizziness without objective nystagmus. The remainder of the otoneurologic examination was normal.

19.2 Differential Diagnosis—Key Points

- The constellation of symptoms is suspicious for superior semicircular canal dehiscence (SSCCD), wherein deficiency of a portion of the arcuate eminence portion of the otic capsule (the bone overlying the superior semicircular canal [SSCC]) results in a communication between the labyrinth and intracranial cavity. It is thought that the dehiscence between the SSCC and the intracranial cavity constitutes a third mobile window to the inner ear (i.e., in addition to the oval and round windows), resulting in a low-impedance pathway for sound and pressure, akin to the round window of the cochlea. The "third window" theory explains the increased sensitivity of the inner ear to sound and pressure stimuli. The pathogenesis of SSCCD is controversial. A developmental theory suggests that SSCCD may result from arrested or failed postnatal bone formation. Another theory proposes the dehiscence may be acquired as a result of trauma or progressive erosion of the middle fossa floor.

Patients with SSCCD may complain of chronic imbalance that worsens when they encounter loud sounds or pressure changes. Sneezing, coughing, or straining may also exacerbate disequilibrium or cause true vertigo. Associated symptoms may include hyperacusis, pulsatile tinnitus, and autophony. Patients may also complain of "hearing" their eye movements or other bodily sounds. These symptoms are thought to be attributable to increased sensitivity to bone-conducted sounds (conductive hyperacusis). Physical examination may reveal Tullio's phenomenon, wherein nystagmus is elicited when the ear is exposed to sound, as well as Hennebert's sign, wherein nystagmus is elicited on insufflation of the ear with pneumatic otoscopy. Tuning fork examination may reveal findings consistent with a conductive hearing loss of the affected ear. In patients with true conductive hyperacusis, a tuning fork placed on the ankle may be readily audible.

For patients with SSCCD, audiometry may show a predominant low-frequency conductive hearing loss distinguishable from otosclerosis by the preservation of an acoustic reflex (which is absent in otosclerosis with stapes footplate fixation). In addition, low-frequency bone conduction thresholds may be supranormal. Cervical vestibular evoked myogenic potential (VEMP) testing may show low thresholds.

High-resolution computed tomography (CT) imaging of the temporal bone is indicated to evaluate the extent of bone between the SSCC and middle intracranial fossa. The SSCCs should be assessed in Stenver's (perpendicular to the canal) and Pöschl's (parallel to the canal) views. Importantly, CT evidence of SSCCD must be interpreted in the context of the patient's symptoms and signs. CT scans performed with 1.0-mm or 1.5-mm collimation may not be specific enough to demonstrate SSCCD. Specificity of CT imaging is enhanced with 0.5-mm collimation. Imaging of patients with unilateral dehiscence often reveals thinning of the contralateral tegmen tympani and tegmen mastoideum. Bilateral SSCCD is also possible.

- Perilymphatic fistula may present with any combination of sensorineural hearing loss, vertigo, tinnitus, and aural fullness; in such patients, symptoms may fluctuate in severity. Causes of pulsatile tinnitus must also be considered.
- Patients with a patulous eustachian tube may also present with autophony. Whereas autophony may be position dependent in patients with patulous eustachian tube, it tends to occur without remittance in the context of SSCCD. Further,

autophony to one's own breathing is common in patulous eustachian tube but atypical in SSCCD. Otologic examination may reveal tympanic membrane excursion that varies with respiration. A thorough history, physical examination, audiometric testing, and imaging studies are useful in identifying a specific cause.

19.3 Test Interpretation

Audiogram showed mild right-sided low-frequency conductive hearing loss. Acoustic reflexes were present. Tympanometry was normal. VEMP testing showed a low right-sided threshold.

CT imaging showed dehiscence of the right SSCC (▶ Fig. 19.1).

19.4 Diagnosis

Superior SSCCD

19.5 Medical Management

Conservative medical management includes avoidance of triggers as well as vestibular physical therapy. For patients with pulsatile oscillopsia, chronic disequilibrium, and autophony, symptoms are unlikely to abate with avoidance of loud noise.

Some otologists have tried pressure-equalizing tube placement with limited success.

19.6 Surgical Management

Surgical correction is considered for patients with severe symptoms that fail to respond to conservative management. Surgical intervention may include plugging of the dehiscent canal with fascia followed by bone wax or bone pate in order to obliterate the canal lumen. Resurfacing the tegmen mastoideum with bone cement and/or cartilage has also been used but is more likely to be associated with recurrence of symptoms. These procedures may be performed via a middle fossa craniotomy or via a postauricular transmastoid approach.

In cases of bilateral dehiscence warranting surgical intervention, staged operations are preferred. Laterality of the first operation is directed to the ear causing severest symptoms. If the first operation is successful, a second operation may be performed 6 to 12 months after the first.

19.7 Rehabilitation and Follow-up

Patients undergoing middle craniotomy approach for repair of SSCCD are closely monitored in an

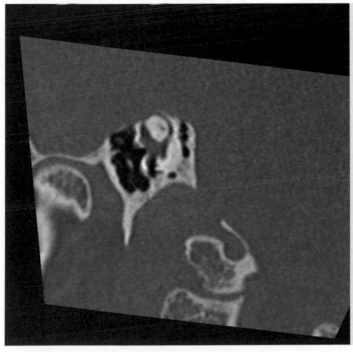

Fig. 19.1 A CT image of the right temporal bone in the plane of the superior semicircular canal, which is dehiscent.

intensive care unit overnight. Frequent neurologic checks are performed due to the risk of intracranial bleeding or temporal lobe injury, although the risk is < 1%. Nausea and vomiting are managed with intravenous promethazine. Equilibrium may be significantly impaired in the immediate postoperative period due to a loss of the superior canal function. Disequilibrium is particularly severe with head motion in the plane of the affected canal. By 4 to 6 postoperative weeks, however, balance is usually significantly improved.

Following surgical intervention, patients generally experience improvement in symptoms of dizziness, autophony, and hyperacusis. Hearing results tend to be much more variable. In one series of 43 patients undergoing superior canal plugging via a middle craniotomy approach, 25% of patients experienced persistent mild sensorineural hearing loss.

19.8 Questions

1. Vestibular evoked myogenic potential (VEMP) thresholds are typically ___ in patients with superior semicircular canal dehiscence (SSCCD).
   a) Low.
   b) High.
   c) Absent.

2. Acoustic reflexes are often _____in otosclerosis but _____ in SSCCD.
   a) Absent, preserved.
   b) Preserved, absent.

3. Which symptom of SSCCD is least likely to improve following surgical intervention?
   a) Autophony.
   b) Hyperacusis.
   c) Hearing loss.

Answers: 1. a 2. a 3. c

Suggested Readings

Merchant SN, Rosowski JJ. Conductive hearing loss caused by third-window lesions of the inner ear. Otol Neurotol. 2008; 29(3):282–289

Minor LB, Solomon D, Zinreich JS, Zee DS. Sound- and/or pressure-induced vertigo due to bone dehiscence of the superior semicircular canal. Arch Otolaryngol Head Neck Surg. 1998; 124(3):249–258

Ward BK, Agrawal Y, Nguyen E, et al. Hearing outcomes after surgical plugging of the superior semicircular canal by a middle cranial fossa approach. Otol Neurotol. 2012; 33(8):1386–1391

Weinreich HM, Crane BT, Carey JP, Minor LB. Superior semicircular canal dehiscence syndrome. In: Brackmann D, Shelton C, Arriaga MA, eds. Otologic Surgery. 4th. 4th ed. Philadelphia, PA: Elsevier Health Sciences; 2015:445–457

20 Cerebrospinal Fluid Otorrhea

Kareem O. Tawfik and Ravi N. Samy

20.1 History

A 63-year-old man presented to the otolaryngology clinic with a 1-month history of right aural fullness and hearing loss. He had no similar episodes in the past. His primary care provider had treated him with a course of amoxicillin for suspected acute otitis media, but his symptoms had not improved. The patient denied a history of recurrent ear infections, otorrhea, otalgia, vertigo, tinnitus, headaches, coughing, rhinorrhea, or sore throat. His past medical history was significant for obesity (body mass index 36.8), hypertension, hyperlipidemia, type 2 diabetes mellitus, and obstructive sleep apnea.

General examination revealed an obese man. Otologic examination showed right middle ear opacification. The left ear appeared normal. Weber's examination with a 512-Hz tuning fork lateralized to the right, and Rinne's testing was negative on the right and positive on the left. Flexible nasopharyngoscopy was performed to rule out nasopharyngeal tumor as a cause of unilateral middle ear effusion, and no masses or abnormalities of the nasopharynx were seen. Audiometry showed a right-sided moderate conductive hearing loss and ipsilateral flat tympanogram.

A right-sided myringotomy was performed and clear fluid drained from the middle ear. Suspicion for cerebrospinal fluid (CSF) otorrhea prompted the otolaryngologist to order high-resolution computed tomography (CT) of the temporal bones, which showed thinning and possible dehiscence of the right tegmen mastoideum. The patient was referred to the otology clinic, where persistent clear right-sided otorrhea through a small perforation at the site of previous myringotomy was noted. Beta-2 transferrin testing was positive. Magnetic resonance imaging (MRI) showed no obvious meningocele or encephalocele (▶ Fig. 20.1). The patient underwent right transmastoid closure of a CSF leak. Intraoperative findings showed a dehiscence of the tegmen mastoideum lateral to the mastoid antrum with an associated small encephalocele. The encephalocele was reduced, the dehiscence repaired with hydroxyapatite, and a lumbar drain placed intraoperatively. The lumbar drain was removed on postoperative day 2, and the patient recovered well.

20.2 Differential Diagnosis—Key Points

- Chronic otitis media with or without cholesteatoma can cause osteitis, progressive thinning and ultimately dehiscence of the tegmen resulting in CSF middle ear effusion or CSF otorrhea if the tympanic membrane is not intact.
- CSF otorrhea is common in patients with a history of head trauma resulting in skull base fractures and occurs in about 1 to 6% of all skull base fractures. In patients who exhibit CSF otorrhea at the time of injury, resolution of otorrhea often occurs within 10 to 14 days if conservative measures such as bed rest, head of bed elevation, and a stool softener are instituted. Acetazolamide has been used to reduce CSF pressure and aid in resolution of the leak. Placement of a lumbar drain is also an option in these patients. Patients who present with middle ear effusion after sustaining a temporal bone fracture warrant a high index of suspicion for CSF effusion. High-resolution CT scan of the temporal bones should be performed to evaluate for defects of the tegmen mastoideum and tegmen tympani.
- Spontaneous CSF otorrhea or effusion may also occur in patients without a history of temporal bone trauma or chronic otitis media/chronic mastoiditis. Possible causes for spontaneous CSF effusion include congenital defects of the lateral skull base and spontaneous dural herniation. During embryologic development, the temporal bone forms at four ossification centers: squamous, mastoid, tympanic, and petrous. After ossification, temporal bone pneumatization occurs, continuing into adulthood. Aberrations in ossification or pneumatization may predispose patients to development of an encephalocele. The roof of the middle ear and mastoid, where encephalocele formation is most likely to occur, is formed by portions of the petrous and squamous ossification centers. Spontaneous CSF leak or encephalocele formation has also been attributed to arachnoid granulations of the temporal bone. Arachnoid granulations that protrude into venous structures are normally involved in CSF resorption. When arachnoid granulations do not terminate in venous structures and blindly end within the temporal bone,

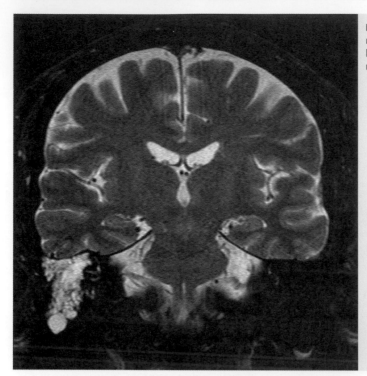

Fig. 20.1 A coronal T2-weighted magnetic resonance image of the temporal lobes showing no obvious right-sided meningoencephalocele.

they may enlarge over time. As they enlarge, the continuous pulsations of CSF in these granulations may lead to tegmen erosion, eventually resulting in a communication into the mastoid or middle ear.

- Idiopathic intracranial hypertension (IIH) has also been associated with spontaneous CSF leak and encephalocele. IIH should be considered in patients with CSF otorrhea or effusion. Patients with IIH may complain of headache, diplopia, dizziness, and pulsatile tinnitus. Fundoscopic examination may reveal papilledema. Lumbar puncture with increased opening pressure is required for formal diagnosis of IIH. Radiographically, IIH may be associated with an empty sella, which itself has been associated with CSF effusion. Additionally, morbid obesity and obstructive sleep apnea have been associated with CSF otorrhea and IIH.

20.3 Test Interpretation

The diagnosis of CSF otorrhea is primarily clinical. Persistent clear otorrhea is considered to be CSF until proven otherwise. Laboratory and radiographic investigations may substantially aid diagnosis. Laboratory studies include immunoelectrophoretic identification of beta-2 transferrin, which is pathognomonic for CSF. This test can be invaluable, but it is not readily available in many laboratories. If enough fluid is collected for testing, chemical analyses may be helpful. CSF chemical analysis reveals glucose value of 60% of serum levels, protein concentration less than 200 mg/dL, and chloride level greater than normal serum levels.

High-resolution CT scan of the temporal bones without contrast with axial and coronal views may be very helpful in localizing potential defects of the tegmen tympani or tegmen mastoideum. CT may also demonstrate soft tissue opacification in either the mastoid or middle ear or demineralization of the ossicles, which may suggest the presence of cholesteatoma or other masses of the temporal bone. MRI allows differentiation of brain tissue from other common causes of opacification, namely, cholesteatoma. CT cisternography with intrathecal radiopaque contrast and/or radionuclide may demonstrate the site of CSF leak. These tests can be falsely negative with either small or intermittent leaks.

In this case, CT scan showed opacification of the right mastoid and a portion of the right middle ear cleft with associated thinning and possible dehiscence of the tegmen mastoideum. MRI showed no definitive evidence of encephalocele (▶ Fig. 20.1), but a small encephalocele was identified intraoperatively.

20.4 Diagnosis

- CSF otorrhea
- Meningoencephalocele

20.5 Medical Management

Although some debate exists in the literature regarding prophylactic antibiotics to prevent bacterial meningitis, we do not feel antibiotics are warranted unless meningitis is suspected. This practice minimizes the risk of selecting resistant organisms. Patients should, however, receive a *Streptococcus pneumoniae* vaccine to reduce the risk of pneumococcal meningitis, such as Pneumovax 23 (Merck) or Prevnar 13 (Pfizer).

20.6 Surgical Management

The surgical approach to a defect in the tegmen of the temporal bone may include middle fossa craniotomy, transmastoid approach, or a combination of the two. The location and size of the defect and patient factors such as age, comorbidities, and personal preferences must be considered. An isolated tegmen mastoideum defect may be suitable for a transmastoid approach if the defect is single and smaller than 2 cm. Middle fossa craniotomy may be preferable for larger defects or multiple defects, either alone or in combination with mastoidectomy. A combined approach is often useful for defects in the tegmen tympani.

After reducing the encephalocele with bipolar cautery and resecting the nonfunctional brain tissue as needed, a multilayered closure offers the best success rate. During this approach, any encephalocele is cauterized and resected from the mastoid or middle ear. Layered closure from the middle fossa may be performed using a variety of materials, including bone, temporalis muscle (as a free graft or rotation flap), fascia, and/or abdominal fat. A typical repair consists of a sandwich of fascia-bone-fascia using temporalis fascia and outer table calvarial bone graft. Fibrin glue can be used to reinforce the repair.

If a craniotomy is medically contraindicated, a useful technique for large or multiple defects is to obliterate the mastoid, middle ear, and eustachian tube with abdominal fat. A lumbar drain is typically placed at the time of surgery and kept in place for up to 5 days postoperatively.

20.7 Rehabilitation and Follow-up

Postoperatively, the patient should be monitored in the hospital for any evidence of CSF leak (via the ear, skin incision, or nose) and for signs and symptoms of meningitis. The head of the bed should be elevated, and the patient should have a bowel regimen to prevent constipation and minimize straining. All of these measures are designed to avoid increases in intracranial pressure. At discharge, the patient should understand that decreased activity and avoidance of straining are critical for operative success. The patient can resume normal activity 1 month postoperatively.

20.8 Questions

1. What protein test can be obtained to assess for the presence of a cerebrospinal fluid (CSF) leak and is considered pathognomonic?
   a) Glycoprotein alpha.
   b) Heat shock protein 70.
   c) Beta-2 transferrin.
   d) Oligoclonal bands.
2. Which two ossification centers give rise to the tegmen tympani and tegmen mastoideum?
   a) Mastoid and petrous.
   b) Tympanic and mastoid.
   c) Tympanic and petrous.
   d) Petrous and squamous.
3. True or false? The brain tissue present in an encephalocele is functional and must not be injured.

Answers: 1. c 2. d 3. False

Suggested Readings

Brown NE, Grundfast KM, Jabre A, Megerian CA, O'Malley BW, Jr, Rosenberg SI. Diagnosis and management of spontaneous cerebrospinal fluid-middle ear effusion and otorrhea. Laryngoscope. 2004; 114(5):800–805

Graham MD, Lundy LB. Dural herniation and cerebrospinal fluid leaks. In: Brackmann DE, Shelton C, Arriaga MA, eds. Otologic Surgery. Philadelphia, PA: WB Saunders Co; 2001: 216–225

Gubbels SP, Selden NR, Delashaw JB, Jr, McMenomey SO. Spontaneous middle fossa encephalocele and cerebrospinal fluid leakage: diagnosis and management. Otol Neurotol. 2007; 28 (8):1131–1139

LeVay AJ, Kveton JF. Relationship between obesity, obstructive sleep apnea, and spontaneous cerebrospinal fluid otorrhea. Laryngoscope. 2008; 118(2):275–278

Nahas Z, Tatlipinar A, Limb CJ, Francis HW. Spontaneous meningoencephalocele of the temporal bone: clinical spectrum and presentation. Arch Otolaryngol Head Neck Surg. 2008; 134(5):509–518

Rao AK, Merenda DM, Wetmore SJ. Diagnosis and management of spontaneous cerebrospinal fluid otorrhea. Otol Neurotol. 2005; 26 (6):1171–1175

Savva A, Taylor MJ, Beatty CW. Management of cerebrospinal fluid leaks involving the temporal bone: report on 92 patients. Laryngoscope. 2003; 113(1):50–56

Scurry WC, Jr, Ort SA, Peterson WM, Sheehan JM, Isaacson JE. Idiopathic temporal bone encephaloceles in the obese patient. Otolaryngol Head Neck Surg. 2007; 136(6):961–965

21 Trigeminal Neuralgia

Shawn M. Stevens and Myles L. Pensak

21.1 History

A 55-year-old woman was referred to your office with a chief complaint of facial pain. She noted this pain came and went intermittently with no symptoms between spells. It only occurred around her left forehead, brow, and periorbital area. The pain was intense and sharp and lasted only a minute or two prior to resolving completely. She denied nasal congestion, discharge, fevers, cough, headache, vision changes, hearing loss, or dizziness. She also denied any periodontal disease or temporomandibular joint (TMJ) pain. She noted having between one and five of these "pain attacks" every day.

The attacks were seemingly random, although she had noticed that a gust of wind or her hair brushing her left cheek had previously triggered episodes. The attacks had been occurring for roughly 8 months, but her job as a local supply chain manager had prevented her from seeing a doctor until now. She was waiting for a consultation with a neurologist the next month. She had tried taking over-the-counter pain medications without reduction in the frequency or severity of the attacks. The remainder of her history was unremarkable. She noted her mother had similar pain attacks prior to passing away in her 70 s.

Her examination revealed a well-appearing Caucasian woman in no distress. On head and neck exam, there was no evidence of masses or lesions, and her oral, oropharyngeal, and nasal exams appeared normal. She had healthy dentition and normal TMJ motion without crepitus. Otomicroscopic exam revealed normal external auditory canals and tympanic membranes bilaterally. Fistula tests were negative. Weber's test with a 512-Hz fork was detected in the midline. Rinne's test was positive bilaterally. Her cranial nerve exam was normal and she had intact sensation in her bilateral V1–3 distributions. Occlusion was class I with strong masseteric function.

21.2 Differential Diagnosis—Key Points

Trigeminal neuralgia (TN) is a facial pain syndrome characterized by unilateral, paroxysmal, shocklike pain attacks located in the somatosensory distribution of the trigeminal nerve. The prevalence of this disorder is 0.015%. It is very uncommon in people under 40 years of age and is primarily a disease of older age. Women are affected more commonly than men, and there is often a positive family history of this disorder. While the pathogenesis of this condition is not fully understood, the classic cases are thought to be related to neurovascular compression of the trigeminal nerve root entry zone in the prepontine cistern. Various other neurophysiologic mechanisms, all poorly understood, are also at play during pain onset and recurrence.

- The International Headache Society recently defined strict clinical criteria for TN diagnosis. Diagnosis is made following ≥ 3 attacks of unilateral facial pain that fulfill the following criteria:
  a) Occurs in one or more trigeminal distributions without radiation beyond this.
  b) The facial pain is associated with at least three of the following:
     1. Paroxysmal, recurrent attacks lasting from 1 second to 2 minutes.
     2. Severe in intensity.
     3. Having an electric shock–like, shooting, stabbing, or sharp quality.
     4. Able to be triggered by innocuous stimuli to the affected side of the face.
- Subtypes of TN have also been proposed.
  a) Type 1 TN fits the classic description shown above, with short bursts of intense pain followed by pain-free intervals between attacks.
  b) Type 2 TN is typified by a lesser aching, throbbing, or burning sensation in the face at most times, punctuated by sharp episodic spells.
- Atypical presentations of facial pain, such as bilateral presentation (only 5% of classic TN cases present bilaterally), lack of a trigger, or absence of a refractory period should raise suspicion for other diagnoses such as multiple sclerosis (MS). In MS, up to 31% of patients will present with bilateral, continuous facial pain. Diabetes mellitus can also rarely present with neuropathic pain in the face.
- Presentations of type 2 TN, as described above, have shown an increased likelihood of being associated with a tumor or vascular malformation or anomaly.
- Tumors of the posterior fossa or Meckel's cave, and petroclival synchondrosis can cause

symptoms similar to TN and may include schwannoma, meningioma, epidermoid cyst, chondroma, chordoma, and various sarcomas. Distant metastases from malignancies of the lung, breast, prostate, colon, and kidney also may affect the petrous temporal bone. In older adults with cancer history and TN symptoms, metastatic disease should be entertained.

• Vascular malformations and anomalies in the prepontine cistern would include a vascular aggregation, arteriovenous malformation, or aneurysm.

• Local regional disorders of the head and neck may also cause fluctuating facial pain including odontogenic inflammatory processes, sinusitis, and TMJ disorders. Directed examination should ensue to rule out such disorders.

21.3 Test Interpretation

TN is primarily diagnosed via thorough history and physical exam. However, neurophysiologic recording of trigeminal reflexes represents a useful and reliable test for confirming the TN diagnosis according to the joint American Academy of Neurology–European Federation of Neurological Societies (AAN-EFNS) guidelines on neuropathic pain assessment. If symptoms of hearing loss, dizziness, or vertigo accompany the facial pain, a baseline audiogram and videonystagmography (VNG) should be considered.

Routine magnetic resonance imaging (MRI) should be considered even in patients with classic TN presentations per the AAN-EFNS guidelines. Unless contraindicated, the key study in this case would be a multiplanar, gadolinium-enhanced MRI with internal auditory canal (IAC) protocol. The addition of three-dimensional fast imaging employing steady-state acquisition (FIESTA) and magnetic resonance angiography (MRA) is also useful, particularly for surgical planning or mapping for stereotactic radiosurgery (SRS). The brainstem, trigeminal root entry zone, prepontine cistern, cerebellopontine angle, petrous apex, and perisellar compartments and Meckel's cave should all be assessed for presence of an occult tumor (▶ Fig. 21.1). MRI may also be useful for detecting demyelination suggestive of MS. High-resolution computed tomography (CT) of the temporal bone would serve as an adjunct to MRI and could be useful for assessing local bone invasion versus expansion if a tumor were detected. CT can also detect microcalcifications, which are suggestive of some tumors such as a meningioma.

The patient in this case did undergo MRI and MRA with FIESTA sequences. An aberrant branch of the vertebrobasilar system was noted to impinge upon the trigeminal root entry zone on the left.

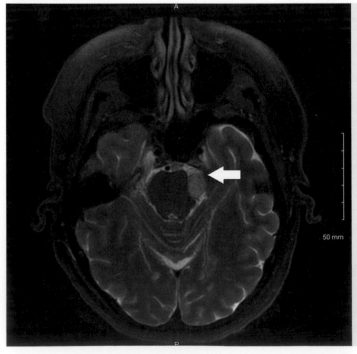

Fig. 21.1 Axial T2-weighted MRI depicting a posterior fossa mass with direct impingement on the trigeminal root entry zone and CNV (arrow). Mass effect with midline shift of the brainstem is noted. MRI is used during the work-up of paroxysmal facial pain to assess for tumors such as this.

21.4 Diagnosis

Trigeminal neuralgia

21.5 Medical Management

TN is principally a medically managed illness. According to the most recent AAN-EFNS guidelines, two antiepileptic drugs are considered to be first-line therapies in TN. Carbamazepine is established as effective in a number of well-randomized controlled trials (Level A evidence). It has been found to reduce both the frequency and the intensity of pain attacks. Unfortunately, numerous adverse effects have been reported with this drug, especially among the elderly population. For this reason, oxcarbazepine has been more often used as initial treatment for TN. While evidence supporting its efficacy is less robust (Level B), it has significantly fewer drug interactions and has greater tolerability when compared to carbamazepine. With either drug, approximately 80% of patients are expected to have a positive response with a reduction in the number of pain attacks and lowering of pain intensity.

Baclofen, lamotrigine, and pimozide may be considered as second-line agents to control pain in patients with TN (Level C evidence). Combinations of medications may also be considered under the discretion of a board-certified neurologist. Experimentation with newer medications is under way for difficult and refractory cases. Combined gabapentin and routine ropivacaine injections has shown some favorable preliminary results. Studies are also currently exploring the safety and efficacy of botulinum toxin injections. Early results using this modality have demonstrated a decrease in pain frequency and intensity in 60 to 80% of patients with no major adverse events. Larger randomized controlled trials to further explore this are currently under way. Finally, it should be noted that use of topical anesthetic ointments, sprays, and ophthalmologic drops is probably ineffective in controlling TN pain (Level B).

SRS is reserved for cases of TN that are refractory to medical management in patients who are poor surgical candidates or refuse surgical intervention. The goal of SRS is to create a radiation-induced rhizotomy at the root entry zone of the trigeminal nerve. Current protocols have delivery goals ranging from 70 to 100 Gy. As the underlying mechanisms for TN are still not fully understood, there remains uncertainty about the exact target and optimum dose. Alternative targets include the trigeminal nuclei in the brainstem or the centromedian nucleus of the thalamus. In general, it has been reported that higher doses of radiation are related to better outcomes, but complications increase at doses greater than 90 Gy.

21.6 Surgical Management

Surgical intervention is typically reserved for refractory cases and those patients who become resistant to pharmaceutical control. Microvascular decompression (MVD) is the gold standard technique and provides the longest duration of pain freedom in TN. It is currently the most common surgical treatment for the disorder. The goal of MVD is to resolve the neurovascular conflict between an abnormal vessel and the trigeminal nerve. For this reason, preoperative radiologic studies are mandatory prior to MVD. FIESTA MRI and MRA are well suited for this task. Unfortunately, not all patients achieve a good outcome after MVD. The reported pain-free duration without medication after MVD can range from 0.6 to 10 years. After 5 years, the percentage of patients who are pain free ranges from 60 to 80%. Patients with classic presentations (type 1 TN) tend to have better outcomes than patients with type 2 or highly refractory presentations.

Described complications after this procedure are infections, facial palsy, facial numbness, cerebrospinal fluid leak, and hearing deficit. Symptoms may also arise secondary to sensory rhizotomy, including neurotrophic keratitis, corneal ulceration, and eating difficulties. Additionally, patients must be counseled that an obvious neurovascular conflict may not be identified at the time of surgery and that the procedure in such a case would result in no changes in symptomatology.

A second group of surgical interventions center around variable degrees of destruction of the gasserian ganglion. These include image-guided injection of glycerol into the trigeminal cistern (glycerol rhizotomy), radiofrequency ablation of the gasserian ganglion rootlets, and percutaneous balloon compression of Meckel's cave. While each option is moderately efficacious, they all are associated with increased adverse effects, sensory deficits, and a shortened duration of effect compared to other treatment modalities. Patients may also experience motor deficits of the trigeminal distribution following these procedures, including masticator weakness.

The patient in this case ultimately opted to start medical therapy with oxcarbazepine. She has noted a decrease in the frequency and intensity of her attacks. She is tolerating the medication well thus far without adverse effects. Her ongoing care has been transferred to a board-certified neurologist.

21.7 Rehabilitation and Follow-up

Unfortunately, pain recurrence following initially successful medical and surgical interventions is common. This likely reflects the lack of understanding of the underlying pathogenesis of this disease process. Patients often require long-term follow-up and counseling regarding second- and third-line management strategies should their primary modality fail.

21.8 Questions

1. The typical presentation of type 1 trigeminal neuralgia (TN) would be expected to include all of the following except
   a) Facial pain attacks lasting minutes followed by silent periods.
   b) Pain attacks associated with retro-orbital pressure.
   c) Facial pain with an electric shock–like quality.
   d) A family history positive for similar symptoms.
2. Which of the following is acknowledged as a first-line therapy for newly diagnosed TN in a healthy 40-year-old woman?
   a) Glycerol rhizotomy.

   b) Botulinum toxin injection.
   c) Carbamazepine.
   d) Gabapentin.
3. What study is mandatory prior to proceeding with surgical microvascular decompression (MVD) for TN?
   a) Magnetic resonance imaging (MRI) and magnetic resonance angiography (MRA), ideally with fast imaging employing steady-state acquisition (FIESTA) sequences.
   b) Trigeminal electromyography.
   c) Fundoscopic examination of the retina.
   d) High-resolution computed tomography (CT) scan of Meckel's cave and the parasellar compartment.

Answers: 1. b 2. c 3. a

Suggested Readings

Al-Quliti KW. Update on neuropathic pain treatment for trigeminal neuralgia. The pharmacological and surgical options. Neurosciences (Riyadh). 2015; 20(2):107–114

Montano N, Conforti G, Di Bonaventura R, Meglio M, Fernandez E, Papacci F. Advances in diagnosis and treatment of trigeminal neuralgia. Ther Clin Risk Manag. 2015; 11:289–299

Günther T, Gerganov VM, Stieglitz L, Ludemann W, Samii A, Samii M. Microvascular decompression for trigeminal neuralgia in the elderly: long-term treatment outcome and comparison with younger patients. Neurosurgery. 2009; 65(3):477–482, discussion 482

Tatli M, Satici O, Kanpolat Y, Sindou M. Various surgical modalities for trigeminal neuralgia: literature study of respective long-term outcomes. Acta Neurochir (Wien). 2008; 150(3):243–255

Gronseth G, Cruccu G, Alksne J, et al. Practice parameter: the diagnostic evaluation and treatment of trigeminal neuralgia (an evidence-based review): report of the Quality Standards Subcommittee of the American Academy of Neurology and the European Federation of Neurological Societies. Neurology. 2008; 71(15):1183–1190

Part IV

The Facial Nerve

IV

22 Congenital Facial Paralysis

Niall D. Jefferson and Daniel I. Choo

22.1 History

A 3-month-old infant was referred for evaluation of feeding difficulties. The infant had been born prematurely and had upper airway obstruction requiring intubation and eventual tracheostomy. She was noted to have micrognathia, microstomia, drooling, a cleft palate, and masklike facies suspicious for congenital facial paralysis (CFP).

In addition to the above features, physical examination revealed bilateral microtia, strabismus, absent lateral gaze with preserved up and down gaze, and an abnormal tongue.

22.2 Differential Diagnosis—Key Points

- CFP is a rare condition that accounts for 8 to 14% of all cases of pediatric facial paralysis. The reported incidence of CFP is 0.8 to 2.1 per 1,000 live births, and 88% of these are associated with a difficult labor.
- CFP is classified as traumatic or developmental, unilateral or bilateral, and complete or incomplete. Partial or complete recovery of function favors a traumatic cause.
- Birth weight more than 3,500 g, forceps delivery, and prematurity are all risk factors for traumatic facial nerve palsy.
- Developmental CFP is associated with other congenital abnormalities including microtia, inner ear abnormalities, facial hypoplasia, cleft palate deformities, other cranial neuropathies, internal organ disorders, and extremity disorders (▶ Table 22.1).
- These abnormalities can result in difficulty feeding and incomplete eye closure. As the child gets older, this can cause problems with speech, mastication, and emotional expression.
- Möbius syndrome (MS) is a form of CFP that is accompanied by absence of the sixth and seventh cranial nerves (CNs). It is estimated that between 2 and 20 cases of MS occur per million births. Because MS is rare, the diagnosis is often delayed. It can, however, be identified by birth by the presence of "masklike" facies and inability to latch on to the breast or bottle when nursing. Also, because of the strabismus, infants with MS cannot follow objects by moving their eyes and

therefore follow by moving their head from side to side.

Multiple other craniofacial, limb, and chest wall anomalies can accompany this diagnosis. The cause remains unknown; however, the predominant theories propose (1) vascular disruption during prenatal brain development, (2) congenital aplasia or hypoplasia of the CN nuclei, (3) association with medications, especially misoprostol and thalidomide, and (4) trauma during the prenatal period.

There are four identified categories of MS based on the radiologic findings:
- Group I: Small or absent brainstem nuclei that control the cranial nerves.
- Group II: Loss and degeneration of neurons in the facial peripheral nerve.
- Group III: Loss and degeneration of neurons and other brain cells is seen with microscopic areas of damage and hardened tissue in the brainstem nuclei.

Table 22.1 Congenital conditions associated with facial nerve paralysis

Hemifacial macrosomia
22q11.2 deletion syndrome
Myotonic dystrophy
Möbius syndrome
Hereditary congenital facial paresis 1
Hereditary congenital facial paresis 2
Hereditary hypertrophic neuropathy
Coloboma of the eye, heart anomaly, choanal atresia, retardation, and genital and ear anomalies (CHARGE) syndrome
Poland syndrome
Teratogenesis (thalidomide and misoprostol)
Osteopetrosis (Albers-Schönberg disease)
Fascioscapulohumeral muscular dystrophy
Trisomy 13, trisomy 18
Congenital unilateral lower lip palsy (CULLP) (asymmetric crying facies)
Branchio-oto-renal syndrome

- Group IV: Characterized by muscular symptoms in spite of a lack of lesions in the cranial nerve.
- A more common disorder that resembles a unilateral partial facial nerve paralysis is congenital unilateral lower lip palsy (CULLP). This condition is also known as neonatal asymmetric crying facies and occurs in 1 in every 160 live births.
- In addition to MS and CULLP, two other types of CFP of developmental origin have been discovered and are designated hereditary CFP 1 and 2 on chromosomes 3q21–22 and 10q21.3–22.1, respectively.

22.3 Test Interpretation

The newborn child with facial paralysis may present with facial asymmetry, incomplete eye closure, and/or feeding problems. To identify the etiology, a complete perinatal and family history, physical examination, and radiographic and neurophysiologic testing may be needed.

When considering the perinatal history, primigravida, high birth weight (> 3,500 g), prolonged labor (especially second stage), and the need for middle forceps delivery all increase the risk of damage to the facial nerve. A positive family history for facial paralysis or other congenital abnormalities increases clinical suspicion for a developmental cause.

Physical examination should involve evaluation of both sides of the face, assessing both the upper and lower divisions of the nerve. Traumatic causes typically affect both divisions and are often unilateral. While many grading systems exist in the evaluation of facial nerve paralysis, the House-Brackmann classification of facial nerve function is the most commonly cited. While it was not developed to examine CFP or early posttraumatic facial paralysis, the classification has intuitive gradings and is generalizable across most facial nerve pathologies. Other clinical findings in keeping with a traumatic origin include mastoid ecchymosis, hemotympanum, and facial swelling.

Electrophysiologic testing can be useful where there is CFP secondary to birth trauma. However, in bilateral facial paralysis secondary to pathologies such as MS, extensive physiologic testing is of little value.

In this case study, middle ear effusions were present bilaterally and the child had failed two newborn hearing screens and had been referred for further work-up. Magnetic resonance imaging (MRI) of the brain revealed a hypoplastic brainstem with straightening of the ventricular floor, an absent CNVI and CNVII, and a hypoplastic CNIX. Electromyography was performed, revealing absent voluntary motor potentials without polyphasic reinnervation potentials.

22.4 Diagnosis

Möbius syndrome

22.5 Medical Management

There is no cure for MS. Therefore, any treatment plans are intended to address the problems related to the neuropathies. Optimal management of CFP requires a multidisciplinary approach. This includes otolaryngologists, plastic surgeons, neurologists, ophthalmologists, speech pathologists, geneticists, and other allied health personnel.

The cranial neuropathies associated with MS can result in dysphagia, dysarthria, drooling, and oral incompetence, as well as possible aspiration risk. A flexible endoscopic evaluation of swallow can evaluate pooling of secretions and vocal fold mobility. A fluoroscopic swallowing evaluation can be a useful adjunct as part of the safe swallowing assessment. Speech therapists and nutritionists can be invaluable in providing education, diet modification, and rehabilitation for the MS patient.

Since many children with MS cannot blink due to the facial nerve involvement, they are at risk of exposure keratitis and corneal ulceration. Artificial tears and ophthalmic ointments are recommended, as well as evaluation and ongoing observation by an ophthalmologist. Additional intervention by the ophthalmologist may be required for strabismus for the abducens nerve palsy typical of MS.

Counseling and psychosocial support can be helpful for patients and their families. Understandably, older children with MS can feel left out because they struggle to communicate fully due to the facial paralysis. They can also be perceived as unfriendly or antisocial by people unfamiliar with their diagnosis.

Dental services should be engaged early owing to the increased risk of developing dental caries, gingivitis, and periodontitis. Establishing good oral hygiene and nutritional habits can reduce the impact of this as the child grows.

22.6 Surgical Management

Surgical options are either to address symptoms related to the diagnosis or to improve cosmesis.

Reanimation techniques can be considered in children with CFP. While these techniques do not restore normal function, they can improve cosmesis and help the child psychologically. Surgical options for reanimation include static and dynamic interventions. These include slings and muscle transfers. Timing of these procedures is ideally in early school age, when the child is old enough to have some understanding of the intervention. Due to the facial motor nerve atresia, some of the other reanimation options are not available. Direct facial nerve anastomosis, interposition grafting, and nerve transposition have no role in the management of the facial paralysis in MS.

Surgery specific to facial paralysis, "smile" surgery has been performed on some affected individuals. This involves a combination of static slings (gracilis) and muscle transfer (temporalis). These treatments are assisted by the fact that CNV is typically spared in MS; affected individuals can then learn to smile using the "chewing" muscles. It should be noted, however, that "smile" surgery should not be considered a surgical cure for MS because it doesn't improve the ability of the patient to form other facial expressions.

Additional reasons for surgical intervention include tarsorrhaphy to protect the cornea if lubrication proves inadequate, cleft palate repair, surgical repair of limb deformities, and orthognathic surgery.

22.7 Rehabilitation and Follow-up

There is little chance for recovery of function in cases of MS. Early recognition and multidisciplinary intervention reduces the likelihood of complications related to the multiple anomalies typical of this diagnosis. While most patients will have normal levels of intelligence, a diagnosis of autism is more common in MS patients; therefore, neuropsychologic evaluation and monitoring may be required.

22.8 Questions

1. The following reanimation procedures can be considered in patients with Möbius syndrome (MS) except
   a) Gracilis muscle transfer.
   b) Interposition grafting.
   c) Temporalis muscle transfer.
   d) Static sling.
2. Risk factors for a traumatic cause to facial paralysis include all of the following except
   a) Birth weight > 3,500 g.
   b) Gestational diabetes.
   c) Forceps extraction.
   d) Prematurity.
3. Which of the following findings is consistent with traumatic facial nerve paralysis?
   a) Bilateral facial nerve involvement.
   b) Only the upper division of the facial nerve is affected.
   c) Hemotympanum.
   d) Absence of facial swelling.

Answers: 1. b 2. b 3. c

Suggested Readings

MacKinnon S, Oystreck DT, Andrews C, Chan WM, Hunter DG, Engle EC. Diagnostic distinctions and genetic analysis of patients diagnosed with moebius syndrome. Ophthalmology. 2014; 121 (7):1461–1468

May M, Schaitkin BM. Facial Nerve Disorders in Newborns and Children. The Facial Nerve. 2nd ed. New York, NY: Thieme New York; 2000: 339–65

Moebius Syndrome Foundation. Available at http://moebiussyndrome.org

23 Bell's Palsy (Idiopathic Facial Palsy)

David F. Smith and John H. Greinwald Jr.

23.1 History

A 40-year-old Caucasian man presented with a 1-week history of a rapidly progressive left-sided facial paralysis. The patient described a recent upper respiratory infection that began as nasal congestion and drainage and progressed to a lower respiratory infection. Approximately 4 days after starting antibiotics, he noticed an acute onset of weakness on the left side of his face.

The patient denied any history of head trauma or neurotologic infections. He complained of difficulty with drooling, especially while drinking liquids, and irritation of the left eye. He also reported left-sided otalgia, aural fullness, and hyperacusis. The only other medical history included mild hypertension controlled with a beta-blocker and allergic rhinitis. The patient denied tinnitus, vertigo, otorrhea, and changes in taste. The patient had not noticed any frequent urination or fatigue. He traveled frequently for work, but he did not like the outdoors and had no recent tick exposures.

On physical examination, the patient appeared to be a well-developed man in no acute distress. The facial nerve function on the left side was a House-Brackmann grade V/VI, with asymmetry at rest and incomplete closure of the left eye. The contralateral facial function was normal with a House-Brackmann of I/VI. The pinna on the affected side was normal. Otoscopic examination of the left external auditory canal revealed normal epithelium without vesicular lesions or areas of ulceration. Further, the tympanic membrane was normal in appearance and mobile, and no effusions were noted in the middle ear space. The remaining cranial nerves were intact, and no other significant findings were noted on the head and neck examination.

23.2 Differential Diagnosis—Key Points

The differential diagnosis for causes of paroxysmal facial paralysis can be organized as described in the following sections.

23.2.1 Central Nervous System Lesions

Cerebellopontine angle masses: Vestibular schwannomas, meningiomas, lipomas, or unusually large lesions associated with the trigeminal nerve or the lower cranial nerves may manifest with facial paralysis. Typically, symptoms associated with other involved structures are also present, as it is rare for such lesions to have facial paralysis as the only presenting symptom.

Facial neuroma: A benign schwannoma that can arise from any segment of the facial nerve.

Stroke: As one of the major causes of morbidity and mortality in the United States, ischemic events that occur from stroke can present with facial paralysis. Based on the most common locations of ischemic or hemorrhagic events, though, patients with stroke routinely have multiple ipsilateral cranial nerve palsies that accompany the facial paralysis. A work-up that includes a complete neurologic examination and imaging will identify the location of strokes.

23.2.2 Infectious Diseases

Bell's palsy: Although a diagnosis of exclusion, Bell's palsy is the most common cause of unilateral facial paralysis. Although bilateral facial paralysis can occur, it is seen in less than 1% of those patients diagnosed with Bell's palsy. Bell's palsy routinely presents with twitching, weakness, or paralysis on one side of the face. Other symptoms can include dryness of the eye or mouth, changes in taste, pain in the ear, ringing in the ear, and sensitivity to loud sounds. Onset is typically rapid, reaching the peak in 48 to 72 hours. Many researchers now attribute Bell's palsy to a reactivation of a latent herpes simplex virus type 1 infection. The ensuing inflammatory process is thought to cause inflammation, edema, and compression of the facial nerve in the fallopian canal.

Lyme disease: Lyme disease is an infectious disease caused by spirochetes from the *Borrelia* genus. The most common organism, *Borrelia burgdorferi*, is carried by the deer tick, *Ixodes scapularis*. Presentation of Lyme disease is highly variable, but it will typically present with the erythema chronicum migrans rash and a flulike illness in the early stages. Lyme disease can affect a number of different body systems and cause a host of symptoms including chills, fevers, headaches, fatigue, muscle and joint pain, cardiac abnormalities, and neurologic dysfunction. Lyme disease should be considered in the differential diagnosis in any patient with a history of exposure to or bite from a tick. Diagnosis is confirmed by specific serologic studies.

Ramsay Hunt syndrome: *Herpes zoster oticus*, also known as *Ramsay Hunt syndrome*, is a viral infection caused by reactivation of the varicella zoster virus. Ramsay Hunt syndrome affects the geniculate ganglion, causing facial nerve inflammation, edema, and compression within the fallopian canal. Patients typically present with severe otalgia, and vesicular lesions of the ipsilateral ear and face are present in up to 80% of those patients with this infection. Varicella zoster infections without concomitant skin lesions, termed *zoster sine herpete*, can occur and are sometimes mistaken for Bell's palsy.

23.2.3 Autoimmune Diseases

Guillain-Barré syndrome: Guillain-Barré syndrome is an acute inflammatory polyradiculoneuropathy that routinely presents as progressive weakness and diminished reflexes. Although facial droop can occur with Guillain-Barré syndrome, paresthesias and weakness typically begin in the distal extremities and rapidly progress proximally. Diagnosis is based on a complete neurologic work-up, biochemical screening, and electromyography (EMG).

Multiple sclerosis (MS): MS is a chronic autoimmune inflammatory disease characterized by demyelination and axonal degeneration of the central nervous system. Symptoms are highly unpredictable and variable, but they can include numbness and tingling of the extremities, fatigue, dizziness, pain, vision problems, bowel and bladder dysfunction, and neurocognitive dysfunction. Peripheral facial nerve palsy as a presenting symptom of MS has only rarely been reported. Diagnosis is made by a combination of serial magnetic resonance imaging (MRI), evoked potential studies, and changes in oligoclonal bands and immunoglobulins in the cerebrospinal fluid (CSF).

23.2.4 Metabolic Diseases

Diabetes: As a disease characterized by glucose metabolism, diabetes does not typically present with facial paralysis. However, Bell's palsy is more common in patients with diabetes. The usual site of facial nerve lesions in patients with diabetes is thought to be distal to the chorda tympani nerve based on the low number of patients with diabetes who have taste disturbances.

23.2.5 Inflammatory and Neurologic Disorders

Chronic otitis media: Chronic otitis media with and without cholesteatoma may manifest with facial paralysis because erosion of the fallopian canal may allow the inflammatory response (e.g., hypertrophic mucosa and granulation tissue) to involve the facial nerve. Rarely, facial paralysis is the sole presenting symptom of a patient with cholesteatoma.

Melkersson-Rosenthal syndrome: Melkersson-Rosenthal syndrome is a rare disorder characterized by recurring facial nerve paralysis, facial and lip swelling, and the development of a furrowed tongue. This syndrome can be associated with unilateral or bilateral facial paralysis. Onset is usually in late childhood or adolescence. Noncaseating granulomas may be seen in lip biopsies of some of these patients, but this is not seen in all patients with the syndrome. The cause is currently unknown, but there may be a genetic predisposition to the disorder.

Sarcoidosis: Sarcoidosis is an inflammatory condition leading to noncaseating granulomas in multiple organs, most commonly the lung and central nervous system. Neurosarcoidosis manifests as cranial neuropathy, with paroxysmal facial paralysis the most common presenting symptom. CSF or serum should be analyzed for angiotensin-converting enzyme to confirm the diagnosis. Further evaluation for systemic sarcoidosis should include chest radiographs, bronchoscopy with biopsy of mediastinal lymph nodes, and contrast-enhanced MRI of the brain. Involvement of the facial nerve may be unilateral or bilateral and relapsing-recurring.

23.2.6 Congenital

Hemifacial microsomia: Hemifacial microsomia is a progressive bony and soft tissue deformity in which half of the lower face fails to form secondary to a developmental malformation of the first and second branchial arches. Facial paralysis is present in a significant portion of these patients, who are diagnosed in early childhood.

Möbius syndrome: Möbius syndrome, also known as congenital facial diplegia, is the congenital agenesis of bilateral facial and abducens cranial nerves. Patients with this disease usually present as infants with complete lack of bilateral mimetic function and bilateral abducens paralysis. Although it occurs less commonly, cranial nerves III and IV, as well as the lower cranial nerves, such as XII, can be additionally affected.

23.2.7 Neoplastic (Benign and Malignant)

Other: Head and neck processes (e.g., squamous cell carcinoma and benign parotid gland neoplasms) may also present with an acute onset of facial paralysis.

23.3 Test Interpretation

Electroneuronography (ENoG), also known as *evoked EMG*, allows for quantitative analysis of facial nerve degeneration and can be obtained as early as 72 hours after the proposed injury. It is the most accurate indicator for prognosis in the first 2 weeks following onset of the facial nerve weakness or paralysis. In general, patients with less than 90% degeneration will have a better outcome and expected partial or complete recovery from the facial paralysis. In the setting of degeneration greater than 90%, the degree of recovery is much less predictable.

EMG may establish the presence or absence of voluntary motor units and is an examination of the muscle activity. EMG is typically used as a complementary study with ENoG because the presence of voluntary motor units in the setting of greater than 90% degeneration is suggestive of good spontaneous recovery of facial function. The presence of fibrillation potentials suggests degeneration of lower motor nerves and is poorly predictive for recovery of function, while polyphasic reinnervation potentials are seen during nerve recovery.

Computed tomography (CT) scan may be obtained if a neoplastic process is suspected. CT scans are also used to evaluate anatomic structures, such as the fallopian canal, in patients that are undergoing surgical decompression as management of the facial paralysis.

The need for imaging is based on the clinical course of each patient. MRI for the initial diagnosis of the patient with Bell's palsy is of limited clinical utility. Patients who do not demonstrate any improvement in 4 to 6 months should undergo MRI with gadolinium to evaluate for possible neoplastic pathology. In the presence of other clinical findings, such as additional cranial neuropathy, or in the setting of recurrent or bilateral facial paralysis, MRI is warranted to rule in or out other more serious pathologies. Additionally, patients who elect to undergo operative intervention as treatment (see discussion of middle fossa approach below) will undergo preoperative MRI to rule out a neoplastic cause.

23.4 Diagnosis

Idiopathic Bell's palsy (idiopathic facial palsy)

23.5 Medical Management

Multiple studies have demonstrated the utility of high-dose systemic corticosteroids for the treatment of Bell's palsy. Current guidelines recommend the use of oral steroids within 72 hours of onset for patients over the age of 16 years. Steroids have been shown to improve facial nerve function as well as speed recovery time. Based on the proposed etiology of facial nerve paralysis, research has recently focused on the use of antiviral therapy for Bell's palsy as well. The additional use of systemic antiviral agents (such as valacyclovir) has generally been considered efficacious, yet data from randomized prospective clinical trials are less clear. Although antiviral monotherapy is not currently recommended, clinicians may offer combination therapy of oral steroids and antivirals that have previously demonstrated small improvements in facial nerve function. Antiviral therapy should always be implemented in the immunocompromised patient with Bell's palsy or herpes zoster oticus.

For patients with incomplete eye closure, attention to eye care is imperative. Ophthalmic lubricants and drops are frequently applied to prevent keratitis. Further, eye patching should be performed while the patient is sleeping, and eye coverage should be used during the daytime to prevent corneal irritation from dust and wind.

23.6 Surgical Management

Surgical management for Bell's palsy remains controversial. Those centers that perform surgical decompression for Bell's palsy routinely use a combination of ENoG and EMG to confirm the absence of recovery and identify those patients that would benefit from surgical decompression. When facial nerve degeneration is found to be greater than 90% on ENoG and no volitional motor units on EMG, surgical decompression can be offered. Due to the low level of confidence based on the small number of patients in previous studies, no academy recommendations can be made regarding surgical decompression in patients with Bell's palsy.

To date, only one multicenter prospective clinical trial examining surgical decompression has been performed. Patients with complete facial nerve paralysis, greater than 90% degeneration on ENoG, and no evidence of intact voluntary motor units on EMG testing were candidates for surgical decompression within 2 weeks of the onset of paralysis. Patients who underwent decompression within 2 weeks of onset exhibited a 91% chance of a House-Brackmann grade I/II facial nerve function versus a 42% chance of obtaining a House-Brackmann grade I/II if treated with steroids only. Considerations against the use of surgical decompression include the risks associated with surgery and the fact that a majority of patients with Bell's palsy improve without surgical intervention.

For patients who elect to undergo facial nerve decompression, a middle cranial fossa approach is used to decompress the labyrinthine segment of the facial nerve (the site of pathology in Bell's palsy). This is performed from the fundus of the internal auditory canal to the meatal foramen and to the proximal tympanic segment. The meatal foramen is the entrance to the labyrinthine segment and represents the anatomically narrowest portion of the fallopian canal. Risks of surgical decompression include dizziness, CSF leaks, seizures, hearing loss, and stroke.

23.7 Rehabilitation and Follow-up

Facial rehabilitation exercises can be used early in the disease process to prevent synkinesis from occurring. Further, electrical nerve stimulation has been proposed as a method of accelerating recovery in patients with Bell's palsy by invoking muscle stimulation. For patients with incomplete eye closure, frequent follow-up is warranted to ensure that keratitis and corneal abrasions are not occurring. For patients in whom return of orbicularis oculi function is anticipated to take longer than 6 months, reversible surgical procedures (such as placement of an upper lid platinum or gold weight) may be performed to optimize corneal protection. In the event that a patient develops synkinesis several months after Bell's palsy, botulinum toxin injections may be performed to reduce hypertonicity and restore facial symmetry.

23.8 Questions

1. True or false? Bilateral facial paralysis is seen in 10% of those patients diagnosed with Bell's palsy.
2. What portion of the facial nerve is involved in the pathophysiology of Bell's palsy?
   a) Intracranial segment.
   b) Meatal segment.
   c) Labyrinthine segment.
   d) Tympanic segment.
   e) Mastoid segment.
3. What is the current recommended therapy for Bell's palsy?
   a) Antiviral monotherapy.
   b) Surgical decompression.
   c) Oral high-dose corticosteroids.
   d) Oral high-dose corticosteroids followed by surgical decompression.

Answers: 1. False 2. c 3. c

Suggested Readings

Baugh RF, Basura GJ, Ishii LE, et al. Clinical practice guideline: Bell's Palsy executive summary. Otolaryngol Head Neck Surg. 2013; 149 (5):656–663

Engström M, Berg T, Stjernquist-Desatnik A, et al. Prednisolone and valaciclovir in Bell's palsy: a randomised, double-blind, placebo-controlled, multicentre trial. Lancet Neurol. 2008; 7(11):993–1000

Gagyor I, Madhok VB, Daly F, et al. Antiviral treatment for Bell's palsy (idiopathic facial paralysis). Cochrane Database Syst Rev. 2015; 11(11):CD001869

Gantz BJ, Rubinstein JT, Gidley P, Woodworth GG. Surgical management of Bell's palsy. Laryngoscope. 1999; 109(8):1177–1188

Gilden DH. Clinical practice. Bell's Palsy. N Engl J Med. 2004; 351 (13):1323–1331

Samy RN, Gantz BJ. Surgery of the facial nerve. In: Glasscock ME, Gulya AJ, eds. Surgery of the Ear.. 5th ed. Hamilton, Ontario, Canada: BC Decker; 2003: 615–639

Sullivan FM, Swan IR, Donnan PT, et al. Early treatment with prednisolone or acyclovir in Bell's palsy. N Engl J Med. 2007; 357 (16):1598–1607

24 Iatrogenic Facial Palsy

Jeffrey J. Harmon and Ravi N. Samy

24.1 History

A 50-year-old woman presented to the operating room with a cholesterol granuloma within the mastoid and an associated right tympanic membrane perforation, chronic otorrhea, and hearing loss. She underwent right canal wall up tympanomastoidectomy with an extended facial recess. In the process of removing bone around the mastoid segment of the facial nerve there was concern about possible facial nerve injury intraoperatively due to stimulation of the nerve as recorded by the nerve monitor. The facial nerve was subsequently decompressed from the midtympanic segment to the midmastoid segment. The nerve was then stimulated in multiple locations to confirm that it was indeed anatomically intact and functional electrically. The patient was a House-Brackmann grade II/VI on the right side in the immediate postoperative period. This weakness resolved at the second follow-up appointment 2 months later.

24.2 Differential Diagnosis—Key Points

- *Epidemiology:* Iatrogenic facial nerve paralysis can be seen following a variety of surgical procedures. A recent single-center review of cases of iatrogenic facial nerve palsy between 2002 and 2012 (total of 1,810 patients) demonstrated that oral and maxillofacial procedures were the most common causes of iatrogenic facial nerve palsy, accounting for 40% of cases. Otologic surgery was the third most common cause with 17% of cases. A large percentage of these patients suffering from facial nerve injury had undergone revision otologic procedures. The case above is an example of iatrogenic facial nerve palsy during a revision otologic procedure. Many cases of iatrogenic facial nerve injury are minor and identified and corrected intraoperatively with little to no long-term postoperative sequelae. The overall rate of iatrogenic facial nerve palsy during otologic cases has been estimated to be less than 4%.
- *Anatomy:* During otologic surgery, the facial nerve is most likely to be damaged at the tympanic segment in transcanal approaches or at the mastoid segment in transmastoid approaches. The tympanic segment is more vulnerable to injury, as it is the most common site of dehiscence in the facial canal, in many cases due to congenital bony dehiscence. Cholesteatoma, granulation tissue, and hypertrophic mucosa can also cause dehiscence. The second most common site of injury is the mastoid segment of the facial nerve, especially at the location of the second genu, where the nerve changes from a horizontal to a vertical direction. Bony malformations or postoperative changes from previous surgeries also increase the risk of facial nerve damage. Finally, heat-induced neuropraxia (from the otologic drill) can cause such palsy.
- *Intraoperative facial nerve monitoring:* Intraoperative facial nerve monitoring has become the standard of care in neurotologic surgery for vestibular schwannoma. It is also beneficial for revision middle ear or mastoid cases, complex cases, and when residents or fellows are involved. Intraoperative nerve monitoring during primary and revision middle ear and mastoid surgeries has been shown to be cost-effective for both primary and revision cases. The facial nerve monitor cannot prevent injury but should be used as an aid to reduce the risk of injury. Knowledge of the temporal bone and facial nerve anatomy is paramount to prevent injury.
- *History:* Concerns in the immediate postoperative period include the effect of local anesthetic or packing. If the facial nerve injury was not identified intraoperatively, the mastoid dressing and packing should be immediately removed to see whether there is any improvement in the function of the facial nerve. It is possible that canal injections with lidocaine may contribute to facial nerve palsy. The effect of lidocaine may persist for several hours. Delayed onset facial weakness is more likely to return than weakness that occurred immediately after surgery. The longer the facial palsy has persisted, the less likely it is that facial nerve function will return to normal. It is important to ask the patient about ocular, nasal, and oral competence. Questions to ask relating to the eye include dryness, pain, or changes in vision. Ask about nasal obstruction, drooling, and dysarthria. Finally, it is important to ask questions about other neurologic deficits.
- *Physical exam:* Physical exam should evaluate each segment of the face. The position and

dynamic movement of the brows and eye closure should be assessed. The position of the nasal base and nasolabial fold should be assessed. Finally, the oral commissure should be evaluated for evidence of incomplete closure.

- *House-Brackmann scale:* Facial nerve function is graded on a scale from I to VI, with a higher grade indicating worse facial nerve function (Table 24.1). A key point to distinguish is the presence or absence of full eye closure. The patient in this case demonstrated a transient House-Brackmann grade II/VI on the right side.
- *Sunderland classification system:* It is important to note that the House-Brackmann scale is utilized for facial nerve injuries proximal to the pes anserinus. This classification system categorizes injuries based on the microanatomic damage done to the nerve. A level 1 injury represents no microanatomic disruption of the nerve (disruption of axoplasmic flow only). Level 2 indicates disruption of axons without damage to the endoneurium. Level 3 indicates damage to the endoneurium. Level 4 indicates damage to the endoneurium and perineurium. Level 5 indicates damage to the endoneurium, perineurium, and epineurium, or complete axonal disruption. Level 3 injury and above guarantees that synkinesis will occur. This classification is associated with the chances that functional recovery can occur. The higher the level the less likely nerve function is to return to a normal or acceptable level of function.
- *Differential diagnosis:* Bell's palsy is an alternative diagnosis when the cause of the

postoperative facial paralysis is not known and/or was not witnessed in the operating room. In fact, it is the most common cause of facial paralysis. It is thought to be related to the reactivation of a virus such as herpes simplex virus in the geniculate ganglion of the facial nerve. However, it could also be due to immunologic or vascular causes. This can occur postoperatively without physical damage to the nerve. See Chapter 23 for a more detailed description of Bell's palsy.
- *Disclosure:* Facial paralysis is a recognized complication in otologic surgery that can be devastating for the patient. This speaks to the importance of a frank and full discussion with the patient of the risk for facial palsy and the consequences of such an injury prior to surgery. In the event of an injury it is important to discuss the cause and prognosis of the injury. It is also important to formulate and offer options for managing the injury postoperatively. Finally, it is important to request assistance from a more senior colleague or have a patient referred to a regional or national expert to address the injury. Facial paralysis due to iatrogenic injury has the potential for adverse medicolegal consequences.

24.3 Test Interpretation

Magnetic resonance imaging (MRI) or computed tomography (CT) can often demonstrate the location of the facial nerve segment involved with the paralysis. An immediate intraoperative complete facial paralysis does not require electrophysiologic

Table 24.1 House-Brackmann grading scale

Grade	Resting function	Gross motor function
I	Normal facial function in all areas	
II	Normal symmetry and tone	Slight weakness noticeable on close inspection, moderate to good function of the forehead, complete closure of the eye with minimal effort, slight asymmetry of the mouth, very slight synkinesis
III	Normal symmetry and tone	Obvious but not disfiguring difference between two sides, slight to moderate movement of the forehead, complete eye closure with effort, slightly weak mouth movement with maximum effort, noticeable but not severe synkinesis
IV	Normal symmetry and tone	Obvious weakness and/or disfiguring asymmetry, no forehead movement, incomplete eye closure, asymmetric mouth movement with maximum effort
V	Asymmetry	Only barely perceptible motion, no forehead movement, incomplete eye closure, slight movement of the mouth
VI	Total paralysis, no movement	

or radiographic studies. Rather, the nerve should be explored immediately and repaired when possible. An immediate or delayed onset partial weakness should be followed similarly to a Bell's palsy.

Complete acute or delayed facial paralysis requires evaluation with electromyography (EMG) and electroneuronography (ENoG). EMG measures the response to a voluntary contraction. ENoG is an evoked EMG. ENoG should be performed > 3 days after the injury to allow wallerian degeneration to occur. Performing this test earlier could provide falsely reassuring results. The key result from ENoG is the percent degeneration measured. If greater than 90%, the chances of recovery of facial function are much lower. EMG is performed following ENoG to provide information regarding the voluntary function of the facial mimetic muscles. If the patient demonstrates myogenic fibrillation potentials and an absence of voluntary motor units, this indicates a poorer prognosis for recovery. A patient with polyphasic motor units demonstrates a regenerating nerve.

24.4 Diagnosis

Iatrogenic facial palsy

24.5 Medical Management

Management of the eye is extremely important, especially with a facial palsy resulting in incomplete eye closure. In fact, the most important issue with facial nerve palsy is eye care. Lubrication with eyedrops during the day and ointment moisturizers at night is most effective. The addition of eye taping or a moisture chamber assists in maintaining a lubricated eye. Finally, an ophthalmology consultation is indicated if there is any concern about vision loss or corneal damage.

In delayed onset facial palsy, steroids are recommended to reduce edema. The regimen for steroid treatment is high-dose prednisone (1 mg/kg) for approximately 1 week as well as a histamine blocker or proton pump inhibitor to prevent gastric ulceration. In the event of suspected Bell's palsy, an antiviral medication such as valacyclovir can be added. The patient should also be monitored with electrophysiologic studies serially if there is no improvement in clinical function.

24.6 Surgical Management

It is important to determine the extent of the facial nerve injury. Damage should be addressed as soon as the injury is recognized. For example, the patient should be taken back to the operating room immediately for exploration of the facial nerve if there is total palsy that is not due to local anesthetic. In the case above, the damage was identified intraoperatively and addressed immediately.

If a return trip to the operative suite is needed, the patient should have a bone-line audiogram performed before surgery to confirm the level of the sensorineural hearing.

If the nerve appears only edematous and hyperemic but still intact, it should be decompressed along its course. If disruption of the nerve is less than 50% in cross-sectional area, the nerve requires decompression alone. In the event that facial nerve function has degraded to less than 10% on ENoG in the first 2 weeks following the injury, then decompression of the facial nerve may be warranted.

Although controversial, disruption of greater than 50% of the nerve should be reanastomosed. This decision also depends on the facial nerve function and whether there is total paralysis or not. The nerve ends are freshened and reapproximated and decompressed. The key to reanastomosis is a tension-free anastomosis. The great auricular and sural nerves can be used as an interposition graft if additional length is needed. The mastoid and tympanic segments should be dissected out and exposed. A middle cranial fossa approach may be warranted to expose the geniculate ganglion region of the nerve. If the patient has profound hearing loss, a translabyrinthine approach would provide excellent exposure of the nerve. It is important to communicate to the patient that if reexploration is required to identify and repair the nerve, in the event of a facial nerve transection, the best outcome possible is restoration of movement to a House-Brackmann III.

24.7 Rehabilitation and Follow-up

After the initial treatment and evaluation, long-term follow-up examinations every 2 to 4 months are appropriate. Facial muscle physical therapy for synkinesis is important, and patients can be referred to a physical therapist for these treatments. There are multiple procedures available to improve function and cosmesis of the face after facial nerve palsy if the patient's facial nerve function does not fully recover. Facial reanimation is discussed in detail in Chapter 25.

24.8 Questions

1. On examination, a patient demonstrates normal facial symmetry and tone at rest with incomplete eye closure. Facial nerve function would be classified as which of the following on the House-Brackmann scale?
   a) Grade II.
   b) Grade III.
   c) Grade IV.
   d) Grade V.

2. A healthy 25-year-old patient awakens in the recovery room following an uncomplicated right tympanoplasty for a tympanic membrane perforation. His facial nerve function is noted to be House-Brackmann II on the right. The next step in management should be
   a) Obtain magnetic resonance imaging (MRI) immediately.
   b) Reexploration of the surgical site with facial nerve reanastomosis as indicated.
   c) High-dose prednisone and valacyclovir.
   d) Reassess facial nerve function in 1 to 2 hours to allow time for the lidocaine injection to wear off.

3. A facial nerve is injured intraoperatively. The endoneurium is disrupted. Which of the following is true?
   a) This is a Sunderland level 3 injury and synkinesis is likely to occur.
   b) This is a Sunderland level 3 injury and synkinesis is unlikely to occur.
   c) This is a Sunderland level 2 injury and synkinesis is likely to occur.
   d) This is a Sunderland level 2 injury and synkinesis is unlikely to occur.

Answers: 1. c 2. d 3. a

Suggested Readings

Danner CJ. Facial nerve paralysis. Otolaryngol Clin North Am. 2008; 41(3):619–632, x

Grosheva M, Wittekindt C, Guntinas-Lichius O. Prognostic value of electroneurography and electromyography in facial palsy. Laryngoscope. 2008; 118(3):394–397

Hadlock T. Evaluation and management of the patient with postoperative facial paralysis. Arch Otolaryngol Head Neck Surg. 2012; 138(5):505–508

Harner SG, Leonetti JP. Iatrogenic facial paralysis prevention. Ear Nose Throat J. 1996; 75(11):715–, 718–719

Hohman MH, Bhama PK, Hadlock TA. Epidemiology of iatrogenic facial nerve injury: a decade of experience. Laryngoscope. 2014; 124(1):260–265

Hohman MH, Hadlock TA. Etiology, diagnosis, and management of facial palsy: 2000 patients at a facial nerve center. Laryngoscope. 2014; 124(7):E283–E293

House JW, Brackmann DE. Facial nerve grading system. Otolaryngol Head Neck Surg. 1985; 93(2):146–147

Wilson L, Lin E, Lalwani A. Cost-effectiveness of intraoperative facial nerve monitoring in middle ear or mastoid surgery. Laryngoscope. 2003; 113(10):1736–1745

25 Facial Reanimation

Jamie L. Welshhans and Ryan M. Collar

25.1 History

A 65-year-old woman presented to your clinic after undergoing a left acoustic neuroma resection 10 years ago. She had complete facial paralysis since the surgery and was under the impression that there was nothing that could be done for her. She was referred to you after her primary care provider pointed out that you could help her facial asymmetry. She complained of the asymmetry at rest (▶ Fig. 25.1) and also of losing some liquids out of the left side of her mouth when she drank. She had been taping her eye shut at night and using drops and had no exposure keratitis or corneal abrasions.

She denied significant medical problems. She did not smoke or drink alcohol. Physical examination revealed a well-nourished, well-developed white woman; a facial photo is shown in ▶ Fig. 25.1. She had good Bell's phenomena with intact extraocular movements. Her pupils were equal and reactive to light and accommodation, and her sclera was without exposure keratopathy. Head and neck examination revealed a well-healed craniotomy incision with House-Brackmann (HB) VI/VI on the left side. She had a ptotic eyebrow,

paralytic lagophthalmos, lack of tone on her lower face, and drooping of her lateral commissure. Her other cranial nerves (CNs) were fully intact, and the remainder of her head and neck examination was unremarkable.

25.2 Differential Diagnosis—Key Points

Facial nerve paralysis can result from trauma, infection, or neoplasm, or it can be idiopathic (Bell's palsy). When patients present for reanimation services, the diagnosis is typically already apparent, but nonetheless, one should always confirm diagnosis with relevant patient history. In terms of differential diagnosis as it pertains to facial reanimation specifically, the clinician should attempt to distinguish the facial paralysis as complete or incomplete, and reversible or irreversible, as these attributes will drive treatment decision making.

Degree of paralysis (i.e., complete versus incomplete): An important system for categorizing degree of paralysis is the House-Brackmann grading system (▶ Table 25.1). HB VI/VI is a complete paralysis, whereas III/VI is incomplete paralysis with full eye closure. An alternative instrument is the Sunnybrook facial grading scale that takes into account function and symmetry by facial level and also incorporates synkinetic motion to arrive at an

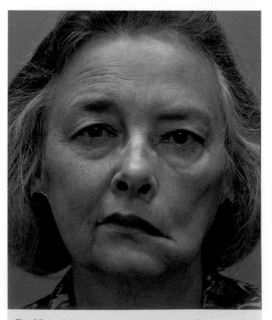

Fig. 25.1 Prior to any operative intervention.

Table 25.1 The House-Brackmann grading system for facial nerve paralysis

House-Brackmann Grade	Description
I	Normal facial function
II	Slight weakness, noticeable only on close inspection
III	Noticeable difference and weakness, complete eye closure, synkinesis
IV	Obvious weakness, normal symmetry at rest, incomplete eye closure
V	Severe weakness, barely perceptible motion, asymmetry at rest
VI	No movement

index for severity of the condition. More invasive procedures for reanimation are typically reserved for complete or near-complete facial paralysis.

Reversibility (i.e., irreversible versus reversible): If new axonal input into the existing mimetic muscles is established, reversible paralysis will improve whereas irreversible paralysis will not. This is a function of the duration of paralysis. Generally speaking, paralysis that is less than 12 to 18 months old may be rehabilitated with new axonal input, whereas long-standing paralysis, such as in this patient, cannot be rehabilitated with new axonal input due to muscle atrophy. This differentiation drives management decision making, specifically, whether nerve transfer procedures can provide benefit, or whether tendon transfers or muscle transplants are required to replace atrophic mimetic musculature to drive motion.

Of immediate importance in the differential diagnosis of patients seeking reanimation services is the status of the eye. Exposure-related keratopathy secondary to paralytic ectropion or lagophthalmos should be immediately identified and managed. Snap and distraction testing should be completed, and if there is concern for corneal ulcer, referral for appropriate ophthalmologic testing (e.g., slit lamp testing with fluorescein) should be completed prior to any intervention.

25.3 Test Interpretation

For patients with complete paralysis after acoustic neuroma surgery, one should establish the likelihood of nerve recovery using well-timed electromyography (EMG) testing. If there is no volitional activity or regeneration potentials present on EMG in the setting of persistent HB VI status approximately 6 months after acoustic neuroma resection, one might consider early intervention with nerve transfer to provide axonal input to mimetic musculature prior to atrophy. Outcomes data have demonstrated poor recovery (i.e., HB V or VI) in this patient group with no intervention, hence leading the clinician to act while the paralysis remains "reversible." In a case such as this, given the 10-year horizon since surgery and persistent HB VI status present since immediately after surgery, EMG generally does not provide actionable information.

Magnetic resonance imaging (MRI) with and without gadolinium is valuable for patients with persistent idiopathic facial paralysis or those patients with new onset paralysis in the setting of known, previously treated neoplasm to rule out new or recurrent tumor. In this case, MRI was obtained and did not show recurrence.

25.4 Diagnosis

Irreversible, complete facial paralysis secondary to acoustic neuroma resection

25.5 Medical Management

The first step in medical management for facial paralysis is eye care. Eye protective measures include an eye ointment at night, followed by taping the eye shut and nonpreservative eyedrops every 2 to 3 hours during the day. Eye patch chamber shields with an elastic strap add comfort to the affected dry eye. Sunglasses that curve around the temples or with side protectors are helpful when it is windy outside.

In addition to eye care, medical management is critical to establish improved symmetry and relief of synkinesis through targeted chemodenervation with botulinum toxin A. Contralateral, normally functioning facial muscles may be targeted with botulinum toxin A to enhance symmetry. For synkinesis, the ipsilateral, involved side may be dramatically improved through careful chemodenervation, especially the orbicularis oculi and lip depressors (which may unlock excursion potential) and the platysma that often causes debilitating neck tightness.

25.6 Surgical Management

Surgical management of facial paralysis is tailored to match the specific goals of the patient. Goals of surgery include eye protection with complete spontaneous blink, resting facial symmetry, volitional smile, nasal valve competency, oral competency, and facial beauty.

As noted above, facial paralysis management is based on the reversibility and degree of paralysis. In the setting of complete paralysis, the timing for surgical intervention is critical. In general the time periods can be classified as *immediate* (0 to 3 weeks), *delayed* (3 weeks to 18 months), and *late* (over 18 months). Procedures that involve nerve-to-nerve reattachment (e.g., nerve transfers) are most successful if performed within 18 months of injury. This is because after prolonged denervation muscular atrophy has likely occurred, preventing new axons from generating action potentials that drive meaningful muscle contraction. In the circumstance of late paralysis, as in the index case, other surgical techniques, such as tendon transfers or muscle transplants, are required for facial movement.

25.6.1 Reversible Complete Paralysis

The optimal method to repair a transected facial nerve is to directly connect its severed ends as soon as possible. Doing so within 3 days is advantageous in that identifying the distal end of the nerve remains possible via electrical stimulation. After neurorrhaphy is complete, axons regenerate along the distal segment at 1 to 3 mm each day. Because the cell body of the facial nerve is located at the brainstem, the more proximal the facial nerve injury, the more time is needed for the regenerating nerve to reinnervate its facial musculature.

If a significant distance between severed nerve ends exists (i.e., resulting from nerve resection from tumor removal or trauma), this gap is bridged with nerve grafts (e.g., the greater auricular nerve or sural nerve).

In scenarios in which the facial nerve cannot be surgically repaired directly or with cable grafts due to the location of the injury (e.g., facial nerve transection near the brainstem from an intracranial injury or tumor), or in the situation of a persistent facial palsy after acoustic neuroma resection in which there is no injury to repair, alternate motor cranial nerves can be recruited through nerve transfer procedures to deliver new axons along the distal facial nerve to still reversible facial mimetic musculature. The hypoglossal nerve may be utilized in an end-to-side configuration preferably distal to the ansa cervicalis with the distal main trunk, or the masseteric nerve may be employed in an end-to-end fashion to either the lower division or main trunk. Both of these maneuvers will create improved facial tone and symmetry, and typically generate volitional nonspontaneous smile. Patients learn to smile either through pushing the tongue against their incisors in the case of the 12–7 transfer or via contracting the masseter with clenching the jaw in the case of the 5–7 transfer. Nerve transfers can be performed alone or in concert with cross-facial nerve grafting. When performed together, the transfers have been coined "babysitter" procedures in that they deliver axons to the mimetic muscles to maintain viability while cross-facial nerves route axons from the contralateral facial nerve that are eventually routed through the involved ipsilateral facial nerve in a second procedure 6 to 12 months later in either an end-to-end or end-to-side fashion. This staged approach may allow production of a smile that is both volitional and spontaneous in that it is partially incited by the contralateral facial nerve, rather than CN V or XII.

25.6.2 Irreversible Complete Paralysis

Eighteen to 24 months after the onset of facial paralysis, denervation atrophy of the facial musculature has likely occurred. In this patient's case it had been 10 years since the initial injury, and hence she had complete irreversible paralysis.

In a situation such as this, additional axonal input through the distal nerve is of no value, and hence new muscle must be supplied for volitional movement, and the temporalis tendon transfer (T3) and the gracilis free flap are the most commonly employed approaches. For patients with functioning temporalis musculature seeking immediate improvement and single-surgery plans, the T3 is an optimal approach. By transferring the temporalis insertion at the medial coronoid process to the modiolus, meaningful volitional yet nonspontaneous (i.e., must be elicited with bite) excursion can be restored. While the gracilis free flap may offer more excursion, this is challenging to objectify given limited continuity of outcomes measure. The procedure may be performed as a single stage using the masseteric nerve, or in a two-staged approach using cross-facial nerve grafting.

Static sling procedures are an additional option to support the oral commissure and are ideal in patients who are medically deconditioned or who have contraindications to the T3 (e.g., CN V palsy) or the gracilis free flap.

25.6.3 Restoring Eyelid Closure and Brow

A patient with facial nerve paralysis is frequently unable to close the eyelids because of paralysis of the orbicularis oculi muscle. In addition, lower eyelid sagging (paralytic ectropion) is often apparent because of the lack of muscular tone of the lower eyelid. With the absence of surface lubrication, these conditions make the cornea very vulnerable to exposure keratitis.

Surgical management for the eyelid includes the placement of gold weight or platinum chain. By having a tailored weight inserted within the upper eyelid, a patient is able to open and close the eyes spontaneously while being upright. Lower lid procedures are designed to position the lower lid at the inferior limbus and include lateral tarsal strip, lateral transorbital canthopexy, medial canthopexy, spacer grafts, and midface lifts. Browlifting is often performed in conjunction with these procedures to improve symmetry and in some cases eliminate temporal hooding that may cause lateral visual field obstruction.

25.7 Rehabilitation and Follow-up

Ultimately this patient had the following procedures: temporalis tendon transfer, facelift, browlift, and platinum chain. Rehabilitation with facial exercises can be beneficial in strengthening and retraining the facial muscle with a physical therapist, speech pathologist, or occupational therapist that is interested in treating patients with facial paralysis.

25.8 Questions

1. What is the House-Brackmann (HB) score of a patient with obvious generalized weakness, complete eye closure, non-disfiguring synkinesis, and asymmetric mouth movement with maximal effort?
   a) II.
   b) III.
   c) IV.
   d) V.
   e) VI.
2. A 40-year-old woman has complete transection of her facial nerve from a transverse temporal bone fracture 2 years ago. What test would be most helpful to determine the best treatment for facial reanimation?

   a) Temporal bone computed tomography scan with contrast.
   b) Electroneuronography.
   c) Electromyography (EMG).
   d) Hilger stimulation test.
   e) Schirmer test.
3. A 55-year-old woman has had complete facial paralysis for 2 years and would like movement of her lower face. EMG shows electrical silence. What would be the best treatment for facial reanimation?
   a) Temporalis muscle sling.
   b) Gracilis free flap.
   c) Hypoglossal nerve transposition to facial nerve.
   d) Facial sling with tensor fascia lata.
   e) Greater auricular cable nerve graft.

Answers: 1. b 2. c 3. b

Suggested Readings

Bascom DA, Schaitkin BM, May M, Klein S. Facial nerve repair: a retrospective review. Facial Plast Surg. 2000; 16(4):309–313

Collar RM, Byrne PJ, Boahene KD. The subzygomatic triangle: rapid, minimally invasive identification of the masseteric nerve for facial reanimation. Plast Reconstr Surg. 2013; 132(1):183–188

Hadlock TA, Greenfield LJ, Wernick-Robinson M, Cheney ML. Multimodality approach to management of the paralyzed face. Laryngoscope. 2006; 116(8):1385–1389

Harris BN, Tollefson TT. Facial reanimation: evolving from static procedures to free tissue transfer in head and neck surgery. Curr Opin Otolaryngol Head Neck Surg. 2015; 23(5):399–406

May M, Schaitkin BM. The Facial Nerve. 2nd ed. New York, NY: Thieme; 2000

Tate JR, Tollefson TT. Advances in facial reanimation. Curr Opin Otolaryngol Head Neck Surg. 2006; 14(4):242–248

Part V

The Oral Cavity and Pharynx

V

26 Benign Cystic Neck Mass

Thomas K. Hamilton and Alfred M. Sassler

26.1 History

A 30-year-old, otherwise healthy man presented with a 2-month history of an enlarging, right-sided, lateral neck mass in the midneck region. The mass was located along the anterior border of the sternocleidomastoid (SCM) and approximately 1 cm inferior to the angle of the mandible. The neck mass fluctuated in size and was minimally tender. It was at least 2 cm in size. No other neck masses or thyroid nodules were palpable.

He denied fevers, chills, and any recent illnesses or sick contacts. He had no dysphagia, odynophagia, shortness of breath, or limitations in neck motion. He denied alcohol, tobacco, and drug use; took no medications; and had no other medical problems. There was no known family history of malignancy. The remainder of the head and neck exam was unremarkable.

26.2 Differential Diagnosis—Key Points

- *General considerations:* The differential for a cystic neck mass will differ based on the age of the patient and the location of the lesion. Congenital neck masses are more common in children and are often further subdivided into lateral and midline masses. Acquired lesions are less age and location specific and can be either benign or malignant.
- *Branchial cleft anomaly:* A branchial cleft anomaly (BCA) occurs when there is an error during the embryologic development of the head and neck. BCAs are classified into four types depending on the embryologic cleft from which they arise, with second BCAs being the most common by a significant margin (~ 70%). While a detailed description of the different types of BCA is outside the scope of this chapter, each type has a characteristic anatomic location of both the cyst itself and its associated tract. BCAs present as *lateral* cystic head/neck masses that are generally otherwise asymptomatic; however, they can become secondarily infected, leading to pain, drainage, and sometimes abscess formation. Although they are congenital masses, BCAs do not always present in childhood; in fact, they oftentimes will not present until the third or

fourth decade. Overall, the age, presentation, mass location, and imaging findings in our patient's case would be most consistent with a noninfected second BCA.
- *Thyroglossal duct cyst:* During development, the thyroid descends from the foramen cecum at the base of the tongue to its normal position in the neck. A thyroglossal duct cyst (TGDC), the most common congenital neck cyst in children, can arise when there is a persistent remnant of this tract along which the developing thyroid travels. A TGDC will generally present as an asymptomatic **midline** cystic neck mass anywhere from the level of the hyoid to the clavicles and will elevate with deglutition and/or tongue protrusion. Both TGDCs and BCAs can become secondarily infected, in which case they can present in a febrile patient with tenderness to palpation, overlying erythema, and potentially purulent drainage. The lateral location of this patient's neck mass made TGDC a less likely diagnosis in this case.
- *Dermoid cyst:* Dermoids can arise either post-traumatically or developmentally as the result of squamous debris entrapment in deeper tissue. In the neck, they are generally nontender, mobile, and found in the midline but **above** the hyoid bone, which can help differentiate them from a TGDC.
- *Cervical lymphadenitis:* It can be difficult to determine whether a neck mass is cystic or solid based on physical exam alone. Although cervical lymphadenitis is characterized by solid rather than cystic masses, because it is so common, it should be considered as a possibility when evaluating any neck mass. Lymphadenitis can present laterally or medially and may therefore be initially confused with a BCA or TGDC, respectively. In contrast to patients with a noninfected congenital mass, however, patients with lymphadenitis will often have a rapid appearance of **multiple** tender masses in characteristic nodal distributions, have symptoms of systemic illness (fevers, chills), and have a history of sick contact exposure and may, depending on the etiology, respond to antibiotics.
- *Other cystic masses:* Other, less common cystic neck masses include laryngocele, plunging ranula, teratoma, thymic cyst, benign skin cyst, and certain vascular neoplasms.

26.3 Test Interpretation

- *Laboratory testing:* If asymptomatic, as in this particular case, no laboratory testing is initially needed. If secondary infection is suspected, baseline complete blood count (CBC) and renal panel may be useful, as well as cultures if there is any purulent drainage.
- *Ultrasound:* Due to lack of ionizing radiation exposure, easy access to the area of interest, and low cost, ultrasound is the initial imaging modality of choice for most neck masses. Ultrasound can be used to determine if the lesion is cystic, solid, or mixed, which can help guide the diagnosis and the next steps in management. BCAs classically appear as thin-walled, lateral, cystic lesions with variable echogenicity whose location will depend on the type of BCA. Second BCAs, as in this case, are most commonly in the lateral midneck, along the anterior border of the SCM. Surrounding inflammatory change may be present if the cyst is secondarily infected.
- CT: *Computed tomography:* Computed tomography (CT) may also be obtained for surgical planning or if there is a concern for something more insidious. BCAs will appear on CT as a homogeneously attenuating lateral lesion with thin walls (▶ Fig. 26.1 &, ▶ Fig. 26.2). The "notch sign," long considered to be pathognomonic for the diagnosis, occurs when the cyst wall extends between the internal and external carotid arteries just above the carotid bifurcation.

26.4 Diagnosis

Second branchial cleft cyst

26.5 Medical Management

The definitive management of a BCA is surgical; however, antecedent medical therapy may be necessary if there is an infection of the cyst. Resection of an infected cyst may increase the chance of recurrence. Incision and drainage is rarely needed and should be reserved for cases that do not respond to antibiotics, as the procedure can cause scarring and ultimately make definitive surgical management more difficult. An empiric antibiotic regimen should be started to cover *Staphylococcus aureus* and respiratory tract anaerobes, such as clindamycin. Once the infection has resolved, the patient should be scheduled for definitive surgical management.

26.6 Surgical Management

Surgery is the mainstay of treatment for symptomatic second BCAs, as they are a nidus for recurrent infections. Care must be taken during the resection to remove not only the cyst, but also the entirety of the cyst tract; otherwise, recurrence will be much more likely. The tract of a second BCA runs between the external and internal carotid arteries, superior to the hypoglossal and glossopharyngeal nerves, and ends in the tonsillar

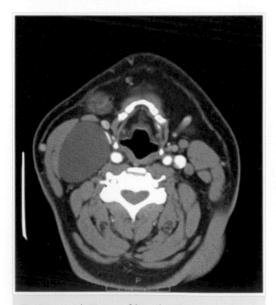

Fig. 26.1 Axial CT scan of lateral neck mass.

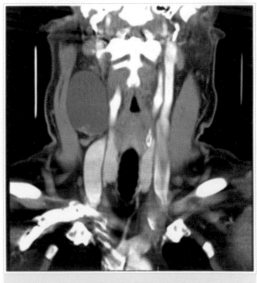

Fig. 26.2 Coronal CT scan of lateral neck mass.

fossa. The resection should include a rim of tissue around the fistulous tract if present, careful dissection of the tract with a cuff of normal tissue, and removal of any cystic structures and the tract up to the tonsillar fossa mucosa. Use of a lacrimal probe throughout the dissection can be helpful to determine the direction of the tract. If the lesion is breached during the course of the dissection, regardless of whether it is currently infected, some authors advocate for prophylactic antibiotics postoperatively. Complications include wound infection, recurrence, and damage to adjacent structures.

26.7 Rehabilitation and Follow-up

The primary complication of not operating on a BCA is recurrent infection. Complications associated with the cyst excision procedure include cyst recurrence, damage to nearby structures, and wound infections. Infections will generally develop between 5 and 7 days after the operation, with erythema, pain, and drainage from the incision. Most recurrences will occur near the initial site, but in theory they can appear anywhere along the original tract. As mentioned previously, if the lesion wall was breached during the course of the dissection, postoperative antibiotics may be helpful to decrease the chance of a wound infection.

26.8 Questions

1. All of the following are possible lateral cystic head/neck masses except
   a) Cystic metastasis.
   b) Thyroglossal duct cyst (TGDC).
   c) First branchial cleft anomaly (BCA).
   d) Dermoid cyst.
2. What are two possible consequences of not surgically removing a BCA?
   a) Hyperthyroidism.
   b) Malignant transformation.
   c) Airway compromise due to mass effect.
   d) Recurrent infections.
3. The most appropriate surgical approach to BCA is
   a) Injection of ethanol to sclerose the cyst.
   b) Excision of the cyst and tract with a cuff of surrounding tissue.
   c) Removal of just the cyst itself.
   d) Excision of the cyst and tract with careful skeletonization.

Answers: 1. b 2. c,d 3. b

Suggested Readings

Koch BL. Cystic malformations of the neck in children. Pediatr Radiol. 2005; 35(5):463–477

Graney DO, Sie KCY. Developmental anatomy. In: Cummings CW, Flint PW, Harker LA, et al., eds. Cummings Otolaryngology Head & Neck Surgery. 4th ed. Philadelphia, PA: Elsevier Mosby; 2005: 3938–3951

Prosser JD, Myer CM, III. Branchial cleft anomalies and thymic cysts. Otolaryngol Clin North Am. 2015, 48(1):1–14

Myer CM III. Congenital neck masses. In: Shumrick Da, Gluckman JL, Myerhoff WL, eds. Otolaryngology. Philadelphia, PA: WB Saunders; 1991:2535–2543

27 Odontogenic Tumors

Alice L. Tang and Keith M. Wilson

27.1 History

A 52-year-old white woman presented to a local dentist when she noticed that her lower jaw had been slowly growing over the last year. She complained of some pain in her lower jaw but mostly was bothered by the sensation that her "bite was off." This discomfort was beginning to cause her to have chewing problems. She was otherwise healthy and had no contributing past medical history. She had no history of smoking, drinking, or previous exposure to radiotherapy.

On physical examination, there was an obvious jaw deformity caused by a firm anterior mandibular mass that was approximately 3 cm × 4 cm in size. Several of her mandibular teeth from tooth 25 to 27 appeared to be loose. There was some dull pain to palpation. The overlying mucosa was intact with normal sensation. Sensation of the lower lip was normal. There was no bruit heard on auscultation of the jaw. The remainder of the head and neck examination was within normal limits.

27.2 Differential Diagnosis—Key Points

- Odontogenic cysts and tumors are a diverse group of lesions, and several classification schemes have been made based on histologic subtypes and clinical behavior. Many of the odontogenic cysts and tumors have similar clinical presentations, and treatment should be tailored to the unique features of the specific lesion based on histopathologic diagnosis.
- Odontogenic tumors are diverse. They arise from epithelial and/or mesenchymal cells. Slow-growing expanding jaw lesions should raise suspicion for odontogenic tumors. The clinical presentation of odontogenic tumors depends, to a certain extent, on the dimensions of the lesion. A small lesion without symptoms will frequently be missed on routine oral examination. However, evaluation of a devitalized or infected tooth will help diagnose smaller lesions. If large, patients will frequently present with obvious deformity, malocclusion, pain, and tooth displacement. Sensory nerve dysfunction is rare.
- Inflammatory and developmental odontogenic cysts include but are not limited to periapical, dentigerous, globulomaxillary, and nasopalatine cysts. The most common is the periapical cyst; the dentigerous cyst, often associated with the crown of an unerupted molar, could give rise to tumors such as ameloblastoma, mucoepidermoid carcinoma, or squamous cell carcinoma (although rare). Keratocystic odontogenic tumor (KCOT, also known as odontogenic keratocyst) is considered a multicystic benign neoplasm that can grow rapidly and be aggressive. Multiple keratocysts with recurrence may occur with basal cell nevus syndrome (BCNS). The diagnosis of BCNS must be entertained in patients with findings of bifid ribs, hypertelorism, widened nasal dorsum, multiple mandibular KCOTs, and early development of basal cell carcinomas of the face and trunk. It is an autosomal dominant disease with high penetration.
- True odontogenic tumors include ameloblastoma, calcifying epithelial odontogenic tumor (Pindborg's tumor), squamous odontogenic tumor, calcifying odontogenic tumor (Gorlin's cyst), adenomatoid odontogenic tumor, odontogenic myxoma, and odontoma. Other rarer tumors occur and are not mentioned here.
- Ameloblastoma is considered the most primitive of the odontogenic tumors and can arise from any of the remnants of tooth development. It is the most common odontogenic neoplasm and is recognized in two main categories: solid/multicystic variant and unicystic variant. When presenting early and as a small lesion, multicystic ameloblastoma can be confused with KCOTs on imaging, as it can appear as a nonspecific ondontogenic radiolucency. However, with time and sufficient growth, ameloblastomas will clinically declare themselves with significant jaw swelling, which is not typical of keratocysts. Usually in the fourth or fifth decade, the slow growth of the lesion forms a new layer of subperiosteum with a cortical outline that is seen on imaging and can be interpreted as an ameloblastoma.
- Vascular malformations (VMs) of the mandible may manifest as slow-growing masses. These lesions are more common in children and are often associated with other physical findings. It is not uncommon for the VM to extend to the tongue with apparent lingual vein distention. A bruit heard on auscultation requires further evaluation with magnetic resonance imaging, magnetic resonance angiography, or

angiography. If embolization is chosen as definitive treatment or before surgical excision, angiography is the best study.

- Metastatic tumor from breast carcinoma, renal cell carcinoma, and other primaries, as well as contiguous involvement of oral cavity and oropharyngeal squamous cell carcinoma, may occur in the jaws. A history of concurrent malignancy may suggest this in the differential diagnosis.

27.3 Test Interpretation

- *Panoramic radiograph:* The most useful radiologic evaluation of the maxilla and mandible is a panoramic radiograph. It can assist with the differential diagnosis of jaw cysts and tumors; however, definitive diagnosis is made on biopsy and histopathologic examination. Slow-growing cysts or benign tumors will have thin, sclerotic bony walls that are well defined. It can cause blunting of tooth roots and displacement of teeth or the inferior alveolar nerve. An aggressive, fast-growing, or malignant lesion will show lysis and resorption of surrounding bone, without tooth displacement. It also has ill-defined margins.
- *Computed tomography (CT) scanning:* CT is indicated in evaluating large lesions with significant anatomy distortion. Also, it is important to identify cortex erosion, especially when malignancy is suspected. CT evaluation with thin cuts through the maxilla and mandible is routine for preexcision and reconstruction of advanced cases. CT is frequently necessary to evaluate the maxillary lesions fully.
- *Incisional biopsy:* Solid tissue biopsy is required to confirm diagnosis for all odontogenic tumors. A large solid biopsy is desirable to include tissue that avoids sampling just simple cystic lining, which will not provide enough information for diagnosis.

- *Panoramic radiograph:* This patient's panoramic radiograph showed a midline lesion with mixed radiolucent and radiopaque lesion most consistent with desmoplastic ameloblastoma. The film also showed swelling of the bone and tooth displacement. Desmoplastic ameloblastomas are most common in the maxilla and anterior portion of the mandible. The classic descriptions of more common histologic variants of a large ameloblastoma (i.e., multicystic/solid) include a "soap bubble" or "honeycomb" appearance. With slow-growing lesions, there can also be evidence of adjacent teeth showing resorption.
  The work-up for the index patient included a panoramic radiograph and CT of the face with three-dimensional reconfiguration (▶ Fig. 27.1) for surgical planning and an incisional biopsy.
- *CT scan:* On CT, there was a heterogeneous expansile mass centered in the left parasymphyseal mandible, extending across midline to the right parasymphyseal region. There were permeative changes centrally with large expansile lucent spaces on the right parasymphyseal region (▶ Fig. 27.1). The mass on CT measured 4.8 cm × 2.8 cm and spanned the entire height of the mandible. There was osteolysis of the anterior overlying mandibular cortex. From the CT imaging alone, the differential diagnosis of this aggressive-appearing mandible lesion included desmoplastic ameloblastoma, odontogenic myxoma, or osseous hemangioma.
- *Biopsy:* The patient was taken to the operating suite, where an incisional biopsy was performed. On high-powered microscopy, the tumor demonstrated dense fibrous stroma with nests of cells in a follicular pattern. Many cells had squamous metaplasia and contained ghost cells. There was bone that was forming within the stroma, which can be misleading on imaging. This biopsy was consistent with desmoplastic ameloblastoma. There were no overt malignant features identified. Solid/multicystic variant

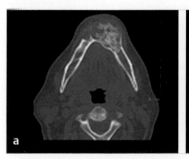 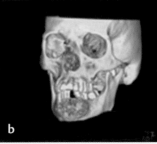

Fig. 27.1 (a,b) Computed tomography of maxilla and mandible preoperatively with three-dimensional reconstruction showing a large expansile lesion of the anterior body of the mandible.

ameloblastomas, which are more common than the desmoplastic variant, have histologic features predominated by two main cell type patterns: peripheral basal cells that are elongated and a multilayered epithelium with few intercellular contacts. The basal cells are palisaded and resemble ameloblasts (for which the tumor is named).

27.4 Diagnosis

Desmoplastic ameloblastoma of the anterior mandible

27.5 Medical Management

Ameloblastomas are relatively resistant to chemotherapy and radiation therapy. Thus there is no role for medical management of this medical problem.

27.6 Surgical Management

Surgical excision is the treatment of choice for ameloblastomas. If left untreated, most ameloblastomas will expand slowly and cause local destruction by infiltrating into adjacent soft tissue. Opinions in the literature vary regarding the appropriate treatment of ameloblastoma. Although it is a benign disease, when inadequately treated with simple enucleation or curettage, ameloblastoma will recur in up to 50% of cases. Thus, simple enucleation for ameloblastomas is not the treatment of choice. Ameloblastomas located near the orbit and cranial base are more difficult to treat and manage, given the proximity to vital structures.

In small and moderately sized tumors on the mandible, a marginal mandibulectomy is performed, leaving a rim of inferior mandible intact. Large, destructive lesions with multiple loculations and obvious bony destruction of the cortices require segmental mandibulectomy for complete removal. One- to 1.5-cm bony margins and one uninvolved overlying anatomic barrier margin are advocated. Ameloblastomas tend to infiltrate into the cancellous bone, and because of this, resections with negative margins will substantially decrease the recurrence rate as compared to enucleation or curettage. Reconstruction after segmental mandibulectomy is best performed with a free tissue transfer. The most commonly used are free fibula and free scapula flaps. The role for radiotherapy in the management of odontogenic

tumors is limited to malignancy, including carcinomas and sarcomas.

Following definitive diagnosis with tissue biopsy, this patient was treated with an anterior segmental mandibulectomy with fibula free flap reconstruction of her jaw. The tumor dimensions were 4.8 × 3.3 × 2.8 cm with margins that were free of neoplasm. On final pathology, the tumor had histopathologic patterns consistent with desmoplastic ameloblastoma.

27.7 Rehabilitation and Follow-up

Close follow-up after surgical treatment of ameloblastoma is required, as recurrence can occur in 10 to 15% of patients with negative margins. Malignant transformation may develop in the recurrence and, although rare, requires extensive revision surgery for treatment. A 5-year follow-up is mandatory, but a 10-year follow-up is prudent.

27.8 Questions

1. Which of the following statements about ameloblastomas is correct?
   a) Enucleation or curettage is an option for medium-sized ameloblastomas.
   b) Ameloblastomas can recur despite having adequate 1-cm negative margins.
   c) The two main categories for ameloblastomas are desmoplastic and unicystic.
   d) Patients who receive radiation after surgical excision have less recurrence.
2. Which of the following is not a reasonable surgical option for ameloblastomas?
   a) Marginal mandibulectomy with preservation of a bony rim.
   b) Segmental mandibulectomy with an iliac crest bone graft.
   c) Removal of 1- to 1.5-cm soft tissue margins abutting the mandible only.
   d) Anterior maxillectomy with 1- to 1.5-cm bony margins around the tumor.
3. Small multicystic/solid ameloblastomas on panoramic radiograph can occasionally be confused with which of the following?
   a) Keratocystic odontogenic tumor.
   b) Odontoma.
   c) Giant Pinborg tumor (calcifying epithelial odontogenic tumor).

Answers: 1. c 2. c 3. a

Suggested Readings

Chung WL, Cox DP, Ochs MW. Odontogenic cysts, tumors, and related jaw lesions. In: Bailey BJ, Johnson JT, et al, eds. Head and Neck Surgery—Otolaryngology. 4th ed. Philadelphia, PA: Lippincott Williams & Wilkins; 2006: 2097-2114

Dunfee BL, Sakai O, Pistey R, Gohel A. Radiologic and pathologic characteristics of benign and malignant lesions of the mandible RSNA Annual Meeting, May 2006

Larsen PL. Odontogenic cysts and tumors. In: Cummings CW, Schuller DE, et al, eds. Otolaryngology—Head and Neck Surgery.. 4th ed. Philadelphia, PA: Elsevier Mosby; 2005:Chapter 93.

Sampson DE, Pogrel MA. Management of mandibular ameloblastoma: the clinical basis for a treatment algorithm. J Oral Maxillofac Surg. 1999; 57(9):1074–1077, discussion 1078–1079

28 Carotid Body Tumor

Brittany A. Leader and Yash J. Patil

28.1 History

A 52-year-old man with diabetes mellitus and hypertension presented to clinic with complaints of a lump in his neck. He had first noticed it 2 years ago and it had been slowly growing since that time. Recently he had developed hoarseness and dysphagia, which caused him to seek evaluation. He denied any history of smoking or unintentional weight loss.

On exam a smooth mass was appreciated in the left anterior neck at the level of the superior thyroid cartilage border. It was mobile laterally, but was fixed rostrocaudally. A bruit was auscultated over the mass. Neurologic exam showed his extraoccular movements were intact and he had no cranial nerve deficits.

A computed tomography (CT) scan of the neck was obtained for further evaluation, which revealed bilateral findings at the level of the carotid bifurcation as shown below (▶ Fig. 28.1).

28.2 Differential Diagnosis—Key Points

Carotid body tumors, also known as paragangliomas, are vascular neuroendocrine tumors, which arise at the carotid bifurcation and involve the carotid body chemoreceptors. While infrequently seen, they may have the ability to secrete catecholamines. The majority are sporadic, while approximately one-third are associated with an inherited syndrome, and the remainder are hyperplastic. The sporadic cases present more commonly in women from age 50 to 70 years old, with familial cases occurring in younger patients. The hyperplastic form occurs in patients with chronic hypoxia; therefore, patients with cyanotic heart disease, those with chronic obstructive pulmonary disease (COPD), and those living at high altitude are at increased risk. Of the carotid body tumors, about 5% are bilateral and 5 to 10% are malignant. Associated symptoms include hoarseness, dysphagia, shoulder drop, palpitations, diaphoresis, and Horner's syndrome.

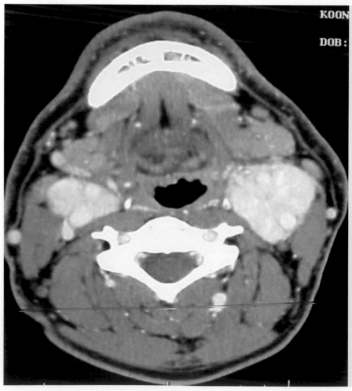

Fig. 28.1 CT of bilateral carotid body tumors.

The differential diagnosis for neck mass in an adult patient is broad and includes cysts, lipomas, salivary gland tumors, thyroid cancer, metastases, infection, and inflammatory lymphadenopathy. In order to narrow this differential, a thorough history and physical exam are essential. In this patient the duration of his symptoms made infection and inflammatory lymphadenopathy less likely. The lack of weight loss and other constitutional symptoms lowered suspicion for malignancy, and the palpable bruit made the mass more likely vascular in origin. Ultimately the diagnosis would be further clarified with diagnostic tests and imaging including ultrasound, which may be performed in clinic.

28.2.1 Test Interpretation

Carotid body tumors can be diagnosed by several imaging studies including ultrasound with color Doppler, CT of the head and neck (▶ Fig. 28.1), digital subtraction angiography, magnetic resonance imaging (MRI), and magnetic resonance angiography (MRA). The gold standard for diagnosing carotid body tumors is arteriography, which will demonstrate a pathognomonic tumor blush and vessels feeding the tumor (▶ Fig. 28.2).

On CT, carotid body tumors characteristically splay the external and internal carotid arteries at their bifurcation by a well-circumscribed mass that displaces the internal carotid artery posterolaterally. The carotid body tumor itself will be contrast enhanced because it is highly vascular. In contrast, a vagal paraganglioma will displace both the internal and external carotid arteries anteriorly and they are associated with erosion and widening of the jugular foramen.

On a T2-weighted MRI, carotid body tumors will have a pathognomonic "salt and pepper" appearance, which is due to the high-flow vascular voids. Use of a fat-suppressed sequence can be useful in further establishing the boundaries of the tumor.

When developing a resection plan for these tumors, angiograms are critical, as they reveal the tumor blood flow dynamics by demonstrating arterial supply and venous drainage. They also detail the surrounding vascular anatomy. Using four-vessel cerebral angiography allows for both qualitative and quantitative studies of the cerebral circulation, and in some cases preoperative embolization of the arteries feeding the tumor may be performed to minimize intraoperative blood loss.

Radionuclide imaging targeting catecholamine synthesis, storage, and secretion by the chromaffin tumor cells can also be useful in the evaluation of carotid body tumors. Different imaging agents target the various activities of the tumor cells. [123]I- and ^{131}I-labeled metaiodobenzylguanidine and ^{18}F-fluorodopamine are actively transported into the catecholamine-producing cells by vesicular monoamine transporters. However, ^{18}F-fluoro-2-deoxyglucose does not target catecholamine

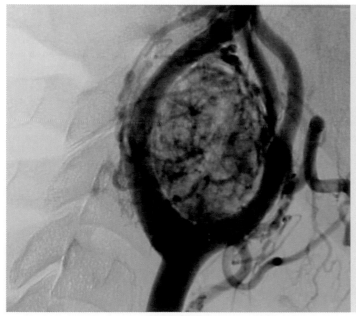

Fig. 28.2 Angiography of carotid body tumor.

pathways but rather enters the cell via glucose transporters and, therefore, indicates glucose metabolism. ^{111}In-octreoscan shows somatostatin type 2 receptors that are expressed in paragangliomas; it is 90% sensitive and specific for head and neck paragangliomas, making it useful postoperatively in scanning for recurrence.

In the work-up of carotid body tumors, it is critical to remember that a small number do secrete catecholamines; therefore, it is essential to screen for a secretory tumor when planning treatment to avoid a catecholamine crisis. Biochemical screening is performed by measuring fractionated plasma metanephrines and/or excretion of urine catecholamines and metabolites in the preoperative evaluation.

28.3 Medical Management

For patients who are poor surgical candidates, radiotherapy is preferred. In patients who are candidates for surgery, it is important to check catecholamine levels preoperatively. If they are elevated, an evaluation for adrenal pheochromocytomas is necessary. If present, the adrenal pheochromocytoma should be removed prior to addressing the carotid body tumor.

28.3.1 Surgical Management

Surgical excision is often indicated, as these can be locally aggressive tumors. When choosing how to treat a carotid body tumor, the presence of multiple tumors as well as the patient's comorbidities guides treatment. Surgical resection is indicated in younger patients healthy enough to undergo surgery. If the tumor is larger than 4 cm, preoperative embolization may be beneficial in reducing intraoperative bleeding. However, this is controversial, as some people believe it may make the subadventitial plane dissection more difficult. Surgical management after resection varies based on the size of the tumor, including a simple suture repair, patching the hole, or a bypass graft. Potential risks of the surgery include injury to cranial nerves IX through XII, hemorrhage, and stroke. The superior laryngeal nerve is most commonly injured.

28.3.2 Rehabilitation and Follow-up

While the risk is rare, patients should be followed for local recurrence by clinical exams.

28.4 Questions

1. Which of the following is not a known risk factor for carotid body tumors?
   a) Genetics.
   b) Cyanotic heart disease.
   c) Smoking.
   d) Living at high altitude.
2. Which of the following is not a common symptom of carotid body tumors?
   a) Palpitations.
   b) Hoarseness.
   c) Dysphagia.
   d) Visual changes.
3. Which of the following is the recommended treatment for carotid body tumors?
   a) Chemotherapy.
   b) Radiation.
   c) Chemotherapy and radiation.
   d) Surgical resection.

Answers: 1. c 2. d 3. d

Suggested Readings

Abu-Ghanem S, Yehuda M, Carmel NN, Abergel A, Fliss DM. Impact of preoperative embolization on the outcomes of carotid body tumor surgery: A meta-analysis and review of the literature. Head Neck. 2016; 38 Suppl 1:E2386–E2394

Amato B, Serra R, Fappiano F, et al. Surgical complications of carotid body tumors surgery: a review. Int Angiol. 2015; 34(6) Suppl 1:15–22

Dixon JL, Atkins MD, Bohannon WT, Buckley CJ, Lairmore TC, et al. Surgical management of carotid body tumors: a 15-year single institution experience employing an interdisciplinary approach. Proc (Bayl Univ Med Cent).–20

Johnson J. Bailey's Head and Neck Surgery Otolaryngology. 5th ed. Baltimore, MD: Lippincott Williams & Wilkins; 2001–2017

29 Nasopharyngeal Carcinoma

Alice L. Tang and Jonathan R. Mark

29.1 History

A 65-year-old man presented with right-sided aural fullness. He had decreased hearing on the right side for 2 weeks and complained of popping and clicking on the same side. He had been on fluticasone nasal spray for 1 year and had recently been treated with multiple courses of antibiotics for acute sinusitis. There was no history of previous otologic problems. An audiogram demonstrated a 40 dB right-sided conductive hearing loss. At the initial visit, a myringotomy was performed on the right side with a large amount of serous fluid evacuated.

The patient returned for follow-up in 1 week with persistent symptoms of the right ear. Upon further questioning, he has intermittent nose bleeds, right-sided tinnitus, and right neck pain. He denied dysphagia, odynophagia, dyspnea, fever, chills, night sweats, and weight loss. He never had head and neck surgery. He denied tobacco and alcohol use. His past medical history was otherwise not contributory. He never had radiation or chemotherapy in the past.

Physical examination revealed right-sided neck fullness and lymphadenopathy in the posterior cervical triangle upon palpation. The left neck was normal. Evaluation of the right ear demonstrated a healed myringotomy site with reaccumulation of fluid. Flexible nasopharyngoscopy was performed, showing a lesion in the fossa of Rosenmüller extending anterior to the right torus tubarius that appeared suspicious. The orifice of the eustachian tube appeared inflamed and friable. The remainder of the cranial nerve and upper aerodigestive tract examination was normal.

29.2 Differential Diagnosis—Key Points

- The finding of unilateral serous otitis media in an adult should make the clinician suspicious for a nasopharyngeal tumor, especially with palpable cervical adenopathy. Presenting symptoms include headache, head pressure, intermittent epistaxis, and aural fullness. Given that presenting symptoms are often nonspecific, they are often dismissed as allergy or sinus issues. These observations may lead the primary care physician to a presumptive diagnosis of upper respiratory infection with acute otitis media leading to one or two courses of antibiotic therapy resulting in a delay in diagnosis. Further tumor growth may result in skull base invasion often characterized by headache and extraocular muscle weakness. A brief list of possible malignancies includes squamous cell carcinoma, lymphoma, adenocarcinoma, adenoid cystic carcinoma, mucoepidermoid carcinoma, plasma cell myeloma, rhabdomyosarcoma, malignant melanoma, fibrosarcoma, chondrosarcoma, and clival chordoma.
- Lymphoma is the second most common tumor to arise in the nasopharynx. Therefore, queries regarding fevers and night sweats, constitutional type B symptoms, should be made.
- Benign nasopharyngeal masses should also be considered, particularly in the absence of cervical lymphadenopathy. Benign processes in this region include Thornwaldt's cyst, squamous papilloma, craniopharyngioma, and angiofibromas.

29.3 Test Interpretation

A patient with a nasopharyngeal mass, cervical adenopathy, and unilateral serous otitis media must undergo several diagnostic tests to be appropriately diagnosed and staged before treatment can be instituted.

- *Computed tomography (CT) scan:* CT scan with contrast from the skull base to the clavicles will delineate the extent of the primary tumor and cervical metastases. Nasopharynx cancer will aggressively metastasize to the cervical lymph nodes, most commonly to the retropharyngeal lymph nodes, followed by level II, III, IV, and V, respectively. If it is possible for the patient to undergo biopsy with minimum morbidity at the initial visit, it should be done. Imaging is obtained subsequently. Skull base invasion occurs in 30% of the cases. CT scan can demonstrate soft tissue extension in the nasopharynx as well as the parapharyngeal space. It is sensitive in detecting any skull base bone erosion. Tumor extension in the region between the foramen rotundum and foramen lacerum may involve the anterior group of cranial nerves (II through VI). Posterior cranial fossa extension may affect the lower cranial nerves (VII through XII).

- *Magnetic resonance imaging (MRI):* In patients with obvious signs of intracranial extension, including cranial neuropathies or other signs suggestive of central nervous system invasion, MRI should be obtained to evaluate the extent of disease. MRI is better in differentiating tumor from inflammation. It is also more sensitive at evaluating parapharyngeal and retropharyngeal extension and deep cervical nodal metastasis. MRI shows bone marrow infiltration even without bone erosion, which may indicate increased risk for distant metastasis.

- *Positron emission tomography/CT (PET/CT):* This imaging modality is more sensitive at detecting persistent and recurrent nasopharyngeal carcinoma (NPC), both locally and in the neck. PET/CT scan may help in detecting nodal and distant metastasis. Suspected lesions may need further study with bone scan, CT of the chest, liver scintigraphy, or bone marrow biopsy. For this patient the PET/CT revealed uptake at the nasopharyngeal primary site and a lateral retropharyngeal lymph node (▶ Fig. 29.1). There was also involvement of the right maxillary sinus; however, there was no extension to parapharyngeal tissues or skull base.

- *Nasal endoscopy and biopsy:* In cooperative patients, a nasopharyngeal mass may be biopsied transnasally in the office after adequate topical anesthesia. This is done under endoscopic guidance. Minimal bleeding occurs that is easily controlled with a light pack of a hemostatic agent. Inspection for Furstenberg's sign and pre-biopsy imaging should be done in lesions where there is the possibility of intracranial connection.

Tumor biopsy specimens suspected to be lymphoma should be placed in saline for fresh specimen preparation. Often the tissue obtained by transnasal biopsy is enough for pathologists to diagnose lymphoma with special stains and immunotyping. Transoral nasopharyngeal biopsy is also an option and is performed under general anesthesia in the operating room. Fine needle biopsies of cervical lymphadenopathy can also be performed to establish the presence of nodal metastasis.

- Histopathologically, there are three distinct forms of NPC. An accurate diagnosis of the subtype offers prognostic guidance. The World Health Organization (WHO) classification is used herein.
  - WHO type I (25% of total NPC cases in the United States): Keratinizing squamous cell carcinoma. These tumors show abundant intercellular bridges and keratin production. Histologically this is similar to other upper aerodigestive tract squamous cancers. It is rare in Southeast Asia. There are three grades in this type: well, moderately, and poorly differentiated.
  - WHO type II (12%): Nonkeratinizing squamous cell carcinoma, with some maturation. Also known as *transitional cell carcinoma* because it resembles this form of bladder malignancy.
  - WHO type III (63%): Undifferentiated carcinomas forming a diverse group of tumors, including lymphoepithelioma, anaplastic, clear cell, and spindle cell variants. This type represents the vast majority of cases (95%) in Southeast Asia.

A transnasal endoscopic evaluation was performed in the patient in question, which demonstrated

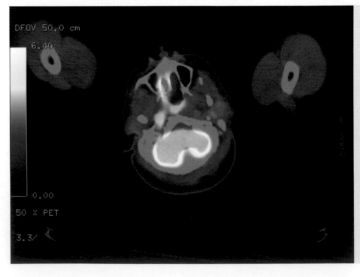

Fig. 29.1 PET/CT demonstrating uptake at primary site and at right lateral retropharyngeal lymph node. There is involvement of the right maxillary sinus but no extension to parapharyngeal tissues or skull base.

extension of the primary tumor into the nasal cavity. On histopathology, the tumor revealed a poorly differentiated keratinizing squamous cell carcinoma of the nasopharynx, WHO type I.

- *Epstein-Barr virus (EBV):* Latent EBV infection seems to be crucial in the pathogenesis of certain types of NPC. Ethnic Chinese people in North America, specifically first-generation immigrants, have the highest incidence of NPC associated with the virus outside of China. It is suspected that a genetic predilection or dietary patterns contribute to the high incidence rates seen in populations originating from southern China. In regions where NPC is endemic, EBV activation is necessary for the pathogenesis of NPC, specifically nonkeratinizing type II and type III, which constitute > 95% of the cases. Thus, screening for EBV in these populations is of value because it can result in early diagnosis leading to better outcomes. EBV DNA titers seem to be an important index for prognostication. In addition, in cases of an unknown primary with metastatic cervical adenopathy, EBV titers may suggest NPC and directed biopsies in the search for the primary tumor. In situ hybridization for EBV was performed on the pathologic specimen of the index patient and was seen to be negative.
- *Human papillomavirus (HPV):* While EBV has been well documented as an etiologic agent for NPC, HPV has been less defined in its role for this disease process. Small-scale studies have indicated that HPV, specifically types 16 and 18, is linked to the pathogenesis of keratinizing and some nonkeratinizing NPC among white people. In nonendemic populations, patients with HPV-positive NPC, as defined by p16 status on histopathology, have been compared to EBV-positive and EBV/HPV-negative patients and were seen to have worse prognosis. HPV testing (p16 staining) was performed on the index patient and was positive.

29.4 Diagnosis

- Nasopharyngeal carcinoma, WHO type I, EBV (–), p16 (+) stage III: T3N1M0. See ▶ Table 29.1 for staging of NPC.
- Right otitis media with effusion.

29.5 Medical Management

Appropriate histopathologic diagnosis and staging are essential before any treatment is initiated. External beam radiotherapy is the primary and curative treatment modality for NPC. The surrounding structures limit the dose of radiation, and thus intensity-modulated radiotherapy (IMRT) is the preferred method of delivery. With IMRT, late radiation toxicity can be reduced as compared to traditional radiation techniques. Additionally, studies have shown that IMRT contributed to an improvement in 5-year locoregional control and disease-specific and overall survival. In general, the dose given to the primary tumor is in the range of 60 to 70 Gy and to the neck, 65 to 70 Gy. In elective neck treatment, the dose can be decreased to 50 to 60 Gy.

Chemotherapy used concurrently with radiotherapy is the treatment of choice in advanced locoregional disease. Combination of cisplatin and 5-fluorouracil is the most widely used and studied.

29.6 Surgical Management

Surgical management is reserved for the development of local recurrences requiring salvage nasopharyngectomy. Neck dissection may be required in patients whose primary tumor has been controlled and residual cervical metastases are palpable. Many surgical approaches to the nasopharynx have been described, and the approach depends on the experience of the surgeon and the extent of the disease. Endoscopic approaches are ideal for small tumors limited to the posterior nasopharyngeal wall. Larger and more extensive tumors require open surgical techniques including lateral rhinotomy and with medial maxillectomy, transpalatal, transmaxillary, and transcervical. The anterolateral approach or the maxillary swing procedure has been used for salvage nasopharyngectomy. The facial translocation approach, which is a temporary removal of the facial skeleton with reinsertion of the segment after resection of tumor, provides an alternative with excellent exposure of the skull base. The success of salvage surgery is impacted by dural and brain involvement. In recurrent NPC, patients that undergo surgery have been shown to have a better survival rate when compared to a re-irradiation group.

A myringotomy with tube insertion should be performed on the patient with serous otitis in the setting of NPC because tumor-induced eustacian tube dysfunction will likely persist during therapy.

29.7 Rehabilitation and Follow-up

After successful treatment of NPC with primary modalities, approximately 5 to 10% of patients will

Table 29.1 Staging of nasopharyngeal carcinoma

Primary tumor (T)			
TX	Primary tumor cannot be assessed		
T0	No evidence of primary tumor		
Tis	Carcinoma in situ		
T1	Tumor confined to the nasopharynx or extends to oropharynx and/or nasal cavity without parapharyngeal extension		
T2	Tumor with parapharyngeal extension denotes posterolateral infiltration of tumor[a]		
T3	Tumor involves bony structures of skull base and/or paranasal sinuses		
T4	Tumor with intracranial extension and/or involvement of cranial nerves, infratemporal fossa, hypopharynx, orbit, or masticator space.		
Regional lymph nodes (N)			
NX	Regional lymph node cannot be assessed		
N0	No regional lymph node metastasis		
N1	Unilateral metastasis in lymph node(s), 6 cm or smaller in greatest dimension, above the supraclavicular fossa and/or unilateral or bilateral, retropharyngeal lymph nodes, 6 cm or less, in greatest dimension		
N2	Bilateral metastasis in lymph node(s), 6 cm or smaller in greatest dimension, above the supraclavicular fossa[b]		
N3	Metastasis in lymph node(s) > 6 cm and/or extension to supraclavicular fossa		
N3a	> 6 cm in dimension		
N3b	Extension to the supraclavicular fossa		
Distant metastasis (M)			
MX	Distant metastasis cannot be assessed		
M0	No distant metastasis		
M1	Distant metastasis		
Stage grouping			
0	Tis	N0	M0
I	T1	N0	M0
IIA	T2a	N0	M0
IIB	T1	N1	M0
	T2	N1	M0
	T2a	N1	M0
	T2b	N0	M0
	T2b	N1	M0
III	T1	N2	M0
	T2a	N2	M0
	T2b	N2	M0

Table 29.1 continued

Primary tumor (T)			
	T3	N0	M0
	T3	N1	M0
	T3	N2	M0
IVA	T4	N0	M0
	T4	N1	M0
	T4	N2	M0
IVB	Any T	N3	M0
IVC	Any T	Any N	M1

Notes: [a]Midline nodes are considered ipsilateral nodes.

[b]The supraclavicular zone/fossa is a triangular region bounded by the superior margin of the sternal end of the clavicle, the superior margin of the lateral end of the clavical, and the point where the neck meets the shoulder. All cases with lymph nodes in the fossa are considered N3b.

have local recurrences. The patient should be evaluated closely after radiation and chemotherapy for any persistent disease and then followed with endoscopic exams every 1 to 3 months for the first year after completion of treatment. Biopsy may be indicated posttreatment to determine if there is persistent disease. Endoscopic examinations occur every 2 to 4 months during the second year of follow-up, with examinations every 3 to 6 months during the third year. Yearly examinations are performed after this time for the duration of the patient's life. PET/CT scan is the most sensitive and specific method for detecting persistence and recurrence.

Long-term sequelae of radiotherapy may develop, including endocrinopathies (from affected pituitary and thyroid dysfunction), auditory, dysfunction cranial neuropathies, Lhermitte's syndrome (described as an electric shock sensation down the neck and extremities caused by neck flexion), xerostomia, and soft tissue fibrosis. Surveillance for late effects is an important part of follow-up in survivors.

29.8 Questions

1. Choose the World Health Organization (WHO) classification of nasopharyngeal carcinoma (NPC) that is consistent with the following histopathologic description: Nonkeratinizing squamous cell carcinoma, with some maturation. Also known as *transitional cell carcinoma*

because it resembles this form of bladder malignancy.
   a) WHO I.
   b) WHO II.
   c) WHO III.
   d) WHO IV.

2. What is the preferred primary definitive treatment modality for a stage III T2N1M0 nasopharynx cancer?
   a) Nasopharyngectomy.
   b) Facial translocation.
   c) Chemoradiation.
   d) Primary radiation.

3. Which imaging modality is the preferred method for detecting persistence or recurrence of NPC?
   a) Magnetic resonance imaging (MRI).
   b) Computed tomography (CT) of maxillary face with contrast.
   c) Positron emission tomography (PET) scan.
   d) PET/CT scan.

Answers: 1. b 2. c 3. d

Suggested Readings

Chan AT, Teo PM, Leung TW, Johnson PJ. The role of chemotherapy in the management of nasopharyngeal carcinoma. Cancer. 1998; 82 (6):1003–1012

Chua ML, Wee JT, Hui EP, Chan AT. Nasopharyngeal carcinoma. Lancet. 2016; 387(10022):1012–1024

Chu EA, Wu JM, Tunkel DE, Ishman SL. Nasopharyngeal carcinoma: the role of the Epstein-Barr virus. Medscape J Med. 2008; 10 (7):165

Hao SP. Facial translocation approach to the skull base: the viability of translocated facial bone graft. Otolaryngol Head Neck Surg. 2001; 124(3):292–296

Tan L, Loh T. Benign and Malignant Tumors of the Naspharynx. In: Cummings CW, Flint PW, Haughey BH, Niparko, JK. Otolaryngology - Head and Neck Surgery, 5th ed. Philadelphia, PA: Elsevier Mosby; 2010, pp 1348-1357.

Stenmark MH, McHugh JB, Schipper M, et al. Nonendemic HPV-positive nasopharyngeal carcinoma: association with poor prognosis. Int J Radiat Oncol Biol Phys. 2014; 88(3):580–588

30 Oropharyngeal Carcinoma

Douglas C. von Allmen and Yash J. Patil

30.1 History

A 55-year-old man presented for 4 months of right-sided otalgia, odynophagia, and weight loss of 30 pounds. He denied significant smoking or alcohol use. He was otherwise healthy but had not seen a physician in several years. A full head and neck exam was performed, which was significant for an irregular asymmetrically enlarged right tonsil that was firm on palpation (▶ Fig. 30.1). A 2-cm level II jugular lymph node was palpable on the right. A nasopharyngeal scope examination was subsequently performed, which revealed normal base of tongue, larynx, and hypopharynx.

30.2 Differential Diagnosis—Key Points

- The boundaries of the oropharynx are as follows:
  a) Anterior: Junction of the hard and soft palate, circumvallate papilla, and anterior tonsillar pillars.
  b) Posterior: Posterior pharyngeal wall.
  c) Lateral: Tonsillar fossa and lateral pharyngeal walls.
  d) Superior: Nasopharynx (at level of hard palate).
  e) Inferior: Level of hyoid.

- The oropharynx is divided into four subsites: base of tongue, soft palate, palatine tonsillar fossa and tonsillar pillars, and pharyngeal walls.
- The clinical scenario above is highly suggestive of squamous cell carcinoma oropharyngeal malignancy with regional metastatic disease. However, other diagnoses that must be considered are lymphoma, sarcoma, adenoid cystic carcinoma, mucoepidermoid carcinoma, adenosquamous carcinoma, papilloma, lymphangioma, and tonsillar hypertrophy. Squamous cell carcinoma and its variants account for greater than 90% of malignant lesions.
- Oropharyngeal squamous cell carcinoma (OPSCC) is now characterized categorically according to etiology as human papillomavirus (HPV)–associated and non–HPV-associated. OPSCC.
  a) HPV-associated OPSCC has increased dramatically in incidence over the past few decades and continues to increase in middle-aged white males. Patients with HPV-positive OPSCC may present without a significant alcohol or tobacco history and may have a higher socioeconomic status.
  b) HPV 16 is the most strongly associated with OPSCC and is responsible for greater than 90% of cases. Vaccination currently exists for males and females ages 9 to 26 covering HPV 6, 11, 16, and 18 and was originally developed to prevent cervical cancer and genital warts, but

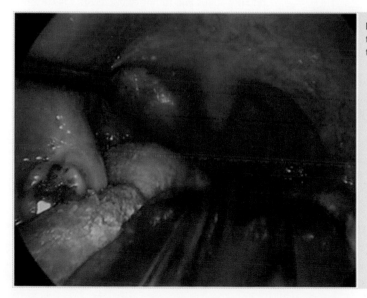

Fig. 30.1 Retraction of the anterior tonsillar pillar reveals a right-sided tonsil mass.

would be beneficial in the prevention of OPSCC.

c) HPV-positive OPSCC has improved survival compared to HPV-negative disease except in those who present with advanced nodal disease.

- HPV-negative OPSCC is associated with smoking and alcohol use and typically presents later in life in the seventh to ninth decade.
- Biopsy of the primary tumor is critical for diagnosis. This can be performed in the office, although not as easily as with biopsy of an oral lesion. More frequently this is performed in the operating room during panendoscopy to thoroughly evaluate the upper aerodigestive tract and assess for the presence of a second primary tumor.
- Imaging plays an important role in staging and surveillance following tumor treatment. Computed tomography (CT) of the neck with contrast and CT of the chest without contrast are common first-line studies to evaluate extent of disease. Magnetic resonance imaging (MRI) is used less commonly but is particularly useful when evaluating for the presence of skull base invasion or neurovascular involvement. Positron emission tomography (PET)/CT can be considered initially in patients with clinically advanced disease at higher risk for distant metastasis. It is also beneficial following treatment to evaluate for residual disease.

30.3 Test Interpretation

- Panendoscopy was performed with biopsy. Biopsy specimens sent for frozen pathology intraoperatively on this patient revealed squamous cell carcinoma.
- CT of the neck with contrast and CT of the chest without contrast revealed a $3.0 \times 3.5 \times 3.0$-cm mass in the right tonsillar fossa. In addition, multiple enlarged right level II lymph nodes were identified. Chest CT scan was unremarkable.

30.4 Diagnosis

Stage IVA (T2N2bM0) squamous cell carcinoma, site: oropharynx, subsite: right tonsil

30.5 Medical Management

Once a diagnosis of OPSCC is made it is important to assess the overall health and functional status of the patient prior to initiation of therapy, whether medical or surgical. Nutritional status is often compromised at the time of patient presentation due to the underlying malignancy, alcoholism, and/or lack of social support. Prealbumin, albumin, C-reactive protein, complete blood count, basic metabolic profile, and liver function tests can help assess the nutritional status of the patient. Alcoholism and lack of social support or transportation may preclude frequent visits for chemotherapy or radiation. As a result, a social worker is a critical member of the treatment team to assess patient support and assist in obtaining resources necessary for treatment. Thyroid function tests are also important to obtain if the patient has a history of prior neck surgery or a history of radiation to the head or neck. Thyroid function also must be monitored in patients after they complete radiation therapy to assess for radiation-induced hypothyroidism. Access to dental care needs to be established both prior to treatment and following the completion of radiation therapy due to the need for possible teeth extraction.

Nonsurgical therapy consists of radiation with or without concurrent chemotherapy. Due to the risk of early metastasis in OPSCC, all but very small primary tumors require treatment to the neck in addition to the primary site. T1 and T2 tumors can be treated with surgery or radiation alone. T3 and T4 tumors require combined-modality treatment (chemoradiation or surgery and postoperative radiation). HPV-associated OPSCCs are more radiosensitive and thus especially conducive to nonsurgical treatment. The consideration for divergent treatment algorithms with de-escalation of therapy based on HPV status and tumor characteristics is currently being investigated. Other tumor markers may also aid in the selection of surgery versus organ-sparing treatment. Low epidermal growth factor receptor (EGFR) and high HPV titer favor a good outcome with chemoradiation treatment alone, while the combination of low p53 and high Bcl-xl expression is unfavorable for organ-sparing therapy. Chemoradiation may also be performed in a palliative setting for incurable disease in an effort to slow tumor growth and alleviate pain. Considering the long-term morbidities associated with radiation therapy, including dysphagia, xerostomia, and the risk of secondary malignancy, patient education and selection is important when discussing treatment modalities.

30.6 Surgical Management

Surgical excision is an option for most oropharyngeal tumors; however, extension into the prevertebral fascia, parapharyngeal space involvement, or carotid artery encasement make surgical control unlikely. Adequate surgical control is dependent on good exposure with a wide margin of excision. Use of frozen section intraoperatively is necessary due to the propensity for submucosal spread of tumor.

Transoral excision is a viable option for many tumors in patients without advanced disease or trismus. The alternative approach of transoral robotic surgery has proven to be a safe alternative for limited tonsil and tongue base cancers; however, patients with trismus or bony involvement or who have failed chemoradiation may require an open approach. Approaches to consider are the mandibular lingual release, suprahyoid pharyngotomy, lateral pharyngotomy, mandibulotomy, or mandibulectomy. At this time, mandibulotomy and segmental mandibulectomy remain the surgical approaches of choice by most head and neck surgeons.

Reconstruction following resection consists of a variety of techniques depending on the nature of the defect, location, and other patient factors. Local flaps have limited use due to the limited amount of tissue they provide and inferior functional results. Regional pedicle flaps are an option for single-staged reconstruction; however, their limited superior reach and bulk are disadvantages that make them difficult to tailor to fill defects involving multiple subsites. Free tissue transfer requires prolonged operating time and a surgeon with microvascular expertise. However, due to its ability to be customized for the defect, the free flap often provides a superior functional outcome for complex defects. The radial forearm free flap is a well-suited myocutaneous flap for soft tissue defects in the mouth and pharynx due to its reduced bulk and pliability. For oropharyngeal defects involving the mandible, the osteocutaneous fibula free flap serves as a good reconstruction option.

Due to the swelling and resulting dysphagia following resection and reconstructive surgery, many of these patients require tracheostomy to provide a secure airway and gastrostomy tubes for long-term enteral access. Adjuvant radiation is frequent following surgical resection unless the surgery is a salvage operation for chemoradiaton failure.

30.7 Rehabilitation and Follow-up

Following completion of treatment, patients require close observation and lifelong follow-up to monitor for recurrence and second primaries. The estimated risk of developing a second primary tumor is 3 to 7% per year. Typically patients are seen every 1 to 2 months for the first year, every 2 to 4 months for the second year, every 4 to 6 months for years 3 through 5, and every 12 months after 5 years. Monitoring consists of physical examination in addition to PET/CT scan beginning 2 to 3 months following the completion of therapy. Three-year overall survival rates for oropharyngeal cancer for low-risk, intermediate-risk, and high-risk groups as defined by the National Institutes of Health (NIH) are 93%, 70%, and 46%, respectively, with smoking history, HPV status, and nodal disease affecting risk stratification.

Treatment of these cancer patients is a multidisciplinary effort. A close relationship with speech therapy is crucial as patients navigate the frequent difficulties with dysphagia resulting from a newly reconstructed oropharynx. Physical therapists also play an important role in the recovery phase. Radiation-induced fibrosis and scarring may cause significantly limited range of motion, and massage and exercises play a key role in reducing the amount of contracture that occurs. Smoking cessation continues to be a challenging obstacle for some patients, and a continued effort to reduce and cease tobacco use in the postoperative setting should remain a focus in follow-up appointments.

30.8 Questions

1. A patient presents with a 4 × 4.5 × 4-cm tumor extending from the left tonsil to the base of tongue involving the palatoglossus and palatopharyngeus. Computed tomography (CT) of the neck identifies bilateral level II 3-cm lymph nodes with necrotic centers. CT of the chest is unremarkable. What is the TNM classification and stage of this tumor?
   a) T2N2cM0.
   b) T3N2bM0.
   c) T3N2cM0.
   d) T4aN2cM0.
   e) T4aN3M0.

2. Which of the following is indicative of a high-risk oropharyngeal squamous cell carcinoma (OPSCC)?
   a) A p16-positive tumor.
   b) Smoking history of < 10 pack years.
   c) A p16-negative tumor.
   d) Absence of metastasis.
   e) Tumor of 1 cm in greatest dimension.

3. A patient has just completed radiation following surgical resection. Which of the following is the appropriate timing of the next positron emission tomography (PET)/computed tomography (CT) scan and follow-up visit?
   a) At completion of the final radiation treatment.
   b) 12 weeks.
   c) 6 months.
   d) 1 year.
   e) Imaging is not indicated.

Answers: 1. d 2. c 3. b

Suggested Readings

Johnson JT, Rosen CA. Bailey's Head and Neck Surgery: Otolaryngology. Lippincott Williams & Wilkins; 2013: 1898–1916

Kumar B, Cordell KG, Lee JS, et al. EGFR, p16, HPV Titer, Bcl-xL and p53, sex, and smoking as indicators of response to therapy and survival in oropharyngeal cancer. J Clin Oncol. 2008; 26(19):3128–3137

Masterson L, Moualed D, Liu ZW, et al. De-escalation treatment protocols for human papillomavirus-associated oropharyngeal squamous cell carcinoma: a systematic review and meta-analysis of current clinical trials. Eur J Cancer. 2014; 50(15):2636–2648

Pytynia KB, Dahlstrom KR, Sturgis EM. Epidemiology of HPV-associated oropharyngeal cancer. Oral Oncol. 2014; 50(5):380–386

31 Lip Cancer

Amy M. Manning and Keith M. Wilson

31.1 History

A 49-year-old woman was seen in the ear, nose, and throat (ENT) head and neck cancer clinic with an ulcerated lower lip lesion. She had a history of wide local excision of invasive squamous cell carcinoma (SCC) of the lip twice in the past. Her most recent wide local excision was 6 months prior, and pathology was consistent with invasive moderately to poorly differentiated SCC, approximately 2 cm in diameter and with a depth of 2 mm invasion into the underlying stroma. Surgical margins were clear but there was an area of invasive SCC < 0.1 cm from the margin of resection. The neck was clinically and radiographically uninvolved at the time of surgery. Following this resection, the patient was treated with 66 Gy adjuvant radiation. One month following the completion of surgery she noted an ulcerated area in the prior surgical bed with increased surrounding edema and induration and presented back to ENT clinic. She reported pain and intermittent drainage from the area. She denied fever, weight loss, dysphagia, odynophagia, or otalgia. She had a 5 pack-year smoking history but had quit approximately 1 year ago.

Physical exam revealed an obese African-American female in no acute distress. She was afebrile with stable vital signs. There was a 2- to 3-cm ulcerated area on the right lower lip approaching midline, with granulation tissue in the wound bed and palpable submucosal extension. The remainder of the intraoral exam was normal. Nasal and ear exams were normal. Facial movement was symmetric and House-Brackmann (HB) grade I/VI bilaterally. Facial sensation was full and equal bilaterally. Neck exam revealed normal range of motion with no palpable lymphadenopathy or mass. An incisional biopsy of the lesion was performed and revealed invasive SCC. The patient was taken to the operating room (OR) for repeated resection followed by reconstruction (▶ Fig. 31.1).

31.2 Differential Diagnosis — Key Points

- Lip cancer is the most common subsite of oral cavity cancer (comprising 20–30% of all oral cancers), and SCC is the most common histologic type of cancer found in the lower lip, while basal cell carcinoma (BCC) is more common in the upper lip. Eighty-eight percent to 95% of neoplasms in the lip occur in the lower lip. Minor salivary gland malignancy is an uncommon type of head and neck cancer, but the lip is the second most common subsite involved, after the hard

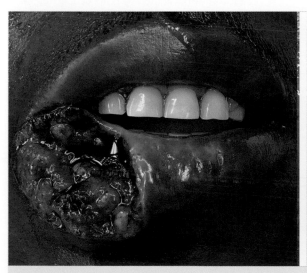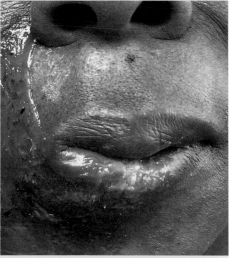

Fig. 31.1 (a,b) A 2- to 3-cm recurrent SCC of the lower lip prior to resection and following resection and Estlander's flap reconstruction. Commissuroplasty is planned for 6 weeks postoperatvely after the first stage of reconstruction.

palate. The most common minor salivary gland malignancies found in the lip are mucoepidermoid and adenoid cystic carcinomas. Other rare malignant lesions found in the lip include melanoma, Merkel's cell carcinoma, malignant fibrous histiocytoma, and malignant granular cell tumors.

- SCC lip cancer occurs most commonly in white males, with a peak incidence in the sixth and seventh decades of life. Risk factors include ultraviolet light exposure, tobacco and alcohol exposure, immunosuppression, poor dental hygiene, and low socioeconomic status. History frequently will reveal a nonhealing ulcer or a crusted lesion that bleeds on removal.
- Lymphatic drainage from the upper lip occurs first to the periparotid, preauricular, and level I neck lymph nodes. Drainage occurs unilaterally, as the embryonic fusion plane of the central frontonasal process separates the neurovascular structures of the two sides. The lower lip lymphatic drainage pattern is bilateral, and the first echelon is the level I neck. The second echelon of lymph node metastasis for both lower and upper lip lesions is level II or occasionally level III. Risk of cervical metastasis increases with tumor size, involvement of the oral commissure, poorly differentiated histology, depth of invasion > 5 mm, or perineural invasion.
- Keratoacanthoma is a benign, self-limiting epithelial neoplasm that can mimic SCC in appearance. It typically has a rapid growth phase over several weeks, then stabilizes and spontaneously involutes. Diagnosis is by incisional biopsy.

31.3 Test Interpretation

1. Diagnosis is established by incisional biopsy. Biopsy specimen should contain a margin of normal tissue, which allows the pathologist to characterize the depth and pattern of invasion or the presence of perineural invasion.
2. Imaging studies including dental panoramic radiograph, computed tomography (CT), or magnetic resonance imaging (MRI) can be helpful in characterizing advanced disease, and are indicated when the tumor extends over the gingival mucosa, adjacent teeth are loose, or there is hypesthesia of the chin.
3. Fewer than 2% of patients with previously untreated lip SCC present with distant metastasis, and 10 to 15% present with regional nodal metastasis. Upper lip and commissure lesions carry a higher risk of regional metastasis.
4. Staging of lip cancer is described by the American Joint Committee on Cancer (▶ Table 31.1).

31.4 Diagnosis

Squamous cell carcinoma of the lip, recurrent, stage T2N0

31.5 Medical Management

1. Primary radiation therapy (either external beam or brachytherapy) has been shown to have similar efficacy as surgery for T1, T2, and T3 disease. If future surgical therapy is needed, history of radiation makes reconstruction more problematic.

Table 31.1 Staging of squamous cell carcinoma of the lip (T stage)

Stage	Description
TX	Primary tumor cannot be assessed
T0	No evidence of primary tumor
Tis	Carcinoma in situ
T1	Primary tumor < /= 2 cm in greatest dimension
T2	Primary tumor > 2 cm but < /= 4 cm in greatest dimension
T3	Primary tumor > 4 cm in greatest dimension
T4a	Moderately advanced local disease; tumor invades through cortical bone, inferior alveolar nerve, floor of mouth, or skin of face
T4b	Very advanced local disease; tumor invades masticator space, pterygoid plates, or skull base and/or encases internal carotid artery

2. Adjuvant postoperative radiation is indicated in cases of T3 or T4 tumors, recurrent tumors, extracapsular spread, nodal metastasis in multiple neck levels or > 2 lymph nodes, and perineural invasion.

3. Potential complications of radiation therapy to the lip include wound contracture ("whistle deformity") and osteoradionecrosis of the mandible.

31.6 Surgical Management

1. The goal of surgical therapy for lip cancer is removal of all malignant tissue as well as reconstruction to allow for adequate oral competence and cosmetic result. Resection should be carefully planned with reconstruction in mind. Reconstructive goals include preservation of oral competence, sensation, and motor function of the lip. Surgery is generally the preferred modality of treatment for small lesions, and provides the advantage of histologic confirmation of clear margins. A resected margin of 1 to 2 cm of normal tissue is generally recommended.

2. Partial-thickness defects can be reconstructed with undermining and advancement of buccal mucosa. Undermining occurs in a plane deep to the minor salivary glands and superficial to the orbicularis oris muscle and labial artery. Small defects of the vermilion may be repaired using a mucosal V-Y advancement flap.

3. Selection of reconstructive techniques for full-thickness defects depends upon both the size and the location of the defect. Defects of one-fourth to one-third of the upper lip and one-third to one-half of the lower lip may be closed primarily. Central defects may be closed via bilateral lip advancement flaps. Important cosmetic considerations include realignment of the vermilion border, placement of scars along relaxed skin tension lines, and preservation of the oral commissure, if possible. The wound is closed in layers, with close approximation of each layer. Consideration of lip subunits is necessary in planning of lip reconstruction.

4. Reconstruction of full-thickness defects of one-third to two-thirds of the lip can be achieved with a Karapandzic's labioplasty or lip switch (Abbe's or Estlander's) flap. The Karapandzic's labioplasty (▶ Fig. 31.2) preserves sensation, mobility, and vascularity to the lips and uses circumoral cutaneous and mucosal incisions and blunt dissection of the muscular layer to reconstruct defects in a single stage. Advantages of this technique include single-stage reconstruction and preservation of oral competence. Disadvantages include microstomia and blunting of the oral commissure. Abbe's and Estlander's techniques transfer full-thickness tissue from one lip to the other, pedicled on the labial artery. The Abbe's flap is typically used to close medial defects and requires a second-stage surgery to divide the pedicle, typically approximately 3 weeks following the first stage of reconstruction. The Estlander's flap (▶ Fig. 31.2) is used to reconstruct defects involving the oral commissure, and tissue is rotated to the opposing lip around the oral commissure. This results in blunting of the oral commissure, and typically requires a secondary commissuroplasty. As a general rule, both the Abbe's and Estlander's techniques employ flaps one-half the size of the defect.

5. Reconstruction of defects of greater than two-thirds of the lip often requires combinations of described techniques, perhaps with the addition of myocutaneous or free tissue transfer flaps. Relatively large midline lower lip defects can be managed with the Webster's modification of the Bernard's cheiloplasty (▶ Fig. 31.2), which employs bilateral cheek advancement flaps and Burow's triangles with the vertical limbs placed in the melolabial and mental creases. More extensive defects require reconstruction with distant flaps; this carries the inherent challenge of reestablishing motor innervation, sensation, and oral competence.

6. Neck dissection is indicated in the presence of clinically evident nodal disease. Sacrifice of the facial artery should be avoided, if possible, to maintain the blood supply to structures used for lip reconstruction. Elective neck dissection is not typically recommended for lip carcinoma, as the incidence of occult metastasis is low.

31.7 Rehabilitation and Follow-up

1. Prognosis for early stage (I and II) lip cancer is good, with 90% 5-year survival. The presence of cervical metastasis decreases the survival rate by 50%.

2. Surveillance of lip cancer following treatment is aided by the highly accessible location of the lips for visualization and palpation.

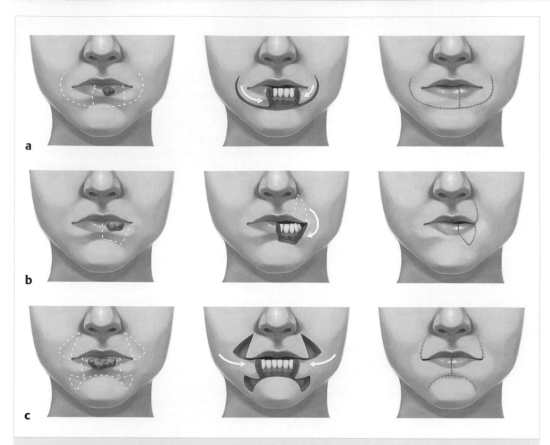

Fig. 31.2 Examples of Karapandzic's labioplasty, Estlander's flap, and Webster's modification of Bernard's cheiloplasty. (a) Karapandzic's labioplasty. Lesion is excised, leaving a full-thickness defect of the lower lip. Circumoral skin incisions are made within the mental and nasolabial creases. Separate incisions are made through the intraoral mucosal layer. The muscular layer is dissected bluntly to identify and preserve neurovascular structures. The skin and mucosa are then advanced and closed. (b) Estlander's flap. Excision of lateral lower lip lesion leaves defect involving the oral commissure. Donor flap is designed such that the donor scar lies in the melolabial crease. The flap is pedicled on the labial artery and rotates about the new commissure. A second-stage commissuroplasty is required to address blunting of the oral commissure. (c) Webster's modification of Bernard's cheiloplasty. A large central lower lip lesion is removed, leaving a large full-thickness defect. Four Burow's triangles are excised such that the scars lie in the melolabial and mental creases. Tissue is then advanced medially and closed in the midline. Mucosal advancement flaps are used laterally to reconstruct the vermilion.

31.8 Questions

1. A patient presents with an expanding ulcerated lesion of the right lower lip, present for the past 6 months. The patient reports progressive hypesthesia of the chin over the past several weeks. Physical examination reveals an indurated area on the right lower lip that is 2.5 cm in diameter. Computed tomography (CT) reveals enlarging of the mental foramen on the right side. Incisional biopsy is positive for squamous cell carcinoma (SCC). What is the T stage?
   a) T1.
   b) T2.
   c) T3.
   d) T4.

2. A patient has a 3-cm SCC in the left upper lip that does not cross the midline. What is the expected first-echelon nodal drainage pattern?
   a) Bilateral periparotid, preauricular and level I lymph nodes.
   b) Left periparotid, preauricular and level I lymph nodes.
   c) Bilateral submental lymph nodes.
   d) Left levels II and III of the neck.

3. A patient has a 3-cm SCC involving the left upper lip that does not cross midline. There is no clinical or radiographic evidence of lymph node involvement. Which of the following is most appropriate in addition to resection of the primary tumor?

a) No neck dissection.
b) Left selective neck dissection.
c) Left modified radical neck dissection.
d) Bilateral selective neck dissection.

Answers: 1. d 2. b 3. a

Suggested Readings

Biasoli ÉR, Valente VB, et al. Lip Cancer: A Clinicopathological Study and Treatment Outcomes in a 25-Year Experience. J Oral Maxillofac Surg. 2016 Jan 30. See comment in PubMed Commons below J Oral Maxillofac Surg. 2016 Jul;74(7):1360-7.

Edge SB, Byrd DR, Compton CC, Fritz AG, Greene FL, Trotti A, editors. AJCC cancer staging manual (7th ed). New York, NY: Springer; 2010.

Faulhaber J, Géraud C, Goerdt S, Koenen W, et al. Functional and aesthetic reconstruction of full-thickness defects of the lower lip after tumor resection: analysis of 59 cases and discussion of a surgical approach. Dermatol Surg. 2010 Jun; 36(6):859–67

Puscas L, Fritz MA, Esclamado RM. Lip Cancer. In Johnson JT, Rosen CA, et al, eds. Bailey's Head and Neck Surgery – Otolaryngology, 5th ed. Philadelphia, PA: Lippencott Williams & Wilkins, 2014.

Renner GJ. Reconstruction of the Lips. In Baker SR, et al. Local Flaps in Facial Reconstruction, 3rd ed. Philadelphia, PA: Elsevier Health Sciences, 2014.

Wein RO, Weber RS. Malignant Neoplasms of the Oral Cavity. In Flint PW, et al. Cummings Otolaryngology: Head and Neck Surgery, 6th ed. London, UK: Elsevier Health Sciences, 2015.

32 Field Cancerization

Brian L. Hendricks and Jonathan R. Mark

32.1 History

A 66-year-old woman presented to establish follow-up and care regarding her prior history of two separate primary head and neck squamous cell carcinomas (SCCs). She was followed at another facility for many years, but relocated to this region several years ago and has not established any follow-up since. She is concerned about gradually worsening dysphagia, odynophagia, and trismus over the past several months. She also reported some right-sided facial pain, nasal congestion, and intermittent self-limited epistaxis from her right nasal cavity.

Her prior head and neck cancer history included a T1N0M0 SCC of the base of tongue for which she underwent primary radiation therapy with completion of treatment 9 years ago. Subsequently, 4 years later, she developed a second T3N0M0 SCC of the base of tongue extending on the larynx, for which she underwent a base of tongue resection and total laryngectomy with neck dissections. The remainder of her past medical history was remarkable for hypertension, coronary artery disease, and chronic obstructive pulmonary disease. She had a 40 pack-year smoking history, as well as prior history of heavy alcohol use.

On physical examination, her oral cavity was dry and subtly hyperemic, and there were small areas of telangectasia along the left anterolateral portion of her tongue. The right buccal mucosa was notable for an area of thickened white tissue near the occlusal surface of her molars. Her oropharynx and neopharynx showed postsurgical and postradiation changes, and the left base of tongue was tender and firm to palpation. There was no palpable cervical lymphadenopathy. Flexible fiberoptic examination revealed a mass that appears to be protruding through the right maxillary sinus wall and beneath the inferior turbinate. Additionally, an area of irregular mucosa and ulceration was noted along the left base of tongue (▶ Fig. 32.1). Her stoma and trachea were unremarkable.

The patient was counseled regarding the possibility of recurrent and new primary malignancies. Computed tomography (CT) of the neck with contrast was ordered, and she was scheduled for panendoscopy with biopsies.

32.2 Differential Diagnosis—Key Points

- The suspicion for neoplasm is higher in patients with prior head and neck malignancies. As there are several areas of concern, this patient is best served by a formal panendoscopy with biopsies. Submucosal recurrence may not be obvious on visual inspection, but persistent pain (localized by the patient) and palpation under general anesthesia aid in directing biopsies. Deep biopsy is often required to detect a submucosal recurrence.

- Leukoplakia in a patient with prior head and neck cancer is concerning. Grossly, dysplasia, carcinoma in situ, SCC, and pseudoepitheliomatous hyperplasia appear similar. Leukoplakia is the result of hyperkeratosis, or a thickening of the epithelial layer related to chronic irritation. Though most patients with leukoplakia report a history of tobacco or alcohol use, it is also commonly found on the tongue or buccal mucosa near the occlusal surface of the molars. When biopsied, approximately 20% of these lesions contain evidence of dysplasia or carcinoma on histology. Of those lesions without dysplasia, approximately 1% undergo malignant transformation. Areas of mucosal irregularity should be closely monitored in all patients, but in particular those with significant risk factors for malignancy.

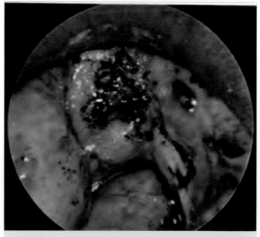

Fig. 32.1 Photograph of left base of tongue mass

- Erythroplakia is a red or pink plaquelike area of mucosa that carries a 90% incidence of dysplasia or malignancy on biopsy. Erythroleukoplakia is a term used to describe lesions with both leukoplakic and erythroplakic components, and these have a reported malignant transformation rate of 23%.
- Carcinoma *in situ* describes cancer confined to the epithelial layer. SCC is the most common malignancy of the oral cavity.
- Field cancerization: In 1953, Slaughter et al described the frequent observation of dysplastic changes in the benign epithelium surrounding the confines of gross resection of malignant oral tumors. Using p53 mutations and loss of heterozygosity at specific chromosomes as markers for dysplasia, research has shown that upward of 35% of oral cavity and oropharyngeal cancers display surrounding genetically altered mucosa. Retrospective studies have shown that these surrounding dysplastic changes play an important role in locoregional recurrence and the development of second primary tumors.

After successful treatment of head and neck cancer with surgery, radiation, and chemotherapy, patients are at an increased risk of metachronous primary tumors at an annual rate of 3 to 10%. In patients, especially both current and former tobacco users, the head and neck mucosa may undergo a process termed field cancerization and manifest multiple additional premalignant and malignant lesions. Field cancerization describes the concept that diffuse injury has occurred in the epithelium from widespread and chronic exposure to carcinogens. The mucosa is broadly affected over large areas, often precluding a limited, localized therapeutic approach. The concept of chemoprevention has been proposed to approach the underlying changes occurring in the condemned mucosa. Proposed agents include retinoids, vitamin E, biologic agents, tyrosine kinase inhibitors, and protease inhibitors.

32.3 Test Interpretation

1. Biopsy is critical to pathologic diagnosis of mucosal lesions of the oral cavity. The clinician should pay special attention to areas that are firm, irregular, painful, or known to previously demonstrate signs of dysplasia or carcinoma.

2. Toluidine blue is a cationic metachromatic dye that has a high affinity for anionic molecules and can be helpful in identifying tissue with evidence of dysplasia or carcinoma. As these tissues generally contain more deoxyribonucleic and ribonucleic acid compared to the surrounding normal epithelium, the use of this acidophilic dye to stain these tissues can allow for easier identification.

3. CT imaging is helpful in evaluating suspicious sites for the area of spread, depth of invasion, and nodal disease. Positron emission tomography (PET) imaging may also be helpful if there is concern for distant metastasis.

32.4 Diagnosis

1. Right buccal mucosa: Hyperkeratosis without evidence of dysplasia.
2. Left anterolateral tongue: Moderately differentiated squamous cell carcinoma.
3. Left base of tongue: Moderately differentiated squamous cell carcinoma.
4. Right maxillary sinus mass: Moderately differentiated, nonkeratinizing squamous cell carcinoma.

32.5 Medical Management

1. Individual treatment algorithms for the management of SCC of the head and neck are beyond the scope of this chapter. Decisions regarding patient care should include consideration of the risks and benefits of surgical resection, radiotherapy, and chemoradiotherapy, as well as any potential combination of these that may be required as adjunctive treatments in the case of recurrence or new primary disease. Unusual or complicated patients should be discussed among a multidisciplinary team that includes expertise from the fields of otolaryngology, medical oncology, radiation oncology, radiology, and pathology.

2. Chemoprevention is currently being studied as a potential strategy for managing high-risk mucosa. It is defined by the use of a wide variety of agents to inhibit or reverse carcinogenesis in at-risk mucosa and lesions. Retinoids, vitamin A, β-carotene, green tea extract, curcumin, Bowman-Birk inhibitor concentrate, black raspberries, and immunomodulators are just some of

the agents that have been tested. Retinoids were one of the first chemopreventative measures studied. Their effect has been attributed to the restoration of retinoic acid receptors, which have been found to be lost in prelmalignant oral lesions. While clinical and/or histologic response has been observed with retinoids and other therapies, long-term reduction in progression to oral cancer after their withdrawal has not yet been shown. Further studies are ongoing.

32.6 Surgical Management

Panendoscopic evaluation in the operating room should involve a thorough examination of the head and neck, including bimanual examination of all subsites of the oral cavity and oropharynx. A combination of direct and telescopic examination is necessary to best evaluate the nasal cavities, nasopharynx, oropharynx, neopharynx, esophagus, and trachea in the patient with a history of a prior laryngectomy. In patients without such a history, the hypopharynx and larynx are examined. Cold steel excision remains an excellent method for biopsy and removal of localized lesions with minimal injury to the tissue architecture and individual cells. CO_2 laser excision may be used to excise localized disease, and ablative techniques can be a useful adjunct for the destruction of superficial lesions.

32.7 Rehabilitation and Follow-up

Frequent follow-up is of the utmost importance in all patients with a history of head and neck SCC. Surveillance should include a full interval history, review of systems, and clinical examination of the head and neck including indirect mirror or flexible fiberoptic examination. For those patients who have not yet ceased the use of tobacco and/or alcohol, they should be counseled extensively regarding the risks of continued use.

The National Comprehensive Cancer Network (NCCN) suggests the following after completion of definitive therapy of head and neck SCC:
- Year 1: Clinical exam every 1 to 3 months, and imaging within 6 months.
- Year 2: Clinical exam every 2 to 6 months.
- Years 3 to 5: Clinical exam every 4 to 8 months.
- > After 5 years: Clinical exam every 12 months.

Beyond the initial posttreatment imaging, additional reimaging is indicated if worrisome signs or symptoms arise, or for surveillance of areas inaccessible to clinical examination. Thyroid-stimulating hormone levels should be checked every 6 to 12 months if the patient has had prior irradiation to the neck.

This particular patient declined palliative/suppressive treatment interventions and continues to be followed for symptom management with the assistance of pain consultants and hospice services.

32.8 Questions

1. Which site of the head and neck displays the highest rate of second primaries?
   a) Oral cavity.
   b) Nasopharynx.
   c) Oropharynx.
   d) Hypopharynx.
   e) Larynx.
2. A 71-year-old white man with a history of heavy tobacco and alcohol use presents for evaluation of multiple painful oral cavity lesions. What is the optimal way to evaluate these lesions after a thorough history and physical exam?
   a) Incisional biopsies from all lesions in clinic.
   b) Fine needle aspiration of these lesions.
   c) Panendoscopy, including laryngoscopy, bronchoscopy, and esophagoscopy, with biopsies under general anesthesia.
   d) Computed tomography scan of the head and neck with contrast.
   e) Magnetic resonance imaging of the head and neck with contrast.
3. Which mucosal lesion has the highest rate of malignant transformation?
   a) Leukoplakia.
   b) Erythroplakia.
   c) Aphthous ulcer.
   d) Hyperkeratosis.
   e) Lichen planus.

Answers: 1. a 2. c 3. e

Suggested Readings

DeVries N, Gluckman JL, Eds. Multiple Primary Tumors of the Head and Neck. New York, NY: Thieme; 1990

Dionne KR, Warnakulasuriya S, Zain RB, Cheong SC. Potentially malignant disorders of the oral cavity: current practice and future directions in the clinic and laboratory. Int J Cancer. 2015; 136 (3):503–515

Leemans CR, Braakhuis BJM, Brakenhoff RH. The molecular biology of head and neck cancer. Nat Rev Cancer. 2011; 11(1):9–22

Licciardello JTW, Spitz MR, Hong WK. Multiple primary cancer in patients with cancer of the head and neck: second cancer of the head and neck, esophagus, and lung. Int J Radiat Oncol Biol Phys. 1989; 17(3):467–476

Slaughter DP, Southwick HW, Smejkal W. Field cancerization in oral stratified squamous epithelium; clinical implications of multicentric origin. Cancer. 1953; 6(5):963–968

Tabor MP, Brakenhoff RH, van Houten VMM, et al. Persistence of genetically altered fields in head and neck cancer patients: biological and clinical implications. Clin Cancer Res. 2001; 7(6):1523–1532

33 Carotid Artery Rupture

Yash J. Patil and Patrick R. Owens

33.1 History

A 72-year-old white man presented to the emergency department (ED) with reports of profuse bleeding at a skilled nursing facility (SNF) after undergoing a total laryngectomy, partial left pharyngectomy, bilateral neck dissection, and left radial forearm free flap 1 month ago, with adequate margins of resection. Radiation and chemotherapy were given 2 years ago as part of a laryngeal preservation protocol. Surgical resection was scheduled after tumor persistence was diagnosed on endoscopy 6 weeks ago. The patient noted worsening dysphagia, weight loss, and right otalgia since the completion of chemoradiotherapy. The postoperative course was complicated by a left pharyngocutaneous fistula. The fistula was located at the inferior aspect of the apron flap 4 cm to the left of the stoma. It had been treated conservatively with packing three times daily during the past 2 weeks. The fistula extended superiorly for 3 to 4 cm. The packing was changed the night before, at which time pulsations were noted to be visible in the open wound (▶ Fig. 33.1).

When the patient arrived in the ED, there was no active bleeding. The patient underwent computed tomography (CT) angiogram of the neck to look for the source of bleed. The results of the scan showed extravasation near the external system. Neurointerventional radiology was then consulted to perform angiogram to determine exact location and possible embolization of the external system if determined to be the source (▶ Fig. 33.2). The patient was also able to undergo balloon occlusion test to assess stroke risk with ligation of the common carotid artery.

33.2 Differential Diagnosis—Key Points

Bleeding from the neck in the postoperative setting is a potentially life-threatening situation. The differential diagnosis for such bleeding includes bleeding from the internal, common, or external carotid artery; jugular vein rupture; tracheoinnominate fistula; or, rarely, upper gastrointestinal bleed. Occasionally, bleeding from granulation

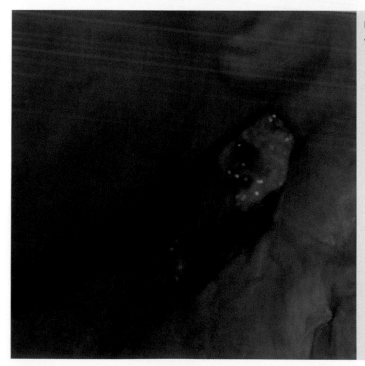

Fig. 33.1 Fistula with exposed carotid artery.

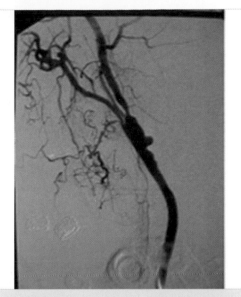

Fig. 33.2 Angiogram of left carotid system demonstrating extravasation of contrast.

tissue or the transverse cervical system can create bleeding, but it is typically less dramatic.

Carotid artery rupture is potentially a life-threatening emergency. Reported mortality varies between 3 and 50%. Severe neurologic deficits are seen in 16 to 50% of survivors. Risk factors for carotid artery rupture include pharyngocutaneous salivary fistula, previous radiation therapy to the head and neck, head and neck ablative surgery, incompletely resected tumor in proximity to the carotid, and local infection. Most patients will have a "herald" bleed hours before carotid artery rupture. Local wound infection plays an important role in carotid artery rupture. Organisms that have been implicated include *Pseudomonas* spp., *Klebsiella* spp., *Staphylococcus aureus*, enterococci, and anaerobes. When a pharyngocutaneous fistula is noted after tumor ablation in a radiated patient, every step should be taken to exclude and cover the vessels from the stream of saliva, prevent desiccation, and prevent local trauma from wound care.

The prevention of carotid artery rupture begins in the preoperative period. Often the size of the primary tumor and neck metastases necessitates extensive resection and neck dissection. Tumors of this nature typically affect oral intake. To maintain an adequate nutritional status, evaluation by a nutritionist, supplementation, and occasionally placement of a feeding tube preoperatively may be used.

Radiotherapy affects postoperative wound healing. Fibrosis, devascularization, and impaired wound healing are commonly seen in the radiated neck and contribute to carotid artery rupture.

Skin flap viability is also compromised in radiated patients. Smoking cessation preoperatively and certainly postoperatively may decrease the risk of skin flap loss. Careful consideration should be given to the placement of surgical incisions. Incision should not overlie the carotid artery and should cross the vessel only once. Trifurcations over the carotid are to be avoided. Typically an apron flap will suffice. If it is necessary to "drop a limb," avoid placing it over the carotid.

Several intraoperative steps may aid in prevention of carotid artery rupture. When neck dissection is performed, the surgeon should avoid stripping the adventitia from the carotid artery. The carotid artery derives 80% of its blood supply from the adventitia, and its removal leads to ischemia. Coverage of the carotid artery with dermal grafts, regional flaps, or free flaps should be performed routinely in cases where the carotid is exposed in continuity with oral cavity or oropharyngeal defects. Watertight mucosal closure is imperative in preventing pharyngocutaneous fistula and wound infection. Once again, regional or free tissue reconstruction should be used to create a tension-free closure.

A sentinel bleed is noted before most carotid artery ruptures. This may be seen as blood-tinged oral secretions, blood clot in the mouth, or bleeding during a dressing change. Typically carotid artery rupture will occur within hours of the sentinel bleed. Once a sentinel bleed is noted, appropriate steps should be taken. The patient should be monitored in a setting where nursing staff are familiar with the care of head and neck patients. Blood should be available in a timely fashion, and the patient should be instructed not to strain or move about unnecessarily. Plans for immediate carotid artery exploration and coverage or endovascular intervention should be made.

33.3 Test Interpretation

Elective cerebral angiogram before carotid rupture may provide insight into collateral circulation across an intact circle of Willis. Patients with no option for coverage of an at-risk carotid should undergo angiography, and a carotid stent should be considered. Use of a stent, even in the presence of tumor, may decrease the incidence of carotid artery blowout and death. Stenting might not decrease the incidence of stroke, especially in patients with recurrent tumor, chronic wounds, and local wound infection. In this setting, the stent may extrude. Despite this, retrospective studies seem to indicate that rupture is much less frequent. If balloon occlusion studies demonstrate collateralization, exclusion of the at-risk carotid may be considered, especially if further wound breakdown is noted. If collateral flow is not present, depending on the patient's prognosis, surgical reconstruction may be considered.

Cerebral angiography has little role in the management of acute carotid artery rupture because brain ischemia cannot be corrected in a timely fashion. Revascularization procedures involving the cervical carotid or as part of an intracranial-extracranial bypass may potentiate a hemorrhagic component to a preexisting ischemic stroke. Once rupture has occurred, control of bleeding is of paramount importance.

33.4 Diagnosis

Impending rupture of the common carotid artery

33.5 Medical Management

Immediate response by physicians and nursing staff is crucial in this life-threatening emergency. Airway, breathing, and circulation should be addressed in a coordinated and calm fashion. It is helpful to have a "crash cart" and tracheostomy tray brought to the room.

Digital pressure should be applied in the wound to control bleeding. Attempting to clamp the carotid artery in this setting is not advisable. Friable tissue and lack of visualization may worsen the bleeding. In general, direct pressure until transfer to the operating room will suffice.

Control of the airway by qualified staff is of paramount importance. A suction setup should be present and functioning. If a tracheotomy is present, a cuffed tracheostomy tube should be used to control and exclude the airway. In laryngectomy patients, the stoma should also be controlled with a cuffed tube. In the case of intraoral rupture, bleeding can be controlled with a tonsil sponge as external digital pressure is applied. If this is not successful, the airway should be kept clear of blood and clot with suction. Oxygen therapy with pulse oximetry should be initiated. In the case of respiratory arrest, the airway is secured with orotracheal intubation or tracheostomy with Ambu bag ventilation.

Simultaneously, large-bore intravenous (IV) access, 14- or 16-gauge peripheral IV catheters, or central venous access should be secured. As this is done, complete blood count and chemistries are sent. A type and cross for 4 units of blood should be drawn at this time. Balanced saline should be rapidly infused to stabilize blood pressure and pulse. Blood products are requested when the operating room is notified. These steps should be performed by physicians and nursing staff simultaneously. Commonly the patient maintains consciousness throughout the ordeal.

33.6 Surgical Management

This patient presented quickly after a sentinel bleeding, allowing time for endovascular studies. The patient passed his balloon occlusion study, allowing ligation of his common carotid artery in a controlled setting.

Acute carotid artery rupture should be transported immediately to the operating room with a physician in attendance. The patient is placed under general anesthesia as fluid resuscitation continues. Hypotension and subsequent cerebral hypoperfusion should be avoided during both the intraoperative and the postoperative period. IV access is finalized and the patient is prepped and draped with continuous digital pressure still controlling the bleeding source. The goal of surgical exploration in this setting is to ligate the carotid and exclude the proximal and distal stumps from the infected wound and salivary fistula. The carotid artery should be isolated and dissected proximally and distally until suitable sites for ligation are identified. Ligation with a vascular stapling device or running Prolene is simple and minimally traumatic. Once ligation is accomplished, it is prudent to cover the arterial ends with a regional flap and attempt closure of the pharyngocutaneous fistula. A pectoralis flap is an excellent source of regional tissue that may be harvested for this purpose. The use of a controlled fistula to direct saliva away from the stumps of the carotid artery should also be considered.

33.7 Rehabilitation and Follow-up

Even after successful management of an acute carotid artery rupture, the patient may require long-term care for neurologic sequelae. In patients with recurrent unresectable malignancy, palliative care, including hospice, should be initiated. When carotid artery rupture occurs after ablative surgery or secondary to soft tissue necrosis after radiotherapy, routine cancer treatment and rehabilitation should be initiated after the patient recovers. In summary, carotid artery rupture is a dreaded complication of head and neck surgery. In general, carotid artery rupture can be prevented with the steps outlined above. When faced with carotid artery rupture, coordinated teamwork directed toward timely surgical intervention can be lifesaving.

33.8 Questions

1. Initial management of carotid artery rupture includes
   a) Applying direct pressure at the bleeding site.
   b) Securing the airway.
   c) Obtaining large-bore intravenous (IV) access.
   d) Notifying the operating room staff.
   e) All of the above.
2. Which of the following is not a risk factor for carotid artery rupture?

a) Pharyngocutaneous fistula.
b) Local wound infection.
c) Previous radiation therapy.
d) Tracheostomy.
e) Neck dissection.
3. Which of the following steps may help prevent carotid artery rupture?
   a) Avoidance of trifurcating neck incisions.
   b) Maintaining a fascial covering over the carotid artery during neck dissection.
   c) Providing adequate nutrition in the perioperative period.
   d) Covering the carotid with vascularized tissue or dermal grafts.
   e) All the above.

Answers: 1. e 2. d 3. e

Suggested Readings

Cohen J, Rad I. Contemporary management of carotid blowout. Curr Opin Otolaryngol Head Neck Surg. 2004; 12(2):110–115

Simental A, Johnson JT, Horowitz M. Delayed complications of endovascular stenting for carotid blowout. Am J Otolaryngol. 2003; 24(6):417–419

Upile T, Triaridis S, Kirkland P, et al. The management of carotid artery rupture. Eur Arch Otorhinolaryngol. 2005; 262(7):555–560

34 Osteoradionecrosis of the Mandible

Amy M. Manning and Yash J. Patil

34.1 History

A 52-year-old man was referred to the ear, nose, and throat (ENT) clinic for management of a 3-year history of progressive right jaw pain and a 2-week history of increased right face, jaw, and neck swelling and erythema. Eight years ago, he underwent excision of the right submandibular gland at an outside institution for myoepithelial carcinoma. He was treated with external beam radiation therapy after surgery. He developed recurrent myoepithelial carcinoma of the right neck 4 years prior to referral to our ENT clinic, at which time he underwent right neck dissection followed by re-irradiation. After his second course of radiation therapy, he noted fracture of multiple right mandibular teeth and subsequently underwent dental extractions. At the time of presentation to our clinic he reported constant oral and jaw pain radiating to the ipsilateral ear as well as xerostomia. He denied dysphagia or odynophagia but reported inability to eat solid food due to pain with chewing.

Physical exam revealed an afebrile, thin man who appeared his stated age. There was significant erythema and soft tissue edema over his right lower face, mandible and upper neck. The area was warm to touch, but there was no associated fluctuance. Nasal and ear exams were normal. Intraoral exam was significant for exposed necrotic bone along the right lingual cortex of the mandible. Intraoral mucosa was dry but otherwise healthy appearing. The neck exam was consistent with postoperative and postradiation changes, with no palpable mass or lymphadenopathy. Flexible fiberoptic laryngoscopy was within normal limits.

Computed tomography (CT) of the neck with contrast was obtained for operative planning purposes and to rule out recurrent disease. The CT showed lytic, moth-eaten bone in the body of the right mandible with associated pathologic fracture (▶ Fig. 34.1). There was significant overlying soft tissue edema and fat stranding. The patient was treated with a course of oral clindamycin for presumed acute cellulitis and subsequently taken to the operating room for right hemimandibulectomy and fibula free flap reconstruction of the mandible. Final pathology revealed osteonecrosis and abscess formation with fibrosis. Tissue Gram stain was consistent with gram-positive cocci in pairs and clusters.

34.2 Differential Diagnosis—Key Points

- The presence of necrotic exposed bone and pathologic fracture in a previously radiated field raises concern for both osteonecrosis and recurrent malignancy. Recurrent disease may coexist with osteonecrosis. Osteoradionecrosis (ORN) is defined as devitalized, exposed irradiated bone tissue that fails to heal over a period of 3 months in the absence of residual or recurrent malignancy.
- There are several theories behind the pathogenesis of ORN of the mandible, including reduced healing ability of hypoxic, hypovascular, hypocellular radiated bone. Recent evidence proposes that ORN occurs due to a radiation-induced fibroatrophic mechanism, including free radical formation, endothelial dysfunction, microvascular thrombosis, fibrosis, remodeling, and tissue necrosis.
- While often associated with postirradiation dental extractions, ORN of the mandible can occur in the context of pre-irradiation dental extractions, spontaneously, following surgery, or from trauma due to prosthetics.
- Microorganisms can typically be cultured from the surface of ORN tissue samples; however, infection appears to play a relatively minor role in the pathogenesis of ORN, and ORN is not synonymous with osteomyelitis. There is no role for

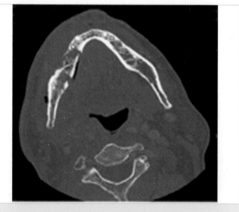

Fig. 34.1 Axial noncontrast CT scan of the neck and face at the level of the body of the mandible, showing lytic, necrotic bone of the right mandible with associated pathologic fracture.

prophylactic antibiotic treatment in preventing ORN.

- The risk of ORN increases with increasing radiation dose, with most cases occurring after > 60 Gy. The incidence of ORN has been decreasing over the last several decades with the advent of more efficient radiation therapy techniques. Pooled studies of patients radiated prior to 1968 showed an incidence of 11.8%, 5.4% from 1968 to 1992, and 3% in patients radiated since 1997. Other risk factors for ORN include malnutrition, immune suppression, peripheral vascular disease, alcohol and tobacco abuse, xerostomia, poor oral hygiene, and poor dentition.

34.3 Test Interpretation

There is no widely agreed upon set of requirements for the diagnosis of ORN or staging system to describe its extent. Various proposed staging systems have classified disease based on duration of symptoms and on extent of bony and soft tissue involvement. Recurrent or residual malignancy must be ruled out, and CT imaging of the face and neck with contrast can assist in this. Histopathologic examination should be done at the time of surgery, if applicable.

34.4 Diagnosis

Osteoradionecrosis of the mandible, complicated by acute cellulitis of surrounding tissues

34.5 Medical Management

Treatment of ORN starts with prevention. Good oral hygiene is paramount in radiated patients, including treatment of xerostomia. A preradiation dental evaluation is valuable. Dental extraction of healthy or restorable teeth is not widely recommended, as both pre- and postradiation extraction can lead to ORN. Additionally, ORN can be incited by ulceration from ill-fitting dentures. Good nutritional status is important in the treatment of any chronic wound.

The role of hyperbaric oxygen (HBO) in the treatment or prevention of ORN is controversial. At this time, multiple studies suggest that it may be useful as an adjunct to surgery but is not an effective treatment alone.

Based on the fibro-atrophic hypothesis of ORN pathogenesis, there is evidence to support the use of pentoxifylline, an antioxidant methylxanthine derivative, along with tocopherol (vitamin E), also with antioxidant effects. Further studies are needed regarding these regimens.

34.6 Surgical Management

Surgical management ranges from sequestrectomy, or removal of small portions of diseased bone with local tissue rearrangement closure, up to segmental resection with microvascular free flap reconstruction. Free tissue transfer reconstruction offers the advantage of bringing nonirradiated healthy tissue into the surgical field. Described flaps for free tissue reconstruction of mandibular defects include the osteocutaneous radial forearm, fibula, scapula, and iliac crest. The osteocutaneous radial forearm free flap provides a limited amount of bone for reconstruction because only one-third of the cross-sectional area of the radius can be harvested without increasing risk for donor site fracture. The fibular free flap is the workhorse of osteocutaneous mandible reconstruction and provides up to 20 to 25 cm of solid bicortical bone stock, generous soft tissue paddle, and large-diameter vascular pedicle. The iliac crest provides robust bone stock, but significant donor site morbidity and limitations in its soft tissue paddle limit its popularity. Fibula and iliac crest bone stock are both adequate for the placement of dental implants. The scapula free flap allows for the most flexible soft tissue paddle design of the described flaps, however, the donor location can make the two-team surgery approach difficult. The harvested bone is thin and is not adequate for the placement of dental implants.

34.7 Rehabilitation and Follow-up

The rates of flap failure and postoperative wound complications, including fistula formation, hardware exposure, and wound infection, may be higher in ORN reconstruction than for primary malignancy resection and reconstruction. Prior surgery and radiation obliterate tissue planes, while fibrotic radiated tissues are predisposed to wound breakdown. Donor vessels may be of poor quality within the radiated field and may have to be dissected from a more distal site, including the contralateral side.

34.8 Questions

1. Which of the following is not a requirement for the diagnosis of osteoradionecrosis (ORN) of the mandible?
   a) Absence of residual or recurrent malignancy.
   b) History of prior dental extractions.
   c) Exposed bone.
   d) Failure to heal over a period of 3 months.
2. Which type of free tissue transfer flap allows for dental implants in a reconstructed mandible?
   a) Osteocutaneous radial forearm.
   b) Iliac crest.
   c) Scapula.
   d) Anterolateral thigh.
3. All of the following are potential components of treatment or prevention of ORN of the mandible except
   a) Hyperbaric oxygen.
   b) Pre-radiation extraction of all remaining teeth.

c) Removal of dead and exposed bone.
d) Prevention of food by mouth (NPO).

Answers: 1. a 2. b 3. d

Suggested Readings

Cannady SB, Wax MK. In: Johnson JT, Rosen CA, et al, eds. Bailey's Head and Neck Surgery – Otolaryngology, 5th ed. Philadelphia, PA: Lippincott Williams & Wilkins; 2014

Marx RE. Osteoradionecrosis: a new concept of its pathophysiology. J Oral Maxillofac Surg. 1983; 41(5):283–288

Wahl MJ. Osteoradionecrosis prevention myths. Int J Radiat Oncol Biol Phys. 2006; 64(3):661–669

Madrid C, Abarca M, Bouferrache K. Osteoradionecrosis: an update. Oral Oncol. 2010; 46(6):471–474

Dhanda J, Pasquier D, Newman L, Shaw R. Current concepts in osteoradionecrosis after head and neck radiotherapy. Clin Oncol (R Coll Radiol). 2016; 28(7):459–466

Lee M, Chin RY, Eslick GD, Sritharan N, Paramaesvaran S. Outcomes of microvascular free flap reconstruction for mandibular osteoradionecrosis: A systematic review. J Craniomaxillofac Surg. 2015; 43 (10):2026–2033

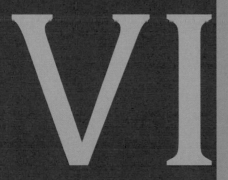

Part VI

The Larynx

VI

35 Laryngopharyngeal Reflux

Brian D. Goico and Rebecca J. Howell

35.1 History

A 45-year-old man presented to clinic with a progressive 3-month history of globus and chronic throat clearing. He denied voice changes, dysphagia, odynophagia, or weight loss. He denied a history of nasal congestion or postnasal drip. He denied epigastric pain but took antacids occasionally for heartburn, especially after he drank orange juice. He frequently ate when he got home from work at around 11:00 p.m. and went to bed 30 minutes later. He had never smoked, but reported one glass of red wine with dinner. On examination, he had no nasal septal deviation, normal-appearing turbinates, intact dentition, 2 + tonsils, and mild cobblestoning of the posterior pharyngeal wall. Fiberoptic examination (▶ Fig. 35.1) demonstrated substantial interarytenoid pachydermia and postcricoid watery edema.

35.2 Differential Diagnosis—Key Points

- Laryngopharyngeal reflux (LPR) has been implicated in many extraesophageal disorders, such as reflux laryngitis, subglottic stenosis, laryngeal carcinomas, vocal process granulomas, vocal nodules, chronic cough, and rhinitis. Esophageal disorders including esophageal dysmotility, Zenker's diverticulum, esophageal candidiasis, esophageal webs/strictures, esophageal adenocarcinoma, reflux, and Barrett's esophagitis are also associated with reflux disease. Although the classic "heartburn" symptoms of intermittent substernal and epigastric chest pain can be present, they occur in less than 40% of patients with LPR. Instead, patients with LPR present with a chronic progression of one or more symptoms including hoarseness, vocal fatigue, pitch breaks, throat clearing, excessive mucus, postnasal drip, dysphagia, coughing, choking, and/or globus pharyngeus. Validated survey instruments such as the Reflux Symptom Index can be useful for both diagnosis and outcome measures (▶ Table 35.1).
- Although they share a similar basic pathogenesis, there are many differences between LPR and gastroesophageal reflux disease (GERD). While GERD is thought to be the consequence of lower esophageal sphincter dysfunction, LPR is believed to result from dysfunction of the upper esophageal sphincter. Patients with LPR tend to be upright (daytime) refluxers, resulting in brief episodic acid exposure. In contrast, those with GERD tend to be supine nocturnal refluxers with prolonged acid exposure, which results from esophageal dysmotility leading to prolonged esophageal acid clearance. Despite these differences, however, it is important to note that there is a subpopulation of patients who experience both LPR and GERD.
- Several factors can predispose to the development of both GERD and LPR, including obesity, prolonged intubation, nasogastric tube placement, late-night meals, and certain types of foods including chocolate, fats, citrus fruits, carbonated beverages, spicy tomato-based products, red wines, and caffeine.

35.3 Test Interpretation

LPR is suspected based upon the history, physical examination, and bedside endoscopic findings. Improvement of symptoms with empiric therapy confirms the diagnosis in most cases. The following are the most common and important test findings associated with the condition:

1. Flexible laryngoscopy should be performed in all suspected cases both to look for signs of reflux and rule out malignancy. Findings most commonly associated with LPR include (1) erythema and edema of the posterior larynx, (2) interarytenoid pachydermia (thickening), (3) contact granulomas, (4) infraglottic edema resulting in a linear indentation of the medial edge of the vocal cord (pseudosulcus vocalis), and (5) pharyngeal cobblestoning (▶ Table 35.2).
2. In cases in which the diagnosis and/or treatment course is not clear, transnasal esophagoscopy (TNE) or esophagogastroduodenoscopy (EGD) are useful adjuncts in detecting signs of reflux esophagitis, Barrett's esophagus, and esophageal malignancy.
3. Videostroboscopy is a useful adjunct in patients presenting with hoarseness who are refractory to medical management of LPR. In this situation, alternative diagnosis should be considered, including benign mucosal lesions, vocal paresis,

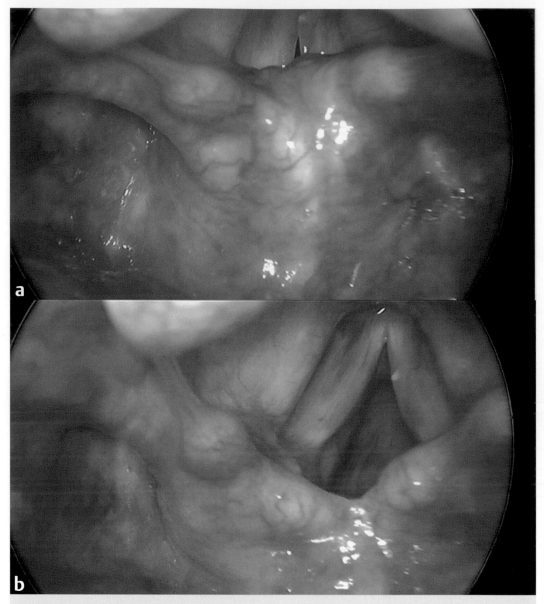

Fig. 35.1 (a) Vocal folds adducted. (b) Vocal folds abducted.

muscle tension dysphonia, vocal fold leukopla-kia, and microinvasive laryngeal carcinoma. All of these conditions have been misdiagnosed as LPR.

4. pH testing with/without impedance is the gold standard to confirm GERD/LPR caused by the reflux of gastric contents (impedance) or acid (pH monitor). pH testing is less reliable for LPR than for GERD because the placement of a dual pH probe (where the upper probe is 2 cm above the upper esophageal sphincter) is considered critical for accuracy. Impedance testing demon-strates the extent of both acid and nonacid reflux events. Testing both on and off reflux medications gives additional information for clinical management. Bile acids and pepsin have been linked to laryngeal cancer development even in the absence of pH abnormalities.

Table 35.1 The Reflux Symptom Index (RSI)

Within the last month, how did the following problems affect you?	0 = No problem 5 = Severe problem				
1. Hoarseness or a problem with your voice	1	2	3	4	5
2. Clearing your throat	1	2	3	4	5
3. Excess throat mucus or postnasal drip	1	2	3	4	5
4. Difficulty swallowing food, liquids, or pills	1	2	3	4	5
5. Coughing after you ate or after lying down	1	2	3	4	5
6. Breathing difficulty or choking episodes	1	2	3	4	5
7. Troublesome or annoying cough	1	2	3	4	5
8. Sensation of something sticking in your throat or a lump in your throat	1	2	3	4	5
9. Heartburn, chest pain, indigestion, or stomach acid coming up	1	2	3	4	5
	Total				

Source: Adapted from Belafsky et al. J Voice 2002;16(2):27277–277.

Table 35.2 Reflux Finding Score (RFS)

Subglottic edema	0—Absent 2—Present
Ventricular obliteration	2—Partial 4—Complete
Erythema/hyperemia	2—Arytenoid only 4—Diffuse
Vocal fold edema	1—Mild 2—Moderate 3—Severe 4—Polypoid
Diffuse laryngeal edema	1—Mild 2—Moderate 3—Severe 4—Obstructing
Posterior commissure hypertrophy	1—Mild 2—Moderate 3—Severe 4—Obstructing
Granuloma/granulation tissue	0—Absent 2—Present
Thick endolaryngeal mucus	0—Absent 2—Present

Source: Adapted from Belafsky et al. Laryngoscope 2001;111(8):1313–1317.

35.4 Diagnosis

Laryngopharyngeal reflux

35.5 Medical Management

The mainstay of treatment should focus on lifestyle modifications and dietary changes. If applicable, patients should be counseled on weight reduction, smoking cessation, head elevation while sleeping, and restricted intake of chocolate, caffeine, fats, citrus fruits, carbonated beverages, spicy tomato-based products, red wines, mints, and late-night meals. In refractory cases, patients may be asked to keep a food diary to identify additional triggers.

In patients for whom lifestyle modification provides inadequate symptom control, medical management is warranted on an empiric basis; however, the optimal drug, dose, and duration of treatment remain controversial. GERD/LPR can be treated with proton pump inhibitors (PPIs), histamine-2 (H2) blockers, and antacids. In PPI-responsive patients, symptoms will typically improve within 2 months, while improvements in laryngeal exam findings may not be evident for greater than 6 months. Patients who improve on reflux medications should have the medication titrated to the lowest dose tolerable. In patients who are refractory to medical management and/or endorse atypical symptoms, further evaluation is warranted.

35.6 Surgical Management

Although surgical indications for GERD are well defined, the indications for surgical management of LPR are not as clear. Nissen's fundoplication and partial fundoplication are the most common antireflux surgeries performed. However, there are increasing data supporting the use of endoscopic procedures (Stretta, Mederi Therapeutics Inc. Esophyx, EndoGastricSolutions Inc.) and lower esophageal sphincter augmentation (Linx, Torax Medical, Inc.). Additionally, in patients with reflux that results from refractory morbid obesity and its associated sequelae, weight loss surgery may be another consideration.

35.7 Questions

1. You are taking care of a 40-year-old patient with chronic hoarseness. Bedside fiberoptic examination demonstrates diffuse glottic erythema and edema. The patient is started on omeprazole 20 mg orally twice a day and instructed on dietary modification. There is no change in symptoms on 3-month follow-up examination. Which of the following is the best next step in management?
   a) Increase omeprazole to 40 mg 40 mg orally twice a day.
   b) Videostroboscopy.
   c) Transnasal esophagoscopy (TNE).
   d) Add ranitidine.
2. After what length of acid suppression therapy will the laryngeal endoscopic findings of laryngopharyngeal reflux (LPR) begin to resolve?

   a) 3 weeks.
   b) 6 weeks.
   c) 3 months.
   d) 6 months.
   e) 3 years.
3. Which of the following is not known to cause reflux of gastric contents?
   a) Tobacco.
   b) Mint.
   c) Ginger.
   d) Lemon juice.
   e) Coffee.

Answers: 1. b 2. d 3. c

Suggested Readings

Belafsky PC, Postma GN, Koufman JA. Validity and reliability of the reflux symptom index (RSI). J Voice. 2002; 16(2):274–277

Belafsky PC, Postma GN, Koufman JA. The validity and reliability of the reflux finding score (RFS). Laryngoscope. 2001; 111(8):1313–1317

Belafsky PC, Postma GN, Koufman JA. Laryngopharyngeal reflux symptoms improve before changes in physical findings. Laryngoscope. 2001; 111(6):979–981

Gooi Z, Ishman SL, Bock JM, Blumin JH, Akst LM. Changing patterns in reflux care: 10-year comparison of ABEA members. Ann Otol Rhinol Laryngol. 2015; 124(12):940–946

Koufman JA, Aviv JE, Casiano RR, Shaw GY. Laryngopharyngeal reflux: position statement of the committee on speech, voice, and swallowing disorders of the American Academy of Otolaryngology-Head and Neck Surgery. Otolaryngol Head Neck Surg. 2002; 127 (1):32–35

Koufman JA. The otolaryngologic manifestations of gastroesophageal reflux disease (GERD): a clinical investigation of 225 patients using ambulatory 24-hour pH monitoring and an experimental investigation of the role of acid and pepsin in the development of laryngeal injury. Laryngoscope. 1991; 101(4 Pt 2) Suppl 53:1–78

36 Reinke's Edema

Hayley L. Born and Rebecca J. Howell

36.1 History

A 64-year-old woman presented with voice changes noticed by her family and her primary care physician (PCP). She reported that her voice had always been rough and deep. She was frequently confused for a man over the telephone. The patient had a history of chronic obstructive pulmonary disease (COPD) and occasional reflux, and she had smoked half a pack of cigarettes per day for 30 years. She denied dysphagia, cough, postnasal drip, or neck masses. She did admit to feeling short of breath, especially with lying flat at night. Her PCP had ordered a chest X-ray, which was normal, and prescribed an inhaled steroid for presumed COPD. However, her positional symptoms had not improved.

On examination, the patient had a low-pitched, rough voice but was breathing comfortably without evidence of stridor or tachypnea. Flexible laryngoscopy demonstrated redundant epithelium and edema of the membranous vocal folds. During inhalation the open space was limited to the posterior glottis (▶ Fig. 36.1). There was slight asymmetry of the left greater than right folds and mild hypervascularity of both folds. There was no leukoplakia and no discrete masses or cysts. The folds moved symmetrically and were able to fully abduct and adduct. The strobe light could not be adequately synchronized due to aperiodicity and irregular mucosal wave bilaterally.

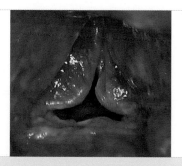

Fig. 36.1 True vocal folds with bilateral polypoid degeneration of the membranous vocal folds consistent with Reinke's edema as seen on inspiration.

36.2 Differential Diagnosis—Key Points

- The superficial layer of the lamina propria (SLP), also known as Reinke's space, is a potential space consisting of loose connective tissue. When fluid collects in this space, it is called Reinke's edema. Generally speaking the fluid extends along the length of the vocal fold, primarily collecting on the superior and medial aspects of the true vocal fold.
- The fluid in Reinke's edema is usually watery and clear but can become more mucoid and cloudy as the disease progresses. It is generally seen bilaterally but is commonly asymmetric.
- The primary association with Reinke's edema is smoking, with longer duration of tobacco use exerting a more negative effect on the histologic lesion. Reinke's edema is more commonly diagnosed in older women (> 39 years old). Vocal abuse and gastroesophageal reflux are other causal factors in Reinke's edema.
- Commonly, patients present with complaints of lower vocal pitch. Mass and fundamental frequency (modal pitch) are inversely proportional, where increasing mass causes a decrease in frequency (i.e., lower pitch). Furthermore, patients with Reinke's edema have increased subglottal pressure and decreased maximum phonation time, clinically resulting in increased effort of voicing.
- Reinke's edema is not a precancerous lesion. Therefore, it is a nonsurgical disease unless it is associated with shortness of breath or stridor without other clinical cause for dyspnea. If the edema becomes severe enough, it can cause static obstruction or dynamic collapse during adduction of the vocal folds.

36.3 Test Interpretation

Flexible laryngoscopy reveals large folds with watery submucosal inclusions without distinct lesions, consistent with Reinke's edema. Stroboscopy can be utilized to evaluate mucosal waves; however, in moderate to severe edema, waves may not be evident and/or the strobe light may be unable to synchronize with the irregularity of the waves.

36.4 Diagnosis

Reinke's edema with hoarseness and mild airway obstruction

36.5 Medical Management

Mild to moderate cases of edema without airway obstruction may be monitored clinically. In patients complaining of dysphonia, treatment options include voice therapy, in-office KTP laser, or microflap surgery. Smoking cessation is critical to prevent recurrence.

36.6 Surgical Management

Absolute indications for surgery in Reinke's edema are
- Airway obstruction.
- Concern for neoplastic lesions underlying the vocal fold abnormality (rare).

Smoking cessation is not a prerequisite for surgery; however, the patient should be informed that recurrence is very likely if smoking continues.

Surgical intervention involves an incision in the superior lateral aspect of the true vocal fold. Mucosal flaps are raised, taking care to leave some of the lamina propria over the ligament to avoid scarring. The fluid is suctioned out of Reinke's space and any excess mucosa is trimmed. The flap is then laid back in place. Special attention should be paid when correcting bilateral edema, as anterior webbing can occur with bilateral vocal fold intervention. Attempts should be made to avoid the anterior commissure during incision and flap formation due to risk of iatrogenic anterior web.

36.7 Rehabilitation and Follow-up

Smoking cessation is essential. No regular monitoring is needed for these patients beyond the immediate postoperative period. Patients should be encouraged to return as needed with increasing symptoms, as recurrence is common.

36.8 Questions

1. The primary risk factor for the development of Reinke's edema is
   a) Gastroesophageal reflux disease (GERD).
   b) Obesity.
   c) Alcohol use/abuse.
   d) Smoking.
   e) Voice use/abuse.
2. Patients with Reinke's edema most commonly complain of which change in their voice?
   a) Decreased pitch.
   b) Decreased volume.
   c) Breathiness.
   d) Increased pitch.
3. Reinke's edema is most likely
   a) Seen in teenagers.
   b) Gradual in onset.
   c) Associated with vocal nodules.
   d) Cured with acid reduction medication such as proton pump inhibitors.

Answers: 1. d 2. a 3. b

Suggested Readings

Zeitels SM, Hillman RE, Bunting GW, Vaughn T. Reinke's edema: phonatory mechanisms and management strategies. Ann Otol Rhinol Laryngol. 1997; 106(7 Pt 1):533–543

Marcotullio D, Magliulo G, Pezone T. Reinke's edema and risk factors: clinical and histopathologic aspects. Am J Otolaryngol. 2002; 23(2):81–84

Zhukhovitskaya A, Battaglia D, Khosla SM, Murry T, Sulica L. Gender and age in benign vocal fold lesions. Laryngoscope. 2015; 125 (1):191–196

Lim JY, Choi JN, Kim KM, Choi HS. Voice analysis of patients with diverse types of Reinke's edema and clinical use of electroglottographic measurements. Acta Otolaryngol. 2006; 126(1):62–69

Martins RH, Fabro AT, Domingues MA, Chi AP, Gregório EA. Is Reinke's edema a precancerous lesion? Histological and electron microscopic aspects. J Voice. 2009; 23(6):721–725

37 Spasmodic Dysphonia

Tasneem A. Shikary and Sid M. Khosla

37.1 History

A 49-year-old woman presented with dysphonia for several years. She described her voice as breaking often and "going in and out." Her symptoms were precipitated by an upper respiratory infection. She stated that her speech was worse when talking on the phone and during stressful situations, but she noted improvement after having an alcoholic beverage. Her voice caused her great personal distress. Her medical history was remarkable only for mild anxiety. She denied smoking, heartburn, hemoptysis, throat clearing, and allergy problems. She had seen several health professionals for her symptoms, and prior treatments included speech therapy, antibiotics, and reflux medication with minimal improvement.

During conversation, the patient's voice was noted to have a strained and strangled quality with abrupt cessation and return of phonation. At times there was a notable tremulousness to her voice. Although she could not count to 10 without intermittent stoppages, she was able to sing her favorite song normally without any voice breaks. Her head and neck examination was otherwise unremarkable. Her neurologic examination was notable only for a fine hand tremor, but cranial nerve exam was normal. Flexible laryngoscopy showed normal-appearing, fully mobile vocal cords without any masses or sulci. During speech, the patient's vocal cords abruptly adducted forcefully corresponding to phonatory stoppages.

37.2 Differential Diagnosis—Key Points

- Spasmodic dysphonia (SD): This neurologic disorder most often manifests in the larynx as a strangled vocal quality with abrupt phonatory stoppages associated with a "choppy" voice. The three forms of laryngeal dystonia consist of adductor SD, abductor SD, and mixed SD. *Adductor SD* is the most common form and is characterized by a strained voice quality with breaks in vocalization. Abductor SD is characterized by a breathy voice quality with intermittent breaks in vocalization. Mixed SD has characteristics of both adductor and abductor laryngeal dystonias. Although many SD patients have a family history of dystonias, which may be associated with chromosome 9, the cause of the underlying SD is largely unknown. SD affects more women than men, with age at presentation usually during the 40 s or 50 s. Occasionally, there is an associated hand tremor. However, it is important to distinguish between essential tremor and SD.

- Essential laryngeal tremor: Essential tremor causes shaking of the head, hands, and voice. The tremor is typically not present at rest and is worse with emotional stress or fatigue. Essential laryngeal tremor manifests as a regular, 4- to 12-Hz tremor seen in the vocal cords during speech and respiration. In contrast, the tremor found in SD is irregular. Vocal tremor can be the only symptom in some patients. The vocal tremor represents rhythmic laryngeal movement, presenting as rhythmic pitch and loudness alterations during speech. Essential tremor can be seen concomitantly with SD.

- Muscle tension dysphonia: Affected individuals are usually unable to sing or whisper without voice breaks. The dysphonia is worse under stressful situations. Unlike SD, intraword phonatory breaks are infrequent. Patients are more likely to exhibit excessive contraction of the intrinsic and extrinsic laryngeal muscles, with an overadduction of the true or false vocal cords or even the supraglottis. Muscle tension dysphonia is most commonly treated with voice therapy. Occasionally botulinum toxin type A is used in conjunction with voice therapy to release the abnormal muscle activation patterns.

- Neurologic disorders: Although not likely to be the initial or sole manifestation, systematic neurologic diseases must be considered during the initial evaluation. Movement disorders such as Parkinson's disease, Huntington's disease, tardive dyskinesia, and cerebellar disorders need to be excluded with a complete neurologic examination. Other neurologic diseases to consider include myoclonus and Meige's syndrome. Oculopalatal myoclonus presents as an involuntary movement of the head and neck region, including the soft palate, pharynx, larynx, and eyes. Laryngeal involvement presents as broken speech. Indirect laryngoscopy would show that the vocal cords have a slow, rhythmic adduction and abduction at the same frequency as the other myoclonic tics. Meige's syndrome consists of myoclonic spasms of the eyelids, pharynx, tongue, floor of the mouth, and larynx.

37.3 Test Interpretation

When no overt laryngeal pathology is found, physiologic tests are indicated to further investigate the cause of the hoarseness.

37.3.1 Speech Evaluation

Patients with SD demonstrate intermittent glottal stops and pitch breaks with speech that are due to excessive and untimely contraction of the adductor laryngeal muscles. This accounts for the strained vocal quality and abrupt stoppages as the glottis squeezes shut. The muscle largely responsible for adductor SD is the thyroarytenoid muscle. Patients are also often unable to carry a constant pitch and exhibit reduced voice loudness. The voice quality may be monotonal with glottal fry and vocal tremor. Characteristic findings of adductor SD can be elicited when the patient is asked to read sentences that have voiced consonants followed by vowels, such as "I eat apples and eggs" or "The dog has a new bone." Interestingly, patients are able to whisper or sing without the usual strangled vocal quality or glottal breaks. Emotional speech and speaking in a falsetto also diminish symptoms.

Abductor SD is characterized by incomplete glottic closure and abrupt glottal openings secondary to hypercontraction of the posterior cricoarytenoid (PCA) muscle, which causes breathy vocal quality and abrupt stoppages. Laryngeal tremor may also be noted. The quality of the abductor SD can be elicited with sentences that alternate between voiceless consonants (h, f, l, p, s, t, th) and vowels, such as "How high is Harry's hat?" and "Did he go to the right or to the left?"

37.3.2 Acoustic Analysis

Adductor SD is characterized by aperiodic segments followed by frequency shifts and phonatory breaks. The location of each of these acoustic events is within the midportion of the vowel production. Patients with SD also exhibit greater jitter and shimmer. Increased perturbations and a reduced signal-to-noise ratio are seen in both SD and essential tremor. Unlike essential tremor patients, tremor analysis does not reveal a laryngeal tremor in SD patients. Also, the signal-to-noise

ratio is even lower with abductor SD because of periods of voicelessness.

SD is a "task-specific" laryngeal dystonia; that is, the severity of dysphonia varies depending on the demands of the vocal task. Voice produced in connected speech as compared with sustained vowels is said to provoke more frequent and severe laryngeal spasms. Reduced dysphonia severity during sustained vowels supports task specificity in adductor SD but not muscle tension dysphonia.

37.3.3 Electromyography

Although electromyography (EMG) is not necessary for the diagnosis of SD, it can be useful to guide therapy. During phonation, EMG would show bursts of electrical activity at rest and enlarged motor unit action potentials in the affected muscle(s). Botulinum toxin injections can be directed to specific muscles using EMG guidance. EMG shows abnormally high resting potential in the thyroarytenoid muscle in adductor SD. There is imbalance between the thyroarytenoid and cricothyroid musculature that contributes to the increased tension in the laryngeal anteroposterior dimension.

37.4 Diagnosis

Adductor spasmodic dysphonia

37.5 Medical Management

Botulinum toxin type A is used to chemically denervate the laryngeal muscles by blocking the release of presynaptic acetylcholine at the neuromuscular junction. EMG-guided injection of botulinum toxin is used widely for the treatment of SD. A monopolar, hollow-bored Teflon-coated EMG needle connected to an EMG recorder is used to inject botulinum toxin. For adductor SD, botulinum toxin is injected transorally or percutaneously into the thyroarytenoid muscle. During percutaneous injection, the needle is passed through the cricothyroid membrane just off midline and directed just lateral to each thyroarytenoid muscle. For abductor SD, botulinum toxin is injected into the PCA muscle. Abductor injection requires grasping the larynx and rotating it to expose the PCA. The patient is asked to sniff, which causes abduction as the EMG indicates action potentials. The effective dose of botulinum toxin to achieve the desired vocal results varies from one individual to another and thus requires titration. The dose can vary from 1 mouse unit to up to 10 mouse units to one or both muscles. Some practitioners stage PCA botulinum toxin injections by 2 weeks after confirming that there is adequate abduction of the previously injected vocal cord. After injection, botulinum toxin can take up to 72 hours to take effect. Patients will note an improvement in their voice within this period. Although the voice is not totally normal, patients are generally satisfied with the improvement in speech following treatment. Side effects include temporary breathiness, possibly mild aspiration, and possibly mild dysphagia for up to 7 days after initial injection. The effects of botulinum toxin may last up to 6 months. Individual titration of botulinum toxin and repeated injections are necessary.

Voice therapy has been used with little success to treat SD primarily. Most techniques attempt to reduce the degree of vocal tightness and the incidence of voice breaks. Biofeedback, inverse phonation (speaking during inspiration), and identification and correction of dysfunctional vocal habits have all been used with low levels of success.

37.6 Surgical Management

A variety of surgical techniques have been used to treat SD. Interventions include recurrent laryngeal nerve denervation alone, selective recurrent laryngeal nerve denervation and reinnervation, thyroplasty type II, and intrinsic laryngeal muscle myectomies. Although recurrent laryngeal nerve section had initially favorable results, long-term results showed recurrence of SD symptoms. More recently, recurrent laryngeal nerve denervation and reinnervation techniques have been used for SD. One method involves the denervation of the adductor branch of the recurrent laryngeal nerve, followed by reanastomosis of distal branches to the ansa cervicalis. Complications include moderate to severe breathiness. Variations in thyroarytenoid myectomies have been applied to adductor SD using microlaryngeal techniques and radiofrequency myothermy. Although novel surgical endeavors may be promising for the amelioration of SD symptoms, the current standard of care consists of botulinum toxin injection to the affected vocal muscles with good results and improved quality of life.

37.7 Rehabilitation and Follow-up

Patients with SD require repeat botulinum toxin injections every 3 to 6 months. They may participate in voice therapy to address any negative compensatory vocal behavior, but it generally plays a minor role in SD treatment.

37.8 Questions

1. A 56-year-old woman has chronic hoarseness of several months' duration. Although she has a slight hand tremor, the remainder of her neurologic examination is normal. What finding would most likely suggest muscle tension dysphonia?
   a) She whispers without voice breaks.
   b) Occasional vocal tremor is detected.
   c) Spectral analysis shows frequent intraword phonatory breaks.
   d) Laryngoscopy shows adduction of false vocal cords and supraglottic squeeze.
   e) Severity of phonation is not task dependent.

2. A 59-year-old woman has chronic hoarseness of several months' duration. Her voice is not raspy or breathy but does have a tremulous quality. On indirect laryngoscopy, her vocal cords are mobile, although mild bowing is present. What finding would most likely exclude a diagnosis of essential tremor?
   a) Absence of a hand tremor.
   b) 12-Hz regular laryngeal tremor.
   c) Acoustic analysis shows reduced signal-to-noise ratio.
   d) Dysphonia worsens during stressful situations.
   e) Tremor analysis does not show a laryngeal tremor.

3. A patient with abductor spasmodic dysphonia (SD) would most likely have a pronounced problem phonating which of the following sentences without breaks?
   a) "I eat apples and eggs."
   b) "The dog has a new bone."
   c) "Did he go to the right or to the left?"
   d) "I went to the store."
   e) "Mary has been there, too."

Answers: 1. d 2. e 3. c

Suggested Readings

Casserly P, Timon C. Botulinum toxin A injection under electromyographic guidance for treatment of spasmodic dysphonia. J Laryngol Otol. 2008; 122(1):52–56

Chan SW, Baxter M, Oates J, Yorston A. Long-term results of type II thyroplasty for adductor spasmodic dysphonia. Laryngoscope. 2004; 114(9):1604–1608

Chang CY, Chabot P, Thomas JP. Relationship of botulinum dosage to duration of side effects and normal voice in adductor spasmodic dysphonia. Otolaryngol Head Neck Surg. 2007; 136(6):894–899

Chhetri DK, Berke GS. Treatment of adductor spasmodic dysphonia with selective laryngeal adductor denervation and reinnervation surgery. Otolaryngol Clin North Am. 2006; 39(1):101–109

Grillone GA, Chan T. Laryngeal dystonia. Otolaryngol Clin North Am. 2006; 39(1):87–100

Merati AL, Heman-Ackah YD, Abaza M, Altman KW, Sulica L, Belamowicz S. Common movement disorders affecting the larynx: a report from the neurolaryngology committee of the AAO-HNS. Otolaryngol Head Neck Surg. 2005; 133(5):654–665

Nakamura K, Muta H, Watanabe Y, Mochizuki R, Yoshida T, Suzuki M. Surgical treatment for adductor spasmodic dysphonia–efficacy of bilateral thyroarytenoid myectomy under microlaryngoscopy. Acta Otolaryngol. 2008; 128(12):1348–1353

Roy N, Whitchurch M, Merrill RM, Houtz D, Smith ME. Differential diagnosis of adductor spasmodic dysphonia and muscle tension dysphonia using phonatory break analysis. Laryngoscope. 2008; 118(12):2245–2253

Sapienza CM, Walton S, Murry T. Acoustic variations in adductor spasmodic dysphonia as a function of speech task. J Speech Lang Hear Res. 1999; 42(1):127–140

38 Unilateral Vocal Fold Paralysis

Andrew J. Redmann and Sid M. Khosla

38.1 History

A 45-year-old woman presented with breathy dysphonia that occurred following an anterior cervical fusion 1 year ago. She underwent an injection laryngoplasty 6 months ago, which helped the quality of her voice. However, over the last month, she had noticed her voice quality decreasing and increasing breathiness. She reported mild dyspnea with exercise, which did not improve after the laryngoplasty. She did not have signs or symptoms of aspiration and denied previous neck surgery.

On physical exam, she was found to have an immobile right vocal cord. The right vocal process was significantly anterior and superior, relative to the normal left side. On inspiration, both the arytenoid mucosa and the right vocal fold moved toward the intraglottal space, producing significant collapse of the airway (▶ Fig. 38.1). This was not seen during expiration. There was a moderate vocal fold gap, and her voice was mildly breathy.

38.2 Differential Diagnosis—Key Points

- Unilateral vocal fold paralysis (UVFP) usually presents with a glottal gap. This gap may increase in the first 6 months if the thyroarytenoid muscle atrophies, or it may improve if there is some reinnervation. If there is reinnervation, this may increase tone and bulk of the vocal fold, but due to synkinesis, there may not be any movement. Many symptoms may result from a membranous vocal fold gap, including a breathy, soft voice; decreased phonation time; and decreased ability to cough. In addition to a vocal fold gap, this patient also demonstrated asymmetry in vocal fold length, height, and tension. If the reinnervation is minimal, the position of the arytenoid will also change. For example, if there is minimal tone in the posterior cricoarytenoid, the arytenoid can tilt anteriorly, producing a vocal process that is anterior and superior to the normal vocal process. The combination of atrophy of the vocalis and thyroarytenoid muscles

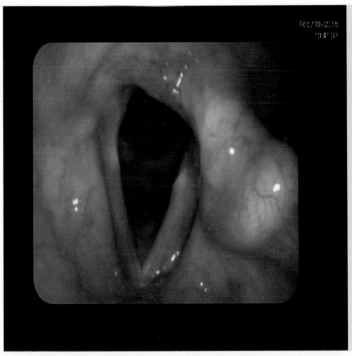

Fec/19/2016
04:37

Fig. 38.1 Left vocal fold paralysis with the left arytenoid prolapsed anteriorly.

and this abnormal positioning results in less tension in the left fold relative to the right. This asymmetric tension may produce an abnormal voice. Unilateral paralysis can be caused by trauma, iatrogenic injury to the recurrent laryngeal nerve (carotid, thyroid, anterior cervical disk, and chest surgery most commonly) and malignant invasion into the vagus or RLN.

- Bilateral vocal fold paralysis (BVFP): In general, stridor is not seen in UVFP, but it can be seen in BVFP. However, in some cases of unilateral paralysis, the anterior position of the arytenoid allows it to be close to the mucosa of the right fold, and the surfaces are close enough that negative pressures, owing to Bernoulli's law, cause a dynamic collapse during inspiration. Collapse is also more likely when the paralyzed fold has little tone and is very floppy. According to Bernoulli's law, the negative pressures increase as the air velocity increases. Thus, if a person is breathing harder, the collapse will worsen.

- Cricoarytenoid fixation must be ruled out through direct palpation of the joint. Arytenoid dislocations can sometimes be recognized by the position of the arytenoid in either an anterior or posterior location, most often after endotracheal intubation. Trauma, previous surgery, or diseases such as rheumatoid arthritis can also cause fixation mimicking vocal fold paralysis.

38.3 Test Interpretation

1. Computed tomography (CT): In this case, it was assumed that the recurrent laryngeal nerve was injured during spine surgery. If the cause is not known, imaging needs to be done along the course of the nerve. A CT scan of the neck (skull base to superior mediastinum) is indicated. A full chest CT scan is not needed so long as the neck CT extends to the aortic arch on the left side due to the path of the recurrent laryngeal nerve (looping under the aorta and then back up into the neck).

2. Video stroboscopy or flexible transnasal laryngoscopy: A recorded examination helps with diagnosis, follow-up, and surgical planning, if needed. If the vocal folds are vibrating, video stroboscopy is necessary to evaluate vibrations.

3. Maximum phonation time (MPT): This measurement can easily be taken in the clinic by measuring how long the patient can sustain a vowel sound. Although MPT can vary depending on the patient's effort, it is a good general measure of air leakage and can be used to monitor progress. Normal MPT is 25 to 35 seconds in adult males and 15 to 25 seconds in adult females. This patient had an MPT of 7 seconds.

4. Patient assessment of the effect of his or her voice problems: Questionnaires such as the Voice Handicap Index can be used for this purpose.

The following tests can be done but are not necessary in all cases.

1. Laryngeal electromyelography (EMG): In this patient, EMG showed spontaneous activity without any voluntary motor units, indicating that return of function was unlikely. Polyphasic action potentials indicate a higher likelihood of recovery. In general, EMG can help predict whether recovery will occur. In addition, it helps differentiate between recurrent laryngeal nerve injury and cricoarytenoid fixation. It is typically performed between 1 and 6 months after the onset of paralysis.

2. Acoustic tests: Acoustic tests will reveal a high amount of broadband noise, which will be reflected by a low signal-to-noise ratio, a low harmonic-to-noise ratio, or a low cepstral peak prominence.

3. Aerodynamic tests: These tests will demonstrate leakage of air during phonation.

4. Modified barium swallow: In instances where there is clinical concern for aspiration, a modified barium swallow may provide additional information for surgical planning, as aspiration of liquids is an indication for arytenoid adduction in patients undergoing medialization thyroplasty.

38.4 Diagnosis

Right vocal fold paralysis secondary to iatrogenic injury to the recurrent laryngeal nerve

38.5 Medical Management

The management of vocal fold paralysis is voice therapy, which can be used to add bulk to the paralyzed fold and to help avoid compensatory habits, such as increased muscle tension or false fold phonation. Many patients with UVFP do well with voice therapy alone, provided the paralyzed vocal fold assumes a median or paramedian position.

38.6 Surgical Management

Management of vocal fold paralysis is based on the length of the paralysis and whether the patient has significant voice or aspiration issues. Treatment is divided into short-term or long-term options. Long-term options should not be attempted before 6 to 12 months after the onset of paralysis.

The most common short-term option is injection laryngoplasty, which involves injecting a filler substance into the paraglottic space. This can be done in the clinic through a variety of approaches: transoral, immediately superior to the thyroid notch, through the thyroid cartilage, or through the cricothyroid membrane. A variety of substances are available for injection, including fat, acellular cadaveric dermis (Cymetra, LifeCell Corp.), aqueous glycerine/carboxymethylcellulose gel (Prolaryn, Merz North America) and calcium hydroxylapatite (Prolaryn Plus, Merz North America). (▶ Table 38.1) Current data suggest that early intervention with injection laryngoplasty may decrease the need for definitive laryngeal framework surgery.

Long-term options include thyroplasty type 1, arytenoid adduction, adduction arytenopexy, and ansa cervicalis–to–recurrent laryngeal nerve reinnervation. Thyroplasty is the most commonly used procedure and will reduce or close the vocal fold gap. This procedure is performed under local anesthesia, usually with intravenous sedation. It can be reversible. Arytenoid adduction mimics the action of the lateral cricoarytenoid and can be used to close a posterior glottic gap and partially restore the prephonatory position of the vocal fold. Adduction arytenopexy mimics the effect of the intrinsic muscles, including the intra-arytenoid. It is also used to stabilize the arytenoid in the anterior-posterior direction, much in the same way that the posterior cricoarytenoid does. A thyroplasty type 1 is always done in addition to an arytenoid repositioning procedure.

The laryngeal reinnervation procedure involves an anastomosis between the recurrent laryngeal nerve and a branch of the ansa cervicalis. It does not produce movement but can result in good muscle tone and bulk and a midline position. This usually takes 3 to 6 months to achieve, so an injection laryngoplasty is often done concurrently.

In this case, a thyroplasty type 1 and an arytenoid adduction were done. The patient's stridor completely resolved, and she was very happy with her voice results.

38.7 Rehabilitation and Follow-up

Following surgery, voice therapy is helpful for two reasons. The first is that many patients develop compensatory techniques when the fold is lateralized, and voice therapy is needed for retraining. The second is to teach patients how to use their voice most efficiently (e.g., teaching proper breath support).

38.8 Questions

1. Which of the following will arytenoid adduction most likely do?
   a) Decrease the maximum phonation time.
   b) Close a posterior gap.
   c) Reduce the amount of asymmetry of the airway.
   d) Result in an improved airway.
2. A patient has a left vocal fold paralysis without history of trauma or recent surgery. What is the most necessary testing?

Table 38.1 Materials for injection laryngoplasty

Material	Length of action	Advantages	Disadvantages
Acellular dermis (Cymetra)	2–4 months	• Low risk of reaction	• Variable length of action • Preparation time
Carboxymethylcellulose (Prolaryn)	1–3 months	• Ease of injection • Good for trial injection	• Minimal
Calcium Hydroxylapatite (Prolaryn Plus)	18 months	• Long lasting	• Unforgiving • VC stiffness with superficial injection
Autologous fat	>2 years	• Autologous material • Forgiving	• Requires harvest • Requires initial overinjection

a) Neck computed tomography (CT).
b) Head and neck CT down to just above the clavicle.
c) Head and neck CT; CT of mediastinum to the level of aortic arch.
d) Chest radiograph.
3. Treatment for unilateral paralysis includes all of the following except which one?
a) Injection of the vocal fold.
b) Reinnervation of recurrent laryngeal nerve.
c) Arytenoid adduction.
d) Reinnervation of superior laryngeal nerve.

Answers: 1. b 2. c 3. d

Suggested Readings

Richardson BE, Bastian RW. Clinical evaluation of vocal fold paralysis. Otolaryngol Clin North Am. 2004; 37(1):45–58

Paniello RC. Laryngeal reinnervation. Otolaryngol Clin North Am. 2004; 37(1):161–181, vii–viii

Zeitels SM. Vocal fold medialization: injection and laryngeal framework surgery. In: Rubin JS, Sataloff RT, Korovin GS, eds. Diagnosis and Treatment of Voice Disorders. San Diego, CA: Plural Publishing; 2006:713–726

Spataro EA, Grindler DJ, Paniello RC. Etiology and Time to Presentation of Unilateral Vocal Fold Paralysis. Otolaryngol Head Neck Surg. 2014; 151(2):286–293

Siu J, Tam S, Fung K. A comparison of outcomes in interventions for unilateral vocal fold paralysis: A systematic review. Laryngoscope. 2016; 126(7):1616–1624

Costello D. Change to earlier surgical interventions: contemporary management of unilateral vocal fold paralysis. Curr Opin Otolaryngol Head Neck Surg. 2015; 23(3):181–184

Munin MC, Heman-Ackah YD, Rosen CA, et al. Consensus statement: Using laryngeal electromyography for the diagnosis and treatment of vocal cord paralysis. Muscle Nerve. 2016; 53(6):850–855

39 Laryngeal Trauma

Ryan A. Crane and Sid M. Khosla

39.1 History

An 18-year-old man presented to the emergency department after a high-speed motor vehicle collision. An emergent cricothyrotomy was performed in the field to establish an airway. Initial trauma survey revealed no penetrating injuries, and abdominal ultrasound showed no evidence of intra-abdominal injury. There was significant swelling and crepitus of the anterior neck. Flexible fiberoptic examination showed a mucosal injury along the left true and false vocal folds. The right vocal fold was intact. The patient was stable and initial imaging was obtained (▶ Fig. 39.1).

39.2 Differential Diagnosis—Key Points

- Resuscitative measures following the advanced trauma life support (ATLS) guidelines are implemented for all serious injuries.
- Presenting symptoms of blunt laryngeal trauma include dyspnea, hoarseness, tenderness, cough, hemoptysis, and dysphagia. Signs of laryngeal trauma are edema, crepitus, subcutaneous emphysema, and flattening of the laryngeal prominence. Laryngotracheal separation can also present in this manner.

- A grading system for laryngeal trauma and management of the acute airway is reviewed in ▶ Table 39.1.
- A complete history of the mechanism of injury should be obtained, as well as any preexisting medical conditions. A thorough physical exam includes both palpation of the neck and a flexible fiberoptic laryngoscopy to evaluate endolaryngeal trauma.
- Concomitant injuries: Cervical spine injuries have been reported in up to 50% of patients with blunt laryngeal trauma. Recurrent laryngeal nerve palsies suggest a possible cricoid crush fracture. Pharyngoesophageal tears must also be evaluated.

39.3 Test Interpretation

Cervical spine and chest X-ray were clear. Neck computed tomography (CT) (▶ Fig. 39.1) revealed a vertical thyroid cartilage fracture just to the left of midline. There was a large amount of subcutaneous emphysema, and a small amount of gas was also noted along the internal aspect of the left thyroid lamina. No other airway injuries were identified. Facial imaging showed no evidence of facial fractures.

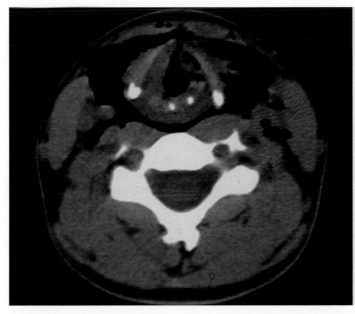

Fig. 39.1 Axial, noncontrasted CT scan of the neck demonstrating severe subcutaneous emphysema and a mildly displaced vertical fracture of the thyroid cartilage.

Table 39.1 Grading laryngeal trauma and managing the acute airway

Group	Features	Management
1	Minimal or no airway compromise; minor endo-layrngeal hematomas or lacerations	Conservative: humidified oxygen, 24-hour observation
2	Moderate edema, hematomas, and airway compromise; minor mucosal lacerations without cartilage exposure and nondisplaced laryngeal cartilage fracture	Tracheotomy under local anesthesia to prevent further damage to the airway by either endotracheal intubation or cricothyrotomy
3	Massive edema, exposed cartilage with large mucosal lacerations, and vocal fold immobility with displaced fractures	Same as group 2
4	Similar findings to group 3, plus more than two fracture lines and a disrupted anterior larynx or an unstable laryngeal skeleton	Same as group 2
5	Full cricotracheal separation	Endotracheal intubation; the distal airway usually retracts into the chest, so tracheotomy may compound the problem

39.4 Diagnosis

Grade 3 blunt laryngeal fracture

39.5 Medical Management

Conservative management is only appropriate for patients in group 1. These patients should be hospitalized for at least 24 hours in a monitored setting because the edema may progress, especially in the 6- to 12-hour period following the injury. Humidified air or oxygen is supplied and voice rest is instituted. The patient can expect a good result in both vocal quality and airway.

39.6 Surgical Management

When he was stabilized, the patient was taken to the operating room. The cricothyrotomy was converted to a formal, low tracheostomy. Midline exploration revealed a displaced vertical fracture of the thyroid cartilage. The fracture was reduced with a miniplate. The endolarynx was then examined endoscopically. A mucosal laceration was again visualized along the left false vocal cord and into the true vocal cord (▶ Fig. 39.2). The laceration extended into but not through the vocalis muscle. The laceration was repaired endoscopically using microlaryngeal instrumentation.

Group 3 or 4 patients should undergo tracheotomy and surgical exploration; group 5 should have immediate exploration and primary repair of the trachea. Indications for open exploration in group 2 patients are as follows:

- Severe upper airway obstructions not from edema or hematoma.
- Displaced laryngeal skeleton fracture.
- Internal (endolaryngeal) derangement and/or exposed cartilage.
- Active hemorrhage.
- Increasing subcutaneous emphysema.

Tracheotomy: Tracheotomy is preferred to reduce the exacerbation of intubating an injured larynx and to provide a more stable airway. For those patients who need general anesthesia and have mild to moderate trauma to the larynx (group 2), but no significant airway distress, tracheotomy is still the preferred method to prevent long-term edema and subsequent airway compromise.

Laryngofissure: When the thyroid cartilage or endolaryngeal mucosa has been severely disrupted or cartilage is exposed, a laryngofissure is needed to gain access to repair the injury. Anterior commissure lacerations and disruption of the free edge of the vocal fold should be approached similarly and repaired primarily. Often, a keel is used to prevent blunting of the anterior commissure. Minor mucosal lacerations and noncomminuted thyroid cartilage fractures do not need a laryngofissure for repair.

Stenting: Stenting is necessary for comminuted thyroid cartilage fractures that are unstable even after open reduction and internal fixation. It is also needed to prevent adhesions in massive endolaryngeal lacerations and to act as a keel in trauma

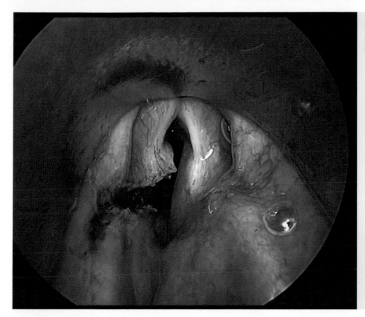

Fig. 39.2 Endoscopic view demonstrating mucosal laceration of the left false and true vocal folds.

resulting in a disrupted anterior commissure. Stents are maintained for a period of 2 to 3 weeks.

39.7 Rehabilitation and Follow-up

In mild (group 1) injuries, normal voice and airway is the standard outcome. With increasing severity of trauma and a delay greater than 24 to 48 hours for operative intervention, the vocal results suffer more than the airway: group 4 patients have a 33% chance of a "fair" voice and a small, but real, possibility of a poor airway.

Long-term follow-up is needed to assist patients who have not returned to their pretraumatic status. Speech therapy, thyroplasty, and laryngotracheoplasty are all possibilities for improving a less than adequate outcome.

39.8 Questions

1. Appropriate treatment for group 1 laryngeal trauma is
   a) Tracheotomy.
   b) Open neck exploration, including tracheotomy.
   c) Close observation.
   d) Tracheotomy and repair of thyroid cartilage fractures.

2. Indications for an open neck exploration in group 2 patients include all of the following except
   a) Displaced thyroid cartilage fracture.
   b) Exposed cartilage.
   c) Aphonia.
   d) Active hemorrhage.
   e) Increasing subcutaneous emphysema.

3. All patients with laryngeal fractures should have
   a) Cricothyrotomy.
   b) Open reduction and internal fixation of the fractures.
   c) Cervical spine X-rays.
   d) Open neck exploration.

Answers: 1. c 2. c 3. c

Suggested Readings

Bent JP, III, Porubsky ES. The management of blunt fractures of the thyroid cartilage. Otolaryngol Head Neck Surg. 1994; 110(2):195–202

Fried MP, Ed. Laryngeal Trauma. In: The Larynx. St. Louis, MO: Mosby-Year Book; 1996:378–396

Schaefer SD. The acute management of external laryngeal trauma. A 27-year experience. Arch Otolaryngol Head Neck Surg. 1992; 118 (6):598–604

Snow JB, Jr. Diagnosis and therapy for acute laryngeal and tracheal trauma. Otolaryngol Clin North Am. 1984; 17(1):101–106

40 Adult Subglottic Stenosis

Alessandro de Alarcon and Michael A. DeMarcantonio

40.1 History

A 43-year-old woman presented with a 5-month history of progressive dyspnea with exertion. She described loud noisy breathing with vigorous exercise. She denied any significant pain, odynophagia, aspiration, or dysphagia but noted mild hoarseness and a strained voice with activity. She reported a history of an uneventful cervical discectomy 6 months ago. At the time of her recent surgery she was informed by the anesthesiologist that she needed a "smaller than normal" endotracheal tube.

The physical examination revealed very mild biphasic stridor detected only upon auscultation. She demonstrated no evidence of retractions while breathing. Her voice was mildly hoarse. The remainder of her head and neck examination is normal with the exception of a right-sided cervical scar consistent with an anterior cervical discectomy and fusion (ACDF). Flexible nasopharyngolaryngoscopy with stroboscopy was performed, revealing normal nasal mucosa, intact septum, and mildly edematous but mobile vocal folds. Stroboscopy demonstrated a normal vibratory pattern and mucosal wave. The subglottis was visualized and appeared stenotic (▶ Fig. 40.1).

The patient was scheduled for a microlaryngoscopy and bronchoscopy with biopsy and possible balloon dilation. A rigid 4-mm Hopkins rod telescopic unit was used for evaluation of the airway.

Both the supraglottis and glottis were found to be normal. The subglottis demonstrated a circumferential stenosis centered at the level of the cricoid cartilage (▶ Fig. 40.2). The airway was sized with 4.0 endotracheal tube with a leak at 15 cm H_2O, indicating a high grade 1 stenosis (▶ Table 40.1). The area of stenosis measured approximately 2 cm in length. The distal trachea and bronchi were normal. The patient was placed in suspension and the site of stenosis was injected with 0.5 mL of 40-mg/mL triamcinolone. Dilation was then performed using a 14-mm balloon. After dilation the airway was sized with a 7.0 endotracheal tube with a leak

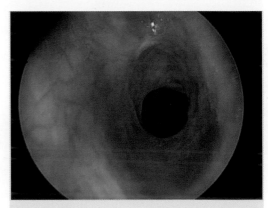

Fig. 40.2 Idiopathic subglottic stenosis seen on rigid bronchoscopy.

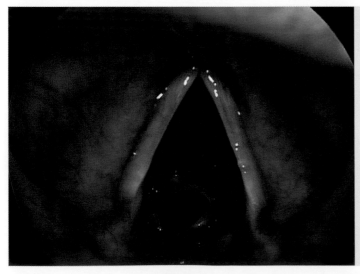

Fig. 40.1 Idiopathic subglottic stenosis viewed on stroboscopy.

Table 40.1 Cotton-Myer Classification of Subglottic Stenosis

Grade	Degree of stenosis
1	0–50%
2	51–70%
3	71–99%
4	100%

Source: Myer CM III, O'Connor DM, Cotton RT. Proposed grading system for subglottic stenosis based on endotracheal tube sizes. Ann Otol Rhinol Laryngol 1994;103(4 pt 1):319–323.

at 10 cm H_2O. She experienced immediate improvement after dilation, but the stenosis recurred after 6 weeks. She desired definitive treatment and underwent cricotracheal resection. At 3 months her airway appeared normal on endoscopy.

40.2 Differential Diagnosis—Key Points

- Intubation, even of a short duration, can place a patient at risk for airway stenosis. Patients with idiopathic subglottic stenosis may be incidentally diagnosed at the time of or after an elective surgical procedure.
- Neck procedures, such as ACDF and thyroid surgery, place the recurrent laryngeal nerve at risk for temporary or permanent paralysis. Given recent ACDF, it was important to evaluate this patient for vocal cord mobility.
- Inflammatory or infectious disorders should be evaluated as possible causes of laryngotracheal stenosis. Sarcoidosis (supraglottic), tuberculosis (glottic), Wegener's granulomatosis (subglottic), and relapsing polychondritis are potential causes.

40.3 Test Interpretation

Erythrocyte sedimentation rate (ESR) and C-reactive protein (CRP) levels were normal. Cytoplasmic-staining antineutrophil cytoplasmic antibody (C-ANCA) and perinuclear-staining antineutrophil cytoplasmic antibody (P-ANCA) were both negative. Angiotensin-converting enzyme (ACE) and calcium levels were normal. A purified protein

derivative skin test was placed and was read as negative.

40.4 Diagnosis

Idiopathic subglottic stenosis

40.5 Medical Management

Idiopathic subglottic stenosis is a diagnosis of exclusion in patients with airway stenosis. Antireflux therapy should be considered given that gastroesophophageal reflux disease (GERD) may worsen subglottic stenosis. Patients that are asymptomatic and have minimal airway stenosis may undergo observation alone.

40.6 Surgical Management

Patients may attain symptomatic relief with balloon dilation ± steroid injection. This may be performed on a repeated basis based on the patient's symptoms. Open surgical management is reserved for patients who fail endoscopic management or for patients who desire permanent surgical treatment. Cricotracheal resection (CTR) and laryngotracheoplasty (LTP) are the two most commonly performed procedures. CTR is more effective in patients with idiopathic subglotic stenosis and patients with high-grade subglottic stenosis. Success rates for CTR are often > 95% for patients with idiopathic subglottic stenosis. In patients with idiopathic subglottic stenosis, removal of the diseased mucosa is crucial to long-term surgical correction and frequently necessitates removal of the anterior cricoid and all of the posterior cricoid mucosa. Tracheal resection alone is not adequate when disease involves the cricoid cartilage and mucosa. LTP will often fail in the long-term management of idiopathic subglottic stenosis, as the disease is not removed.

40.7 Rehabilitation and Follow-up

Following dilation the patient should be followed up in 1 to 2 weeks for evaluation of clinical symptoms. If symptoms resolve most patients may return to clinic/operating room on an as-needed basis. Some patients may prefer undergoing repeat dilations every 1 to 2 years in lieu of open surgical therapy. Should symptoms fail to resolve, a series of 3 to 4 balloon dilations may be scheduled at 2-week intervals. If the patient continues to have symptoms, open airway reconstruction should be discussed. Risks of open airway reconstruction, including infection, scarring, need for additional endoscopic procedures, vocal cord paralysis, decreased voice pitch, dysphonia, dehiscence, and need for tracheostomy, should be reviewed thoroughly with the patient. Patients should be aware that voice therapy may be required postoperatively. Following airway reconstruction, the patient may require repeat airway evaluations to assess for the development of recurrent stenosis.

40.8 Questions

1. Surgical options for the treatment of idiopathic subglottic stenosis include all the following except
   a) Pericardial patch tracheoplasty.
   b) Cricotracheal resection.
   c) Laryngotracheoplasty.
   d) Observation.
2. What laboratory finding is usually seen in Wegener's granulomatosis?
   a) Positive purified protein derivative.
   b) Increased angiotensin-converting enzyme (ACE) level.
   c) Increased cytoplasmic-staining antineutrophil cytoplasmic antibody (C-ANCA).
   d) Increased antinuclear antibody (ANA) titers.
3. Which study must be performed prior to operative intervention?
   a) Flexible fiberoptic laryngoscopy.
   b) Magnetic resonance imaging (MRI) of neck.
   c) Computed tomography (CT) of neck.
   d) Pulmonary function tests (PFTs).

Answers: 1. a 2. c 3. a

Suggested Readings

Ching HH, Mendelsohn AH, Liu IY, Long J, Chhetri DK, Berke GS. A comparative study of cricotracheal resection and staged laryngotracheoplasty for adult subglottic stenosis. Ann Otol Rhinol Laryngol. 2015; 124(4):326–333

Colice GL, Stukel TA, Dain B. Laryngeal complications of prolonged intubation. Chest. 1989; 96(4):877–884

Lebovics RS, Hoffman GS, Leavitt RY, et al. The management of subglottic stenosis in patients with Wegener's granulomatosis. Laryngoscope. 1992; 102(12)(Pt 1):1341–1345

Wang H, Wright CD, Wain JC, Ott HC, Mathisen DJ. Idiopathic Subglottic Stenosis: Factors Affecting Outcome After Single-Stage Repair. Ann Thorac Surg. 2015; 100(5):1804–1811

41 Supraglottic Cancer

Jeffrey J. Harmon and Keith M. Wilson

41.1 History

A 67-year-old male veteran with a 125 pack-year smoking history presented with 3 months of sore throat, odynophagia, and 20 pounds of unintentional weight loss over the past 5 months. Palpation of the neck demonstrated a 2-cm left level II neck mass. Flexible laryngoscopy demonstrated a fungating mass on the laryngeal surface of epiglottis with normal vocal cord mobility. A computed tomography (CT) scan of the neck with contrast demonstrated a 1.5-cm mass on one subsite of the supraglottis without invasion of the preepiglottic space or cartilage and a 1.5-cm left neck level II node with central necrosis. CT of the chest without contrast demonstrated no concerning lung masses. The patient was taken to the operating room 3 days later for panendoscopy and multiple biopsies. The biopsies revealed squamous cell carcinoma of the supraglottis. He underwent radiation therapy of the tumor, as well as radiation therapy of the neck bilaterally.

41.2 Differential Diagnosis—Key Points

- *History of present illness:* Presenting symptoms include cervical lymphadenopathy, sore throat, hemoptysis, dysphagia, odynophagia, otalgia, unintentional weight loss, and globus sensation. The supraglottis has more extensive lymphatics than the glottis. Therefore, the rate of spread to cervical lymph nodes is higher than with cancer of the glottis. Also, supraglottic cancer does not present with symptoms as early as glottic cancer. As a result, supraglottic cancer is more often diagnosed at a late stage. Therefore, the only presenting symptom may be cervical lymphadenopathy.
- *Physical exam:* A full head and neck exam is necessary for every patient who presents with symptoms concerning for cancer. Flexible laryngoscopy is also indicated to evaluate for gross anatomic changes associated with the larynx and pharynx.
- *Anatomy:* The supraglottis extends from the superior border of the epiglottis and aryepiglottic folds to the laryngeal ventricle. It is composed of five subsides including the lingual surface of the epiglottis, laryngeal surface of the epiglottis, laryngeal surface of the aryepiglottic folds (the opposite surface is the hypopharynx), arytenoids, and false vocal folds.
- *Imaging:* There are multiple imaging modalities used to diagnose and monitor supraglottic cancer. A contrast-enhanced CT of the neck can help identify tumors in the larynx and whether there is cartilage and preepiglottic space involvement or extralaryngeal extension. It can also identify concerning lymphadenopathy based on size criteria and nodal characteristics. Malignant nodes tend to be round and may have central necrosis, as was the case for the example above. Ultrasound is also used to identify concerning lymphadenopathy, as well as to serve as a guide for fine needle aspiration (FNA) in an effort to find cytologic evidence of cancer. A positron emission tomography (PET)/CT scan can identify nodal or metastatic disease as well as cancer recurrence posttreatment.
- *Panendoscopy:* Evaluation of the upper aerodigestive tract is commonly performed under general anesthesia and primarily allows for tissue sampling of the tumor. It also facilitates the search for a synchronous cancer, for which the risk is approximately 10%. Therefore, it is important to perform a complete, systematic examination of the oral cavity, oropharynx, larynx, hypopharynx, and esophagus to ensure that no other lesions are present.
- *Pathology:* Histologic verification is a critical part of the oncologic work-up of a primary tumor. There are two options for acquiring tissue for pathologic evaluation. One is through biopsy during panendoscopy. Another option is to perform an FNA on suspicious lymphadenopathy, especially if there is no clear primary tumor or the tumor has been treated and there is concern for neck recurrence.
- *Staging:* See ▶ Table 41.1 for the T staging system for supraglottic cancer.
- *Differential diagnosis:* The most common malignancy is squamous cell carcinoma. However, the differential diagnosis for a mass includes infectious causes such as tuberculosis or fungal infections, autoimmune disease such as sarcoidosis and malignancies including but not limited to squamous cell carcinoma. Non–squamous cell carcinoma malignancies include salivary gland

Table 41.1 T staging for supraglottic cancer

T stage	Description
T1	Primary tumor limited to one subsite of the supraglottis with normal true vocal fold mobility
T2	Primary tumor invades mucosa of more than one adjacent subsite of the supraglottis, glottis, base of tongue, vallecula, or medial wall of the piriform sinuses without true vocal fold fixation
T3	Primary tumor invades postcricoid area, preepiglottic space, paraglottic space, or inner cortex of the thyroid cartilage or causes true vocal fold fixation
T4a	Primary tumor invades through the thyroid cartilage or tissues beyond the larynx
T4b	Primary tumor invades the prevertebral space, encases the carotid artery, or invades mediastinal structures

tumors such as adenoid cystic carcinoma and mucoepidermoid carcinoma, adenocarcinoma, neuroendocrine tumors, and sarcomas.

41.3 Diagnosis

T1N1M0 squamous cell carcinoma of the supraglottis

41.4 Medical and Surgical Management

Early stage supraglottic squamous cell carcinomas (Tis, T1, T2) are most often treated with a single modality. Late stage supraglottic squamous cell carcinoma (T3, T4) often require a multimodality approach. The treatment chosen also factors in the cervical nodal status of the patient and whether there is metastatic disease. Other factors include the cost, time commitment, and posttreatment morbidity associated with the treatment including the treatment's effects on swallowing and speech.

Single-modality treatment with a goal of laryngeal preservation is indicated in early stage supraglottic squamous cell carcinoma. The options for treatment include radiation therapy, transoral laser microsurgery, transcervical partial laryngectomy, and transoral robotic supraglottic laryngectomy.

The benefit of radiation therapy is that the structure of the larynx is preserved. The disadvantages of radiation therapy are that it can only be used once, it may preclude treatment with a partial laryngectomy in the future if the cancer were to recur, and the near-term and long-term morbidity can be debilitating. In fact, long-term morbidity includes the possibility of developing a nonfunctional larynx that can result in chronic aspiration requiring a total laryngectomy.

Surgery is often better for younger patients because it leaves the option of using radiation for a recurrence and reduces the risk of long-term sequelae of radiation therapy.

Laryngeal conservation surgery is an option when an appropriate resection preserves the functional integrity of the cricoid cartilage and at least one cricoarytenoid unit. The patient must also have sufficient pulmonary reserve. Contraindications for laryngeal conservation surgery include invasion of a significant portion of the subglottis, the preepiglottic space, the pharynx and/or base-of-tongue, the postcricoid or interarytenoid tissue, the cricoid cartilage, and extralaryngeal extension.

Transoral laser microsurgery is one surgical option. The limits to transoral laser surgery include anatomic problems that prevent adequate exposure. The procedure differs from other surgical options in that the tumor is transected to assess depth and then removed in multiple blocks as opposed to an *en bloc* resection. The European Laryngological Society has developed guidelines for transoral laser microsurgery excision of supraglottic tumors.

A transcervical horizontal partial laryngectomy is a second surgical option. The options for resection of a supraglottic tumor include a supraglottic partial laryngectomy and supracricoid partial laryngectomy. A supraglottic partial laryngectomy involves the excision of the preepiglottic space, epiglottis, vestibular folds, and superior portion of the thyroid cartilage. Of note, the supraglottic partial laryngectomy can be performed transorally using a robot in some cases. A supracricoid partial laryngectomy, on the other hand, involves excision of the bilateral paraglottic spaces, preepiglottic space (although extensive preepiglottic space involvement is a contradindication), bilateral vocal folds, bilateral vestibular folds, the thyroid cartilage, and up to one arytenoid. A partial laryngectomy leaves radiation as a possible future treatment in the event of a recurrence.

Late stage supraglottic squamous cell carcinomas (T3, T4) require a multimodality approach. The treatment options are total laryngectomy followed by radiation and concurrent chemotherapy and radiation with the possibility of a salvage laryngectomy if this treatment fails. The principle behind concurrent chemotherapy and radiation is that chemotherapy serves as a radiosensitizer that augments the effect of radiation therapy. Unfortunately, it also increases the toxic effects of radiation. In the case of late stage laryngeal cancer, quality of life for patients who underwent concurrent chemotherapy and radiation versus total laryngectomy with/without concurrent chemotherapy and radiation is higher. However, morbidity is greater for patients who require a salvage total laryngectomy after the failure of concurrent chemotherapy and radiation. Also, the risk of an incompetent larynx resulting in aspiration and eventual loss of speech is not insignificant in patients treated with concurrent chemotherapy and radiation. Current evidence suggests that for late stage supraglottic squamous cell carcinomas without distant metastases, a total laryngectomy followed by radiation is significantly superior to concurrent chemotherapy and radiation. However, laryngeal preservation is better with a nonsurgical approach.

One must consider the nodal status of the cancer when considering treatments. A clinically negative neck should be treated if the risk of subclinical neck disease is 20% or greater. Supraglottic cancer has a higher rate of cervical metastases compared with glottic and subglottic cancer due to extensive lymphatics (4–35%). Therefore, a neck dissection is warranted in supraglottic squamous cell carcinoma. Moreover, because the rate of bilateral metastases to the cervical lymph nodes is high due to the embryologic origin of the supraglottis as a single midline structure, bilateral neck dissection is indicated.

41.5 Rehabilitation and Follow-up

The frequency of the follow-up is proportional to the patient's risk of recurrence. Most recurrences occur during the first 2 years following completion of treatment. The standard follow-up schedule is every 1 to 2 months for the first 2 years and every 3 to 6 months for the next 3 years. Annual visits are encouraged starting 5 years after completion of treatment. Symptoms including otalgia, dysphagia, odynophagia, unintentional weight loss, and increasing fatigue should be concerning for possible recurrence. Most recurrences occur in the neck. A PET/CT, if utilized, is performed no sooner than 3 months following completion of treatment. The 3-month time frame is important because residual uptake can still occur regardless of recurrence up to this time point after completion of treatment.

Dysphagia occurs in 50 to 60% of patients who undergo radiation therapy. Most improvement occurs in the first 6 months following completion of treatment.

Voice outcomes can be good for transoral endoscopic excision and partial laryngectomy if one vocal cord generates a mucosal wave. Even a cordectomy can result in vocalization once tissue has regenerated. In fact, quality of life outcomes for voice after transoral laser microsurgery is comparable to radiotherapy with the caveat that the postoperative recovery from transoral laser microsurgery occurs after 3 to 6 months.

The ability to speak is significantly affected in patients who have undergone a total laryngectomy. There are three options for restoring voice after laryngectomy. The goal of all three is to simulate the mechanisms of normal voice generation. The three options are esophageal speech, electrolarynx, and a tracheoesophageal fistula device. All patients should be evaluated by a speech-language pathologist if they are to undergo speech rehabilitation, preferably preoperatively. Esophageal speech is produced by swallowing air and releasing it in a manner that allows voice to be generated by the vibration of the neopharynx. The advantages of this technique are that it requires no additional devices and it requires no additional surgery. The disadvantages are that it can be difficult to learn esophageal speech and the voice quality can be poor. The electrolarynx utilizes an external device to generate vibrations in the oral cavity or the pharyngeal mucosa. The advantages of the electrolarynx are that there is no need for surgery and it is easy to learn to use. The disadvantages are that it requires purchasing an expensive device and the voice quality is mechanical. Tracheoesophageal puncture utilizes a fistula created between the trachea and the esophagus so that air generated in the lungs can be forced through the pharynx and oral cavity to generate speech. The advantages of a tracheoesophageal puncture are that it is the easiest to learn and the voice quality is the best out of all the procedures. The disadvantages are that it requires an additional procedure with all of its associated morbidities and there may be additional costs associated with the prosthesis. Alternatively, the puncture can be placed at the time of total laryngectomy and the device inserted by a speech-language pathologist on an outpatient basis at a later date.

41.6 Questions

1. A 57-year-old woman is being evaluated with a positron emission tomography (PET)/computed tomography (CT) scan at 3 months postoperatively for supraglottic laryngeal carcinoma for which she underwent an endoscopic laser procedure and bilateral neck dissection. There is mild positive uptake in the region of the larynx. What is the next best step in management?
   a) Operative biopsy of the area.
   b) Magnetic resonance imaging (MRI).
   c) Evaluate clinically followed by repeat imaging in 1 month.
   d) Radiation therapy.
   e) Open total or partial laryngectomy.
2. A 63-year-old man with a long-standing history of tobacco and heavy alcohol use is diagnosed with supraglottic squamous cell carcinoma staged as T2N0M0. Of the following, which is not an appropriate method of management?
   a) External beam radiation to the larynx and neck.
   b) Open partial laryngectomy with bilateral selective neck dissection.
   c) Transoral laser microsurgery with bilateral neck dissection.
   d) All of the above are appropriate.
3. How would the tumor in the original case have been staged if there were fixation of one vocal fold?
   a) T1N1M0.
   b) T2N1M0.
   c) T3N1M0.
   d) T4N1M0.

Answers: 1. a 2. d 3. c

Suggested Readings

Mor N, Blitzer A. Functional Anatomy and Oncologic Barriers of the Larynx. Otolaryngol Clin North Am. 2015; 48(4):533–545

Mourad M, Sadoughi B. Transcervical Conservation Laryngeal Surgery: An Anatomic Understanding to Enhance Functional and Oncologic Outcomes. Otolaryngol Clin North Am. 2015; 48(4):703–715

Sadoughi B. Quality of Life After Conservation Surgery for Laryngeal Cancer. Otolaryngol Clin North Am. 2015; 48(4):655–665

Tang CG, Sinclair CF. Voice Restoration After Total Laryngectomy. Otolaryngol Clin North Am. 2015; 48(4):687–702

42 Glottic Cancer

Jeffrey J. Harmon and Keith M. Wilson

42.1 History

A 52-year-old man presented with hoarseness, otalgia, neck pain, and 20 pounds of unintentional weight loss in the context of an approximately 50 pack-year smoking history. Flexible laryngoscopy demonstrated a mass on the right true vocal fold. The right vocal fold was immobile. A computed tomography (CT) scan of the neck with contrast demonstrated a mass originating in the glottis and extending to the paraglottic space. The patient underwent panendoscopy and biopsy. The biopsies confirmed the diagnosis of squamous cell carcinoma of the glottis. There was no concerning cervical lymphadenopathy on a CT of the neck with contrast or on physical exam. There was no indication of lung nodules on a CT of the chest without contrast. He was diagnosed with T3N0M0 squamous cell carcinoma of the glottis and treated with chemotherapy using cisplatin with concurrent radiotherapy. Positron emission tomography (PET)/CT 3 months after completion of therapy demonstrated uptake in the right laryngeal tissues. He underwent a second endoscopy and biopsy. Biopsies revealed squamous cell carcinoma. He subsequently underwent total laryngectomy, a latissimus dorsi pharyngeal interposition free flap, and bilateral neck dissection. Final pathology demonstrated invasion of the thyroid cartilage. All dissected cervical lymph nodes were negative for malignancy indicating a T4aN0M0 squamous cell carcinoma of the glottis.

42.2 Differential Diagnosis—Key Points

- *History of present illness:* Unlike supraglottic or subglottic cancers, glottic cancer presents earlier with symptoms of hoarseness. Also, cervical lymphatic metastases are infrequent due to cartilaginous and ligamentous anatomic barriers and sparse lymphatics. Presenting symptoms include hoarseness, dysphagia, aspiration, sore throat, stridor, otalgia, or unintentional weight loss.
- *Physical exam:* A full head and neck exam is necessary for every patient who presents with symptoms concerning for malignancy. Flexible laryngoscopy is also indicated to evaluate for gross anatomic changes associated with the larynx including abnormalities of vocal fold movement or spread of malignancy to the pharynx.
- *Anatomy:* Vocal fold immobility, involvement of the anterior commissure, and subglottic extension are three important factors to consider when evaluating the severity of a glottic cancer. These factors affect prognosis and treatment options. The glottis extends from the laryngeal ventricle to 1 cm below the inferior border of the true vocal fold. The true vocal folds consist of a stratified squamous epithelium, a three-layered lamina propria, and the vocalis muscle. The layers of the lamina propria are a superficial layer consisting of soft gelatin-like tissue whose vibration generates voice and intermediate and deep layers that form the vocal ligament. The glottis derives a lymphatic and vascular supply independent of the supraglottis and subglottis. Moreover, the glottis has less extensive lymphatics than other subunits of the larynx, resulting in a reduced risk of spread to cervical lymph nodes. Other barriers to the spread of glottic cancer include ligamentous membranes and perichondrium. For example, the thyroglottic ligament helps prevent the spread of cancer from the glottis to supraglottis and vice versa. On the other hand, the anterior commissure ligament, Broyles's ligament, can both be a barrier to spread in early stage cancers and facilitate cartilaginous involvement in advanced laryngeal cancers.
- *Imaging:* There are multiple imaging modalities that can be used to help stage and survey for recurrent glottic cancer. Videostroboscopy is an important modality that can evaluate glottic cancers during staging and monitor for early recurrence. While most helpful to diagnose benign midmembranous lesions, stiffening of the vocal fold suggests deeper invasion of the true vocal folds and, possibly, malignancy. The mechanism by which vocal fold fixation may occur is through invasion of the cricoarytenoid unit, infiltration of the laryngeal musculature, or fixation of the true vocal fold itself.
- *Contrast:*enhanced CT can help identify tumors in the larynx. It can also identify concerning lymphadenopathy based on size criteria. Ultrasound is used to identify concerning lymphadenopathy, as well as to serve as a guide for fine

needle aspiration (FNA). PET/CT can identify recurrent disease in the posttreatment setting.

- *Panendoscopy:* Evaluation of the upper aerodigestive tract is commonly performed under general anesthesia and primarily allows for tissue sampling. It also facilitates the search for synchronous cancers, which occur in 10% of cases. Therefore, it is important to perform a complete, systematic examination of the oral cavity, oropharynx, larynx, hypopharynx, and esophagus to ensure that no other lesions are present.
- *Pathology:* Histologic verification is a critical part of the oncologic work-up. There are two options for acquiring tissue for pathologic evaluation. One is through biopsy during panendoscopy. Another option is to perform an FNA on suspicious lymphadenopathy, especially if there no clear primary tumor or the tumor has been treated and there is concern for neck recurrence.
- *Staging:* See ▶ Table 42.1 for T staging of glottic cancer.
- *Differential diagnosis:* The most common malignancy of the upper aerodigestive tract is squamous cell carcinoma. However, the differential diagnosis for a mass concerning for cancer includes infectious causes such as tuberculosis or fungal infections, autoimmune disease such as sarcoidosis, and malignancies including but not limited to squamous cell carcinoma. Nonsquamous cell carcinoma malignancies include salivary gland tumors such as adenoid cystic carcinoma and mucoepidermoid carcinoma, adenocarcinoma, neuroendocrine tumors, and sarcomas.

42.3 Diagnosis

pT4aN0M0 squamous cell carcinoma of the glottis

42.4 Medical and Surgical Management

Early stage glottic squamous cell carcinomas (Tis, T1, T2) are most often treated with a single-modality therapy. Late stage glottis squamous cell carcinomas (T3, T4) often require a multimodality approach. The treatment chosen also factors in the cervical nodal status of the patient and whether there is metastatic disease. Other factors include the cost, time commitment, and posttreatment morbidity, including effects on swallowing and speech.

Single-modality treatment with a goal of laryngeal preservation is common in early stage glottic squamous cell carcinoma. In other words, the goal of therapy is for the patient to maintain voice and swallowing function. The options for treatment include radiation therapy, transoral laser microsurgery, and transcervical partial laryngectomy. Radiation and transoral endoscopic laser surgery are equally efficacious options for Tis and T1a glottic squamous cell carcinomas. Surgery is more often the choice for T1a and T2 cancers that involve the anterior commissure. Finally, surgery is often chosen in younger patients, because radiation is withheld to treat a recurrence and there is reduced risk of long-term sequelae of radiation therapy.

The benefit of radiation therapy is that the entire structure of the larynx is preserved. The disadvantages of radiation therapy are that it can only be used once, it precludes treatment with a partial laryngectomy in the future for cancer recurrence, and the near- and long-term morbidity can be debilitating. In fact, long-term morbidity includes the possibility of developing a nonfunctional larynx that can result in chronic aspiration requiring a total laryngectomy.

Table 42.1 T staging for glottic cancer	
T stage	**Description**
T1a	Primary tumor limited to the true vocal folds with normal mobility, one true vocal fold involved
T1b	Primary tumor limited to the true vocal folds with normal mobility, both true vocal folds involved
T2	Primary tumor extends to the subglottis or supraglottis, or impaired true vocal fold mobility
T3	Primary tumor with true vocal fold fixation, invasion of the paraglottic space, or invasion of the inner cortex of thyroid cartilage
T4a	Primary tumor has invaded the outer cortex of the thyroid cartilage or tissues beyond the larynx
T4b	Primary tumor has invaded the prevertebral space, encases the carotid artery, or invades mediastinal structures

Laryngeal conservation surgery is possible for tumors when an oncologically sound resection spares the functional integrity of the cricoid cartilage and at least one cricoarytenoid unit. The patient must also have sufficient pulmonary reserve.

Transoral endoscopic excision is a surgical option. The limits of transoral laser surgery include anatomic problems that prevent adequate exposure or advanced tumors. The European Laryngological Society classification for transoral laser microsurgery resection of glottic tumors is widely used as a guideline for resection. Margins of 2 mm for a glottis squamous cell carcinoma are indicated.

A transcervical partial laryngectomy is another surgical option. A partial laryngectomy offers the best initial local control. It is useful in the event that inadequate exposure is achieved during an attempted transoral procedure. And like transoral laser microsurgery, it leaves radiation as a possible future treatment in the event of a recurrence. However, it is more expensive, is associated with more immediate postoperative morbidity than transoral laser microsurgery, and is contraindicated when both cricoarytenoid units are involved. The options for a transcervical partial laryngectomy include a vertical partial laryngectomy and supracricoid partial laryngectomy. A vertical partial laryngectomy involves resection of the involved vocal fold, the anterior commissure, and a portion of the thyroid cartilage. A supracricoid partial laryngectomy involves en bloc resection of the paraglottic spaces, the preepiglottic space, bilateral vocal folds, a portion of the thyroid cartilage and one cricoarytenoid unit. These procedures are infrequently indicated in late stage glottic squamous cell carcinomas.

Late stage glottic squamous cell carcinomas require a multimodality approach. The treatment options are total laryngectomy followed by radiation and concurrent chemotherapy and radiation with the possibility of a salvage laryngectomy. The principle behind concurrent chemotherapy and radiation is that chemotherapy serves as a radiosensitizer that augments the effect of radiation therapy. Unfortunately, it also increases the toxic effects. In the case of late stage laryngeal cancer, quality of life for patients who underwent chemoradiation versus total laryngectomy with/without chemoradiation is higher. However, morbidity is greater for patients who require a salvage total laryngectomy after the failure of concurrent chemotherapy and radiation. Also, the risk of an incompetent larynx resulting in aspiration and eventual loss of speech is not insignificant in patients treated with concurrent chemotherapy and radiation. Current evidence suggests that for late stage glottic squamous cell carcinomas without metastases, a total laryngectomy followed by radiation is superior to concurrent chemotherapy and radiation, but laryngeal preservation is approximately 66% with concurrent chemotherapy and radiation therapy.

One must consider the nodal status of the cancer when considering treatments. A clinically negative neck should be treated if the risk of subclinical neck disease is 20% or greater. In early glottic cancer, observation of the clinically negative neck is warranted. There is no evidence to support a prophylactic neck dissection for T1 and T2 cancer without clinical evidence of nodal metastases. All clinically positive necks should be treated.

It is important to consider not only the oncologic outcomes of glottic cancer but also the quality of life outcomes and "hidden costs" including time lost and administrative costs associated with the treatment pathway. Smith et al looked at such costs for a group of 101 patients with Tis or T1 glottic squamous cell carcinoma treated with either surgery or radiation therapy between January 1990 and December 2000. For this group the hidden costs included traveling time, traveling distance, and work missed by the patient, friends, and family. They utilized a modified University of Washington Quality of Life Questionnaire (UW-QOL-R), the Performance Status Scale for Head and Neck Cancer Patients (PSS-HN), and a self-developed questionnaire to assess the hidden costs previously described. There was no statistical difference between groups treated with radiation primarily and endoscopic surgery primarily based on the UW-QOL-R questionnaire. All responders reported no limitations on the PSS-HN domains. The radiation therapy cohort had high hidden costs in terms of travel distance and travel time. Patients undergoing radiation therapy missed three times as much work as those who underwent endoscopic surgery. This study demonstrated that in early glottis cancer the quality of life outcomes are good in radiation and endoscopic surgery treatment groups, with higher hidden costs in the radiation therapy group.

42.5 Rehabilitation and Follow-up

The intensity of the follow-up is proportional to the patient's risk of recurrence. Most recurrences occur during the first 2 years following completion of treatment. The standard follow-up schedule is every 1 to 2 months for the first 2 years and every 3 to 6 months for the next 3 years. Annual visits are encouraged starting 5 years after completion of treatment. The appearance of or worsening of symptoms including otalgia, dysphagia, odynophagia, unintentional weight loss, and increasing fatigue should alert the clinician as symptoms of recurrence. Most recurrences occur in the neck or stoma. A PET/CT is performed approximately 3 months following completion of treatment. The 3-month time frame is particularly important for nonsurgical treatment protocols where acute phase reactions can take up to 12 weeks to resolve.

Dysphagia occurs in 50 to 60% of patients who undergo radiation therapy, with most improvement in dysphagia occurring in the first 6 months following completion of treatment. Voice outcomes can be good for transoral endoscopic excision and partial laryngectomy even if one vocal cord generates a mucosal wave. Even a cordectomy can result in vocalization once tissue has regenerated, typically over a 6-month time frame.

In the case of a total laryngectomy, however, new forms of speech generation are required. There are three options for alaryngeal speech: esophageal speech, electrolarynx, and a tracheoesophageal fistula device. The goal of all three is to simulate the mechanisms of normal voice generation. All patients should be evaluated by a speech-language pathologist if they are to undergo speech rehabilitation, preferably preoperatively. Esophageal speech is produced by swallowing and releasing air in a manner that allows voice to be generated by vibration of the neopharynx. The advantages of this technique are that it requires no additional devices and it requires no additional surgery. The disadvantages are that it can be difficult to learn esophageal speech and the voice quality can be poor. The electrolarynx utilizes an external device to generate vibrations in the oral cavity or the pharyngeal mucosa. The advantages of the electrolarynx are that there is no need for surgery and it is easy to learn to use. The disadvantages are that it requires purchasing an expensive device and the voice quality is mechanical. Tracheoesophageal puncture utilizes a fistula created between the trachea and the esophagus so that air generated in the lungs can be forced through the pharynx and oral cavity to generate speech. The advantages of a tracheoesophageal puncture are that it is the easiest to learn and the voice quality

is the best out of all the procedures. The disadvantages are that it requires an additional procedure with all of its associated morbidities and there may be additional costs associated with the prosthesis. Alternatively, the puncture can be placed at the time of total laryngectomy and the device inserted by a speech-language pathologist on an outpatient basis at a later date.

42.6 Questions

1. A patient arrives in your clinic with 3 months of progressively worsening hoarseness, odynophagia, otalgia, unintentional weight loss, and a 100 pack-year smoking history. What is the next step in the work-up for this patient?
   a) Computed tomography (CT) of the neck with contrast.
   b) Panendoscopy with biopsy.
   c) Flexible laryngoscopy.
   d) None of the above.
2. In which patient would transoral laser microsurgical excision be the best treatment option?
   a) A 50-year-old man with a T1a squamous cell carcinoma of the right glottis without other comorbidities.
   b) A 65-year-old obese man with a T2 squamous cell carcinoma of the left glottis who has severe chronic obstructive pulmonary disease (COPD) and a history of cervical spinal disease requiring surgical stabilization.
   c) An 85-year-old man with a T2 squamous cell carcinoma of the right glottis with a history of multiple myocardial infarctions requiring multivessel bypass surgery.
   d) None of the above.
3. In which situation does the patient not require treatment (either radiation or surgery) of the neck?
   a) T2N0M0 glottic squamous cell carcinoma.
   b) T2N0M0 squamous cell carcinoma of the left aryepiglottic fold.
   c) T2N0M0 squamous cell carcinoma of the subglottis.
   d) None of the above.

Answers: 1. c 2. a 3. a

Suggested Readings

Hartl DM. Evidence-based practice: management of glottic cancer. Otolaryngol Clin North Am. 2012; 45(5):1143–1161
Hartl DM, Brasnu DF. Contemporary Surgical Management of Early Glottic Cancer. Otolaryngol Clin North Am. 2015; 48(4):611–625

Jamal N, Sofer E, Chhetri DK. Treatment considerations for early glottic carcinoma: lessons learned and a primer for the general otolaryngologist. Otolaryngol Head Neck Surg. 2014; 150(2):169–173

Jamal N, Sofer E, Chhetri DK. Treatment considerations for early glottic carcinoma: lessons learned and a primer for the general otolaryngologist. Otolaryngol Head Neck Surg. 2014; 150(2):169–173

Karatzanis AD, Psychogios G, Zenk J, et al. Comparison among different available surgical approaches in T1 glottic cancer. Laryngoscope. 2009; 119(9):1704–1708

Mor N, Blitzer A. Functional Anatomy and Oncologic Barriers of the Larynx. Otolaryngol Clin North Am. 2015; 48(4):533–545

Mourad M, Sadoughi B. Transcervical Conservation Laryngeal Surgery: An Anatomic Understanding to Enhance Functional and Oncologic Outcomes. Otolaryngol Clin North Am. 2015; 48(4):703–715

Smith JC, Johnson JT, Cognetti DM, et al. Quality of life, functional outcome, and costs of early glottic cancer. Laryngoscope. 2003; 113 (1):68–76

Tang CG, Sinclair CF. Voice Restoration After Total Laryngectomy. Otolaryngol Clin North Am. 2015; 48(4):687–702

Tibbetts KM, Tan M. Role of Advanced Laryngeal Imaging in Glottic Cancer: Early Detection and Evaluation of Glottic Neoplasms. Otolaryngol Clin North Am. 2015; 48(4):565–584

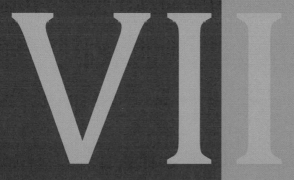

43 Multinodular Goiter

Tasneem A. Shikary and Reena Dhanda Patil

43.1 History

A 62-year-old man with a long-standing palpable neck mass was referred by his primary care physician for evaluation. The mass was nontender, but the patient did report some gradual enlargement over the last several months. He endorsed a family history of goiter and thyroid surgery but no family history of thyroid cancer or personal history of radiation exposure. He reported mild dysphagia to solids worse than liquids, but denied dyspnea, hoarseness, or symptoms of hypothyroidism or hyperthyroidism. He was a nonsmoker and consumed alcohol occasionally.

Physical examination revealed a diffusely enlarged, nodular midline neck mass above the sternal notch that was nontender to palpation and moved when the patient was asked to swallow. Indirect laryngoscopy using a mirror revealed normal vocal cord function. No other masses or evidence of adenopathy were noted.

43.2 Differential Diagnosis—Key Points

Multinodular goiter is common and often hereditary and/or related to environmental factors. Three main questions should arise in a clinician's mind when evaluating patient findings consistent with a multinodular goiter: (1) Could the mass be malignant? (2) Is it related to an endocrine dysfunction? (3) Is there evidence of compression of surrounding structures as a result of its size?

43.3 Test Interpretation

Work-up for multinodular goiter initially includes ultrasonography with fine needle aspiration of any suspicious or enlarged nodules and thyroid function tests. In this patient, the thyroid-stimulating hormone (TSH) level was 0.4, which is subnormal, but the free T4 level was in the normal range at 1.2, suggestive of subclinical hyperthyroidism. Radioactive iodine uptake scan was performed and showed a cold nodule on the right side. Ultrasound confirmed a multinodular goiter with solid dominant hypoechoic nodules bilaterally: a 3.2 × 2.4 × 5.1-cm dominant nodule on the right and a 3.3 × 2.1 × 2.8-cm dominant nodule on the left. Numerous nonpalpable smaller nodules were noted as well. There was no evidence of nodal disease or extrathyroidal extension, but substernal extension was present. None of the nodules were noted to have features suspicious for malignancy. Fine needle aspiration of the cold right nodule was performed and follicular lesion of undetermined significance was reported. Given the substernal extension, a computed tomography (CT) scan of the chest was performed for further evaluation and showed extension substernally, but above the level of the aortic arch (▶ Fig. 43.1). After counseling, the patient elected for total thyroidectomy, given compressive symptoms and biopsy results.

Ultrasound is the best imaging modality for evaluation of the thyroid to assess the presence of nodules, for accurate sizing, to identify features suspicious for malignancy, and to guide fine needle aspiration biopsy. Suspicious sonographic features of thyroid nodules are 80% sensitive for malignancy, such as papillary thyroid cancer. Size alone is nondiscriminatory, but larger nodules (> 1.5–2 cm) are often biopsied to exclude malignancy even in the absence of suspicious features. In the presence of multiple nodules, biopsy of suspicious nodules should be preferentially performed over benign-appearing larger ones. In a multinodular goiter, often the largest "dominant" nodule on each side is biopsied along with any sonographically suspicious nodules, requiring biopsy of as many as four nodules to exclude malignancy (see papillary thyroid carcinoma case in chapter 46 for further description of ultrasound-guided fine needle biopsy and cytologic findings).

Screening TSH should be done to exclude subclinical hyperthyroidism, which is common in multinodular goiter. If the TSH is low, then follow-up testing of free triiodothyronine (T_3) and free thyroxine (T_4) is necessary to monitor for the development of future hyperthyroidism. Radioactive iodine uptake scans are generally not needed as part of work-up for multinodular goiter, but in the setting of hyperthyroidism it can assist in determining if hyperthyroidism is caused by a toxic adenoma within a multinodular goiter. Nodules that have increased uptake are consistent with toxic adenoma and do not require additional investigation; however, cold nodules warrant further work-up with fine needle aspiration biopsy.

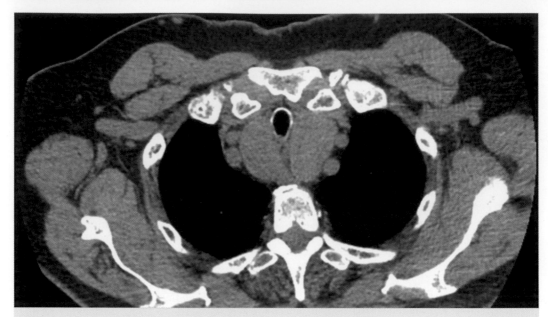

Fig. 43.1 CT scan demonstrating large multinodular goiter with substernal extension.

Slowly growing multinodular goiters confined to the neck are often asymptomatic to the patient, as the neck musculature and skin expand with growth. Goiters that extend into the thoracic inlet and mediastinum more commonly cause tracheal deviation and compression. If the inferior extent of the goiter is not visualized on ultrasound, then chest CT is indicated for further evaluation and preoperative planning. Pulmonary function tests in the sitting and supine position or with flexion and extension may be helpful to assess dyspnea. Barium swallow to evaluate dysphagia rarely demonstrates extrinsic compression but may be helpful to exclude other causes of dysphagia, such as esophageal dysmotility or strictures, especially in older individuals.

43.4 Diagnosis

Multinodular goiter

43.5 Medical Management

Medical management primarily consists of thyroid hormone suppression therapy or ablative radio-iodine treatment. Thyroid hormone replacement therapy to keep TSH levels in the low normal range is indicated for patients with hypothyroidism. Thyroid hormone suppression therapy with levothyroxine to suppress TSH to subnormal values may

reduce goiter size for some patients but is associated with increased risk of cardiac arrhythmia and osteoporosis, and goiter recurs following discontinuation of suppressive therapy. Thus, routine suppression is not recommended.

Radio-iodine treatment may be more effective than TSH suppression, but requires higher doses of radio-iodine for euthyroid multinodular goiter compared with hyperthyroid patients. Radio-iodine may reduce volume size by 20 to 40% over a 1- to 2-year period but is associated with a small risk of malignancy and is not recommended routinely. However, it may be an option in patients who are poor surgical candidates but are experiencing significant compressive symptoms. TSH-stimulated radio-iodine therapy may improve radio-iodine uptake and subsequent volume reduction with lower radio-iodine doses and should be considered if this mode of therapy is undertaken.

43.6 Surgical Management

Total thyroidectomy is curative for bilateral multinodular goiter. In unilateral nodular goiter, fine-needle biopsy to exclude malignancy followed by hemithyroidectomy will be sufficient for most patients but may require completion thyroidectomy if occult malignancy is discovered or subsequent enlarging nodular disease develops in the remaining lobe. Partial lobectomy, subtotal thyroidectomy, and bilateral subtotal thyroidectomy should be avoided because of the likelihood of recurrent nodular disease requiring reoperative surgery in a prior operative field with increased risk to the parathyroid glands and recurrent laryngeal nerve. Surgery should be reserved for cases suspicious for malignancy or for large or enlarging goiters, especially in younger patients. Involvement of the thoracic inlet or superior mediastinum or evidence of tracheal compression or significant deviation is an indication for surgery. If there is substernal extension, most goiters can be removed with a traditional cervical incision without the need for sternotomy. If there is extension to the level of the aortic arch, then sternotomy may be required.

43.7 Rehabilitation and Follow-up

If observation is elected, annual TSH testing and ultrasound are reasonable to evaluate for progression of nodular disease, development of new nodules, and/or development of thyroid dysfunction. Repeat fine needle biopsy to exclude malignancy in previously cytologically benign nodules without significant change on ultrasound is not necessary but should be considered if suspicious sonographic features appear or significant growth occurs.

43.8 Questions

1. What is the best imaging modality for a euthyroid patient suspected of having a thyroid nodule?
a) Ultrasound.
b) Computed tomography (CT) scan.
c) Magnetic resonance imaging (MRI) scan.
d) Radio-iodine uptake and scan.
e) Positron emission tomography (PET) scan.
2. What biochemical screening test is indicated for a patient suspected of having a multinodular goiter?
a) Thyroglobulin.
b) Calcitonin.
c) Thyroid-stimulating hormone (TSH).
d) Free thyroxine.
e) Free thyronine.
3. What surgical procedure is indicated for management of an enlarging bilateral multinodular goiter with compressive symptoms?
a) Bilateral subtotal thyroidectomy.
b) Unilateral subtotal thyroidectomy.
c) Total thyroidectomy.
d) Hemithyroidectomy (lobectomy).
e) Isthmusectomy.

Answers: 1. a 2. c 3. c

Suggested Readings

Haugen BR, Alexander EK, Bible KC, et al. American Thyroid Association Guidelines Taskforce. Management guidelines for adult patients with thyroid nodules and differentiated thyroid cancer. Thyroid. 2016; 26(1):1–133

Netterville JL, Coleman SC, Smith JC, Smith MM, Day TA, Burkey BB. Management of substernal goiter. Laryngoscope. 1998; 108(11 Pt 1):1611–1617

Management of substernal goiter. Laryngoscope. 1998; 108(11 Pt 1):1611–1617

44 Graves Disease

Alice L. Tang and David L. Steward

44.1 History

A 43-year-old woman presented with a 25-pound weight loss in the past year despite having a good appetite. She complained of heat intolerance, excessive sweating, tremor, and palpitations. She denied cold intolerance, dysphagia, constipation, or any compression or tenderness in her neck. She specifically denied vision changes. She was otherwise healthy and took no medication. There was no history of thyroid cancer in first-degree relatives, but she did have a sister with thyroid problems requiring thyroid hormone.

On physical exam, her vitals were normal except that her pulse was 110. Her skin was warm and moist to the touch. Her head and neck exam revealed bilateral exophthalmos with preserved extraocular motion. She had a mildly enlarged thyroid that was diffusely palpable and non-tender.

44.2 Differential Diagnosis—Key Points

The history and physical in this case are suggestive of hyperthyroidism. The differential diagnosis for hyperthyroidism includes Graves disease, subacute or early chronic lymphocytic thyroiditis, or toxic nodular goiter. The presentation of ophthalmopathy with a diffusely enlarged nontender thyroid gland strongly suggests Graves disease, which is responsible for 70 to 80% of endogenous hyperthyroidism. This disease can occur at any age and is more common in females than males. The family history suggests both hyperthyroidism and hypothyroidism, and current understanding of autoimmune thyroid disease suggests that Hashimoto's thyroiditis and Graves disease are genetically related and can coexist in the same patient.

Initial work-up should focus on biochemical confirmation of the hyperthyroidism and amelioration of symptoms, with further work-up focused upon the etiology of the hyperthyroidism. The treatment and prognosis depend upon the etiology of the hyperthyroidism.

44.3 Test Interpretation

Biochemical diagnosis includes thyroid-stimulating hormone (TSH), free T_3, and free T_4 levels, with low TSH and high free T_3 and/or free T_4 levels diagnostic for hyperthyroidism. Subclinical hyperthyroidism is associated with low TSH with normal free T_3 and free T_4 levels. Without further testing, thyroid function tests alone are insufficient for diagnosing Graves disease.

Other serologic results are required to support the diagnosis of autoimmune thyroid disease. Graves disease is an autoimmune disease classically caused by thyrotropin receptor antibodies (TRAb) stimulating the thyrotropin receptor, which acts to increase thyroid hormone synthesis and secretion and causes enlargement of the gland. Elevated TRAb levels are diagnostic of Graves disease. In contrast, elevated thyroglobulin (Tg) and/or anti–thyroid peroxidase (anti-TPO) antibodies are consistent with chronic lymphocytic thyroiditis (Hashimoto's disease), which causes gland destruction and transient release of stored thyroid hormone that can mimic Graves disease but usually results in hypothyroidism with time. In the absence of positive antibody testing and an elevated erythrocyte sedimentation rate (ESR) (>60), a tender thyroid is consistent with viral subacute thyroiditis (de Quervain's disease), which causes transient thyrotoxicosis that is self-limited.

To further delineate other causes of hyperthyroidism, radio-iodine uptake (RAIU) and scanning is useful in differentiating toxic nodular goiters (patchy uptake) from Graves disease (diffuse uptake) (▶ Fig. 44.1). Specifically, RAIU will demonstrate marked elevated 24-hour iodine uptake (>35%) and a diffuse and intense positive scan in Graves disease. The presence of a cold area within a background of Graves disease suggests a nodule that requires work-up to exclude malignancy. RAIU is usually high normal or mildly elevated to 25 to 30% in toxic adenoma or toxic multinodular goiter. RAIU will be low (<5–10%) in hyperthyroid patients with thyroiditis. Other causes of low RAIU in hyperthyroidism include iodine-induced thyrotoxicosis, exogenous thyrotoxicosis (factitia), and ectopic functional thyroid tissue.

Thyroid ultrasound will demonstrate characteristic diffuse thyroid enlargement with hypervascularity in Graves disease and occasionally will demonstrate nodular disease requiring further evaluation. Ultrasound will show a characteristic heterogeneously hypoechoic thyroid in thyroiditis, sometimes with intrathyroidal reactive lymph

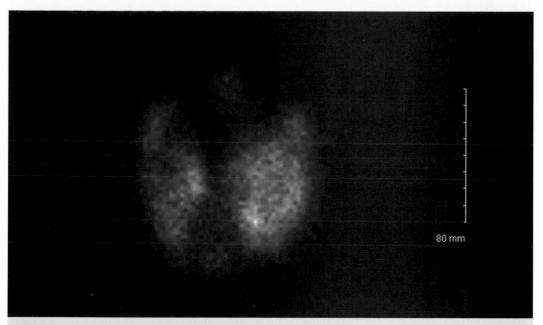

Fig. 44.1 Radioactive iodine scan with diffuse uptake characteristic of Graves disease.

Table 44.1 Lab results of this patient's biochemical tests

	Result	Reference range
Thyroid-stimulating hormone	<0.02	0.45–4.50 mIU/L
T_3, free	9.0	2.8–5.3 pg/mL
Free T_4	1.93	0.61–1.76 ng/dL
Thyroglobulin antibody	<20.0	0.0–39 IU/mL
Thyroid peroxidase antibody	12	0–34 IU/mL
Thyrotropin receptor antibody	5.78	0.0–1.75 IU/L

nodes. Toxic adenomas will appear as a solitary solid possibly hypervascular nodule but may require radio-iodine scanning to assess the function of the nodule to differentiate Graves disease with a cold nodule from a hot nodule within a background of suppressed thyroid. Toxic multinodular goiter on ultrasound alone will be indistinguishable from nontoxic multinodular goiter and requires radio-iodine scanning to identify the hyperfunctional nodule(s) and those that are hypofunctional possibly requiring further work-up (biopsy) (▶ Table 44.1).

Additionally, the neck ultrasound revealed a diffusely enlarged hypervascular thyroid without nodules. The radioactive uptake and scan showed a left thyroid lobe that was larger in comparison to the right with no discrete hyperfunctioning nodule noted. The 24-hour uptake was 45.9%.

In summary, the patient had a positive TRAb with elevated uptake consistent with Graves disease.

44.4 Diagnosis

Hyperthyroidism and Graves disease

44.5 Medical Management

Initial medical management includes use of a beta-blocker for symptomatic treatment of thyrotoxicosis. If left untreated, hyperthyroidism can cause decreased quality of life and significant cardiovascular disease (i.e., atrial fibrillation, cardiomyopathy, and congestive heart failure). Propranolol is beneficial for blocking T_4 to T_3 conversion in severe cases. Alternatively, atenolol may be used in less severe cases.

Antithyroid medical therapy is the first-line treatment for Graves disease. Medical management with thioamides (methimazole or propylthiouracil) will inhibit synthesis of thyroid hormone and result in euthyroidism within 4 to 6 weeks in most patients. Production of TSH by the pituitary may remain suppressed for several months, which necessitates regular measurements of free T_3 and T_4 levels to assess the effectiveness of thioamides. Long-term use of thioamides is associated with a low risk of agranulocytosis and hepatotoxicity and is less desirable than definitive treatment with radio-iodine or surgery for most patients. Furthermore, there is a high relapse rate with antithyroid drugs when used as a primary therapy; therefore, it is more often used as an adjunct to radio-iodine therapy and/or surgery.

Corticosteroids are effective in medically refractory patients during acute toxic crisis or in preparation for surgery. The steroids inhibit the autoimmune stimulation of the TSH receptor by the TRAb and also inhibit peripheral conversion of T_4 to T_3.

Radio-iodine therapy is the preferred definitive treatment for Graves disease in the United States, especially for those who are not good surgical candidates. For patients in Europe and Asia, antithyroid drugs and/or surgery are the more preferred treatments. This treatment modality is aimed at abolishing sufficient thyroid gland to effectively cause the patient to be euthyroid or hypothyroid. Radio-iodine therapy will render most patients with Graves disease hypothyroid (10–24%), and it may take months for the effects to manifest. For some patients with very large thyroid glands or those for those for whom a single treatment fails to resolve the hyperthyroidism, radio-iodine may need to be repeated. Radio-iodine is associated with risk for worsening Graves orbitopathy (especially in smokers), and thus the presence of ocular symptoms is a relative contraindication to RAIU. If planned, concomitant corticosteroids may reduce this risk. Radio-iodine is teratogenic and absolutely contraindicated in pregnancy, and pregnancy should be deferred for 6 to 12 months following radio-iodine treatment. It is not recommended during breastfeeding due to significant radio-iodine uptake in lactating breast tissue.

Radio-iodine may be associated with a very small absolute risk of subsequent development of radiation-induced malignancy, which should be discussed with the patient.

Exophthalmos will improve with beta-blockers and when the patient becomes euthyroid. Referral of the patient to an ophthalmologist is recommended for evaluation of possible corneal or other complications of opthalmopathy. Adequate moisturization of the eye is important.

This patient in our index case underwent radio-iodine therapy. However, despite adequate radio-iodine therapy, she remained hyperthyroid despite concurrent therapy with antithyroid drugs.

44.6 Surgical Management

Total thyroidectomy is curative of hyperthyroidism. Thyroid surgery for Graves disease is more difficult than other cases due to the large and hypervascular nature of the gland. Preoperatively, patients should be rendered euthyroid with thioamide therapy and/or corticosteroids to reduce the risk of postoperative thyrotoxic crisis. Treatment with supersaturated potassium iodide (SSKI) 1 week preoperatively may further reduce thyroid vascularity and reduce risk of thyroid storm. Perioperative beta-blocker therapy is recommended to protect the heart and should be continued for 1 week postoperatively. Thyroid hormone replacement with levothyroxine should be initiated after surgery and all antithyroid drugs should be discontinued. Attempts to perform subtotal thyroidectomy to avoid postoperative hypothyroidism are misguided and associated with risk for recurrence of hyperthyroidism.

Orbital decompression of the medial and inferior walls to allow decompression of the medial and inferior rectus muscles into the ethmoid and maxillary sinus can improve worsening exophthalmos but causes diplopia and is not indicated for mild orbitopathy. The eye disease may improve slowly 1 to 2 years following total thyroidectomy, presumably because removal of the thyroid reduces the overall antigen load presented to the immune system despite the fact that the antibodies reacting to the extraocular muscles may be different from the TSH receptor antibodies causing hyperthyroidism.

Our patient subsequently underwent total thyroidectomy for Graves disease and remains euthyroid on lifelong thyroid replacement hormone. She had no complications from radio-iodine therapy or surgery. Her exophthalmos resolved within months of her surgery.

44.7 Rehabilitation and Follow-up

Long-term thyroid hormone replacement is necessary for patients treated with thyroidectomy or radio-iodine therapy. Serial thyroid function testing and possibly complete blood counts should be performed for patients on thioamide therapy.

44.8 Questions

1. Which of the following are possible side effects of thioamide therapy?
   a) Hepatoxicity, rash, agranulocytosis.
   b) Cardiomyopathy, hepatotoxicity.
   c) Renal dysfunction, hearing loss.
   d) Hyperthyroidism, hypocalcemia.
2. Which of the following is not typically elevated in Graves disease?
   a) Free T3.
   b) Free T4.
   c) Anti–thyroid peroxidase (anti-TPO) antibody.
   d) Thyrotropin receptor antibody (TRAb).
   e) Radio-iodine uptake.
3. Which of the following is not an appropriate preoperative medical therapy regimen for patients with Graves disease?
   a) Propanolol
   b) Potassium iodide.
   c) Atenolol.
   d) Levothyroxine.
   e) Prednisone.

Answers: 1. a 2. c 3. d

Suggested Readings

Randolph G. Surgery of the Thyroid and Parathyroid Glands. Elsevier Saunders, Philadelphia, PA; 2012: 52–57

Singer PA, Cooper DS, Levy EG, et al. Treatment guidelines for patients with hyperthyroidism and hypothyroidism. Standards of Care Committee, American Thyroid Association. JAMA. 1995; 273 (10):808–812

45 Hashimoto's Thyroiditis

Alice L. Tang and David L. Steward

45.1 History

A 40-year-old woman presented with symmetric swelling of her neck that had been slowly enlarging for 1 year. She complained of difficulty losing weight and felt fatigued. She also had a history of cold intolerance. She denied dysphagia or pressure sensation in her neck. She denied a personal history of radiation and otherwise had no significant past medical history. Her mother had Graves disease and she had a sister who took thyroid medication.

Physical examination revealed an overweight woman with coarse hair. Her skin was cold to touch. On neck exam, she had a diffusely firm thyroid gland that was nontender. There was no evidence of cervical lymphadenopathy. She did not have any ocular changes.

45.2 Differential Diagnosis—Key Points

Symptoms of hypothyroidism can be vague and diverse given the broad systemic function of thyroid hormone. Patients can clinically present with no symptoms or with a range of nonspecific complaints including weight gain, lethargy, constipation, muscle aches, and neck fullness. Compressive symptoms such as dysphagia and dyspnea can occasionally be the presenting symptom if the thyroid gland is especially enlarged, causing nearby structures to be affected.

This patient presented with symptoms of hypothyroidism that would need to be confirmed with thyroid function tests. The most common cause of hypothyroidism in the United States is chronic lymphocytic thyroiditis or Hashimoto's thyroiditis. There are other less common causes of thyroiditis including subacute lymphocytic thyroiditis (i.e., postpartum thyroiditis, sporadic thyroiditis), de Quervain's thyroiditis, drug-induced thyroiditis, radiation thyroiditis, or very rarely, Riedel's thyroiditis. In older patients, hypothyroidism may not be the result of thyroiditis but rather a consequence of aging. Outside the United States in iodine-deficient areas, hypothyroidism may be due to endemic iodine deficiency.

Hashimoto's thyroiditis classically presents in a young woman (peak 30–50 years old) with a non-painful but persistent goiter. Patients usually present in a euthyroid or hypothyroid state. Occasionally, hyperthyroidism is observed if it is early in the disease process as a result of transient release of stored hormones from gland destruction, which can mimic Graves disease. There is evidence that autoimmune thyroid diseases have a genetic predisposition associated with certain human leukocyte antigens (HLAs). Although the relationship remains unclear, Hashimoto's disease and Graves disease are genetically linked, and it is not uncommon for families to have members with both disease processes.

45.3 Test Interpretation

Hypothyroidism is confirmed with thyroid function tests showing a high thyroid-stimulating hormone (TSH) level and normal or low free T_4. Free T_3 testing has limited utility in confirming hypothyroidism as opposed to hyperthyroidism. The hallmark of Hashimoto's disease is the presence of antithyroid antibodies. Antithyroid peroxidase (anti-TPO) antibodies are found in > 90% of patients with Hashimoto's disease and are considered the best serologic marker to establish diagnosis. A less sensitive and specific marker is antithyroglobulin (anti-Tg), which is only positive in 60 to 80% of patients with this disease.

Neck ultrasound is indicated to rule out discrete nodules in the presence of a firm palpable thyroid gland. Thyroiditis and hypothyroidism may increase the risk of malignancy. Ultrasound commonly reveals a hypoechoic heterogeneous thyroid gland in thyroiditis and occasionally benign-appearing intrathyroidal lymph nodes, especially in younger patients. Discrete nodules, if present within the thyroid, require fine needle biopsy to exclude malignancy if the nodules appear sonographically suspicious or are greater than 1.5 cm in size. However, interpretation of cytology to establish malignancy can be difficult, as it can show the presence of lymphocytes along with Hürthle cells showing metaplasia. If aspirates are predominantly Hürthle cells, cytopathologists may diagnose "atypia of undetermined significance" or Hürthle cell neoplasm according to the Bethesda system for reporting thyroid cytopathology, indicating neither a definitely benign nor a malignant process.

Rapidly enlarging diffuse enlargement should raise suspicion for thyroid lymphoma, which is rare but has relatively increased risk (67x) in patients with thyroiditis. This requires a core or incisional biopsy.

This patient's TSH level was high at 33 (ref 0.4–4.5) with a low free T_4 at 0.7 (ref 0.9–1.8) confirming hypothyroidism. Anti-TPO serologic testing revealed a value of 309 (ref 0–34). Neck ultrasound demonstrated a diffusely enlarged hypoechogenic thyroid that was consistent with thyroiditis without discrete nodules.

45.4 Diagnosis

Hypothyroidism with Hashimoto's thyroiditis

45.5 Medical Management

The mainstay treatment for Hashimoto's disease is primarily medical management. Thyroid hormone replacement therapy with levothyroxine is instituted. The initial dose is proportional to elevation of the TSH, requiring higher dosing for higher TSH. Due to the profound symptoms and high TSH and free T_4, this patient was started on near-full replacement dosing (1.5 µg/kg/day). A TSH level was obtained 4 to 6 weeks later with titration of levothyroxine therapy to a target TSH of between 1 and 3. In older patients or those with known coronary artery disease, initiation of therapy should be at lower dosing (i.e., 25 µg daily), with slow incremental increases ultimately to the same target TSH level.

Some studies have suggested improved cognitive function with combined levothyroxine (LT_4) and liothyronine (LT_3) therapy, but most studies have failed to demonstrate a benefit. Further, LT_3 has a short half-life, requiring dosing at two or three times per day, and results in supraphysiologic T_3 levels transiently, potentially increasing the risk for cardiac and skeletal effects of hyperthyroidism. As T_4 is peripherally converted to T_3, LT_3 is not necessary for the vast majority of patients and discouraged for routine use. For patients who continue to feel fatigued with target TSH between 1 and 2 and normal free T_4 levels, obtaining a free T_3 to ensure adequate peripheral conversion will usually prove normal, suggesting no need for LT_3 therapy.

45.6 Surgical Management

Surgical management is generally not indicated for hypothyroidism or thyroiditis unless there is suspicion for malignancy based upon fine needle biopsy of discrete nodules. Thyroidectomy may be an option for patients experiencing compressive symptoms from progressive enlargement of the thyroid gland refractory to thyroid hormone replacement therapy, but this is a small minority of patients. Surgery is often more difficult in patients with thyroiditis due to fibrosis of the gland to surrounding structures. Further, Hashimoto's thyroiditis is usually self-limited with progressive gland atrophy precluding need for surgical intervention.

45.7 Rehabilitation and Follow-up

Semiannual to annual TSH testing to confirm adequacy of thyroid hormone replacement therapy is important, with more frequent testing earlier in the disease course. This patient was rendered euthyroid with levothyroxine with improvement in symptoms.

45.8 Questions

1. When is the most appropriate time frame for rechecking thyroid-stimulating hormone (TSH) after instituting full thyroid hormone replacement therapy?
   a) 1 to 2 weeks.
   b) 2 to 3 weeks.
   c) 4 to 6 weeks.
   d) 10 to 12 weeks.
2. Patients with Hashimoto's disease have a 67x increased risk for developing which of the following?
   a) Anaplastic thyroid cancer.
   b) Thyroid lymphoma.
   c) Clear cell carcinoma.
   d) Papillary thyroid cancer.
3. Which of the following is the most sensitive marker for diagnosing Hashimoto's disease?
   a) Anti–thyroid peroxidase (anti-TPO).
   b) Antithyroglobulin.
   c) Anti-TSH receptors.
   d) TSH.
   e) Free T_4.

Answers: 1. c 2. b 3. a

Suggested Readings

Singer PA, Cooper DS, Levy EG, et al. Treatment guidelines for patients with hyperthyroidism and hypothyroidism. Standards of Care Committee, American Thyroid Association. JAMA. 1995; 273 (10):808–812

Randolph G. Surgery of the Thyroid and Parathyroid Glands. Elsevier Saunders, Philadelphia, PA; 2012: 41–43

Caturegli P, De Remigis A, Rose NR. Hashimoto thyroiditis: clinical and diagnostic criteria. Autoimmun Rev. 2014; 13(4–5):391–397

46 Papillary Thyroid Carcinoma

Alice L. Tang and David L. Steward

46.1 History

A 25-year-old woman was referred by her primary care doctor for a prominent right thyroid nodule and a right neck mass during a routine visit. She denied any history of childhood radiation exposure or family history of thyroid cancer. She had no significant past medical history. She denied hoarseness, weight change, fatigue, or palpitations.

On physical examination, it was evident that she had a firm 2-cm palpable right thyroid nodule. In her right lateral neck exam, there were two obvious neck masses in level IV, each approximately 2 to 3 cm in size. These lymph nodes were hard and fixed. She did not have a hoarse voice. Her primary care physician had ordered a computed tomography (CT) scan that demonstrated the neck and thyroid disease (► Fig. 46.1).

46.2 Differential Diagnosis—Key Points

Palpable thyroid nodules are present in approximately 5% of women and 1% of men. The risk of malignancy in thyroid nodules is approximately 7 to 15% in patients without significant risk factors. Age (young or old), male sex, childhood radiation exposure, whole body radiation for bone marrow transplantation, and a strong family history of thyroid cancer are factors that would increase the risk of malignancy. Many nonpalpable nodules are discovered incidentally on anatomic imaging, and generally, only nodules that are > 1 cm should be evaluated, although smaller nodules can be further evaluated in the presence of clinical suspicion or associated lymphadenopathy. Ultrasound is the most sensitive and cost-effective imaging modality for thyroid nodules that do not extend into the chest. The sensitivity for malignancy based upon sonographic features exceeds 80%.

The patient had no symptoms to suggest hyperthyroidism or hypothyroidism but should undergo screening thyroid-stimulating hormone (TSH) measurement to assess thyroid function, as the results may affect management of the patient. For example, a solitary toxic adenoma has an extremely low risk (0.1%) of malignancy and likely does not require biopsy. In contrast, a nonfunctional nodule within a background of Graves disease requires biopsy to exclude malignancy prior to consideration for radio-iodine therapy.

46.3 Test Interpretation

Screening TSH is the initial evaluation and is indicated for all patients with nodular thyroid disease. If normal no further thyroid function tests are necessary and the work-up proceeds to exclude malignancy. If the TSH is high, suggestive of hypothyroidism, a free T4 level should be obtained to confirm the diagnosis and treatment with levothyroxine (LT4) should be initiated and the

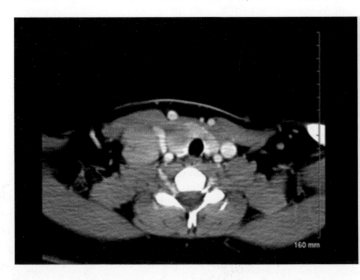

Fig. 46.1 CT scan demonstrating thyroid and nodal disease.

work-up proceeds to exclude malignancy as in euthyroid patients. If the TSH is low, suggestive of hyperthyroidism, free thyronine (T_3) and free thyroxine (T_4) levels should both be obtained. In hyperthyroid patients with thyroid nodules, a radio-iodine uptake and scan is helpful to determine the etiology of the hyperthyroidism, which impacts management. The radio-iodine uptake and scan is not indicated and not helpful in the routine evaluation of euthyroid and hypothyroid patients.

Thyroglobulin, a precursor to thyroid hormone, is produced by benign thyroid follicular cells as well as well-differentiated thyroid carcinomas (papillary, follicular, and Hürthle cell carcinoma). It is a very sensitive postoperative and postablative marker for persistent or recurrent malignancy but is not helpful preoperatively to screen for malignancy and is not indicated.

Ultrasound is the best imaging modality for thyroid nodules contained within the neck or thoracic inlet. Sonographic features suggestive of malignancy are stratified into high, intermediate, low, and very low suspicious patterns. High-risk patterns (> 70–90% risk of malignancy) include microcalcifications, hypoechogenicity, irregular margins, extrathyroidal extension, a shape taller than wide as seen on a transverse view, and/or suspicious lymphadenopathy. Intermediate-risk patterns (10–20%) include hypoechoic solid nodule with regular margins. Nodules that are ≥ 1 cm with high or intermediate suspicious sonographic pattern should be biopsied. Low-risk nodules, described as solid hyperechoic or isoechoic with regular margins and/or partially cystic, can be 1.5 cm in size before biopsy is recommended. Observation without fine needle aspiration (FNA) is a reasonable option for nodules that are ≤ 2 cm with very low suspicious sonographic pattern (e.g., spongiform). Additionally, ultrasound should be performed to look for associated lymphadenopathy. If present, suspicious lymph nodes should undergo ultrasound FNA for cytology and thyroglobulin rinse.

Neck CT or magnetic resonance imaging (MRI) is rarely necessary unless there is clinical concern for invasive malignancy or in centers without experience in neck ultrasound for nodal disease in biopsy-proven malignancy. Chest CT is indicated in cases of thyroid extension below the thoracic inlet for evaluation of inferior extent of the goiter and degree of tracheal deviation or compression. Chest CT may also be indicated preoperatively or postoperatively to assess for pulmonary or mediastinal metastatic disease in biopsy proven malignancy with bulky nodal disease.

[18]FDG-PET scan is not indicated for routine evaluation of thyroid nodules. Focal uptake seen incidentally on [18]FDG-PET scan for other reasons that is confirmed by an ultrasound to be a discrete nodule carries an approximate 35% risk of malignancy. These nodules, if greater than 1 cm, should be biopsied. However, if diffuse uptake is seen in the thyroid gland with clinical and sonographic correlation of chronic lymphocytic thyroiditis without discrete or suspicious nodules, no biopsy is indicated.

Ultrasound-guided fine needle biopsy is the best test to exclude malignancy in thyroid nodules, with false negative rates of 1 to 2% in experienced centers. Fine needle biopsy sensitivity and specificity are significantly improved with ultrasound guidance to confirm the needle tip in the target nodule and avoid sampling error from normal thyroid tissue. Palpation-guided fine needle biopsy has insufficient negative predictive value and should not be performed unless ultrasound guidance is unavailable and the nodule is anteriorly located and discretely palpable. Ultrasound-guided fine needle biopsy requires a minimum of two separate needle passes to sample the nodule. The nondiagnostic rate can be reduced by utilizing three to four separate needles for each nodule.

Biopsy results should be reported using the six categories outlined in the Bethesda System for Reporting Thyroid Cytopathology: nondiagnostic/unsatisfactory, benign, atypia of undetermined significance or follicular lesion of undetermined significance (AUS/FLUS), follicular neoplasm or suspicious for a follicular neoplasm, suspicious for malignancy, and malignant. Each category conveys a risk assessment based upon literature review of 5 to 10%, < 5%, 10 to 50%, 20 to 30%, 50 to 90%, and > 95%, respectively.

Interpretation of the results of fine needle biopsy requires an understanding of the limitations of cytologic evaluation. Nondiagnostic specimens contain less than 6 to 8 follicular cell clusters and must be repeated to exclude malignancy. Repeatedly nondiagnostic biopsy may require surgery to exclude malignancy. Benign follicular and/or Hürthle cells are the most common finding and do not require further biopsy or surgery in the absence of clinical indications, but should be followed with ultrasound to assess for significant interval growth, which, if present, may warrant repeat biopsy or surgery. Cytopathology determined to be AUS/FLUS or follicular neoplasm/Hürthle cell neoplasm may be seen in follicular adenoma, follicular carcinoma, and follicular-variant papillary carcinoma and therefore classically requires diagnostic surgery to exclude malignancy. Pathology suspicious for malignancy is usually papillary thyroid cancer, though occasionally it could be medullary thyroid cancer, which then would require surgical excision for therapeutic intent. Malignant cytology is most commonly seen in classic papillary thyroid carcinoma and requires surgery for definitive therapy rather than diagnostic purposes.

Cytomolecular testing has recently been introduced to facilitate surgical decision making for indeterminate cytology results. Prior to the advent of molecular testing, standard of care is to perform diagnostic surgery for FNA results that were indeterminate. Several molecular markers have been proposed to complement FNA results in efforts to avoid unnecessary diagnostic surgery for benign nodules or second surgical procedure in cases where malignancy was diagnosed postoperatively (completion thyroidectomy). Current investigations are under way in validating which platforms and mutation panels are most optimal in complementing cytology for routine clinical practice. Careful consideration of patient preference, clinical and sonographic suspicion, and test performance (negative predictive value/positive predictive value) are important.

For this patient, screening TSH, diagnostic ultrasound, and ultrasound-guided fine needle biopsy of thyroid nodule and lateral neck node were necessary. A CT scan of the neck with contrast was also obtained, given the suspicion of bulky nodal metastatic disease on ultrasonography. The use of iodinated contrast will result in delay of radioactive-iodine (RAI) therapy but was deemed necessary to adequately plan definitive surgery.

Testing in this patient revealed a normal TSH and the patient biochemically euthyroid. Ultrasound demonstrated a $0.9 \times 1.8 \times 1.0$-cm hypoechoic right nodule with irregular borders and microcalcifications. Additionally, there was a mass along the lateral margin of the right lobe of the thyroid gland that measured $4.0 \times 2.6 \times 3.0$ cm containing internal vascular flow and areas of calcifications. Ultrasound-guided fine needle biopsy of the thyroid nodule resulted in papillary thyroid carcinoma. The lateral neck lymph node demonstrated malignant follicular cells confirming metastatic papillary thyroid carcinoma. Given a malignant pathologic result on cytology, molecular testing was unnecessary. The CT scan of the neck demonstrated multiple suspicious nodes in bilateral lateral neck compartments.

46.4 Diagnosis

Metastatic papillary thyroid carcinoma

46.5 Medical Management

Thyroid hormone suppressive therapy with levothyroxine to suppress TSH levels to low normal or subnormal levels has been shown to reduce recurrence and morbidity. The degree of TSH suppression is based upon risk of recurrence. For low-risk patients, TSH suppression to 0.1 to 1.5 or 2.0 is recommended. Higher-risk patients or those with known persistent disease should have TSH suppression to < 0.1. TSH suppression may result in atrial arrhythmia and osteoporosis, which can be reduced with less aggressive TSH suppression and adjunctive medical therapy when indicated.

Radio-iodine therapy may reduce risk of recurrence and mortality, especially in more advanced disease. Remnant ablation may facilitate long-term surveillance with thyroglobulin levels in lower-risk patients. Repeated radio-iodine treatment may increase risk of second malignancy and may cause salivary or lacrimal gland dysfunction. Radio-iodine is teratogenic and contraindicated in pregnancy.

46.6 Surgical Management

Total thyroidectomy is indicated based upon the cytologic and imaging results. In general, total thyroidectomy has been shown to reduce recurrence of advanced thyroid cancer or in the presence of multicentricity when compared to hemithyroidectomy alone. The recurrent and superior laryngeal nerves should be identified and preserved along with the parathyroid glands in situ with blood supply intact. Parathyroid autotransplantation is performed if parathyroid devascularization occurs during dissection. Confirmation of parathyroid with biopsy and frozen section is recommended to avoid transplantation of tumor.

Due to the presence of bilateral clinically detectable lateral nodal metastasis (cN1b), central (level VI) neck dissection and lateral (levels IIa–Vb) neck dissections are performed with preservation of all vital structures not involved with cancer, including the internal jugular vein, sternocleidomastoid muscle, spinal accessory nerve, and preferably with preservation of cervical sensory nerves as well.

Well-differentiated thyroid cancers that are > 1 cm but < 4 cm without evidence of metastasis or extrathyroidal extension can be managed with thyroid lobectomy and close surveillance of the contralateral lobe after surgery. However, this option would prohibit the use of postoperative radioactive iodine treatment. For cancers that are < 1 cm without other significant risk factors (extrathyroidal extension, multifocality nodule involvement), patients can be counseled on thyroid lobectomy alone or active surveillance for older patients.

Postoperative complications of thyroidectomy include transient or permanent recurrent or superior laryngeal nerve injury with resultant dysphonia for unilateral injury and rare but possible airway obstruction from bilateral recurrent nerve injury. Hypoparathyroidism, transient or permanent, with resultant hypocalcemia can be diagnosed with rapid intact parathyroid hormone (PTH) measurement in recovery room (< 8–15 pg/mL) or by serial calcium measurement in recovery, evening of surgery, and morning of postoperative day 1 (< 8.0 mg/dL). Treatment of hypoparathyroidism includes frequent oral calcium supplementation (three or four times daily) along with early and aggressive 1,25-dihydroxy vitamin D supplementation (calcitriol). The risk of hypoparathyroidism increases with central neck dissections.

Postoperative hematoma can result in airway obstruction requiring urgent opening of the wound to decompress the neck and return to the operating room for hematoma evacuation and control of bleeding. Use of neck drains does not prevent postoperative bleeding but may facilitate management if this complication occurs.

Postoperative hypothyroidism is an expected consequence of total thyroidectomy requiring lifelong thyroid hormone replacement therapy. Long-term therapy with levothyroxine sodium (LT4) is initiated at approximately 1.5 µg/kg/day with subsequent dose titration based upon TSH levels obtained 5 to 6 weeks after initiation of therapy. Short-term therapy with liothyronine (LT3) is an alternative in the early postoperative period when thyroid hormone withdrawal is planned for physiologic TSH elevation to facilitate radio-iodine 4 to 6 weeks postoperatively. Liothyronine therapy at 25 µg daily in divided doses can be started 1 week postoperatively to limit severity and duration of symptoms from hypothyroidism during this period. Recombinant human TSH is more commonly given intramuscularly as an alternative to physiologic TSH elevation from thyroid hormone withdrawal to prepare for radio-iodine remnant ablation, avoiding the need for postoperative hypothyroidism or short-term liothyronine therapy.

46.7 Rehabilitation and Follow-up

Radio-iodine whole body scans had traditionally been the mainstay of scanning for recurrent or persistent cancer, but have been shown to have low sensitivity (20%) in more recent studies. Serum thyroglobulin and neck ultrasound have been shown to have combined sensitivity of greater than 90% in most studies and have become the mainstay of well-differentiated thyroid cancer surveillance. The presence of antithyroglobulin antibodies, common in thyroiditis and in approximately 25% of thyroid cancer patients, severely limits the measurement and interpretation of serum thyroglobulin levels and should always be measured along with thyroglobulin. Rising thyroglobulin antibodies postoperatively and after RAI are concerning for recurrent disease. Further, the presence of persistent benign thyroid tissue following surgery without postoperative radio-iodine ablation precludes discrimination of benign from malignant disease with low detectable levels of thyroglobulin. TSH-stimulated thyroglobulin measurement with recombinant human TSH injection improves the sensitivity of thyroglobulin to detect persistent/recurrent disease in patients who have undergone total thyroidectomy and RAI.

46.8 Questions

1. When is molecular testing for thyroid nodules considered?
   a) All nodules.
   b) Biopsy-proven metastasis in the lateral neck.
   c) Suspicious for malignancy on cytology.
   d) Cytologically indeterminate nodules or follicular neoplasm.
2. What is an appropriate treatment option for a papillary thyroid cancer that is 3.5 cm without evidence of extrathyroidal extension and without evidence of positive neck nodes?
   a) Radioactive iodine ablation.
   b) Hemithyroidectomy (lobectomy).
   c) Thyroid-stimulating hormone (TSH) suppression therapy.
   d) Close surveillance.

3. What is the next step in management in the evaluation of a patient with a thyroid nodule found to have a low TSH?
   a) Supplementation with levothyroxine.
   b) TSH suppression therapy.
   c) Radioactive iodine uptake scan.
   d) Computed tomography (CT) scan of the neck with contrast.

Answers: 1. d 2. b 3. c

Suggested Readings

Haugen BR, Alexander EK, Bible KC, et al. 2015 American Thyroid Association Management Guidelines for Adult Patients with Thyroid Nodules and Differentiated Thyroid Cancer: The American Thyroid Association Guidelines Task Force on Thyroid Nodules and Differentiated Thyroid Cancer. Thyroid. 2016; 26(1):1–133

47 Medullary Thyroid Carcinoma

Nathan D. Wiebracht and David L. Steward

47.1 History

A 78-year-old man with history of hypertension presented with a palpable left thyroid mass. He reported slow growing of the mass over the last several months. His primary care physician ordered a computed tomography (CT) scan (▶ Fig. 47.1). He denied any symptoms of hyper- or hypothyroidism, as well as any voice changes or dysphagia. His family history was remarkable for thyroid cancer in his mother, but he was unsure of the histologic type. He denied any history of radiation exposure. The physical exam was remarkable for a large, firm, nontender, unilateral left goiter. Flexible laryngoscopy revealed bilateral normal true vocal cord motion. The remainder of the physical exam was unremarkable.

Ultrasonography was remarkable for a left 9-cm solid, hypoechoic nodule. Additionally, a 2-cm suspicious left level 3 node was noted. Fine needle aspiration (FNA) was cytologically suspicious for medullary thyroid carcinoma. (MTC) Laboratory studies were significant for Calcitonin 11,426 pg/mL (norm 0–8.4), carcinoembryonic antigen (CEA) 99.5 ng/mL (0–3.0), Calcium 10 mg/dL (8.6–10.3), parathyroid hormone (PTH) 32 pg/mL (12–38), thyroid-stimulating hormone (TSH) 0.91 /mL (0.34–5.6), and normal urine metanephrines.

47.2 Differential Diagnosis—Key Points

The patient had a large thyroid nodule suspicious for MTC with a family history of thyroid cancer and was at risk for familial MTC, multiple endocrine neoplasia (MEN) 2A, or MEN2B. Genetic testing for the *Ret* proto-oncogene is diagnostic and required for this autosomal dominant hereditary disease. If this reveals the proto-oncogene, then all the patient's siblings and offspring require the same testing, and therapeutic or prophylactic thyroidectomy if positive. In addition, MEN2A is associated with primary hyperparathyroidism and pheochromocytoma; MEN2B is associated with pheochromocytoma, mucosal neuromas, gastrinomas, and marfanoid body habitus. Biochemical screening for these associated disorders is important preoperatively to identify hyperparathyroidism, which should be addressed concomitantly at

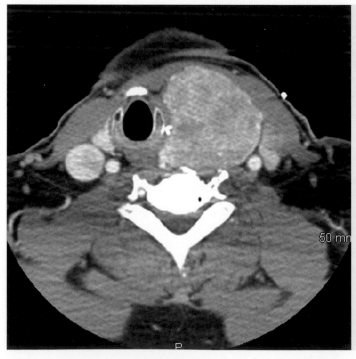

Fig. 47.1 Axial CT scan demonstrating a large thyroid mass.

the time of thyroidectomy. Because of the risk for perioperative hypertensive crisis, screening for pheochromocytoma should be performed before addressing the MTC.

47.2.1 Diagnostic Tests

The work-up of a thyroid nodule is reviewed in Chapter 46 and includes screening TSH, ultrasound, and ultrasound-guided fine needle biopsy if indicated. The cytology specimen should be sent for immunohistochemical staining for calcitonin in addition to standard hematoxylin and eosin staining, if MTC is suspected.

Calcitonin is produced by parafollicular c-cells within the thyroid. After malignant transformation, these cells continue to produce calcitonin, although they do so at much higher levels. Therefore, serum calcitonin is a reasonable screening test in patients with thyroid nodules and suspicion for MTC because of greater sensitivity than fine needle biopsy. However, due to low disease prevalence, false positives limit the utility of this test. In patients with a family history of MTC, it is mandatory. Slight elevation of serum calcitonin may be normal or may represent c-cell hyperplasia. Elevation above 100 is more specific for medullary cancer. If the calcitonin is greater than 1,000, a chest and abdominal CT should be considered to look for pulmonary, mediastinal, and liver metastases.

Genetic testing for the *RET* proto-oncogene is commercially available and indicated in all patients diagnosed with medullary carcinoma because 25% of apparently sporadic cases (no family history) are found to have the genetic alteration. If the index patient with medullary carcinoma is negative, then no further family members require genetic testing. If the index patient is positive, then all surviving biologic parents, siblings, and offspring require testing. Furthermore, genetic counseling is strongly recommended. The specific codon affected will diagnose MEN2A versus MEN2B with important clinical implications regarding the aggressiveness of MTC(codon 918 MEN2B generally more aggressive and earlier presentation), as well as associated endocrine neoplasias. Overall, the prognosis of MEN2A and familial MTC (FMTC) is better than that of sporadic cases. MEN2B, which has the worst prognosis. *RET*-positive family members have an approximate 90% risk of the development of MTC and require biochemical work-up and therapeutic or prophylactic thyroidectomy. Prophylactic removal of other endocrine glands is not recommended.

Pheochromocytomas are seen in ~50% of patients with MEN2A, but the risk may be codon specific. These benign adrenal tumors produce epinephrine, norepinephrine, and its precursors and metabolites, causing poorly controlled hypertension. All patients diagnosed with or suspected of having hereditary MTC should have preoperative screening. Plasma and 24-hour urinary catecholamines and metanephrines are the most sensitive and specific tests. If these are abnormally elevated, imaging is indicated and removal of the pheochromocytoma before thyroidectomy is important.

Primary hyperparathyroidism, usually from multiple parathyroid adenomas or hyperplasia, is seen in around 20% of patients with MEN2A. Biochemical screening should include serum calcium and intact parathyroid hormone levels. If elevated, then concomitant parathyroidectomy at the time of thyroidectomy is indicated.

47.3 Test Interpretation

Serum TSH was normal and the patient was euthyroid. Ultrasound revealed a 9-cm left-sided hypoechoic nodule with suspicious 2-cm left level 3 lymph node. Ultrasound-guided fine needle biopsy revealed cytologically suspicious cells that stained positive for calcitonin, diagnostic of MTC. Serum calcitonin was elevated at 11,426 pg/mL, suggesting likely distant metastatic disease. The *RET* proto-oncogene test was negative, thereby ruling out FMTC, MEN2A, and MEN2B. Plasma and 24-hour urinary catecholamines and metanephrines were normal. Calcium and parathyroid hormone levels were also normal.

47.4 Diagnosis

Medullary thyroid carcinoma, sporadic, with regional and possible distant metastases

47.5 Medical Management

Postoperative thyroid hormone replacement therapy with levothyroxine sodium should be initiated immediately postoperatively at 1.6 mg/kg/day, with titration of levothyroxine to keep TSH levels within the normal range, ideally between 1 and 3. Because the cellular lineage of MTC is from the parafollicular c-cells, thyroid hormone suppression and radio-iodine have no role in therapy.

Calcitonin doubling time less than 6 months has higher mortality risk. Two tyrosine kinase inhibitors, vandetanib and cabozantinib, have been approved for treatment for patients with rapidly progressive disease. Both agents target VEGFR and *RET*.

47.6 Surgical Management

Total thyroidectomy remains the gold standard for treatment of MTC. For small cT1N0 sporadic unifocal cases, hemithyroidectomy may be sufficient. Prophylactic comprehensive central compartment (level VI) dissection with care to include prelaryngeal (Delphian), pretracheal, and bilateral paratracheal lymph nodes medial to the carotid arteries and extending inferiorly to the innominate artery in the superior mediastinum (level VII) is important to reduce recurrent or persistent disease. This is important even in the absence of clinically apparent nodal metastases. All efforts should be made to preserve grossly normal parathyroid glands in situ with blood supply intact in the absence of biochemical evidence of hyperparathyroidism. Therapeutic central and lateral neck dissection (levels II–V) is indicated in the presence of clinically or radiographically suspicious lymph nodes. Resection in the presence of distant metastases requires balancing surgical morbidity with disease risk. In the case presented for this chapter, the patient had total thyroidectomy with central and lateral (IIa-Vb) neck dissection.

47.7 Rehabilitation and Follow-up

Serum calcitonin and CEA levels are the mainstay of long-term MTC surveillance. Undetectable calcitonin and CEA levels are suggestive of no persistent or recurrent disease. In low-risk patients these should be monitored semiannually to annually. In patients with a MEN2 syndrome, annual biochemical screening for associated endocrine neoplasias is indicated. Neck ultrasound is also a clinically useful tool in local and regional surveillance.

Persistently elevated calcitonin and CEA levels for more than 1 month postoperatively are consistent with persistent disease. The greater the calcitonin, the higher likelihood there is of distant metastases. Depending on calcitonin levels, structural imaging of the neck, chest, liver, and brain using ultrasonography, CT, and magnetic resonance imaging (MRI) to localize disease is performed. Lower calcitonin levels are associated with regional disease, whereas higher levels are associated with distant metastatic disease. Bone metastasis is best localized with bone scintigraphy. Radionuclide imaging using octreotide or fluoro-deoxyglucose positron emission tomography may occasionally be helpful to localize disease if structural imaging is nonlocalizing.

Rapidly doubling calcitonin levels are worrisome for progressive disease. Radiation therapy is generally not indicated for MTC after thyroidectomy, except when the risk of local recurrence is perceived to be high, for example, with a T4 tumor with positive margins. As mentioned previously, the tyrosine kinase inhibitors vandetanib and cabozantinib may be considered as adjuvant therapy in cases of rapidly progressive disease. Doubling times less than 2 years are associated with reduced 10-year survival compared with greater than 2-year doubling times. Very rapid doubling times of less than 6 months are associated with poor 5- and 10-year survival. In this case, a patient may consider involvement in a clinical trial.

47.8 Questions

1. Which of the following is the proto-oncogene diagnostic for an multiple endocrine neoplasia 2 (MEN2) syndrome?
   a) Menin.
   b) *RET*.
   c) p53.
   d) Carcinoembryonic antigen (CEA).
2. Which hormone, when elevated, is most concerning for medullary thyroid carcinoma? (MTC)
   a) Thyroid-stimulating hormone (TSH).
   b) Parathyroid hormone (PTH).
   c) Glucagon.
   d) Calcitonin.
3. True or false? In a patient with pheochromocytoma and MTC, it is recommended to address the pheochromocytoma first in order to prevent hypertensive crisis.

Answers: 1. b 2. d 3. True

Suggested Readings

Wells SA, Jr, Asa SL, Dralle H, et al. American Thyroid Association Guidelines Task Force on Medullary Thyroid Carcinoma. Revised American Thyroid Association guidelines for the management of medullary thyroid carcinoma. Thyroid. 2015; 25(6):567–610

48 Postthyroidectomy Hypocalcemia

David R. Lee and David L. Steward

48.1 History

A 53-year-old man presented to the emergency department complaining of numbness and muscle spasms that began 2 days ago when he was discharged home following a total thyroidectomy. His postoperative stay was uncomplicated, and his serum calcium on postoperative day 1 was 7.9. He was sent home with a calcium supplementation of 1 g three times a day. On physical exam, he confirmed perioral and bilateral upper and lower extremity paresthesias. He also had positive Chvostek's sign (facial twitching after tapping on the main trunk of the facial nerve) and Trousseau's sign (spasms of the muscles of the hand and forearm after a blood pressure cuff is inflated above systolic pressure). His incision was clean, dry, and intact with surgical Steri-Strips in place. His voice was normal. The remaining physical exam was unremarkable.

48.2 Differential Diagnosis—Key Points

Total thyroidectomy or completion thyroidectomy can inadvertently result in postthyroidectomy hypoparathyroidism via devascularization or resection of the parathyroid glands and subsequent hypocalcemia. The parathyroid glands regulate the body calcium levels via bone mobilization, renal concentration, and vitamin D activation for gut absorption of calcium. Transient or permanent hypoparathyroidism with subsequent hypocalcemia is a risk for any patient undergoing bilateral thyroid surgery, even if performed initially as a lobectomy or hemithyroidectomy with later completion thyroidectomy for the contralateral lobe. Concomitant central node dissection increases this risk.

Early detection of postthyroidectomy hypoparathyroidism can be made in the recovery room with rapid intact parathyroid hormone (PTH) testing; however, this ability is institution dependent. This is made possible due to the rapid half-life of PTH (~5 minutes). PTH levels less than 15 pg/dL are associated with significantly increased risk for hypocalcemia. Exact methods and timing to detect hypocalcemia vary for each surgeon. Hypocalcemia can be detected by serial calcium measurements performed in recovery, the evening of surgery, and in the early morning on postoperative day 1. Corrected serum calcium levels below 8.0 mg/dL (reference range 8.4–10.4) are diagnostic. Patients will often become symptomatic with corrected calcium levels below 7.5 to 8.0, and perioral numbness is an early and specific complaint. Extremity paresthesias may be more sensitive but less specific. Chvostek's sign has a fairly high false positive rate. Trousseau's sign is considered to be more specific for hypocalcemia. Muscle spasm and rigidity is a late and worrying sign of tetany and corrected calcium levels below 7.0.

48.2.1 Diagnostic Tests

An immediate repeat renal panel including low calcium level and elevated phosphorus level is diagnostic for hypoparathyroidism-related hypocalcemia. Ionized calcium may be more accurate but is less reliable due to pH dependence. In the early postthyroidectomy setting, hypoparathyroidism is etiologic, and PTH testing is rarely needed for diagnosis once hypocalcemia develops. The novel use of early and rapid PTH testing in the operating room—or immediately in the recovery room—can diagnose hypoparathyroidism prior to development of hypocalcemia, allowing for early intervention and prevention of its sequelae. Checking serum magnesium levels may be helpful, as it is also a divalent cation and low levels may exacerbate hypocalcemic signs and symptoms.

48.3 Test Interpretation

Calcium level was measured at 6.5 mg/dL (normal range 8.4–10.4) in the emergency room. A renal panel showed a slightly low albumin at 3.7 g/dL with a corrected calcium of 6.7 mg/dL and elevated serum phosphorus of 5.5 (range 3.5–5.0). Intact PTH levels were sent but not available for several days. Based on these lab values, the diagnosis of hypocalcemia from postthyroidectomy hypoparathyroidism was confirmed.

48.4 Diagnosis

Hypocalcemia from postthyroidectomy hypoparathyroidism

48.5 Medical Management

Oral calcium supplementation is the mainstay of therapy for hypocalcemia but requires vitamin D supplementation in order for calcium to be adequately absorbed. PTH converts 25-OH vitamin D into the active 1,25-OH vitamin D. Patients with hypoparathyroidism require treatment with 1,25-OH vitamin D, available as calcitriol. Many patients have previously unknown vitamin D deficiency and require load dosing with calcitriol in order to adequately absorb calcium.

Severely symptomatic patients with critically low calcium levels such as this patient require intravenous calcium to bring the calcium level into the low normal range. The preferable method of replacement is continuous infusion of calcium gluconate in saline run over several hours until the calcium levels can be maintained within the low normal range. Alternatively, intravenous boluses may be utilized, but this can prolong the time to normalization. Oral supplementation with calcium should be instituted immediately, with the frequency of dosing more important than the dose. Oral calcium can be calcium carbonate or calcium citrate; however, calcium citrate is better absorbed and often better tolerated. Severe hypocalcemia may require 1 to 2 g calcium orally four to five times daily. Calcitriol should be given with a load dose of 2 to 3 µg and then 1 µg daily.

48.6 Surgical Management

There is no surgical treatment for postthyroidectomy hypocalcemia. The best treatment is prevention and correct parathyroid gland management during thyroidectomy. Parathyroid glands should be left with the blood supply from the inferior thyroid artery intact. When branches of the inferior thyroid artery are taken during thyroidectomy, they should be taken medial to the parathyroid glands.

If inadvertently a parathyroid gland becomes devascularized, it should be minced and autotransplanted into a nearby muscle, most commonly the sternocleidomastoid or sternohyoid. Prior to passing the thyroid specimen from the field, it should be inspected to ensure no parathyroid glands have been removed. If parathyroid glands are found on the specimen, they are autotransplanted. Confirmation of parathyroid tissue with a frozen biopsy prior to autotransplantation may prevent transplantation of tumor in the presence of malignancy.

48.7 Rehabilitation and Follow-up

Oral supplementation with calcium and calcitriol is continued until the hypoparathyroidism resolves, with target calcium between 8.0 and 9.0 mg/dL. If not resolved within 1 year, it is likely permanent. However, the majority of reported postthyroidectomy hypoparathyroidism is transient and will resolve within 1 month, whereas < 2% of these cases are permanent. Parathyroid glands that are autotransplanted may take longer to become functional.

This patient was admitted and treated with intravenous calcium until oral supplementation stabilized the serum calcium in the low normal range at 8.5 mg/dL. The patient was discharged on hospital day 2, on calcium carbonate four times daily along with calcitriol daily. The PTH level in the emergency room was undetectable. Renal panel obtained 3 days after discharge showed a corrected calcium of 9.7 mg/dL with an elevated phosphorus consistent with adequately treated hypoparathyroidism. Weekly renal panels were obtained with a slow wean of calcium supplements from initial four times daily dosing to three times daily, then twice daily, then once daily tapered weekly based upon the serum calcium levels. At 1 month, the patient's calcium was 8.5 mg/dL and intact PTH was 24 pg/nL, suggesting partial recovery of parathyroid function. By 3 months postoperatively, serum calcium, phosphorus, and PTH levels had normalized without supplements, suggesting transient hypoparathyroidism with adequate resolution.

48.8 Questions

1. Which of the following patient signs or symptoms is not a common sequelae of postoperative hypocalcemia?
   a) Tetany.
   b) Extremity paresthesia.
   c) Perioral paresthesia.
   d) Nausea.
   e) Chvostek's sign.
2. What is the single most important biochemical test to order in a patient suspected of having postthyroidectomy hypocalcemia?
   a) Serum calcium.
   b) Magnesium.
   c) Parathyroid hormone (PTH).
   d) 24-hour urinary calcium.
   e) Calcitonin.

3. What percentage of patients undergoing total or completion thyroidectomy will undergo postoperative hypocalcemia (either transient or permanent)?
   a) 5%.
   b) 10%.
   c) 30%.
   d) 70%.
   e) 95%.

Answers: 1. d 2. a 3. c

Suggested Readings

Jameson MJ, Levine PA. Chapter 20 - Complications of Thyroid Surgery. Terris and Gourin editors. Thyroid and Parathyroid Diseases. 2008

Reeve T, Thompson NW. Complications of thyroid surgery: how to avoid them, how to manage them, and observations on their possible effect on the whole patient. World J Surg. 2000; 24(8):971–975

Terris DJ, Snyder S, Carneiro-Pla D, et al. American Thyroid Association Surgical Affairs Committee Writing Task Force. American Thyroid Association statement on outpatient thyroidectomy. Thyroid. 2013; 23(10):1193–1202

49 Hyperparathyroidism

David R. Lee and David L. Steward

49.1 History

A 57-year-old woman with a history of hypertension and migraines was found to have hypercalcemia on routine screening by her primary care provider. She had three episodes of nephrolithiasis in the past 2 years, but had never had any previous fractures. She had no family history of recurrent kidney stones or hypercalcemia. She denied psychiatric symptoms but noted that she had worsening bone pain over the past several years. Her physical exam was noncontributory.

49.2 Differential Diagnosis—Key Points

Isolated asymptomatic hypercalcemia is most likely primary hyperparathyroidism and is most commonly seen in women above the age of 50. Primary hyperparathyroidism is most often sporadic. Approximately 90% of patients will have a solitary parathyroid adenoma, and 10% will have multigland disease, primarily four-gland hyperplasia and occasionally multiple adenomas. Familial primary hyperparathyroidism is seen with the multiple endocrine neoplasia (MEN) syndromes, specifically MEN1 and MEN2A. MEN1 is associated with a menin gene mutation resulting in parathyroid hyperplasia that is challenging to surgically treat. MEN2A is associated with a *RET* proto-oncogene mutation and is often associated with multiple parathyroid adenomas when accompanied by primary hyperparathyroidism. In MEN2A, biochemical screening for medullary thyroid carcinoma and pheochromocytoma is indicated (see Chapter 47).

Other causes of isolated hypercalcemia are less common but can include malignancy, milk-alkali syndrome, granulomatous disease, familial hypocalciuric hypercalcemia (FHH), and medications. Severe hypercalcemia can be secondary to malignancy through tumor production of parathyroid hormone (PTH)–related peptide (PTHrP), most commonly seen in small cell lung cancer. Similarly, extensive metastatic disease, such as is seen in multiple myeloma, may cause hypercalcemia and fractures. Milk-alkali syndrome is excessive calcium or vitamin D ingestion and can cause isolated hypercalcemia. Hypercalcemia may also be seen in granulomatous disease such as tuberculosis or sarcoidosis resulting from extrarenal vitamin D production in macrophages. In theses cases, intact PTH levels will be low, essentially ruling out asymptomatic primary hyperparathyroidism. FHH can present similarly to primary hyperparathyroidism and is excluded with a 24-hour urinary calcium level in or above the reference range or a fractional excretion of calcium > 1%. Medications such as lithium or thiazide diuretics can alter calcium metabolism. Lithium may cause or mimic primary hyperparathyroidism via alteration in the calcium-sensing receptor, while thiazide diuretics may exacerbate or unmask primary hyperthyroidism and can cause hypercalcemia through renal tubular absorption.

49.2.1 Diagnostic Tests

Confirmation of primary hyperparathyroidism in this patient can be made by checking an intact PTH and repeated calcium level. If both are elevated, primary hyperparathyroidism is the most likely diagnosis. Phosphorus, creatinine, and albumin will aid in the diagnosis, and can be found along with calcium in a full renal panel. Calcium in serum is bound to proteins, principally albumin. The serum calcium can be corrected for albumin using the formula where corrected Ca = measured Ca + (4.0– albumin) x (0.8). Reduced phosphorus levels can confirm primary hyperparathyroidism. Creatinine clearance is a property of renal function, and can affect calcium levels. However, it is essential to understand that the diagnosis of primary hyperparathyroidism is biochemical and is not based upon imaging.

Bone density scanning, such as dual-energy X-ray absorptiometry (DEXA), should be performed to assess for osteopenia or osteoporosis. This test generally includes the spine and hip, but distal radius should also be checked. Primary hyperparathyroidism can selectively affect the cortical long bones, such as the radius.

Further testing can include a 24-hour urinary calcium level and a 25-OH vitamin D level. A 24-hour urinary calcium and creatinine should accompany a renal panel to exclude FHH. Patients on diuretics, especially thiazide diuretics, should discontinue use for about a month prior to testing. In a patient with osteoporosis and suspected primary hyperparathyroidism, a 25-OH vitamin D level should be checked to look for associated secondary hyperparathyroidism, which may exacerbate osteoporosis if unrecognized.

49.3 Test Interpretation

This patient's serum calcium was elevated at 10.8 mg/dL (reference range 8.4–10.4) with a normal albumin and simultaneously elevated intact PTH level of 81 pg/nL (reference range 20–65). Twenty-four hour urine calcium was elevated at 400 mg, and 25-OH vitamin D level was low normal at 22 ng/mL (reference range 20–100). Her bone density was reduced at all sites with DEXA scan revealing a T-score of < -2.5 (diagnostic for osteoporosis). These findings are all consistent with primary hyperparathyroidism complicated by nephrolithiasis and osteoporosis. Normal reference ranges may vary depending on hospital and lab facility.

49.4 Diagnosis

Primary hyperparathyroidism with hypercalcemia complicated by nephrolithiasis and osteoporosis

49.5 Medical Management

Medical management of primary hyperparathyroidism is challenging. Bisphosphonate therapy may improve or prevent progression of osteoporosis, but has less effect on serum calcium. Long-term therapy with bisphosphonates is associated with many adverse effects, including osteonecrosis of the jaw. Vitamin D therapy may help prevent progression of osteoporosis and improve hyperparathyroidism without significant worsening of hypercalcemia. In this patient with significant osteoporosis, both bisphosphonate and vitamin D therapy may be indicated.

Calcium intake should not be restricted below 1,200 mg daily, as this will likely drive progression of osteoporosis. The patient should be advised to have adequate fluid intake, both to help prevent further kidney stones and because poor hydration can further exacerbate hypercalcemia. As discussed, thiazide diuretics exacerbate hypercalcemia and are generally discouraged, unless used to prevent hypercalciuria and nephrolithiasis. Calcimimetics, such as cinacalcet, are calcium agonists routinely used in the treatment of secondary hyperparathyroidism and can reduce serum calcium in primary hyperparathyroidism. However,

these drugs are costly and are primarily used in patients who have previously failed surgery or are not medically cleared to undergo surgery.

49.6 Surgical Management

Surgery is the most effective way to treat primary hyperparathyroidism. Historically, four gland explorations with removal of all enlarged parathyroid glands was the gold standard, and remains so in hereditary disease and secondary or tertiary hyperparathyroidism. Increasingly, for sporadic primary hyperparathyroidism, unilateral or focused parathyroidectomy with removal of only an enlarged gland localized preoperatively by imaging is performed, often with intraoperative measurement of PTH levels to confirm resolution of the hyperparathyroidism. PTH levels after removal of the suspected adenoma that have fallen at least 50% from preincision baseline while remaining within the reference range are considered consistent with successful resolution of hyperparathyroidism. In these cases, further surgical exploration is not warranted. Obtaining a second baseline at the time of removal of the suspected adenoma may be helpful.

49.6.1 Preoperative Imaging

The options for preoperative imaging include parathyroid scintigraphy with technetium 99 m sestamibi, single photon emission computed tomography (SPECT) or computed tomography (CT) fusion, high-resolution neck ultrasound, and recently, 4D CT.

Parathyroid scintigraphy with technetium 99 m sestamibi has consistently been the most sensitive parathyroid localization study, but it lacks anatomic detail and is less sensitive for smaller adenomas. This is performed using a dual-phase technique with early images showing both the thyroid and parathyroid tissue and delayed images showing the enlarged parathyroid after the thyroid washes out. SPECT sestamibi and CT fused sestamibi provide additional anatomic detail compared to standard anterior imaging alone. Nuclear medicine subtraction studies with sestamibi technetium 99 m and radioactive iodine-123 are less commonly used.

High-resolution neck ultrasound has been shown to provide equal or greater sensitivity for parathyroid adenoma localization in experienced centers at lower cost and with greater anatomic detail than typical sestamibi scanning. The two are complementary and are often both obtained. However, the accuracy of neck ultrasound is highly operator dependent.

Recently, 4D CT has been a useful modality to localize parathyroid adenomas. The "fourth" dimension is time between repeated CT scans, during which the radiographic changes can be seen in parathyroid adenomas. The adenomas undergo rapid iodine contrast uptake and washout compared to surrounding thyroid, which remains enhancing on venous phase. The use of 4D CT is nonstandardized and institution dependent, and it results in significant radiographic exposure from the multiple timed phases.

Regular CT and magnetic resonance imaging (MRI) are generally less sensitive and are primarily useful for nonlocalized adenomas after previously failed surgery or for those suspected of being intrathoracic where ultrasound is not helpful.

49.7 Rehabilitation and Follow-up

This patient underwent high-resolution neck ultrasound with localization of a small left inferior parathyroid adenoma confirmed with intraoperative resolution of the hyperparathyroidism and postoperative resolution of the hypercalcemia. Serum calcium should be measured 6 to 12 months postoperatively to ensure no recurrence and annually thereafter. It is essential to stress the importance of adequate calcium and vitamin D intake in the management of the osteoporosis. Bone density testing should be repeated 2 to 3 years postoperatively.

49.8 Questions

1. Which of the following biochemical tests is consistent with primary hyperparathyroidism?
   a) High calcium, low parathyroid hormone (PTH), low phosphorus.
   b) Low calcium, high PTH, high phosphorus.
   c) Low calcium, low PTH, high phosphorus.
   d) High calcium, high PTH, low phosphorus.

2. Which of the following bone density measurements is consistent with osteoporosis?
   a) T-score > 2.5.
   b) T-score > 1.0 and < 2.5.
   c) T-score > –1.0 and < 1.0.
   d) T-score < –1.5 and > –2.5.
   e) T-score < –2.5.

3. During unilateral parathyroid exploration with removal of a single enlarged parathyroid gland, which of the following intraoperative PTH test results would most accurately suggest surgical resolution of primary hyperparathyroidism?
   a) Postremoval PTH < 50% of preremoval PTH.
   b) Postremoval PTH > 50% of preremoval PTH.
   c) Postremoval PTH > 70 pg/dL.

Answers 1. d 2. e 3. a

Suggested Readings

Bilezikian JP, Potts JT, Jr, Fuleihan Gel-H, et al. Summary statement from a workshop on asymptomatic primary hyperparathyroidism: a perspective for the 21st century. J Clin Endocrinol Metab. 2002; 87(12):5353–5361

Rodgers SE, Hunter GJ, Hamberg LM, et al. Improved preoperative planning for directed parathyroidectomy with 4-dimensional computed tomography. Surgery. 2006; 140(6):932–940, discussion 940–941

Terris DJ, Gourin CG. Parathyroid Diseases. In: Thyroid and Parathyroid Diseases: Medical and Surgical Management. New York, NY: Thieme; 2008

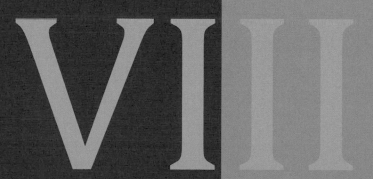

Part VIII

The Salivary Gland

VIII

50 Parapharyngeal Mass

Brian D. Goico and Yash J. Patil

50.1 History

A 55-year-old woman with a history of cervical spine degenerative disk disease underwent a magnetic resonance imaging (MRI) scan of the cervical spine that incidentally demonstrated a right parapharyngeal space mass (▶ Fig. 50.1). A contrast computed tomography (CT) scan of her neck was performed, which confirmed a 3.8 × 2.1-cm parapharyngeal mass (▶ Fig. 50.2), prompting referral to an otolaryngologist for further evaluation and treatment. The patient denied a history of alcohol or tobacco use, had no significant sexual history for human papillomavirus (HPV) infection, and noted no recent odontogenic or respiratory infections. She denied a history of salivary gland swelling or pain and denied any focal sensory or muscle weakness, fevers, chills, or night sweats. Her physical examination indicated no focal cranial nerve weakness, no intraoral or palpable neck masses or lesions, and symmetric vocal cord motion with intact pharyngeal sensation on flexible fiberoptic laryngoscopy. The patient subsequently underwent excision of the mass through a transcervical approach in

conjunction with a deep lobe parotidectomy. Her final pathology demonstrated a pleomorphic adenoma. She recovered well from surgery without focal nerve deficits or specific complaints other than a pain with her first bite of a meal.

50.2 Differential Diagnosis—Key Points

- The parapharyngeal space is an inverted pyramid bordered by the skull base superiorly, the pterygomandibular raphe and pterygoid fascia anteriorly, the cervical vertebrae and prevertebral muscles posteriorly, the pharynx medially, and the ramus of the mandible, medial pterygoid, and deep lobe of parotid, and lateral belly of the digastric laterally. It is divided into the prestyloid and retrostyloid spaces by the fascia from the styloid process to the tensor veli palatini. The prestyloid space contains fat, a variable portion of the deep lobe of the parotid, the internal maxillary artery, and the lingual, auriculotemporal, and inferior alveolar nerves. The

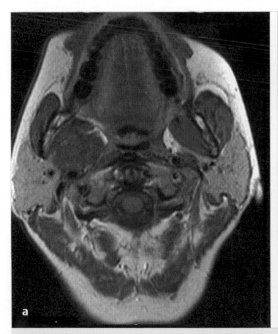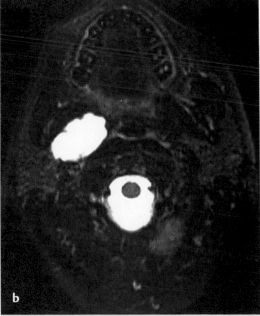

Fig. 50.1 (a,b) Axial T1 noncontrast MRI scan demonstrating isointense parapharyngeal mass and axial T2 noncontrast MRI scan demonstrating hyperintense parapharyngeal mass.

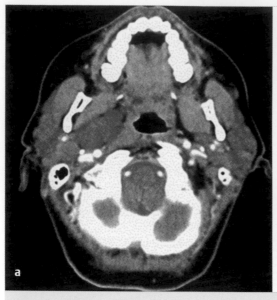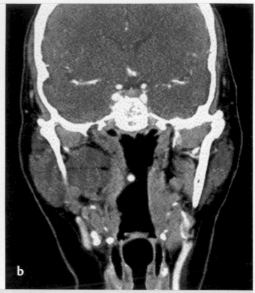

Fig. 50.2 (a,b) Axial and coronal CT with contrast demonstrating right parapharyngeal mass.

retrostyloid space contains the carotid, jugular vein, cranial nerves IX through XII, the sympathetic chain, and lymph nodes.

- The differential diagnosis for masses of the parapharyngeal space can be divided based upon their occurrence in the prestyloid or retrostyloid spaces. Prestyloid tumors are most likely to be salivary gland tumors, lipomas, or lymphomas. Poststyloid tumors are more likely to be paragangliomas, nerve sheath tumors, or connective tissue tumors. Based on a large-scale systematic review, around 80% of parapharyngeal tumors are benign. The most common lesion is a pleomorphic adenoma, occurring in around 30%. The most common malignant lesion is adenoid cystic carcinoma (3%). The two most common origins of tumors are salivary gland (45%) and neurogenic (40%). Salivary gland tumors may arise from the parotid or minor salivary glands in the lateral pharyngeal wall or ectopic tissue rests. Multiple other types of lesions have been noted, including aneurysms, hemangiomas, cystic hygromas, branchial cleft cysts, connective tissue tumors, lymphomas, metastatic tumors, and undifferentiated carcinomas.
- Despite the significant number of important structures in this anatomic region, patients frequently present with few, subtle symptoms. In fact, these masses can present as incidental findings on imaging obtained for other reasons, as was the case in our patient. Patients who do

present symptomatically frequently endorse pain and/or cranial nerve palsies.

- A thorough history should include any episodes of syncope or hemodynamic instability as well as any alcohol or tobacco use and a sexual history to evaluate for risk factors of HPV-associated pharyngeal cancers. In addition, a history of any upper respiratory or odontogenic infections should be obtained. Physical exam should include a thorough examination of cranial nerves IX, X, and XI, as well as a detailed oropharyngeal exam and an endoscopic examination with documentation of any mass effects or cranial nerve deficits in pharyngeal sensation or vocal cord motion. Further evaluation with diagnostic imaging is necessary as outlined below.

50.3 Test Interpretation

1. The primary study for preoperative evaluation of the parapharyngeal space is contrast-enhanced CT. This modality offers good anatomic delineation of mass characteristics that is essential for further classification of the mass and operative planning, such as differentiation between prestyloid and retrostyloid tumors, deep lobe parotid versus extraparotid tumors, and evidence of malignant characteristics such as skull base erosion or vascular invasion. In cases of suspected malignancy, this imaging modality can also assess for nodal metastases.

2. Further evaluation with MRI and magnetic resonance angiography (MRA) may be necessary, depending on the findings on the CT scan. These studies are especially helpful for delineation of soft tissue invasion and vascular involvement, respectively. Furthermore, angiography may be needed if a lesion is thought to require preoperative embolization.

3. There is ambivalence in the literature about the role of fine needle aspiration (FNA) with CT or ultrasound guidance in the diagnosis of parapharyngeal space tumors, with some authors endorsing a high rate of diagnosis and others demonstrating highly inconclusive samples and difficulty in interpretation. Similarly, some authors endorse core needle biopsy, while others indicate this might lead to tumor seeding and higher rates of complications.

4. Urinary catecholamines should be obtained for any suspected paraganglioma to plan for medical management of hypertension or arrhythmias intraoperatively.

50.4 Diagnosis

Parapharyngeal space pleomorphic adenoma

50.5 Medical Management

Although the mainstay of treatment is surgical, there are a few situations in which medical therapy is indicated. Catecholamine-secreting paragangliomas require preoperative medication with an alpha-adrenergic antagonist. Perioperatively, these patients should be managed with rapid-acting agents to control blood pressure and heart rate variations. Medical management with antibiotics is indicated in situations that suggest an infectious etiology.

50.6 Surgical Management

Surgical excision is typically required for definitive diagnosis and treatment of parapharyngeal space masses. Because the exact procedure that is required may be unclear preoperatively, a thorough discussion must be had with the patient regarding possible approaches and risks of cranial nerve and vascular injury. The following approaches have been used for parapharyngeal space tumors: transcervical, mandibular split, transparotid, transoral, and infratemporal fossa. Additionally, combinations of the above approaches have been described. The most common approach for resection is transcervical. If the tumor arises from the parotid gland, a superficial parotidectomy may be simultaneously performed, as was necessary in this case. The possibility of a mandibular osteotomy for expanded access should be discussed with patients prior to surgery. For appropriately positioned tumors, transoral robotic surgery has been described with good results. For vascular lesions such as paragangliomas, preoperative embolization may be indicated. The most common complications of surgery are nerve injuries, especially to the vagus nerve. This also is an expected outcome of excision in certain masses, such as vagal paragangliomas.

50.7 Rehabilitation and Follow-up

All cases should be followed for recurrence; however, the recurrence of benign parapharyngeal space lesions is quite low, around 3%. Further procedures such as gastrostomy and thyroplasty may be indicated if a nerve is sacrificed or damaged during resection. A frequent sequela of parapharyngeal space surgery, which was noted by this patient, is the "first bite syndrome," or pain that is felt in the region of the parotid following the first bite of a meal. This pain is thought to be due to disruption of sympathetic nerve function to the parotid. Treatments that have demonstrated efficacy include intraparotid botulinum toxin injections; anticonvulsants such as carbamazepine, pregabalin, and gabapentin; and tricyclic antidepressants such as amitriptyline.

50.8 Questions

1. What is the most common malignant tumor of the parapharyngeal space?
   a) Squamous cell carcinoma.
   b) Adenoid cystic carcinoma.
   c) Rhabdomyosarcoma.
   d) Acinic cell carcinoma.
2. What compartment of the parapharyngeal space is more likely to contain a paraganglioma?
   a) Prestyloid.
   b) Poststyloid.
   c) Prevertebral.
   d) Infratemporal fossa.
3. What causes first bite syndrome?
   a) Disruption of sympathetic nerve function to the parotid.

b) Disruption of parasympathetic nerve function to the parotid.
c) Disruption of sympathetic nerve function to the submandibular gland.
d) Disruption of parasympathetic nerve function to the submandibular gland.

Answers: 1. b 2. b 3. a

Suggested Readings

Colen TY, Mihm FG, Mason TP, Roberson JB. Catecholamine-secreting paragangliomas: recent progress in diagnosis and perioperative management. Skull Base. 2009; 19(6):377–385

Kuet ML, Kasbekar AV, Masterson L, Jani P. Management of tumors arising from the parapharyngeal space: systematic review of 1,293 cases reported over 25 years. Laryngoscope. 2015; 125(6):1372

Laccourreye O, Werner A, Garcia D, Malinvaud D, Tran Ba Huy P, Bonfils P. First bite syndrome. Eur Ann Otorhinolaryngol Head Neck Dis. 2013; 130(5):269–273

Olsen KD. Tumors and surgery of the parapharyngeal space. Laryngoscope. 1994; 104(5 Pt 2) Suppl 63:1–28

51 Recurrent Pleomorphic Adenoma

Adam D. Goodale and Jonathan R. Mark

51.1 History

A 62-year-old man presented for evaluation of a left parapharyngeal space mass. He reported having two previous surgeries on his left salivary gland. The first surgery was a superficial parotidectomy for pleomorphic adenoma performed 10 years ago, and he had no facial weakness after surgery. He described similar surgery 4 years ago for the same pathology with close margins. Postoperatively he developed synkinesis and required eyelid weight placement for lagopthalmos. He did receive radiation therapy to the area after his second surgery. The parapharyngeal mass was noted incidentally during imaging of his head for an unrelated issue.

On physical examination there was a well-healed preauricular scar consistent with previous parotidectomy. No masses were palpated over his parotid gland. Intraoral examination showed three-finger jaw opening and a normal-appearing pharynx. There was no palpable lesion along his lateral pharyngeal wall. The rest of his head and neck exam was normal. Magnetic resonance imaging (MRI) was obtained to better define the lesion and demonstrated two masses in the parapharyngeal space that were high intensity on T2- and homogeneously enhancing on T1-weighted images with gadolinium (▶ Fig. 51.1). Surgical excision was undertaken via lip split and mandibulotomy with facial nerve preservation. Complete excision of multifocal disease was noted on final pathology, with two microscopic foci of carcinoma ex pleomorphic adenoma arising within the pleomorphic adenoma (▶ Fig. 51.2).

51.2 Differential Diagnosis—Key Points

- Pleomorphic adenomas are the most common salivary gland tumor, accounting for

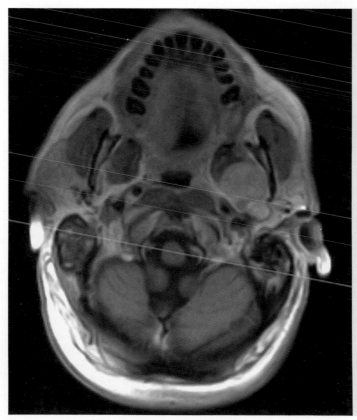

Fig. 51.1 T1-weighted MRI with gadolinium scan showing an isointense left parapharyngeal mass.

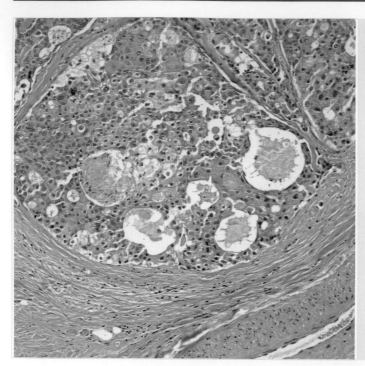

Fig. 51.2 High-powered photomicrograph of carcinoma ex pleomorphic adenoma arising within a background of pleomorphic adenoma; the carcinoma component in the center shows pleomorphic tumor cells with vacuolated cytoplasm.

approximately 50% of all salivary gland neoplasms. They are the most common salivary neoplasm in all salivary glands, but are most commonly found in the parotid gland.

- Also called benign mixed tumors, pleomorphic adenomas contain both epithelial and mesenchymal components, with varying predominance of either component. The gross appearance shows a well-encapsulated tumor; however, microscopic visualization may show incomplete encapsulation or pseudopod extension. Incomplete excision of these pseudopod extensions is thought to contribute to the recurrent nature of pleomorphic adenomas. Other reasons for recurrence include capsule rupture, tumor spillage, satellite lesions, and grossly positive margins.

- When pleomorphic adenomas are removed by simple tumor enucleation, recurrence rates range from 20% to 45%. Performing a superficial parotidectomy with adequate margins reduces recurrence rates to 1% to 4%. Recurrent pleomorphic adenomas are almost always multifocal and recur at a mean of 7 to 10 years after initial surgical excision. Surgical excision remains the treatment of choice for recurrent pleomorphic adenomas. Adjuvant radiotherapy is beneficial in certain cases and has been shown to limit locoregional recurrence.

- Malignant transformation to carcinoma ex pleomorphic adenoma is uncommon but does occur in approximately 1.5% of patients within 5 years of diagnosis and 10% within 15 years of diagnosis. The risk of malignant transformation is higher in cases of multiple recurrences, reportedly as high as 15%. Thus, long-term follow-up is warranted for patients with pleomorphic adenomas.

- Other benign tumors of the parotid gland include Warthin's tumor, oncocytoma, and basal cell adenoma. Warthin's tumors account for 23% of all benign parotid lesions and are more common in men and smokers. These lesions can be bilateral in 12% of patients.

- Malignant lesions of the parotid gland include mucoepidermoid carcinoma, adenoid cystic carcinoma, carcinoma ex pleomorphic adenoma, and acinic cell carcinoma. Facial nerve involvement and rapid enlargement are concerning for malignancy. Primary lymphoma of the salivary glands accounts for 5% of extranodal lymphomas and is most commonly large B-cell lymphoma, follicular lymphoma, or mucosa-associated lymphoid tissue (MALT) type.

- Nonneoplastic causes of parotid gland enlargement should also be considered. This includes viral sialadenitis, bacterial sialadenitis, granulomatous infections, sialadenosis, and cystic lesions.

51.3 Test Interpretation

Patients with a parotid mass should undergo a complete work-up with close evaluation of the nature of the lesion as well as the status of the facial nerve. For all parotid lesions, a fine needle aspiration should be performed with or without ultrasound guidance. Obtaining tissue helps guide surgical management and has been shown to change the clinical approach in 35% of cases. Clinicians should be aware that parotid biopsies have a relatively high false negative rate of 4% to 7%.

Imaging options include ultrasound, computed tomography (CT), and MRI. For small, well-defined masses limited to the superficial lobe, imaging may not be warranted. All other lesions, particularly large tumors, tumors involving the deep lobe, or tumors extending into the parapharyngeal space, should be imaged. MRI is the preferred imaging modality for parotid lesions due to its superior soft tissue differentiation. MRI is particularly useful in cases of recurrent pleomorphic adenomas to characterize the location and amount of residual parotid gland, as well as the presence of multiple lesions. Despite the improving resolution of MRI, studies have shown that MRI often misses microscopic recurrent foci. The retromandibular vein is a radiographic surrogate reference for the position of the facial nerve.

51.4 Diagnosis

Recurrent pleomorphic adenoma, carcinoma ex pleomorphic adenoma

51.5 Medical Management

Although management for recurrent pleomorphic adenoma is primarily surgical, observation and radiotherapy should be considered in certain cases. Considerations for treatment include location and number of masses, previous treatment, number of recurrences, facial nerve status, patient preference, patient age, and patient comorbidities. Observation may be a reasonable option for medically complex and elderly patients. Additionally, patients in whom tumor removal would greatly put the facial nerve at risk can be observed if the risk of malignancy is acceptable. These patients should be closely followed with serial clinic visits and ultrasound. Patients should be educated on the risk of malignant conversion, cosmetic changes, and the potential for facial nerve weakness.

Radiotherapy can be considered in patients that are poor surgical candidates or those with tumor location unfavorable for surgical resection. Definitive radiosurgery has been shown to obtain a 75% locoregional control at 15 years; however, there is concern that administering radiation increases the risk of malignant conversion. In addition, radiotherapy has been shown to be less effective for large tumor burden.

51.6 Surgical Management

Surgical excision is the preferred treatment for both primary and recurrent pleomorphic adenomas. Previously, pleomorphic adenomas were excised with simple tumor enucleation with high recurrence rates. The current recommendation is to perform a superficial parotidectomy or partial superficial parotidectomy with an adequate cuff of surrounding normal tissue. This change in technique decreased recurrence rates from 20% to 45% to less than 4%. Surgical excision for recurrent pleomorphic adenomas depends on several issues, including the location and amount of residual parotid tissue, the location of recurrence, and the number of recurrent tumor foci. In cases where a partial superficial parotidectomy was initially performed, a completion superficial parotidectomy can be considered. However, many authors advocate performing a total parotidectomy for recurrent disease due to the multifocal nature and high rate of secondary recurrence. The surgical approach should be tailored to each patient and the nature of their disease (▶ Fig. 51.3).

Postoperative facial nerve paralysis is significantly higher following excision of recurrent pleomorphic adenomas compared to primary tumor excision. The incidence of temporary facial nerve paralysis increases from 9.1% to 64% after primary parotid tumor excision to 90% to 100% for recurrent pleomorphic adenomas, and permanent facial nerve paralysis increases from 0% to 3.9% for primary resection to 11.3% to 40%. Facial nerve dysfunction rates continue to increase with each additional surgery. The use of intraoperative facial nerve monitoring has been shown to decrease the incidence of facial nerve injury for recurrent cases, as well as decrease operative time. Patients should be appropriately counseled on the risk of facial nerve damage prior to surgery.

Adjuvant radiotherapy should be considered to limit secondary recurrences. In particular, adjuvant radiotherapy should be considered in cases when complete tumor removal is not possible, when facial nerve sacrifice would have been necessary, or after multiple recurrences. Numerous studies have evaluated the benefit of adjuvant

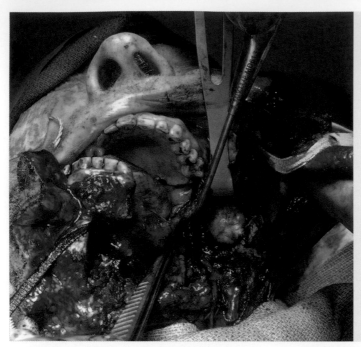

Fig. 51.3 Mandibulotomy approach to a recurrent pleomorphic adenoma in the parapharyngeal space at the skull base.

radiotherapy following surgery. Collectively, these studies showed an improvement in local tumor control from 63% after surgery alone to 91% when radiotherapy was given after surgical excision.

51.7 Rehabilitation and Follow-up

Given the high rate of recurrence, patients with pleomorphic adenomas should be followed for many years after surgical resection. Of patients with a primary recurrence, 43% to 45% have a second recurrence within 10 years after surgical resection. Patients should be followed with close clinical examination with the option of serial ultrasounds, depending upon physician preference. Ultrasound may assist in identifying subclinical recurrent disease. MRI and CT can also be used for surveillance and provide better imaging of deep lobe recurrences.

Facial nerve function should be closely evaluated following surgery for recurrent disease. In cases of incomplete recovery, adequate eye care and appropriate facial nerve rehabilitation measures should be considered.

51.8 Questions

1. What is the most common benign salivary gland tumor in children?
   a) Pleomorphic adenoma.
   b) Hemangioma.
   c) Lymphangioma.
   d) Warthin's tumor.
2. Which of the following is not thought to contribute to the high rate of recurrence of pleomorphic adenomas?
   a) Incomplete tumor removal.
   b) Tumor spillage.
   c) Multifocal primary tumors.
   d) Incomplete excision of pseudopod extensions.
3. What is the overall survival at 5 years for patients diagnosed with carcinoma ex pleomorphic adenoma?
   a) 12%.
   b) 28%.
   c) 48%.
   d) 70%.

Answers: 1. b 2. b 3. c

Suggested Readings

Larian B. Parotidectomy for Benign Parotid Tumors. Otolaryngol Clin North Am. 2016; 49(2):395–413

Witt RL, Eisele DW, Morton RP, Nicolai P, Poorten VV, Zbären P. Etiology and management of recurrent parotid pleomorphic adenoma. Laryngoscope. 2015; 125(4):888–893

52 Submandibular Gland Adenoid Cystic Carcinoma

Brian D. Goico and Yash J. Patil

52.1 History

A 53-year-old man presented with a slowly enlarging mass below his right jaw of several months' duration. The patient was initially treated with antibiotics without improvement of symptoms. He denied any associated symptoms including weight loss, dysphagia, odynophagia, neck masses, or odontogenic infections. He was not regularly followed by a physician but had no documented past medical conditions. He smoked one pack of cigarettes per day, which he had done for 30 years. He had a tonsillectomy in childhood but denied any other surgeries of the head or neck. On physical examination, a large, firm, immobile right submandibular mass was noted. No associated neck masses were appreciated. He had no weakness of the right marginal mandibular nerve. He had a contrast computed tomography (CT) scan of the neck (▶ Fig. 52.1), and then underwent submandibular gland excision, with pathology shown below (▶ Fig. 52.2).

52.2 Differential Diagnosis—Key Points

- Salivary gland enlargement has a multitude of causes, which can be grouped as neoplastic or nonneoplastic. Neoplastic causes can be further divided into benign and malignant lesions. Benign tumors include pleomorphic adenoma, papillary cystadenoma lymphomatosum (Warthin's tumor), oncocytoma, monomorphic adenoma, and basal cell adenoma, whereas malignant tumors include mucoepidermoid carcinoma, adenoid cystic carcinoma, (ACC), acinic cell carcinoma, carcinoma ex pleomorphic adenoma, adenocarcinoma, polymorphous low-grade adenocarcinoma, salivary duct carcinoma, and squamous cell carcinoma. Excessive caution must be used when diagnosing a primary squamous cell carcinoma of the salivary gland, as both metastatic spread to intraglandular lymph nodes and high-grade mucoepidermoid cancer

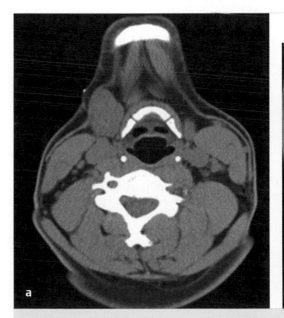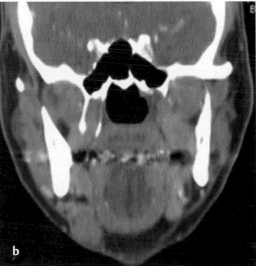

Fig. 52.1 (a,b) Axial and coronal contrast CT scan of the neck demonstrating a large right submandibular mass.

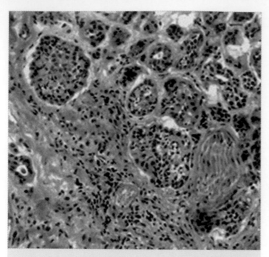

Fig. 52.2 Pathology slide showing basaloid epithelium in cylindric formations, as well as perineural invasion.

are far more common causes of very similar pathology. Nonneoplastic causes can be classified as infectious and noninfectious. Infectious causes include bacterial infections, especially *Staphylococcus*, but also *Streptococcus*, *Haemophilus*, *Escherichia coli*, *Bartonella*, *Mycobacterium*, syphilis (*Treponema pallidum*), and Lyme disease (*Borrelia*). Other infectious causes include viruses, most classically mumps (paramyxovirus), but also cytomegalovirus and Epstein-Barr virus, and fungal agents such as histoplasmosis and coccidioidomycosis. Noninfectious causes include autoimmune diseases such as Sjögren's syndrome, rheumatic diseases such as granulomatosis with polyangiitis and sarcoidosis, radiation injury, sialolithiasis, sialadenosis, and traumatic injury.

- While sialadenitis, sialadenosis, and sialolithiasis frequently present quite suddenly, salivary gland masses, autoimmune diseases, and rheumatic diseases tend to present subacutely or chronically. In the absence of trauma, radiation, or systemic signs of an autoimmune or rheumatic disease, neoplasm should be at the top of the differential diagnosis. A comprehensive physical exam, ultrasound, and fine needle aspiration (FNA) would be helpful in verifying the diagnosis.
- About 50% of submandibular gland neoplasms are benign. The most common benign neoplasm of the parotid and submandibular glands is pleomorphic adenoma. The most common malignant

neoplasm of the parotid gland and minor salivary glands is mucoepidermoid carcinoma, and the second most common is ACC, while the most common malignant neoplasm of the submandibular gland is ACC and the second most common is mucoepidermoid carcinoma. Pain and paralysis of the facial or hypoglossal nerves are signs that a mass is more likely to be malignan or, exhibit perineural spread, and indicate a worse prognosis. ACC is frequently associated with perineural spread.

52.3 Test Interpretation

- FNA is the mainstay of diagnosis in most cases. Traditionally this test was done with the aid of manual palpation; however, more recently ultrasound or CT guidance has become more commonly utilized to verify correct needle placement. FNA has been demonstrated to have a sensitivity of 92% and specificity of 100% in the diagnosis of salivary gland lesions. As FNA is easily done and frequently makes a diagnosis, if the initial FNA is nondiagnostic, most authors advise a second FNA in lieu of a core needle biopsy or incisional biopsy, as the latter two may result in tumor seeding. In this case, with a solitary mass confined to the submandibular gland, FNA was not necessary. Final pathology demonstrated a "Swiss cheese" pattern with glandlike spaces filled with eosinophilic hyaline stroma surrounded by a basaloid epithelium consistent with ACC. Among the other common types of salivary gland neoplasms, pleomorphic adenoma demonstrates an epithelial component within a mesenchymal stroma that may be myxoid, chondroid, fibroid, or osteoid; Warthin's tumor has a papillary double-layer epithelium and a lymphoid stroma that frequently demonstrates germinal centers, and mucoepidermoid carcinoma is composed of aggregates of mucoid cells separated by strands of epidermal cells. As mucoepidermoid carcinoma becomes higher grade, more of the tumor is made up of these epidermal cells and less of the mucinous debris and mucoid cells.
- Basic imaging: Ultrasound may be used to determine if a mass near a salivary gland is actually within the substance of the gland, differentiate cystic and solid lesions, and demonstrate reassuring features such as regular margins and a lack of extraglandular spread. Additionally, ultrasound can facilitate needle localization during

FNA. The sensitivity of ultrasound is 0.629 and its specificity is 0.920. CT scanning is helpful to determine tumor extent, relationship to bony and vascular structures, and concomitant lymphadenopathy. CT scan has a sensitivity of 0.830 and a specificity of 0.851. Magnetic resonance imaging (MRI) gives an excellent assessment of soft tissue involvement, perineural involvement, and intracranial extension and has a sensitivity of 0.807 and a specificity of 0.903.

52.4 Diagnosis

Adenoid cystic carcinoma

52.5 Medical Management

Radiation therapy demonstrates a good initial response; however, most tumors will recur with time. Chemotherapy is only for locoregional recurrences and distant metastases that are not amenable to surgical resection or radiation therapy. Several trials have demonstrated responses to chemotherapeutic agents either alone or as combination therapy.

52.6 Surgical Management

Surgery is the standard treatment for ACC, with postoperative radiation therapy to treat perineural invasion, which is frequently present. The surgery performed involves excision of the submandibular gland with surrounding lymph node contents of the submandibular triangle as well as any surrounding gross tumor spread with a margin. Elective neck dissection is not indicated, as ACC demonstrates no significant tendency for lymphatic metastasis. ACC frequency demonstrates long-term recurrence and distant metastasis, so long-term follow-up is indicated.

52.7 Rehabilitation and Follow-up

Several reports have documented the long-term recurrence of ACC both locally and distantly. As a result, patients require lifetime follow-up to monitor for recurrence. Although there is no established surveillance protocol, routine follow-up with chest radiographs has been recommended. Positron

emission tomography (PET) scans may be helpful if recurrence is suspected. The patient in this case underwent resection with postoperative radiation therapy with no documented recurrence at 8 years' follow-up.

52.8 Questions

1. What is the most common type of malignancy of the submandibular gland?
   a) Adenoid cystic carcinoma (ACC).
   b) Mucoepidermoid carcinoma.
   c) Acinic cell carcinoma.
   d) Adenocarcinoma.
2. Which salivary gland tumor demonstrates a papillary double-layer epithelium?
   a) ACC.
   b) Mucoepidermoid carcinoma.
   c) Papillary cystadenoma lymphomatosum.
   d) Pleomorphic adenoma.
3. Why is neoadjuvant radiation indicated for ACC?
   a) Lymphovascular invasion.
   b) Perineural spread.
   c) In-transit metastases.
   d) All of the above.

Answers: 1. a 2. c 3. b

Suggested Readings

Chen AM, Bucci MK, Weinberg V, et al. Adenoid cystic carcinoma of the head and neck treated by surgery with or without postoperative radiation therapy: prognostic features of recurrence. Int J Radiat Oncol Biol Phys. 2006; 66(1):152–159

Chen AM, Garcia J, Granchi PJ, Johnson J, Eisele DW. Late recurrence from salivary gland cancer: when does "cure" mean cure? Cancer. 2008; 112(2):340–344

Khafif A, Anavi Y, Haviv J, Fienmesser R, Calderon S, Marshak G. Adenoid cystic carcinoma of the salivary glands: a 20-year review with long-term follow-up. Ear Nose Throat J. 2005; 84(10):662–664, 664–667

Laurie SA, Licitra L. Systemic therapy in the palliative management of advanced salivary gland cancers. J Clin Oncol 2006; 24 (17):2673–2678

Liu Y, Li J, Tan YR, Xiong P, Zhong LP. Accuracy of diagnosis of salivary gland tumors with the use of ultrasonography, computed tomography, and magnetic resonance imaging: a meta-analysis. Oral Surg Oral Med Oral Pathol Oral Radiol. 2015; 119(2):238–245–e2

Stewart CJR, MacKenzie K, McGarry GW, Mowat A. Fine-needle aspiration cytology of salivary gland: a review of 341 cases. Diagn Cytopathol. 2000; 22(3):139–146

Westra WH. The surgical pathology of salivary gland neoplasms. Otolaryngol Clin North Am. 1999; 32(5):919–943

Part IX

The Skin

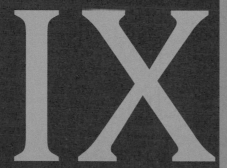

53 Cutaneous Squamous Cell Carcinoma

Jamie L. Welshhans and Ryan M. Collar

53.1 History

A 79-year-old man presented with a large, fungating mass at the left temporal/preauricular area (► Fig. 53.1). He came at the urging of his daughter, but otherwise had not sought medical care in his adult life and therefore had no medical history. The mass had been present for about 6 months. It occasionally bled but was not very painful. He did smoke two packs of cigarettes per day and drank a six-pack of beer (minimum) per day. He lived on a farm and still did much of the land work himself.

On physical exam there was a large, fungating mass in the left temporal/preauricular area that was 3.5 × 3.5 cm in size. The most superficial aspect of the tumor was ulcerated and crusting. There was no palpable lymphadenopathy in the parotid or in the cervical lymph nodes. He had other sun damage skin changes on the skin of his head and neck, but the exam was otherwise normal.

53.2 Differential Diagnosis—Key Points

The following lesions should be considered in a patient with suspected cutaneous squamous cell carcinoma. The first consideration is actinic keratosis (AK) versus invasive squamous cell carcinoma. AK lesions are erythematous, scaly macules or papules and are precursors to invasive squamous cell carcinoma. Other considerations include seborrheic keratosis, basal cell carcinoma, Merkel's cell carcinoma, atypical fibroxanthoma, or cutaneous metastasis from another primary tumor.

A squamous cell carcinoma typically presents as an erythematous, ulcerated, crusting lesion with a very friable base. There is usually an inflamed and indurated area at the lesion's base, as well. Persistent ulceration at the area of previous scar or trauma is another concerning finding to indicate squamous cell carcinoma, and if present this is known as a Marjolin's ulcer.

Physical exam is essential in determining if the lesion may be benign or malignant. If concerning features are present as noted above, then the lesion should be biopsied.

53.3 Test Interpretation

After physical examination, the next step in diagnosis of any skin cancer is biopsy. This patient underwent punch biopsy, which demonstrated irregular masses of epidermal cells proliferating down toward and invading the dermis, consistent with cutaneous squamous cell carcinoma. There were also keratin pearls seen on histology.

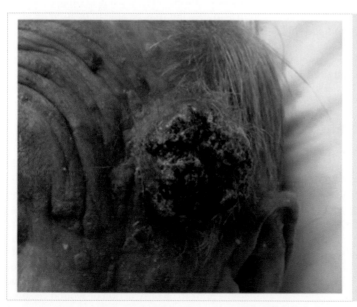

Fig. 53.1 This patient's lesion is seen in the left temporal/preauricular area (an example of cutaneous squamous cell carcinoma)

Table 53.1 TNM staging system for nonmelanoma skin cancer

T stage	Characteristics
Tis	Carcinoma in situ, tumor is still in the epidermis
T1	Less than or equal to 2 cm in size or has none or only one high-risk feature
T2	Greater than 2 cm but not more than 4 cm in size, or two or more high-risk features
T3	Locally invasive, into mandible, maxilla, orbit, or temporal bone
T4	Invades skull base, invasion into axial or appendicular skeleton
N stage	Characteristics
N1	Single, ipsilateral node, 3 cm or less
N2a	Single, ipsilateral node, more than 3 cm but not more than 6 cm
N2b	Multiple ipsilateral nodes, none more than 6 cm
N2c	Bilateral or contralateral nodes, none more than 6 cm in size
N3	Any lymph node greater than 6 cm in size
M stage	Characteristics
0	No metastatic disease
1	Metastatic disease present

The patient also underwent computed tomography (CT) of the neck with contrast and CT of the chest without contrast to look for metastatic disease. There was no abnormal lymphadenopathy present and no lung masses.

The TNM staging system for nonmelanoma skin cancers is shown in ▶ Table 53.1. The high-risk features used to differentiate T1 and T2 tumors in this system are tumor thickness > 2 mm or invasion into Clark's level IV or V, perineural invasion, location on ear or lip (non–hair bearing), and poor histologic differentiation.

This patient had no high-risk features on biopsy and the lesion was 3.5 cm in size, making the clinical stage for this patient T2N0M0

53.4 Medical Management

Multiple treatment modalities exist for cutaneous squamous cell carcinoma. As far as nonsurgical treatment, radiotherapy is an option as an adjuvant treatment for patients with advanced disease or as a primary modality for patients who are poor surgical candidates. There is also a role for palliation for painful or bleeding lesions. As adjuvant therapy for patients with advanced disease (T3-T4) or high-risk features (T2), radiotherapy has been shown to decrease local recurrence and increase disease-free survival.

Immunotherapy can be used to treat some squamous cell lesions as well. Imiquimod can be used topically in select carcinoma in situ (CIS) patients (low-risk individuals or patients who are poor surgical candidates).

Diclofenac is a nonsteroidal anti-inflammatory drug that works to inhibit the cyclooxygenase-2 enzyme thought to be up-regulated in nonmelanoma skin cancer. This topical gel is approved only for use in AKs, but may be able to be used for clearance in CIS lesions (reported in a few case series).

Drugs like cetuximab (or erlotinib or gefitinib), which work via epidermal growth factor receptor (EGFR) inhibition, can be used for treatment of recurrent or metastatic head and neck squamous cell carcinoma. These are typically used with concurrent radiotherapy.

53.5 Surgical Management

Surgical management for cutaneous squamous cell carcinoma includes wide local excision (WLE) and Mohs micrographic surgery (MMS).

WLE is typically used with margins of ~1 cm, though in cosmetic areas the initial margin may be less with frozen section to determine adequate resection. After WLE tumor margins are sent for frozen section analysis as well to ensure negative margins prior to reconstruction or wound closure.

MMS is another option for patients and is an excellent choice for smaller lesions in cosmetic areas of the face. MMS first begins with a topical agent that fixes the lesion in situ and allows for careful serial excisions. Excisions continue until all pockets of carcinoma are removed. The margins in MMS are resected in entirety rather than a random sampling, as with WLE. This is a significant benefit. Also, it allows removal of neoplasm with maximal preservation of normal tissue. The biggest disadvantage is the expertise required to perform MMS. Cure rates with MMS are 96 to 99%.

This patient did undergo a WLE with reconstruction. There was no lymphadenopathy and so no elective neck dissection was performed. However, the risk of lymph node metastasis in cutaneous squamous cell carcinoma is 12.5%. Regional lymph node dissection including parotid nodes and upper cervical nodes should always be discussed, especially in tumors over 3 cm in size.

53.6 Rehabilitation and Follow-up

The patient underwent surgery as noted above and is not a candidate for adjuvant therapy, given his T2 lesion and the fact that he refused to return to the local treatment facility for radiation treatments.

He will need to establish care with a dermatologist for at least yearly skin checks. Ear, nose, and throat (ENT) will follow him several times a year for the first several years and then decrease the frequency if he does well. Recommendations for follow-up are typically every 3 to 6 months for the first 2 years and then annually after that for at least 5 years, with lifetime skin checks. Second skin cancer development is very likely in patients who have already had one.

Prevention is of utmost importance. Patients should be counseled on sun protection, including sunscreen and protective clothing.

53.7 Questions

1. Sun exposure is associated with which of the following skin cancers?
   a) Melanoma.
   b) Cutaneous squamous cell carcinoma.
   c) Basal cell carcinoma.
   d) All of the above.
2. Which of the following are high-risk features of cutaneous carcinoma?
   a) Thickness > 1 mm.
   b) Clark's level III or deeper.
   c) Lesion on ear.
   d) Lesion on hair-bearing lip.
3. A patient presents with a 1-cm lesion on the left ala, with erythema and ulcerations. She notes that it bleeds often and has been present for 3 weeks. Biopsy is consistent with squamous cell carcinoma without high-risk features. There is no metastatic disease present (by computed tomography [CT] scan). What is the best treatment regimen?
   a) Wide local excision (WLE) with 1-cm margins and reconstruction.
   b) Mohs micrographic surgery (MMS) with reconstruction.
   c) MMS with reconstruction and elective parotidectomy and selective neck dissection.
   d) WLE with 2-cm margins and reconstruction.

Answers: 1. d 2. c 3. b

Suggested Readings

Cherpelis BS, Marcusen C, Lang PG. Prognostic factors for metastasis in squamous cell carcinoma of the skin. Dermatol Surg. 2002; 28 (3):268–273

Dubas LE, Ingraffea A. Nonmelanoma skin cancer. Facial Plast Surg Clin North Am. 2013; 21(1):43–53

Han A, Ratner D. What is the role of adjuvant radiotherapy in the treatment of cutaneous squamous cell carcinoma with perineural invasion? Cancer. 2007; 109(6):1053–1059

Madan V, Lear JT, Szeimies RM. Non-melanoma skin cancer. Lancet. 2010; 375(9715):673–685

54 Basal Cell Carcinoma

Brittany A. Leader and David B. Hom

54.1 History

A 75-year-old man in good health presented with a 1-year history of a growing skin lesion on his left temple (▶ Fig. 54.1). It bled occasionally. There was no previous history of skin cancer and he denied pain or weight loss. His past occupation was as a truck driver for 40 years. On physical exam, the 1-cm plaque lesion was slightly raised and friable. His facial nerve was fully intact. He had no parotid or cervical adenopathy. He had Fitzpatrick's 2 skin type. The remaining head and neck exam was within normal limits. A punch biopsy was performed (▶ Fig. 54.2).

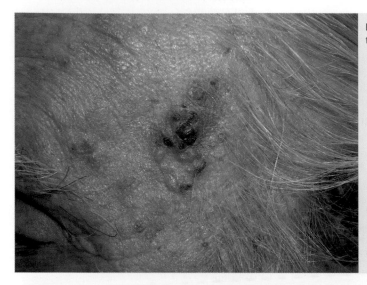

Fig. 54.1 Left temple lesion with features of basal cell carcinoma.

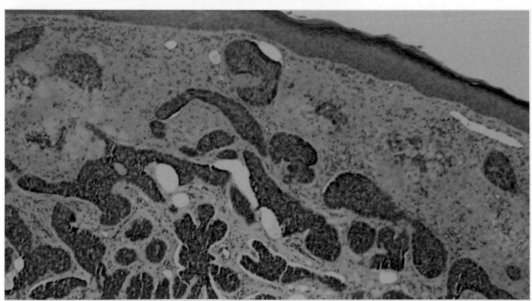

Fig. 54.2 Hematoxylin and eosin stain of left temple biopsy demonstrating histology consistent with basal cell carcinoma.

54.2 Differential Diagnosis—Key Points

Basal cell carcinoma (BCC) is a malignant neoplasm of keratinocytes that is correlated with both genetic and environmental factors. Significant sun exposure is the most significant risk factor, with a majority occurring on the face and scalp. Other risk factors include radiation therapy, long-term immunosuppression, and basal cell nevus syndrome. Almost 90% of BCCs have a mutation in the Hedgehog signaling pathway.

- Nodular BCC, the most common subtype, is commonly found on sun-exposed areas such as the head and neck. It classically appears as a telangiectatic pearly papule with rolled borders, which will often ulcerate in the center as it progresses. The differential diagnosis includes dermal nevus, seborrheic keratosis, amelanotic melanoma, and sebaceous carcinoma.
- Superficial BCC, the second most common, appears most commonly as an erythematous patch or plaque on the trunk. The differential diagnosis includes eczema, dermatophytosis, psoriasis, Bowen's disease, Paget's disease, tinea corporis, and squamous cell carcinoma.
- Morpheaform (sclerosing) BCC is an aggressive variant that appears as a white or pink plaque, which is often indurated with poorly defined borders. Differential diagnosis includes scar tissue and morphea.
- Pigmented BCC appears as a hyperpigmented, sometimes pearly papule. Differential diagnosis includes malignant melanoma, compound nevus, blue nevus, appendageal tumor, seborrheic keratosis, and nodular melanoma.

54.3 Test Interpretation

A biopsy is the diagnostic procedure of choice. Biopsy can be performed either by shave biopsy, incisional (punch) biopsy, or excisional biopsy with primary closure. A shave biopsy can be performed, with the exception of morpheaform BCC or recurrent BCC in a scar, in which a punch biopsy is more effective. If an incisional biopsy is performed, it is important to include the thickest portion of the nodule and the periphery, including an edge of normal skin to show maturation, the deepest area of invasion, and skin transition.

A complete otolaryngology exam should be performed prior to the removal of the primary tumor so that an estimate of the tumor size and possible spread can be evaluated.

54.4 Diagnosis

Nodular basal cell carcinoma. Histopathology shows basaloid, basophilic staining cells emanating downward from the epidermis with palisading of peripheral cells and clefting.

54.5 Medical Management

Treatment of BCC is guided by the location of the lesion, the size, the depth, and the histopathologic subtype. While treatment is often surgical, several medical options are available, with radiation therapy being the treatment of choice for poor surgical candidates. Other options include topical imiquimod, photodynamic therapy, ingenol mebutate, and vismodegib. Topical imiquimod is approved for nonfacial superficial BCC. Photodynamic therapy and ingenol mebutate have also demonstrated benefits in patients with superficial BCC. Vismodegib, which targets a protein in the Hedgehog intracellular signaling pathway, is approved for treatment of both locally advanced and metastatic BCC.

This patient had a BCC in a cosmetic area. The patient should have a complete cutaneous exam to rule out other cutaneous malignancies.

54.6 Surgical Management

The various modalities of surgical treatment include wide local excision with frozen section control, Mohs micrographic surgery, cryosurgery, and curettage. The cure rates with each of these techniques exceed 90% in most large series, depending on the subtype and location of the BCC. Excision with frozen section control is the historical and conventional standard. However, this technique has been criticized by some for not providing adequate control due to the difficulty in obtaining good frozen sections in functionally crucial and delicate facial areas. The concern is that in order to gain adequate frozen section control, more sacrifice of normal tissue may be required (up to 1 cm from the skin lesion). Therefore, Mohs micrographic surgery can be performed for BCC occurring on the head and neck because it allows for histopathologic evaluation of all margins and maximally preserves uninvolved tissue. Mohs surgery has the lowest 5-year BCC recurrence rates compared to other types of treatment.

Mohs micrographic surgery has the advantage of using a microscopic sampling technique to enable better preservation of normal tissues. Most studies have suggested less than a 1% recurrence rate for primary BCCs treated by Mohs surgery. In addition, Mohs surgery is the treatment of choice for morpheaform and infiltrating BCCs, recurrent BCCs, and other high-risk BCCs (nasal, ocular, and postauricular regions) where tissue conservation is of the utmost importance. The disadvantages of Mohs surgery are that it is more time-consuming and may possibly require two separate sittings for removal and reconstruction. Finally, radiation therapy offers advantages that include less patient discomfort and a nonsurgical option for patients in poor health who are not good surgical candidates. However, in large BCCs the cure rates are lower than for surgical resection. In addition, cosmesis is often rated inferior to surgical excision and may actually worsen over time. Curettage and cryosurgery are primarily reserved for the treatment of low-risk BCCs and are not appropriate treatment modalities for large, aggressive, deeply invasive tumors.

Surgical reconstruction may entail primary closure, skin grafts (full or split), or local tissue rearrangement. This patient underwent Mohs microrgraphic excision and primary closure. No undermining was done toward the eyebrow to prevent brow distortion and to maintain brow symmetry.

54.7 Rehabilitation and Follow-up

Patients diagnosed with sun-related skin cancer have a 30% to 40% chance of developing another cutaneous malignancy. Thus, routine follow-up is important for tumor surveillance. Furthermore, patients must be closely followed to guard against local recurrence. The earliest sign of recurrence should be biopsied and resected if positive. In addition, the avoidance of sun exposure and the use of sunscreens should be recommended.

54.8 Questions

1. The most common type of basal cell carcinoma (BCC) is
   a) Superficial.
   b) Morpheaform.
   c) Nodular.
   d) Pigmented.
   e) Amelonotic.
2. The approved treatment for metastatic BCC is
   a) Imiquimod.
   b) Mohs micrographic surgery.
   c) Vismodegib.
   d) Ingenol mebutate.
   e) Cyclosporine.
3. The treatment option with the lowest recurrence rate is
   a) Mohs micrographic surgery.
   b) Vismodegib.
   c) Wide local excision.
   d) Photodynamic therapy.
   e) CO_2 laser therapy.

Answers: 1. c 2. c 3. a

Suggested Readings

Boyd CM, Baker SR, Fader DJ, Wang TS, Johnson TM. The forehead flap for nasal reconstruction. Arch Dermatol. 2000; 136(11):1365–1370

Burget GC, Walton RL. Optimal use of microvascular free flaps, cartilage grafts, and a paramedian forehead flap for aesthetic reconstruction of the nose and adjacent facial units. Plast Reconstr Surg. 2007; 120(5):1171–1207, discussion 1208–1216

Chiummariello S, Dessy LA, Buccheri EM, et al. An approach to managing non-melanoma skin cancer of the nose with mucosal invasion: our experience. Acta Otolaryngol. 2008; 128(8):915–919

Dubas LE, Ingraffea A. Nonmelanoma skin cancer. Facial Plast Surg Clin North Am. 2013; 21(1):43–53

Mureau MA, Moolenburgh SE, Levendag PC, Hofer SO. Aesthetic and functional outcome following nasal reconstruction. Plast Reconstr Surg. 2007; 120(5):1217–1227, discussion 1228–1230

Schulze HJ, Cribier B, Requena L, et al. Imiquimod 5% cream for the treatment of superficial basal cell carcinoma: results from a randomized vehicle-controlled phase III study in Europe. Br J Dermatol. 2005; 152(5):939–947

55 Malignant Melanoma

Jamie L. Welshhans and Ryan M. Collar

55.1 History

An 89-year-old male presented to the clinic with a pigmented lesion on the right cheek present for ~6 months. The lesion had been growing in size. The patient had dementia and did not seek medical care for this lesion. He was otherwise healthy. He complained of new back pain.

On physical examination there was a 1.7 × 1-cm lesion on the patient's right cheek that was slightly raised and ulcerated in some areas. It was dark brown, had irregular borders, and had been getting larger and more ulcerated with time (▶ Fig. 55.1). The patient had several other lesions on his skin from sun exposure that looked like actinic keratosis. There was no palpable lymphadenopathy in the bilateral parotid, perifacial region, or neck. The remainder of a complete head and neck examination was normal

55.2 Differential Diagnosis—Key Points

Benign lesions in the differential diagnosis may include benign melanocytic nevus, dysplastic melanocytic nevus, seborrheic keratosis, and actinic keratosis. Malignant lesions in the differential diagnosis may include pigmented basal cell carcinoma, squamous cell carcinoma, Merkel's cell carcinoma, atypical fibroxanthoma, or cutaneous metastasis from another primary.

There are several characteristics of the lesion that may help one determine the diagnosis. The ABCDE rule is useful in differentiating benign acquired nevi from melanoma: A, asymmetry; B, irregular borders; C, variegated color; D, diameter greater than 6 mm; E, evolution. Lesions that satisfy one or more ABCDE criteria should be considered for biopsy. Full skin examination (including intertriginous regions, palms, soles, and nail beds) and lymph node palpation to rule out other lesions and metastatic disease is critical to the evaluation.

Risk factors for melanoma are as follows: having fair skin (Fitzpatrick's 1–2), excessive sun exposure, history of severe sunburn, having many nevi, and a family history of melanoma. Patients with dysplastic nevi have a 2 to 12% lifetime increased risk of melanoma. Removing these does not decrease risk, as it is only a marker for increased risk of developing melanoma; however, they should be removed if moderate to severe atypia is present. Sending the patient to a dermatologist may also be helpful if you are not sure if the lesion appears malignant or benign, as they are well versed in dermoscopy, which can help differentiate.

55.3 Test Interpretation

The first step in diagnosis of any skin cancer, including melanoma, is biopsy. This patient underwent punch biopsy that demonstrated melanoma with 4.4-mm Breslow's depth into the reticular

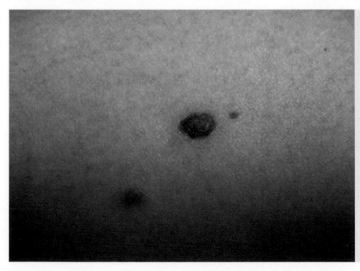

Fig. 55.1 An example of nodular melanoma

Table 55.1 2009 AJCC melanoma staging system.

Classification	Thickness (mm)	Ulceration state/mitoses
T		
Tis	NA	NA
T1	≤ 1.00	a) Without ulceration and mitosis < 1/mm^2 b) With ulceration or mitoses ≥ 1/mm^2
T2	1.01–2.00	a) Without ulceration b) With ulceration
T3	2.01–4.00	a) Without ulceration b) With ulceration
T4	> 4.00	a) Without ulceration b) With ulceration
N	No. of metastatic nodes	Nodal metastatic burden
N0	0	NA
N1	1	a) Micrometastasis b) Macrometastasis
N2	2–3	a) Micrometastasis b) Macrometastasis c) In-transit metastases/satellites without metastatic nodes
N3	4 + nodes, or matted nodes, or in-transit metastases/satellites with metastatic nodes	
M	Site	Serum LDH
M0	No distant metastasis	NA
M1a	Distant skin, subcutaneous, or nodal metastases	Normal
M1b	Lung metastases	Normal
M1c	All other visceral metastases	Normal
	Any distant metastasis	Elevated

Abbreviations: NA, not applicable; LDH, lactate dehydrogenase.

dermis, Clark's level IV, with ulceration. Imaging is recommended to evaluate specific signs and symptoms. In this case, the patient underwent positron emission tomography (PET)/computed tomography (CT) that demonstrated uptake at the primary site only.

Biopsy is very important in melanoma because the depth of the lesion is essential for proper staging and treatment. A shave biopsy is inadequate because it will not elucidate depth. An incision or excisional biopsy or a punch biopsy including skin and subcutaneous fat is the appropriate course of action.

The American Joint Committee on Cancer (AJCC) melanoma staging system may be found in ▶ Table 55.1. Aggressive features in this staging system include presence of mitoses, ulceration, lymph nodes (both micro- and macrometastases), satellite lesions, and distant metastases. T stage is based on Breslow's thickness. Breslow's thickness is measured from the granular layer of the epidermis to the deepest portion of the tumor. Clark's level (level of dermal involvement) is often reported but is not of prognostic significance. Using this staging system, the patient's stage is T4bN0M0.

55.4 Medical Management

Melanoma is primarily a surgical disease, but there may be a role for radiotherapy for lesions that may not be amenable to surgical resection (i.e., sinonasal melanoma and palliative treatment). Immunotherapy can be used to treat malignant melanoma, as well, including interleukin-2 (IL-2) and interferon. There are also multiple biologic medicines with approval by the Food and Drug Administration (FDA) for unresectable or metastatic melanoma; they include trametinib, dabrafenib, ipilimumab, vemurafenib, pembrolizumab, and nivolumab. Very recently, the FDA approved talimogene laherparepvec, which is a live attenuated oncolytic herpes virus.

55.5 Surgical Management

Treatment of choice for melanoma is wide local excision with appropriate treatment of lymph nodes in the draining nodal basin. Margins for excision depend on tumor depth (▶ Table 55.2). After wide local excision, lymph nodes need to be addressed. In patients with macrometastasis (e.g. those palpable and otherwise known prior to primary resection), the drainage basins should be excised completely through appropriate selective neck dissection plus or minus parotidectomy. In patients with no evidence of nodal disease but Breslow's depth greater than 0.75 mm, the clinician should consider and discuss sentinel lymph node (SLN) biopsy. SLN status has been shown to be the single most prognostic factor in head and neck melanoma. The rate of late regional recurrence after a negative SLN biopsy has been

reported to be 4% in large head and neck–specific reviews.

This patient did undergo a wide local excision with reconstruction and an SLN biopsy, which was negative (▶ Fig. 55.2).

55.6 Rehabilitation and Follow-up

The patient underwent surgery as noted above and is not a candidate for adjuvant therapy, given the low efficacy and his history of dementia. He is healing well from surgery.

He will need to establish care with a dermatologist for at least yearly skin checks. Ear, nose, and throat (ENT) will follow him several times a year for the first several years and then decrease the frequency if he does well. There are no official follow-up guidelines. Checking lactate dehydrogenase (LDH) may be helpful because it is elevated in distant metastatic disease.

Prevention is of utmost importance. Patients should be counseled on sun protection including

Table 55.2 Recommended surgical margins based on Breslow's thickness for malignant melanoma

Tumor Depth	Margin
In situ	0.5–1 cm
< 1 mm	1 cm
>1 mm	2 cm

Note: No benefit has been seen with margins larger than 2 cm.

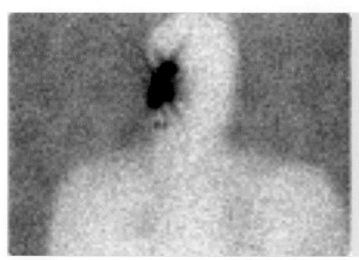

Fig. 55.2 Lymphoscintigraphy image from prior to sentinel lymph node biopsy

sunscreen and protective clothing. Evidence suggests that the patient or the patient's family members discover most recurrences or metastases; hence, self-awareness and examination are important.

55.7 Questions

1. A 52-year-old woman presents with a pigmented lesion on her left cheek. Melanoma is suspected. Which of the following is the most appropriate biopsy?
   a) An incisional biopsy of the lesion taking skin only.
   b) A punch biopsy.
   c) A shave biopsy.
   d) An excisional biopsy of the lesion with narrow margins.
2. A 34-year-old woman presents with a 1-cm lesion on her right ear. Biopsy is positive for superficial spreading melanoma. Breslow's depth is 0.4 mm, with ulceration. She had positron emission tomography (PET)/computed tomography (CT) done, which demonstrated uptake at the primary site only. What is the best surgical management?
   a) Wide local excision (WLE) with 1-cm margins and no sentinel lymph node (SLN) biopsy.
   b) WLE with 0.1-cm margins and SLN biopsy.
   c) WLE with 1-cm margins and elective radical neck dissection and parotidectomy.

d) WLE with 0.5-cm margins only, consider adjuvant treatment.
3. Which of the following is true regarding melanoma?
   a) Depth of invasion is the single most important prognostic factor.
   b) Radiation therapy is the gold standard adjuvant therapy for malignant melanoma.
   c) SLN biopsy should be performed on all patients with N0 neck and malignant melanoma.
   d) High mitotic rate upstages a patient from T2a to T2b.

Answers: 1. b 2. b 3. a

Suggested Readings

Balch CM, Gershenwald JE, Soong SJ, et al. Final version of 2009 AJCC melanoma staging and classification. J Clin Oncol. 2009; 27 (36):6199–6206

Erman AB, Collar RM, Griffith KA, et al. Sentinel lymph node biopsy is accurate and prognostic in head and neck melanoma. Cancer. 2012; 118(4):1040–1047

Gogas H, Polyzos A, Kirkwood J. Immunotherapy for advanced melanoma: fulfilling the promise. Cancer Treat Rev. 2013; 39(8):879–885

Ingraffea A.Melanoma. Facial Plast Surg Clin North Am. 2013; 21 (1):33–42

Mahadevan A, Patel VL, Dagoglu N. Radiation Therapy in the Management of Malignant Melanoma. Oncology (Williston Park). 2015; 29(10):743–751

Roy JM, Whitfield RJ, Gill PG. Review of the role of sentinel node biopsy in cutaneous head and neck melanoma. ANZ J Surg. 2016; 86(5):348–355

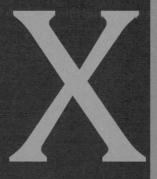

56 Epistaxis

David R. Lee and Reena Dhanda Patil

56.1 History

A 47-year-old man presented to the emergency department with epistaxis that had been intermittent since he sustained blunt facial trauma during an assault 3 days ago. He stated that immediately after the trauma the blood was bright red and quickly stopped. However, he reported intermittent slow dark red epistaxis for the past 3 days that had been persistent for the past 6 hours. At the time of the trauma he was evaluated at an outside hospital, where maxillofacial computed tomography (CT) was reportedly negative for acute fracture. His past medical history was significant for poorly controlled hypertension and coronary artery disease. His vital signs were within normal ranges, except for a blood pressure of 165/95. On physical exam he had slow drainage of dark red blood from his left nare. Anterior rhinoscopy of the left nare revealed blood posterior and superior to the inferior turbinate, with no apparent pulsations. Examination of the right nare on anterior rhinoscopy did not reveal bleeding. The remainder of the physical exam was noncontributory.

56.2 Differential Diagnosis—Key Points

The blood supply to the nose originates from both the external and internal carotid systems. The external carotid artery supplies the facial and internal maxillary arteries, the latter of which terminates in the sphenopalatine artery, which enters the nasal cavity through the posterior lateral nasal wall. The posterior septal nasal artery, a branch of the sphenopalatine artery, is a common source of posterior epistaxis. The internal carotid artery supplies the ophthalmic artery, which branches into anterior and posterior ethmoidal arteries that supply the upper lateral nasal wall and septum. However, the source of most nosebleeds and almost all anterior bleeds is the anteroinferior nasal septum, in an area known as Kiesselbach's plexus. This is where terminal branches of five arteries anastomose to form a vascular plexus—the sphenopalatine, greater palatine, superior labial, and anterior and posterior ethmoid arteries.

The lifetime incidence of epistaxis is approximately 60% in the general population, with less than 10% of all cases requiring medical attention. The condition has a bimodal distribution, commonly seen in children younger than 10 years of age and adults over 50 years old. The majority (80%) of all cases of epistaxis are from an anterior source. Minor bleeds, which are usually found on the anterior septum, are more frequently encountered in the pediatric population. Severe episodes of epistaxis that require invasive intervention often originate posteriorly and are seen more commonly in adults.

The differential diagnosis of epistaxis is very broad. As with all clinical presentations, a directed history and physical should be obtained. The most common cause of epistaxis in any age group is digital trauma (nose picking). Mucosal dryness, maxillofacial trauma (including nasal bone fracture or septal deviation), active inflammation or infection (including nasal polyps), and previously undiagnosed benign and malignant tumors (e.g., inverting papilloma, juvenile nasopharyngeal angiofibroma, squamous cell carcinoma, and melanoma) are all potential causes of epistaxis. In adults, medications such as aspirin, nonsteroidal anti-inflammatory drugs (NSAIDs), warfarin, or newer anticoagulants such as rivaroxaban have been implicated in epistaxis. Hypertension is not firmly established as an independent risk factor for epistaxis, but it may make control of epistaxis more challenging.

Excessive use of intranasal corticosteroids, especially when directed against the nasal septum, may contribute to nosebleeds as well. Systemic conditions that predispose individuals to epistaxis include von Willebrand's disease, hemophilia, and leukemia, all of which contribute to either poor platelet function or thrombocytopenia (low platelet counts). Hereditary hemorrhagic telangiectasia (also known as HHT or Osler-Weber-Rendu syndrome) is an autosomal dominant condition that presents with arteriovenous malformations (AVMs) and telangiectasias in the nasal mucosa, lungs, and brain, and very commonly will present with epistaxis.

56.3 Test Interpretation

A complete blood count should be ordered on any patient presenting with recurrent or active epistaxis. A low hemoglobin may imply that a patient either has suffered massive acute blood loss or has had gradual blood loss from intermittent epistaxis. In most cases, platelet levels will be normal, although thrombocytopenia could be a factor in recurrent epistaxis. A platelet count of less than 20,000/mm^3 significantly increases the difficulty of controlling an episode of epistaxis. Prothrombin time or partial thromboplastin time may be helpful if an underlying bleeding dyscrasia is present or suspected, which might warrant further work-up.

56.4 Diagnosis

Recurrent epistaxis secondary to facial trauma

56.5 Medical Management

The first step in treating minor epistaxis is conservative medical management. Most uncomplicated epistaxis will self-resolve with no or minimal intervention. This may include direct pressure applied to both nares for 15 to 20 minutes with or without topical application of oxymetazoline or phenylephrine solution for vasoconstriction. Long-term prevention can be achieved by reducing mucosal dryness, which may be achieved with saline nasal sprays, application of petrolatum or antibiotic ointment, or use of humidifiers at home.

A patient presenting with severe nasal hemorrhage is at risk for both airway compromise from aspiration of blood and hemodynamic instability from acute blood loss. In these instances, following an acute care protocol is critical. If necessary, an artificial airway can be placed first, under controlled circumstances if at all possible. Typically this can be achieved by rapid sequence induction, followed by orotracheal intubation. A surgical airway may be necessary but should only be performed if intubation cannot be performed owing to an inability to visualize the airway as a result of the hemorrhage. If the patient is seen in an emergency department setting, recruiting medical assistance to manage the patient's airway and hemodynamic resuscitation may be immensely helpful while the otolaryngologist attempts to control the source of epistaxis.

In this patient, pressure was held for 15 minutes and topical oxymetazoline was liberally applied, with persistence of slow epistaxis despite these conservative measures. His airway remained patent and uncompromised.

56.6 Surgical Management

There are multiple options for surgical management of epistaxis, depending on both the severity of the hemorrhage and the familiarity of the treating physician with the numerous tools available to control nosebleeds. Localized anterior mucosal bleeds may respond well to topical application of silver nitrate cautery. However, silver nitrate causes local chemical damage to bleeding tissues, so care must be taken to avoid aggressive cautery of both sides of the nasal septum to decrease risk of septal perforation. Other methods of controlling anterior epistaxis include anterior nasal packing devices such as Rhino Rocket (Shippert Medical Technologies) sponges, Rapid Rhino (ArthroCare Corporation) inflatable packs, or in more severe cases, formal packing using ribbon gauze covered with petroleum jelly. If further bleeding is seen, packing in the opposite (nonbleeding) nasal passage before removing the already placed pack may be attempted to further stablize the septum and allow for more efficient pressure hemostasis.

Posterior epistaxis can be difficult to treat owing to its location and often its greater severity. Several specially designed balloon systems and packs are available for posterior nosebleeds, including the EpiStax (Summit Medical) and a longer anterior-posterior version of the Rapid Rhino. A simple readily available alternative method involves placement of a 12 or 14 French Foley's catheter into the nasal cavity, inflation of the balloon with 10 mL of saline, and pulling of the catheter anteriorly until the balloon lodges in the posterior choanae. The anterior nasal passage is then packed tightly with layered petrolatum gauze. Up to 70% of posterior packing procedures are successful in stopping epistaxis. It is important to note that many patients do not tolerate posterior nasal packing while awake, and thus elective endotracheal intubation and sedation can be performed for comfort and to protect the airway prior to packing.

In patients refractory to formal anterior and/or posterior packing, operative intervention may be required. The initial action is generally electrocautery of the affected area under nasal endoscopy. If unsuccessful, septoplasty and ligation of the anterior ethmoidal or sphenopalatine arteries can be attempted. A nonoperative approach to controlling severe intractable epistaxis includes catheterization and embolization of selected arteries from the external carotid circulation and may be preferentially performed in unstable patients or those considered unsuitable for general anesthesia.

Every patient undergoing posterior packing or other intervention for a posterior nosebleed should be admitted and their oxygen saturation monitored, due to the potential for hypoxia and cardiac arrhythmias. Complications that can arise from prolonged packing include ulceration and necrosis of the mucosa, skin, and cartilage of the nasal tip, septum, and nasopharynx. Other complications include septal perforation, sinusitis, and synechiae. Antibiotic therapy should be initiated in patients with nasal packing in place to prevent toxic shock syndrome or the development of secondary bacterial sinusitis. Nasal packs may be removed after 48 to 72 hours if no further bleeding is seen.

This patient was refractory to conservative medical measures. Initially, a Rapid Rhino was placed in the left nare and inflated with 5 mL of saline. This, in conjunction with medical management of the patient's hypertension, temporarily stalled the epistaxis. However, his bleeding returned and required both an anterior-posterior Rapid Rhino in the left nare and a second Rapid Rhino in the right nare to provide additional pressure. He was then admitted for antibiotics, pain management, and hypertension control, and after 48 hours both nasal packs were removed without further bleeding.

56.7 Rehabilitation and Follow-up

Patients with a history of previous epistaxis are at a higher risk of recurrence. Preventive measures are strongly recommended for all patients. These include refraining from nose blowing or picking; abstinence from alcohol or hot drinks that can vasodilate nasal vessels; regular use of saline nasal sprays; petrolatum ointments and humidification to moisturize the nasal passages; and appropriate management of comorbidities that can contribute to epistaxis, including hypertension. Use of specific medications such as aspirin or warfarin should be closely monitored. All patients with severe or recurrent epistaxis should have a formal evaluation of the nasal cavity performed, either while hospitalized or in an outpatient setting, to rule out a neoplastic process or anatomic abnormalities.

56.8 Questions

1. Most cases of epistaxis arise from where?
   a) Kiesselbach's plexus.
   b) Woodruff's plexus.
   c) The sphenopalatine artery.
   d) The anterior ethmoid artery.
2. Kiesselbach's plexus is supplied by each of the following arteries except which one?
   a) Sphenopalatine.
   b) Greater palatine.
   c) Anterior ethmoid.
   d) Superior labial.
   e) Inferior labial.
3. Potential complications from nasal packing include which of the following?
   a) Hypoxia.
   b) Toxic shock syndrome.
   c) Nasal adhesions.
   d) Septal perforation.
   e) All of the above.

Answers: 1. a 2. e 3. e

Suggested Readings

Awan MS, Iqbal M, Imam SZ. Epistaxis: when are coagulation studies justified? Emerg Med J. 2008; 25(3):156–157
Douglas R, Wormald PJ. Update on epistaxis. Curr Opin Otolaryngol Head Neck Surg. 2007; 15(3):180–183
Villwock JA, Jones K. Recent trends in epistaxis management in the United States: 2008–2010. JAMA Otolaryngol Head Neck Surg. 2013; 139(12):1279–1284

57 Granulomatosis with Polyangiitis (Wegener's Granulomatosis)

Brian L. Hendricks and Lee A. Zimmer

57.1 History

A 55-year-old Caucasian man presented for evaluation of suspected chronic sinusitis. He reported a constellation of signs and symptoms including chronic nasal obstruction, hyposmia, intermittent self-limited epistaxis, and thick rhinorrhea. His primary care provider had prescribed a combination of antibiotics, nasal steroids, saline irrigations, and topical decongestants without improvement. He had developed symptoms over the last 2 years, but they had significantly affected his quality of life over the last several months. He reported no prior history of significant sinonasal complaints.

On further questioning, the patient endorsed a chronic cough and slowly progressive hearing loss. He denied dyspnea, stridor, vertigo, or tinnitus. He reported a history of mild renal insufficiency but no other diagnosed medical problems. He denied any known history of nasal trauma, surgery, seasonal allergies, reflux, or illicit drug use. He reported a family history of hypertension and diabetes.

On physical examination, remarkable findings included nasal crusting and ulceration (▶ Fig. 57.1), as well as a small-sized clot abutting the nasal septum. After removal of the clot, a septal perforation was discovered. Endoscopy was performed, and the ostiomeatal complex appeared reasonably patent on both sides. The larynx was unremarkable on

flexible fiberoptic examination. Oral examination revealed mild mucosal hyperplasia, but no ulcerations or lesions. Otologic exam was notable for a serous effusion on the left, and tuning fork tests corresponded with a conductive hearing loss on this side.

An audiogram was obtained during this visit and confirmed an approximate 20-dB conductive hearing loss on the left and a bilaterally symmetric mild high-frequency hearing loss. An endoscopic nasal septal biopsy was performed under local anesthesia, and the patient was sent to phlebotomy to draw a blood sample for an antineutrophil cytoplasmic antibodies (ANCA) panel.

57.2 Differential Diagnosis—Key Points

- This patient's clinical history was suggestive of chronic rhinosinusitis. Common etiologies include allergic rhinitis, mucociliary dysfunction, systemic inflammatory conditions, immunologic disorders, microbial colonization, nasal polyposis, and anatomic abnormalities resulting in mechanical obstruction.
- On physical examination, the most significant findings included nasal crusting, ulceration, and a septal perforation. The differential diagnosis

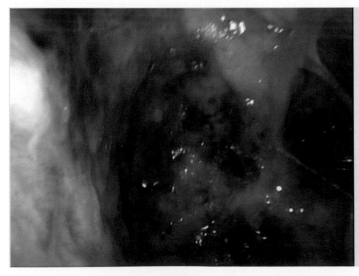

Fig. 57.1 Nasal cavity of a patient with granulomatosis with polyangiitis. Note the dried nasal mucus crusting to the lateral and posterior nasal walls.

for the patient's septal perforation included prior nasal trauma, prior sinonasal surgery, cocaine use, neoplasm, infection, and autoimmune disorders. Because the patient denied any history related to many of these causes, the starting differential was narrowed.

- The absence of a mass or other suspicious findings reduced the likelihood of neoplasm. Infectious processes were also considered less likely given the lack of evidence of an obstructed middle meatus or purulence on examination. Nasal polyposis was also eliminated based on physical exam.

- Given the presence of a septal perforation without any clear etiology by patient history, the suspicion for an autoimmune or inflammatory condition must be raised. While this patient's other reported history of hearing loss, chronic cough, and renal insufficiency may be unrelated, they could also be explained by granulomatosis with polyangiitis (GPA), which is a disease that affects small- and medium-sized blood vessels. This patient also fit the demographic profile, as most patients diagnosed with GPA are Caucasian and between the ages of 40 and 65. Nasal symptoms often present early in the disease process, and can include crusting, obstruction, epistaxis, and rhinorrhea. Saddle nose deformity is generally a late finding after the disease has had time to progress. Otitis media, gingival hyperplasia, mucosal ulcers, and subglottic stenosis are among the other possible findings in patients with GPA.

57.3 Test Interpretation

In a patient with an unexplained perforation or ulcerative lesion, biopsies should be performed to evaluate for neoplasm. Biopsy also plays a role in evaluating for possible GPA, though multiple biopsies may be required to reach a diagnosis. Histopathologic findings include granulomatous inflammation, scattered giant cells, vasculitis, and extravascular necrosis.

An elevated erythrocyte sedimentation rate can support the presence of an inflammatory condition, but is nonspecific and does not provide a diagnosis. Relevant laboratory studies include cytoplasmic and perinuclear ANCA (C-ANCA and P-ANCA). In patients with systemic GPA, C-ANCA levels are elevated in over 90% of patients. In disease localized only to the head and neck, elevated C-ANCA levels are detected in approximately 50 to 70% of patients.

Urinalysis and chest radiographs can also be helpful in evaluation for suspected GPA, but our preference is to defer this portion of the work-up to rheumatology.

57.4 Diagnosis

Granulomatosis with polyangiitis (Wegener's granulomatosis)

57.5 Medical Management

Medical therapy for the disease is based partially on severity. In patients with minor symptoms limited to the head and neck, therapy may be directed only at the chief complaints. This may include topical ointments, saline sprays, and irrigations to reduce crusting and epistaxis. In patients with functional obstruction and evidence of rhinosinusitis, additional therapy may include steroids and antibiotics when necessary. Refractory disease should be treated with culture-directed antibiotic therapy, keeping in mind that *Staphylococcus aureus* and *Pseudomonas aeruginosa* are two frequently found organisms.

For patients with more advanced or systemic disease, the mainstays of treatment include corticosteroids and immunosuppressants. Disease progression can be monitored with serial C-ANCA titers. These patients should generally be referred to and managed by rheumatology for their systemic disease.

57.6 Surgical Management

There is a limited role for surgical management of sinonasal GPA. In particular, it should be noted that patients with GPA who undergo sinonasal surgery can experience a multitude of complications postoperatively, including extensive synechiae, scarring, crusting, and lack of symptomatic improvement compared with their presurgical status.

In patients whose disease has advanced enough to develop a saddle nose deformity, open rhinoplasty can be offered for both improved function and cosmesis. However, surgical intervention should generally be delayed until the patient's disease process has been adequately treated to reduce the chance of failure or recurrent deformity. Many clinicians advise against attempted septal perforation repair in patients with GPA, as inflammation involving the nasal septal vasculature can complicate postoperative wound healing and reduce the likelihood of success.

57.7 Rehabilitation and Follow-up

Long-term remission can be achieved with medical therapy. The mean survival time of untreated systemic GPA is 5 months, and approximately 90% of untreated patients are deceased within 1 year due to severe renal or pulmonary involvement. With the advent of modern immunosuppressive regimens, patients with systemic GPA now have a median survival of 21.7 years after diagnosis.

Nasal saline irrigations or sprays should be used long-term. Acute exacerbations of bacterial rhinosinusitis should ideally be treated with culture-directed antimicrobial therapy.

57.8 Questions

1. Sinusitis associated with Wegener's granulomatosis is often difficult to treat. What organism is most commonly cultured from these patients?
   a) *Streptococcus pneumoniae*.
   b) *Staphylococcus aureus*.
   c) *Haemophilus influenzae*.
   d) Fungal species such as *Alternaria*, *Fusarium*, and *Aspergillus*.
2. Which type of vessels are affected by Wegener's granulomatosis vasculitis?
   a) Small vessels.
   b) Medium vessels.
   c) Large vessels.
   d) Small- and medium-sized vessels.
3. Which of the following is the most commonly reported early symptom in patients with head and neck involvement of granulomatosis with polyangiitis?
   a) Difficulty breathing.
   b) Hearing loss.
   c) Nasal crusting.
   d) Saddle nose deformity.

Answers: 1. b 2. d 3. c

Suggested Readings

Gubbels SP, Barkhuizen A, Hwang PH. Head and neck manifestations of Wegener's granulomatosis. Otolaryngol Clin North Am. 2003; 36(4):685–705

Rasmussen N. Management of the ear, nose, and throat manifestations of Wegener granulomatosis: an otorhinolaryngologist's perspective. Curr Opin Rheumatol. 2001; 13(1):3–11

Trimarchi M, Sinico RA, Teggi R, Bussi M, Specks U, Meroni PL. Otorhinolaryngological manifestations in granulomatosis with polyangiitis (Wegener's). Autoimmun Rev. 2013; 12(4):501–505

Tsuzuki K, Fukazawa K, Takebayashi H, Hashimoto K, Sakagami M. Difficulty of diagnosing Wegener's granulomatosis in the head and neck region. Auris Nasus Larynx. 2009; 36(1):64–70

58 Anosmia

Thomas K. Hamilton and Allen M. Seiden

58.1 History

A 26-year-old man presented with a referral from his primary care physician complaining of a decreased ability to smell and taste. He first noticed the symptoms about 2 weeks ago when foods seemed to taste more bland than usual, and he began to realize he could not smell anything. When questioned, he said he had noted no olfactory or gustatory distortions, and he felt he could distinguish salt, sweet, and maybe sour, although these seemed to be less intense. He had a recent history of an altercation at a bar about a month ago where he sustained blunt head trauma. He was brought to the emergency department (ED) at that time and was sent home after evaluation without the need for any acute intervention. No X-rays were done, but he did not suffer any facial fractures. He denied any history of sinusitis and had not had any symptoms of an upper respiratory tract infection or recent sick contacts. He had no other medical problems and there was no family history of any genetic conditions.

Physical examination of the head and neck revealed no abnormalities. Specifically, the external nose was not deviated, the nares were patent, the nasal septum was midline, the nasal mucosa was pink and nonedematous, and there was no evidence of polyps or other masses within the nasal cavities. Olfactory testing was administered using the University of Pennsylvania Smell Identification Test, confirming a complete loss of smell.

58.2 Differential Diagnosis — Key Points

- Olfactory loss has significant implications, both by its impact on quality of life and safety concerns related to fire, gas leak, and spoiled foods. Anosmia is a complete loss of smell, whereas hyposmia is a diminished sense of smell. Disturbances in the sense of smell are not uncommon. It is estimated that 19% of individuals over 20 and 25% of those over the age of 53 have at least some loss of smell.
- Overall, the three most common causes of anosmia/hyposmia are the following:
  - Head trauma.
    Even relatively minor head trauma that is without associated fractures can cause a loss of smell. Often, the symptom is noticed late after the incident due to other, more pressing injuries or concerns that can accompany head injury.
    Posttraumatic olfactory loss is believed to be due either to direct injury to the olfactory nerve or to a concussive injury to olfactory structures. It most commonly occurs after a frontal or occipital blow, due to coup-contrecoup forces. Direct injury to the olfactory nerve is not likely to recover. Concussive injuries can lead to recovery of function, most often within a year of injury. Improvement is seen in 10 to 35% of cases.
  - Chronic rhinosinusitis (CRS).
    The olfactory neuroepithelial receptors are located within the nasal vault, and olfactory perception occurs when odors reach this area to combine with those receptors. CRS causes inflammatory changes in the nose that can obstruct this area and lead to olfactory loss. There are also data to suggest that inflammatory changes actually occur on a molecular level within the olfactory neuroepithelium. Many patients with olfactory loss secondary to CRS report that their loss fluctuates. Some patients may have no other nasal symptoms other than the loss of smell.
    Olfactory loss secondary to rhinosinusitis usually is responsive to treatment aimed at reducing nasal inflammation and obstruction to the nasal vault.
  - Upper respiratory tract infection (URI).
    A viral URI can cause a temporary loss of smell during its acute phase due to nasal congestion. However, the virus can directly cause degenerative changes within the olfactory neuroepithelium in some patients, leading to a persistent loss of smell. As the congestion of the acute phase resolves, patients will become aware that their sense of smell does not return.
    This type of loss is often associated with olfactory distortions, both in response to actual odors (parosmia) and occurring spontaneously (phantosmia).
    Over time, some spontaneous recovery may occur. The likelihood of such recovery is inversely related to the severity of the initial loss.

- Congenital anosmia is a consideration in younger individuals who report a lifelong inability to smell. While a congenital olfactory loss is reported in association with a variety of congenital syndromes, for example, Kallman's syndrome (hypogonadotropic hypogonadism), most patients with congenital olfactory loss have no such syndrome.
- Loss of smell can also be an early symptom of a neurodegenerative disease, such as Parkinson's disease or Alzheimer's disease. Schizophrenia has also been associated with difficulty identifying particular smells.
- Certain environmental toxins have been implicated in anosmia, including cadmium, mercury, and formaldehyde. Additionally, nasal zinc preparations, formerly available over the counter, have also been associated with a diminished sense of smell.
- This patient also complained of a loss of taste. More specifically he noted that foods tasted bland. The fact that he could detect salt and sweet indicated that his taste was actually intact. Our taste buds respond to the five basic tastes of salt, sour, sweet, bitter, and umami, and a true loss of taste is very uncommon. However, the flavor of food is perceived via retronasal olfactory stimulation while we eat. Patients who lose their smell immediately notice this loss of flavor and misinterpret that as a loss of taste.

When taking a history, more accurate information can be gathered by asking patients whether they can distinguish salt and sweet rather than simply asking them if they can taste.

58.3 Test Interpretation

The most important component of working up a patient with anosmia is a detailed history and physical exam with an emphasis on recent head injuries, current illnesses, and chronic sinus problems. A family history of congenital diseases may be relevant. A detailed social history may uncover environmental exposures that could be contributing factors. Other than active nasal and sinus disease, the etiology of a loss of smell is based largely on a historical trigger preceding the loss. If no such event can be determined from the history, the loss is labeled as idiopathic.

If available, objective testing is appropriate, as the patient's subjective complaint often correlates poorly with objective testing. The most commonly utilized test in this country is the University of Pennsylvania Smell Identification Test. This includes 40 odors, each on a microencapsulated scratch and sniff pad. The score is based upon the number correct: 35 to 40, normosmia; 20 to 34, hyposmia; and < 20, anosmia. The Sniffin' Sticks test is the most widely utilized in Europe and includes an identification test, discrimination test (odor present or not), and a threshold test. The result of these three is then combined into a composite score.

Physical examination should include nasal endoscopy to rule out nasal or sinus inflammatory disease as the possible etiology. Such inflammatory disease may not be apparent from the history and may not be easily visible on anterior rhinoscopy.

Laboratory testing is rarely needed in the evaluation of anosmia. If a congenital etiology is suspected and possible syndromic characteristics are noted, then testing for other laboratory abnormalities, such as with hormone testing for suspected Kallman's syndrome, may be appropriate. Similarly, imaging is usually not required. If CRS is suspected as the cause of anosmia, a computed tomography scan of the sinuses may be helpful to confirm the extent of disease. If the olfactory loss is idiopathic, a magnetic resonance imaging scan of the brain to rule out intracranial pathology is indicated.

58.4 Diagnosis

Anosmia secondary to head trauma

58.5 Medical Management

Medical therapy is only effective when there is a treatable underlying inflammatory cause of anosmia. In these cases, treating any bacterial infection or allergic component is important, but steroids will generally be the most helpful in reversing the loss. For other causes of anosmia, there is generally no effective medical therapy. Enhancing other aspects of flavor can help make food more palatable, such as varying the textures and temperatures of the food or adding hot sauce to foods. Also, it is important to emphasize the importance of using smoke detectors in the home, as these patients are less able to detect the presence of something burning.

58.6 Surgical Management

Surgical therapy is generally helpful when the olfactory loss is secondary to CRS. While prednisone can reverse the loss in such cases, its long-term use carries many risks. Endoscopic sinus surgery has been shown to be effective in cases of obstructive anosmia, combined with ongoing topical treatment as appropriate.

58.7 Rehabilitation and Follow-up

Patients who have lost their smell secondary to CRS will require ongoing follow-up based upon their response to treatment. There are some recent data to suggest that olfactory training, or exercise, can improve the incidence of recovery in patients suffering a postviral or posttraumatic loss.

58.8 Questions

1. True or false? Most patients with anosmia following a head injury will recover spontaneously.
   a) b.
2. Which of the following is true regarding recovery after posttraumatic olfactory loss?
   a) Occurs in 10 to 35% of cases and generally within a year.
   b) Occurs in 80 to 90% of cases within the first 3 months.
   c) Occurs in 80 to 90% of cases and generally within a year.
   d) Occurs in 10 to 35% of cases within the first 3 months.
3. Of the following statements regarding smell, which is true?
   a) Our sense of smell improves with age.
   b) Smell does not affect the ability to enjoy food.
   c) A quantitative test exists to test a patient's ability to smell.
   d) Congenital anosmia is the most common cause of diminished smell.

Answers: 1. False 2. a 3. c

Suggested Readings

Harless L, Liang J. Pharmacologic treatment for postviral olfactory dysfunction: a systematic review. Int Forum Allergy Rhinol. 2016; 6 (7):760–767

Hoekman PK, Houlton JJ, Seiden AM. The utility of magnetic resonance imaging in the diagnostic evaluation of idiopathic olfactory loss. Laryngoscope. 2014; 124(2):365–368

Coelho DH, Costanzo RM. Posttraumatic olfactory dysfunction. Auris Nasus Larynx. 2016; 43(2):137–143

Stuck BA, Hummel T. Olfaction in allergic rhinitis: A systematic review. J Allergy Clin Immunol. 2015; 136(6):1460–1470

Ottaviano G, Frasson G, Nardello E, Martini A. Olfaction deterioration in cognitive disorders in the elderly. Aging Clin Exp Res. 2016; 28(1):37–45

Konstantinidis I, Tsakiropoulou E, Bekiaridou P, Kazantzidou C, Constantinidis J. Use of olfactory training in post-traumatic and postinfectious olfactory dysfunction. Laryngoscope. 2013; 123(12):E85–E90

59 Allergic Fungal Sinusitis

Brittany A. Leader and Alfred M. Sassler

59.1 History

A 19-year-old woman was referred to clinic for chronic nasal congestion that had been refractory to previous treatment by her primary care physician. It was associated with postnasal drainage, occasional dark nasal crusting, and frequent headaches. Her symptoms had been gradually worsening over 12 months. Previously she had tried daily saline rinses, oral antihistamines, and intranasal steroids without improvement. A 2-week course of oral prednisone gave some symptomatic relief, but her symptoms recurred within weeks of completing treatment. A course of antibiotics provided no improvement. Allergy testing had not been performed, but she denied a history of asthma or sensitivity to aspirin. The headaches were frontal, without associated sensitivity to light or sound, and she had not identified any triggers. She denied any history of diabetes or chronic steroid use, and was otherwise healthy without any other medical conditions.

On focused physical examination there was slight left-sided proptosis with intact extraocular movements. Anterior rhinoscopy revealed a minimally deviated septum to the left, bilateral turbinate hypertrophy, and bilateral nasal polyps.

59.2 Differential Diagnosis—Key Points

- On the differential was aspirin-exacerbated respiratory disease, which is a triad of aspirin sensitivity, asthma, and nasal polyposis. However, given that she did not have a history of asthma or aspirin sensitivity, this diagnosis was unlikely.
- Aspergilloma, mycetoma, or a fungus ball of the sinuses were also possible, but these tend to involve a single sinus, most often the maxillary antrum or sphenoid sinus.
- Invasive fungal sinusitis was very unlikely, as she did not have diabetes and was not immunocompromised.
- The differential diagnosis for headaches includes migraines and tension headaches. The diagnostic criteria for migraines are at least five headache episodes lasting 4 to 72 hours, with at least two of the following characteristics:
  - Unilateral location.

- Pulsating quality.
  - Moderate or severe pain intensity.
  - Aggravated by or contributing to avoidance of routine activities such as walking.
- and at least one of the following:
  - Nausea and/or vomiting.
  - Photophobia and phonophobia.
- Migraines may also be associated with auras. Tension headaches are often associated with neck muscle tension, and stress usually triggers these symptoms later in the school day or workday.
- Allergic fungal sinusitis (AFS) is a type of chronic rhinosinusitis due to a localized allergic inflammation in response to noninvasive fungi in areas with poor mucous drainage. It is characterized by thick eosinophil-laden mucin, which contains fungal hyphae and eosinophils, as well as characteristic radiographic findings.
- While the pathogenesis is controversial, AFS is thought to be a result of a Gell and Coombs type I T-helper cell hypersensitivity in response to inhaled fungal antigens, usually of the dematiaceous species, leading to its characteristic features of allergic fungal mucin.
- The diagnostic criteria for AFS are chronic rhinosinusitis with nasal polyposis (unless previously treated medically or surgically removed), eosinophilic mucin with histologic findings of noninvasive fungal hyphae and degranulating eosinophils, and characteristic computed tomography (CT) findings. AFS is neither confirmed by a positive fungal culture nor excluded by a negative fungal culture. Definitive diagnosis requires a specimen and is normally made after sinus surgery.
- AFS is most common in young adults and adolescents and is often seen in the southern United States, which may be related to increased exposure to mold spores.
- AFS is distinguished from chronic rhinosinusitis by histology with mucin-containing eosinophils and fungal hyphae, as well as characteristic CT findings.

59.3 Diagnosis

Allergic fungal sinusitis

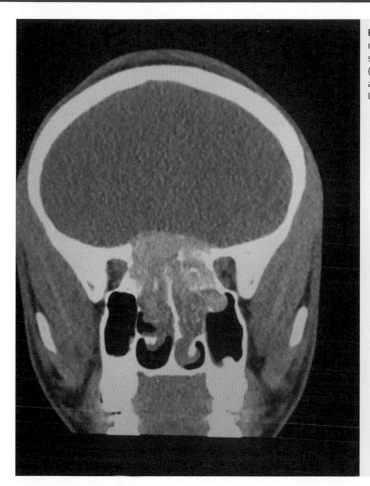

Fig. 59.1 CT demonstrating heterogeneous intrasinus densities with expansion and erosion of the bony skull base. (Image courtesy of Sarah K. Wise, MD, and Patricia A. Loftus, MD, Emory University School of Medicine..)

59.4 Test Interpretation

Radiology: CT of the sinuses demonstrates a heterogeneous signal intensity that is characteristic of allergic fungal mucin (▶ Fig. 59.1). Often one or more sinuses are involved, and it can be either unilateral or bilateral. Nasal polyposis is also frequently seen. On magnetic resonance imaging (MRI), AFS is demonstrated by a hypointense signal and mucosal thickening.

59.4.1 Histology

Hematoxylin-eosin staining of the mucosa will reveal an inflammatory infiltrate of eosinophils, lymphocytes, and plasma cells, and will lack necrosis and granulomas (▶ Fig. 59.2). The mucus is thick, and under microscopy it shows sheets of eosinophils with broken down eosinophils known as Charcot-Leyden crystals. The mucin will also contain noninvasive fungal hyphae that can be demonstrated on GMS stain (▶ Fig. 59.3), which are by definition absent from the mucosa and other tissues.

59.5 Medical Management

While the definitive treatment is surgical, medical management may be used both preoperatively to optimize a patient and after surgery to reduce further recurrences. Many surgeons utilize preoperative systemic glucocorticoids to shrink polyps, reduce swelling, and minimize bleeding. Postoperatively, systemic glucocorticoids are given for several weeks with a taper. Topical and systemic steroids are often used in conjunction. The use of systemic and/or topical antifungals is controversial, and they are typically reserved for high-risk patients. Additionally, patients are advised to receive allergy immunotherapy if a fungal allergy is demonstrated on specific serum immunoglobulin E (IgE) or skin testing.

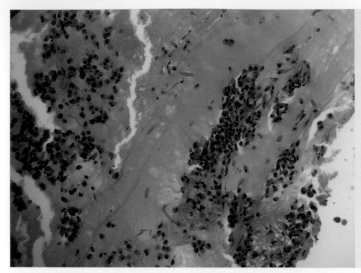

Fig. 59.2 Hematoxylin-eosin stain with Charcot-Leyden crystals. (Image courtesy of Sarah K. Wise, MD, and Patricia A. Loftus, MD, Emory University School of Medicine.)

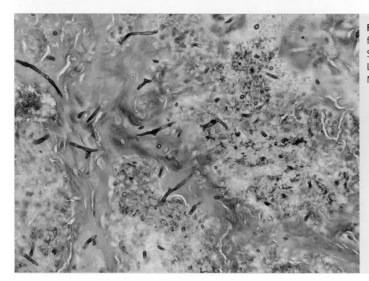

Fig. 59.3 GMS stain with noninvasive fungal hyphae. (Image courtesy of Sarah K. Wise, MD, and Patricia A. Loftus, MD, Emory University School of Medicine.)

59.6 Surgical Management

Endoscopic sinus surgery is the mainstay of treatment. Complete removal of allergic fungal debris, mucinous secretions, and polyps is essential, which requires widely patent sinusotomies and vigorous irrigation of the sinuses in the operating room. In addition to debridement, mucin removal allows for a histologic diagnosis. The other goal of surgery is to improve drainage by optimizing the sinus outflow tracts to minimize future mucus accumulation, which allows rinses and sprays to have improved efficacy. Symptom recurrence is more frequent if patients are not compliant with therapy or if they do not receive postoperative steroids.

59.7 Rehabilitation and Follow-up

Patients may benefit from allergy testing and immunotherapy to reduce the severity of their hypersensitivity reaction. Nasal steroid use and leukotriene antagonists may help to delay the formation of new polyps. It is important to continue to follow patients with endoscopy to ensure patency of their sinuses.

59.8 Questions

1. All of the following are diagnostic criteria for allergic fungal sinusitis (AFS) except

a) Characteristic radiographic findings.
b) Chronic rhinosinusitis.
c) Immunodeficiency.
d) Mucin with degranulating eosinophils and fungal hyphae.

2. The following are mainstays of AFS treatment except
a) Endoscopic sinus surgery.
b) Systemic antifungals.
c) Systemic postoperative glucocorticoids.
d) Topical postoperative glucocorticoids.

3. All of the following regarding AFS are true except
a) AFS is frequently seen in the southern United States.
b) Patients may present with reduction of or loss of the sense of smell.
c) Patients have an aspirin sensitivity.
d) Patients may present with facial dysmorphia.

Answers: 1. c 2. b 3. c

Suggested Readings

Folker RJ, Marple BF, Mabry RL, Mabry CS. Treatment of allergic fungal sinusitis: a comparison trial of postoperative immunotherapy with specific fungal antigens. Laryngoscope. 1998; 108(11 Pt 1):1623–1627

Glass D, Amedee RG. Allergic fungal rhinosinusitis: a review. Ochsner J. 2011; 11(3):271–275

Jen A, Kacker A, Huang C, Anand V. Fluconazole nasal spray in the treatment of allergic fungal sinusitis: a pilot study. Ear Nose Throat J. 2004; 83(10):692–695, 694–695

Krouse JH. Allergic and non-allergic rhinitis. In: Bailey BJ, Johnson JT, Newlands SD, et al, eds. Bailey's Head and Neck Surgery—Otolaryngology 4th ed. Philadelphia, PA: Lippincott Williams & Wilkins; 2004

Lanza DC, Dhong HJ, Tantilipikorn P, Tanabodee J, Nadel DM, Kennedy DW. Fungus and chronic rhinosinusitis: from bench to clinical understanding. Ann Otol Rhinol Laryngol Suppl. 2006; 196:27–34; 460–488

Simon-Nobbe B, Denk U, Pöll V, Rid R, Breitenbach M. The spectrum of fungal allergy. Int Arch Allergy Immunol. 2008; 145(1):58–86

60 Sinus Mucocele

Ryan A. Crane and Lee A. Zimmer

60.1 History

A 37-year-old woman was referred for evaluation of retro-orbital pain, greater on the left than the right, with pressure between her eyes. She was previously seen by the referring otolaryngologist for intermittent left eye exophthalmos with associated headache. She denied any fevers, chills, unintended weight loss, epistaxis, or nasal obstruction. She denied pain with eye movement, blurred vision, or purulent drainage from her eyes or nose. She was a nonsmoker. Her past medical history was significant for seasonal allergies and chronic rhinosinusitis. She underwent uncomplicated functional endoscopic sinus surgery at the age of 19.

Physical examination showed a well-appearing woman in no distress. Her left eye was slightly proptotic. Extraocular movements were intact. There was no periorbital edema or erythema. There was no drainage from the eyes and the conjunctiva appeared normal. There was no cervical lymphadenopathy. Nasal endoscopy showed a large, smooth, cystic mass in the left ethmoid sinus that was soft to palpation and a smaller, similar lesion in the right ethmoid.

60.2 Differential Diagnosis—Key Points

- A thorough history regarding the patient's headache was important to create a differential diagnosis. The differential diagnosis of headaches includes, but is not limited to, tension headache, cluster headache, migraine, meningitis, intracranial mass, sinusitis, fungus ball, and temporomandibular joint (TMJ) syndrome. This patient described her headaches as retro-orbital and between the eyes. The patient denied aura symptoms such as visual changes (transient blind spots, shimmering lights) or temporary paresthesias of the face, tongue, or hand. She also had no family history of migraine, making the diagnosis of migraine less likely. Because there was no history of trauma and the headaches had been present for an extended period, the possibility of a space-occupying lesion was more concerning.
- The symptom of left eye proptosis was consistent with a mass lesion of the sinuses. In the

appropriate clinical setting, this could also be suggestive of a postseptal infectious process including subperiosteal abscess or orbital cellulitis/abscess. The lack of infectious signs (fever, erythema, pain with eye movement) and the fluctuating course of her proptosis made this diagnosis unlikely. In a traumatic or postoperative setting, orbital hematoma should be considered.
- Imaging studies were crucial to this diagnosis. The computed tomography (CT) maxillofacial scan showed a homogeneous, smooth-walled lesion involving the left ethmoid sinus with erosion of the lamina papyracea and lateral displacement of the medial rectus muscle (▶ Fig. 60.1). The lesion extends superiorly into the ipsilateral frontal sinus, and a smaller, similar lesion is noted in the right ethmoid sinus with erosion of the lamina papyracea.

60.3 Test Interpretation

Nasal endoscopy typically shows smooth cystic swelling in the bilateral ethmoid sinuses with no ulcerations. A maxillofacial CT scan is ordered to look for bone erosion. If a space-occupying lesion is identified on CT, magnetic resonance imaging (MRI) can be performed to provide additional detail. The CT characteristics of mucocele include a homogeneous, nonenhancing, expansile sinus mass that fills the potential sinus cavity, expanding or remodeling surrounding bone. MRI is superior for demonstrating the connection of the mucocele with surrounding cranial or orbital structures. MRI findings will vary depending on the contents of the mucocele. However, the typical mucocele has low signal intensity on T1-weighted images and high signal intensity on T2-weighted images.

60.4 Diagnosis

Frontoethmoid sinus mucocele

60.5 Medical Management

Frontoethmoid sinus mucoceles are managed surgically. A course of preoperative steroids may reduce the size of the lesion or decrease the

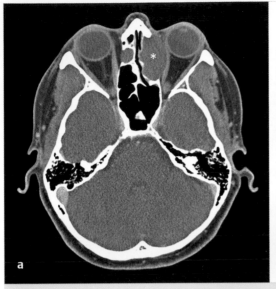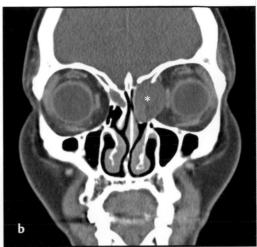

Fig. 60.1 (a) Axial, noncontrasted computed tomography image showing a homogeneous lesion (asterisk) involving the left ethmoid sinus with associated erosion of the lamina papyracea. The lesion encroaches on the left medial rectus, and the eye is slightly proptotic. It also extends superiorly to involve the frontal sinus (not shown). A smaller lesion is also noted in the right ethmoid sinus. (b) Coronal, noncontrasted computed tomography image from the same patient, again demonstrating the lesion involving the left ethmoid sinus and extending into the left frontal sinus.(asterisk). The globe is slightly displaced laterally.

associated swelling, providing temporary symptom relief. Evaluation by medicine or anesthesia may be warranted if the patient has significant comorbidities.

60.6 Surgical Management

The gold standard for surgical treatment is transnasal endoscopic frontoethmoidectomy with mucocele marsupialization. The procedure allows excellent visualization of the frontal and ethmoid sinuses and provides better restoration of normal sinus function.

60.7 Rehabilitation and Follow-up

Patients are treated with nasal saline rinses in the immediate postoperative period. Symptoms related to mass effect from the mucocele are expected to resolve after marsupialization of the mucocele. Some physicians may choose to get repeat imaging after surgery, and others follow the patient clinically. Currently no published studies address the need for postoperative imaging.

60.8 Questions

1. All the signs and symptoms listed below are associated with frontoethmoid mucocele except
   a) Diplopia.
   b) Pain.
   c) Epistaxis.
   d) Proptosis.
   e) Visual loss.
2. What is the appropriate management of symptomatic frontoethmoid sinus mucoceles?
   a) Observation.
   b) Steroid burst and saline irrigation.
   c) External frontoethmoidectomy (Lynch's procedure) with resection of the mucocele.
   d) Transnasal endoscopic marsupialization of the mucocele.
3. The presence of proptosis is consistent with all of the following except
   a) Mass lesion involving the sinuses.
   b) Orbital abscess.
   c) Orbital hematoma.
   d) Cerebrospinal fluid leak.

Answers: 1. c 2. d 3. d

Suggested Readings

Dhepnorrarat RC, Subramaniam S, Sethi DS. Endoscopic surgery for fronto-ethmoidal mucoceles: a 15-year experience. Otolaryngol Head Neck Surg. 2012; 147(2):345–350

Kang IG, Kim ST, Jung JH, et al. Effect of endoscopic marsupialization of paranasal sinus mucoceles involving the orbit: a review of 27 cases. Eur Arch Otorhinolaryngol. 2014; 271(2):293–297

Khong JJ, Malhotra R, Wormald PJ, Selva D. Endoscopic sinus surgery for paranasal sinus mucocoele with orbital involvement. Eye (Lond). 2004; 18(9):877–881

Picavet V, Jorissen M. Risk factors for recurrence of paranasal sinus mucoceles after ESS. B-ENT. 2005; 1(1):31–37

61 Inverting Papilloma

Patrick R. Owens and Allen M. Seiden

61.1 History

A 49-year-old man presented with a chief complaint of difficulty breathing through his right nasal cavity for longer than a year, with frequent nasal drainage and occasional epistaxis. He was referred after being thoroughly treated for chronic sinusitis with antibiotics and nasal steroid sprays without resolution of his symptoms. He denied any previous history of nasal surgery. The patient was a social drinker with no smoking history.

On physical examination he appeared to have decreased movement of air through his right nasal cavity. Anterior rhinoscopy was clear, but on nasal endoscopy a fairly large polypoid mass could be seen projecting from beneath the right middle turbinate (▶ Fig. 61.1). The mass was not erythematous, friable, firm, or vascular appearing. Endoscopic examination of the left nasal cavity was clear, demonstrating no evidence of polyps or ostiomeatal disease. A subsequent computed tomography (CT) scan of the sinuses was obtained.

61.2 Differential Diagnosis—Key Points

- The most common nasal mass is a benign inflammatory polyp. However, these tend to be bilateral and have a gray, translucent appearance. The finding of a unilateral nasal mass opens a broad differential that includes infectious processes as well as benign and malignant tumors. Antrochoanal polyps can present as unilateral polypoid masses filling the middle meatus. Benign tumors include osteomas, chondromas, ossifying fibromas, schwannomas, neurofibromas, meningiomas, vascular tumors, hamartomas including ameloblastomas, and most commonly, papillomas. Malignant tumors of the nasal cavity are most commonly squamous cell cancer but can include adenocarcinoma, esthesioneuroblastoma, lymphoma, and melanoma.
- Inverting papilloma is a lesion arising from the schneiderian membrane. This is the transition between the endoderm-derived respiratory epithelium and the ectodermally derived squamous epithelium. Other lesions can arise from this membrane, including fungiform papillomas, which are often found on the nasal septum and are human papillomavirus (HPV) related, and cylindric papillomas, which appear different but act similar to inverting papillomas. Debate exists as to whether these are different entities or expressions of the same process in different locations.
- Inverting papillomas histologically have an epithelium that inverts into the underlying connective tissue stroma. They often appear exophytic, polypoid, more vascular than an inflammatory polyp, and with a gray to pink appearance. In contrast to the lesion in this case, they may

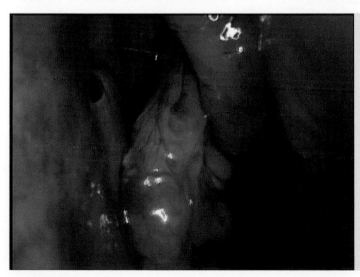

Fig. 61.1 Right nasal polypoid mass protruding from beneath the middle turbinate.

Table 61.1 Staging system for inverting papilloma

Stage	Description
T1	Tumor confined to the nasal cavity
T2	Tumor involving the ostiomeatal complex, ethmoid sinus, and/or medial wall of maxillary sinus
T3	Tumor involving lateral, inferior, superior, anterior, or posterior walls of maxillary sinus, sphenoid sinus, and/or frontal sinus
T4	Tumors with extranasal and extrasinus extension and all malignant tumors

Source: Adapted from Krouse JH. Development of a staging system for inverted papilloma. Laryngoscope 2000;110:965–968.

sometimes appear more fibrous and friable. No mucus cells or eosinophils are present. Koilocytes can be present. This is in contradistinction to inflammatory nasal polyps. The basement membrane remains intact. Although invasion into surrounding structures such as occurs with malignancy is not present, pressure and mass effect can cause bone remodeling and destruction.

- Inverting papilloma is the most common benign epithelial tumor of the nose and paranasal sinuses. Incidence is in the range of 0.2 to 0.6% per 100,000 people per year, making up 0.5 to 4% of primary nasal tumors. The male-to-female ratio is 3:1, and predominance in white patients is suggested in the literature. The most common sites of origin include the lateral nasal wall at the root of the middle turbinate and the maxillary sinus.
- There is no widely accepted cause, but there may be an association with HPV. Various types, including 6, 11, 16, and 18, have been found in these lesions, but no clear causative factor has been found. Further study is needed in this area and in establishing a possible link with smoking. Allergy does not appear to have any association with inverting papillomas.
- A universally accepted staging system does not exist, but the one by Krouse is often used (▶ Table 61.1).
- Malignancy, usually squamous cell cancer, may develop as a focus in an inverting papilloma, as a separate lesion, or as a metachronous lesion presenting after an inverting papilloma resection. Metachronous lesions may present years later. Malignancy risk has been quoted as anywhere between 1 and 53%, but 10% is a more likely rate. This risk, along with the tendency to recur and cause local destruction, is what creates the indication for aggressive surgical removal.

61.3 Test Interpretation

Confirmative diagnosis lies in biopsy. This is best done before plans are made for definitive surgical management. This patient underwent biopsy in the clinical setting, with minor bleeding controlled with silver nitrate. On hematoxylin and eosin staining, fronds of epithelium inverting into the surrounding stroma were demonstrated (▶ Fig. 61.2). In such cases, the epithelium can be squamous, transitional, or respiratory.

If a vascular tumor such as a hemangioma, hemangiopericytoma, juvenile nasopharyngeal angiofibroma, or pyogenic granulama is suspected, an office biopsy may be contraindicated because it may cause extensive bleeding. With this in mind, any biopsy of a nasal mass should be approached cautiously in a controlled environment with resources available to manage epistaxis.

Imaging studies are important to define the extent of the lesion. A friable, vascular-looking lesion whose upper extent cannot be visualized raises the concern for a possible encephalocele or other intracranial pathology. In such situations, it is helpful to obtain imaging studies prior to biopsy.

CT is the imaging modality of choice, depicting both soft tissue and bony changes. A CT scan will often support a diagnosis of inverting papilloma versus benign respiratory polyps by demonstrating an expansile appearance with surrounding bone destruction. However, it is important to note that benign polypoid disease associated with allergic fungal sinusitis, antrochoanal polyp, and other conditions can cause bony destruction of the uncinate process and medial wall of the maxillary sinus.

Magnetic resonance imaging is valuable in selected cases to distinguish tumor from retained secretions and to differentiate from other soft tissue structures in the event of extension beyond the sinus.

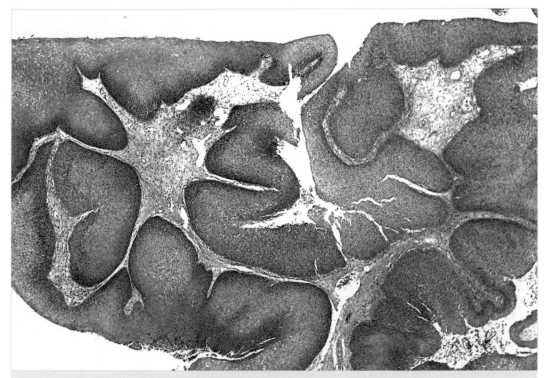

Fig. 61.2 Histologic examination reveals hyperplastic epithelium invaginating into the fibrovascular connective tissue stroma.

61.4 Diagnosis

Inverting papilloma

61.5 Medical Management

Both radiation and chemotherapy have been used in the treatment of inverting papillomas. There are no clear guidelines for when these are indicated, but these modalities are usually considered when there is either an associated malignancy or an incomplete resection. Steroids and antibiotics have also been used to alleviate any inflammatory or infectious component before surgery, which can allow the extent of the papilloma to be more clearly visualized.

61.6 Surgical Management

Surgery is the modality of choice for treating inverting papilloma. Before the pathology of these lesions was fully understood, an intranasal polypectomy was associated with recurrence rates greater than 70%, leading to the development of more aggressive, en bloc resections. In the 1980s, a lateral rhinotomy with medial maxillectomy became the standard of care to remove completely the lateral nasal wall, with recurrence rates less than 15%. Complications include epiphora, a misplaced medial canthus, and a large facial scar. An alternative approach that spares an external incision is the midface degloving technique.

With the advent of endoscopic surgical techniques, many inverting papillomas are now being addressed in this manner. Recurrence rates have been comparable to traditional approaches. Initially only patients with small tumors were selected, but this has now been expanded to include most cases. Limited tumors can be addressed by limited resections, but if necessary a medial maxillectomy can also be performed endoscopically. A Caldwell-Luc approach, in which a sublabial incision with maxillary puncture is performed, may aid in access to the lateral, anterior, and inferior aspects of the maxillary sinus. En bloc resection via an endoscopic approach is possible and may be beneficial in cases associated with malignancy. However, a diagnosis of cancer often necessitates an external approach, as well as adjunctive therapy. The most important aspect of inverting papilloma surgery is that the site of tumor attachment must be adequately addressed, often with removal or drilling of the underlying bone. Even though the inverting papilloma may be large at presentation, the site of attachment is often quite localized, but it may be beyond the confines of the lateral nasal wall. If the attachment site is not addressed, recurrence is likely. After surgery, endoscopic surveillance can usually be performed.

61.7 Rehabilitation and Follow-up

The risk of recurrence of inverting papilloma can approach 13%, even with aggressive surgery. The risk of malignancy also makes monitoring an important aspect of care. It has been shown that lesions can occur 1 to 24 years later, but most present within 24 months. Therefore, regular follow-up with a thorough endoscopic examination and imaging when appropriate is important.

61.8 Questions

1. Why does inverting papilloma need to be treated aggressively?
   a) It can cause severe bleeding.
   b) It is malignant.
   c) It may cause local destruction.
   d) It can metastasize.
   e) All of the above are correct.
2. Along with the middle turbinate and middle meatus, what is the most common site of origin of inverting papilloma?

a) Frontal sinus.
b) Ethmoid sinus.
c) Maxillary sinus.
d) Sphenoid sinus.
3. What is the rate of associated malignancy with inverting papilloma?
   a) 10%.
   b) 15%.
   c) 20%.
   d) 25%.

Answers: 1. e 2. c 3. a

Suggested Readings

Cannady SB, Batra PS, Sautter NB, Roh HJ, Citardi MJ. New staging system for sinonasal inverted papilloma in the endoscopic era. Laryngoscope. 2007; 117(7):1283–1287

Eggers G, Mühling J, Hassfeld S. Inverted papilloma of paranasal sinuses. J Craniomaxillofac Surg. 2007; 35(1):21–29

Karkos PD, Fyrmpas G, Carrie SC, Swift AC. Endoscopic versus open surgical interventions for inverted nasal papilloma: a systematic review. Clin Otolaryngol. 2006; 31(6):499–503

Krouse JH. Development of a staging system for inverted papilloma. Laryngoscope. 2000; 110(6):965–968

Landsberg R, Cavel O, Segev Y, Khafif A, Fliss DM. Attachment-oriented endoscopic surgical strategy for sinonasal inverted papilloma. Am J Rhinol. 2008; 22(6):629–634

Busquets JM, Hwang PH. Endoscopic resection of sinonasal inverted papilloma: a meta-analysis. Otolaryngol Head Neck Surg. 2006; 134(3):476–482

Myers EN. Operative Otolaryngology—Head and Neck Surgery, 2nd ed. Philadelphia, PA: WB Saunders; 2008

Philpott CM, Dharamsi A, Witheford M, Javer AR. Endoscopic management of inverted papillomas: long-term results–the St. Paul's Sinus Centre experience. Rhinology. 2010; 48(3):358–363

62 Esthesioneuroblastoma

Tasneem A. Shikary and Allen M. Seiden

62.1 History

A 46-year-old man presented with a 3-month history of right nasal congestion and recurrent self-limited epistaxis. He also reported headaches that were mild. He endorsed a history of allergic rhinitis, but denied purulent rhinorrhea or changes in smell. He did not ordinarily take any medication for his allergies, or any antiplatelet agents or anticoagulants.

Examination revealed anterior deviation of the nasal septum to the right with slight crusting, making the right posterior and superior nasal cavity somewhat difficult to visualize. However, no other lesions were noted on anterior rhinoscopy. His basic head and neck examination was otherwise unremarkable. Visual acuity and extraocular movements were intact. Pupils were equal, round, and reactive.

On nasopharyngoscopy the left side appeared unremarkable apart from inflammation of the inferior and middle turbinates suggestive of mild allergic disease. Examination of the right side demonstrated a polypoid, friable irregular mass in the superior nasal vault, medial to the middle turbinate. Maxillofacial computed tomography (CT) confirmed a soft tissue mass filling the right nasal vault, involving bilateral ethmoids, right sphenoid, and right maxillary sinus with no apparent erosion of the cribriform plate or lamina papyracea (▶ Fig. 62.1). A subsequent magnetic resonance imaging (MRI) scan of the head and neck with contrast also revealed a large homogeneously enhancing mass filling bilateral ethmoid sinus and right sphenoid sinus with postobstructive maxillary sinus disease with intracranial, no orbital extension (▶ Fig. 62.2). The patient was scheduled for nasal endoscopy and nasopharyngoscopy with biopsy in the operating room.

62.2 Differential Diagnosis—Key Points

- Although the patient's symptoms could have been attributed to a deviated nasal septum, unilateral nasal obstruction and persistent epistaxis warranted further examination with nasal endoscopy, and a unilateral mass should raise suspicion for neoplasm, benign or malignant.

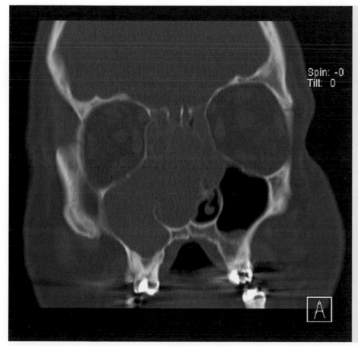

Fig. 62.1 Computed tomography scan of an advanced esthesioneuroblastoma, with erosion of the skull base and bilateral lamina papyracea.

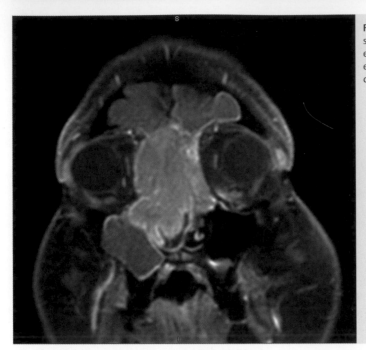

Fig. 62.2 Magnetic resonance imaging scan of a patient with an advanced esthesioneuroblastoma. Intracranial extension is demonstrated, with clear delineation between tumor and brain.

Nasal obstruction, localized pain, and epistaxis are the three most common presenting symptoms for sinonasal malignancy.

- Benign neoplasms include inverting papilloma, hemangioma, schwannoma, benign inflammatory polyp, and meningocele or meningoencephalocele. Squamous cell carcinoma, both within the setting of a preexisting inverting papilloma and as an isolated neoplasm, is the most common malignant sinonasal mass, followed by sinonasal undifferentiated carcinoma (SNUC) and adenoid cystic carincoma. Other malignancies include adenocarcinoma, mucoepidermoid carcinoma, hemangiopericytoma, and blue cell tumors such as esthesioneuroblastoma (ENB), rhabdomyosarcoma, plasmacytoma, malignant mucosal melanoma, lymphoma, and nasopharyngeal carcinoma.
- Nasal masses should generally be biopsied in the operating room under controlled conditions if there is concern for bleeding. Imaging should be performed prior to biopsy to rule out intracranial mass lesion and typically includes both CT and MRI with contrast.

62.3 Test Interpretation

- Imaging is necessary to assess the extent of sinonasal masses and can also facilitate tumor staging for malignant lesions. A direct coronal CT scan with cuts 3 mm or less is the preferred initial radiologic exam for sinonasal masses.
(▶ Fig. 62.1). Tumors will appear as a homogeneous soft tissue mass with uniform moderate contrast enhancement. Bony erosion can also occur, so it is important to evaluate the cribriform plate, fovea ethmoidalis, or lamina papyracea, as these are barriers to the orbit and intracranial structures.
- If there is obstruction of the sinus ostia, it can be difficult to differentiate tumor from accumulated secretions on a CT scan, and MRI can be useful in this situation. MRI is also necessary to delineate tumor spread into the cranium and orbit, perineural invasion, and dural involvement, and it thus is usually complementary to the CT
(▶ Fig. 62.2).
- Biopsy: Histologic analysis revealed discrete nests of cells with dense stromal blood vessels. The tumor cells were of the small blue cell type, showing small dark round or oval nuclei, absence of nucleoli, and little cytoplasm, and they exhibited pseudorosette configurations around a fibrillary eosinophilic material that stained positively with S100.

62.4 Diagnosis

Esthesioneuroblastoma

62.5 Medical Management

ENB or olfactory neuroblastoma is a rare malignant neoplasm of olfactory and neuroectodermal origin. Patients typically present at an advanced stage, as it arises high in the nasal vault, and nonspecific symptoms such as nasal obstruction, epistaxis, rhinorrhea, pain, or headache may delay further investigation until the symptoms become severe. Interestingly, anosmia is a rare symptom, although the tumor arises from olfactory epithelium. It is important to histologically distinguish ENB from other non-ENB neuroendocrine tumors such as SNUC and sinonasal neuroendocrine carcinoma because non-ENB tumors are typically more advanced and treated with systemic therapy.

The most widely used staging system is Kadish's classification, which has been modified to include lymph node status: A, confined to the nasal cavity; B, extension to the paranasal sinuses: C, extending beyond these limits; and D, regional lymph nodes or metastasis. Dulguerov's staging system or the University of California, Los Angeles (UCLA) staging system has also been developed more recently. It is based on the TNM classification (Classification of Malignant Tumours) and may have more implications for prognosis since it provides more detail regarding local disease spread, cervical involvement, and metastatic disease.

Treatment is generally surgical, followed by postoperative radiation for most cases. Although evidence is limited, reports have shown improved survival outcomes with adjuvant therapy, especially if there are close or positive margins or advanced disease. There is less evidence for chemotherapy use, but it is generally indicated for high-grade lesions, positive margins, unresectable disease, or distant metastases. Chemotherapeutic agents such as cisplatin, vincristine, and etoposide have shown efficacy when combined with radiation. Generally radiation regimens consist of 40 to 60 Gy over 4 to 6 weeks.

62.6 Surgical Management

Wide resection of the tumor is usually achieved through anterior craniofacial resection, which is the standard of care. However, with the advent of endoscopic sinus surgery, purely endoscopic or endoscopically assisted techniques have been described in the literature with comparable oncologic outcomes. Orbital exenteration should be undertaken when periorbital soft tissues are involved, followed by adjuvant chemoradiation. Cervical lymph node involvement is present in 5 to 8% of cases at diagnosis, and spread will occur in up to 30% of patients. Levels I to III and retropharyngeal lymph nodes are most commonly involved. Neck dissection for clinically positive neck disease is undertaken at the time of primary resection, but the role of elective neck dissection in N0 disease remains controversial. Some advocate elective neck dissection for advanced (Kadish B or C) disease, while others support observation with close surveillance, as the incidence of neck metastasis is generally low.

62.7 Rehabilitation and Follow-up

Postoperative complications include those associated with sinus and skull base surgeries, such as infection, cerebrospinal fluid leak, meningitis, pneumocephalus, and seizures. Nasal crusting may be a significant problem that requires daily maintenance. Long-term follow-up surveillance for recurrence requires regular office evaluation and radiologic study. Average reported survival rates based upon Kadish's stages A, B, and C are 72%, 59%, and 47%, respectively. Recurrence is most often local and may not occur until many years (10 +) after initial therapy.

62.8 Questions

1. Symptoms that might be consistent with a neoplastic process in the nose include
   a) Unilateral nasal obstruction.
   b) Epistaxis.
   c) Purulent nasal discharge.
   d) Unilateral facial pain.
   e) All of the above.
2. Physical findings that raise concern for a neoplastic process in the nose include
   a) Unilateral nasal mass.
   b) Generalized turbinate congestion.
   c) Purulent nasal discharge.
   d) Generalized nasal crusting.
   e) All of the above.
3. The lesion described in this case would be Kadish's classification stage
   a) A.
   b) B.
   c) C.

Answers: 1. e 2. a 3. c

Suggested Readings

Castelnuovo PG, Delù G, Sberze F, et al. Esthesioneuroblastoma: endonasal endoscopic treatment. Skull Base. 2006; 16(1):25–30

Devaiah AK, Larsen C, Tawfik O, O'Boynick P, Hoover LA. Esthesioneuroblastoma: endoscopic nasal and anterior craniotomy resection. Laryngoscope. 2003; 113(12):2086–2090

Turakhia S, Patel K. Esthesioneuroblastoma. Indian J Radiol Imaging. 2006; 16(4):669–672

Komotar RJ, Starke RM, Raper DMS, Anand VK, Schwartz TH. Endoscopic endonasal compared with anterior craniofacial and combined cranionasal resection of esthesioneuroblastomas. World Neurosurg. 2013; 80(1)(-)(2):148–159

Schwartz JS, Palmer JN, Adappa ND. Contemporary management of esthesioneuroblastoma. Curr Opin Otolaryngol Head Neck Surg. 2016; 24(1):63–69

63 Orbital Complications of Sinusitis

Amy M. Manning and Alfred M. Sassler

63.1 History

A 14-year-old boy presented to the emergency department with a 1-day history of progressive left eye and eyelid swelling and redness, as well as a 1-week history of headache and upper respiratory infection symptoms. He reported worsening pain with extraocular motion and diplopia, as well as photophobia.

Physical examination revealed a well-nourished adolescent boy with fever of 101.5 and otherwise normal vital signs. Ear exam was normal. Intranasal exam demonstrated edema but no obvious purulent secretions. Tonsils were surgically absent. Ophthalmologic evaluation revealed bilateral 20/20 vision but limitation of left eye motion, especially with adduction and upward gaze. There was chemosis of the left upper and lower eyelids, and the eye itself was firm to the touch. He was found to have elevated intraocular pressure of 29 mm H_2O and 8 mm of left eye proptosis. Pupillary exam was normal. Due to his presentation, a computed tomography (CT) scan of the sinuses and orbits with contrast was performed. This scan revealed left-sided maxillary, ethmoid, and frontal sinus opacification, proptosis, and edema of the left medial and superior rectus and superior oblique muscles. There was a left medial orbital fluid collection with a single bubble of gas present (▶ Fig. 63.1).

63.2 Differential Diagnosis— Key Points

- Swelling of the upper and lower eyelids should prompt the clinician to consider intrinsic abnormalities of the eye and orbit, as well as orbital complications of periorbital processes. Swelling of the eye can occur due to trauma, insect bite, the presence of a foreign body, bacteremia, or spread from a regional infection, including sinusitis, conjunctivitis, dacryocystitis, or dental disease.

- It is important to distinguish between preseptal and postseptal involvement. This is differentiated by the presence of inflammation posterior to the orbital septum, a fibrous sheet of tissue extending from the periosteum of the orbital rim that blends superiorly with the levator palpebrae superioris and inserts inferiorly into the tarsal plate. Preseptal cellulitis will often present with eyelids that are swollen shut, but extraocular movements and visual acuity will be intact. Limitation of globe movement, proptosis, chemosis and decreased visual acuity are signs concerning for inflammatory involvement of postseptal structures. Findings of postseptal involvement are concerning due to the possibility of spread of infection intracranially via valveless veins, as well as long-term vision loss due to elevated intraocular pressure. This patient had findings concerning

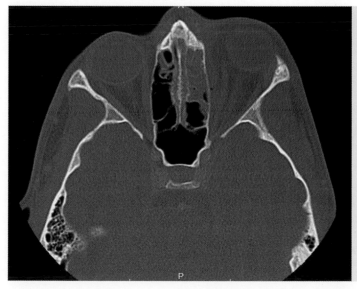

Fig. 63.1 Axial computed tomography scan of a patient with a subperiosteal abscess.

Table 63.1 Modified Chandler's staging system for orbital inflammation

Stage	Description
I	Preseptal cellulitis
II	Orbital cellulitis
III	Subperiosteal abscess
IV	Orbital abscess
V	Cavernous sinus thrombosis

for postseptal involvement, and CT imaging was concerning for subperiosteal abscess.

- The modified Chandler's staging system for orbital inflammation (▶ Table 63.1) groups orbital complications of sinusitis into five groups: preseptal cellulitis, orbital cellulitis, subperiosteal abscess, orbital abscess, and cavernous sinus thrombosis. The latter four groups are postseptal. Cavernous sinus thrombosis can present with bilateral ocular findings.
- The most common cause of periorbital and orbital cellulitis in children is sinus disease, most commonly ethmoid disease; however, there is a peak in incidence of complications of sinusitis in adolescents due to the enlarging presence of frontal and sphenoid sinuses, as these become pneumatized throughout late childhood and adolescence. Some cases may respond to treatment with intravenous antibiotics and may not require surgical intervention. Orbital complications of sinusitis are more common in children.
- Causative organisms of complicated sinusitis are similar in adults and children and include mainly *Staphylococcus* and *Streptococcus* species. These infections are often polymicrobial and can include anaerobes as well.

63.3 Test Interpretation

- A CT of the sinus with contrast is the study of choice to evaluate the paranasal sinuses and to determine the presence or absence of orbital cellulitis, subperiosteal phlegmon or abscess, or intracranial involvement. In some cases it can be difficult to differentiate subperiosteal inflammation and edema (phlegmon) from discrete abscess on the basis of imaging. Attention should be paid to the cavernous sinus for asymmetric enhancement or the absence of signal, which may indicate the spread of infection to this area and presence of thrombosis.

- Magnetic resonance imaging (MRI) should be performed when intracranial complications, including cavernous sinus thrombosis, are suspected due to the presence of ominous physical findings or bilateral ocular findings.
- Complete blood count (CBC) with differential should be obtained to establish a baseline and help to monitor the response to medical therapy. Additionally, a CBC may raise concern for an underlying immunodeficiency.
- Blood cultures should be obtained to rule out the presence of bacteremia.

63.4 Diagnosis

Subperiosteal abscess

63.5 Medical Management

Most orbital infections respond to medical management with intravenous (IV) antibiotics. If CT imaging does not indicate the presence of a drainable fluid collection and if there is no ophthalmoplegia or decrease in visual acuity on examination, admission and treatment with broad-spectrum IV antibiotics is reasonable. Additionally, patients who have a small (less than 4 mm), uncomplicated subperiosteal abscess may respond to medical treatment only. Choice of antibiotics should be directed at the most common offending organisms (i.e., ampicillin plus sulbactam or vancomycin in combination with a second- or third-generation cephalosporin if index of suspicion is high for methicillin-resistant *Staphylococcus aureus*). In addition, nasal hygiene with nasal saline irrigations and both topical and systemic decongestants can help promote sinus drainage. Topical and/or systemic steroid treatment can help to decrease periorbital and nasal edema, though systemic steroid treatment renders the use of CBC as a clinical marker of infection meaningless. Systemic anticoagulation should be considered in cases of cavernous sinus thrombosis. Ophthalmology consultation should be obtained in any child with ocular findings. Improvement of symptoms should occur within 48 hours; failure to improve should prompt reimaging and possible surgical intervention.

63.6 Surgical Management

Imaging that indicates a clearly drainable fluid collection, the presence of ocular findings (including decreased visual acuity, proptosis, and ophthalmoplegia), and failure to respond to medical therapy are indications for surgical treatment. Functional endoscopic sinus surgery is now the mainstay of surgical treatment for sinus drainage in patients with infectious complications. Open approaches may be used in addition to endoscopic approaches; these include Lynch's incision or oculoplastic techniques such as the transconjunctival or transcaruncular approach. The presence of acute inflammation and bleeding in an acutely infected sinus make endoscopic drainage more challenging. A more superior or superolateral location of the abscess may make it less amenable to endoscopic drainage alone.

63.7 Rehabilitation and Follow-up

The postoperative course should include continued IV antibiotics, as well as follow-up of culture specimens obtained at the time of drainage to tailor appropriate medical therapy. Follow-up should be multidisciplinary, including frequent ophthalmologic examinations. Clinical improvement is expected within 48 hours, and again, failure to improve sufficiently should prompt reimaging and reoperation if indicated.

63.8 Questions

1. Which of the following is indicative of postseptal involvement of infection?
   a) Erythema of eyelid.
   b) Edema of eyelid.
   c) Chemosis.
   d) Tenderness to palpation.
2. A child is admitted from the emergency department with eyelid edema after a computed tomography (CT) scan indicated preseptal cellulitis. He is placed on intravenous (IV) ampicillin/sulbactam. Forty-eight hours after the initiation of treatment, the patient continues to be febrile. Additionally, he has begun to have proptosis on the involved side. What is the appropriate next course of action?
   a) Change antibiotic therapy to vancomycin and a second- or third-generation cephalosporin because the causative organism is likely methicillin-resistant *Staphylococcus aureus* (MRSA).
   b) Repeat CT of the sinuses.
   c) Proceed directly to the operating room for endoscopic sinus surgery.
   d) Add systemic steroids with the goal of reducing intranasal edema and enhancing clearance of the sinuses.
3. Periorbital cellulitis may occur secondary to
   a) Ethmoid sinusitis.
   b) Dacryocystitis.
   c) Trauma.
   d) Insect bite.
   e) All of the above.

Answers: 1. c 2. b 3. e

Suggested Readings

Giannoni CM. Complications of Rhinosinusitis. In: Johnson JT, Rosen CA, Bailey BJ, et al, eds. Bailey's Head and Neck Surgery—Otolaryngology 5th ed. Philadelphia, PA: Lippencott Williams & Wilkins; 2014. pp: 573-585.
Oxford LE, McClay J. Medical and surgical management of subperiosteal orbital abscess secondary to acute sinusitis in children. Int J Pediatr Otorhinolaryngol. 2006; 70(11):1853–1861
Pelton RW, Smith ME, Patel BC, Kelly SM. Cosmetic considerations in surgery for orbital subperiosteal abscess in children: experience with a combined transcaruncular and transnasal endoscopic approach. Arch Otolaryngol Head Neck Surg. 2003; 129(6):652–655

64 Cerebrospinal Fluid Rhinorrhea

Douglas C. von Allmen and Lee A. Zimmer

64.1 History

A 51-year-old woman presented with a history of prior meningitis and intermittent clear rhinorrhea. She stated the rhinorrhea got worse when bending over, and she endorsed an occasional metallic taste in her mouth. She denied headache, fevers, photophobia, or limited neck range of motion at that time. There was no history of trauma. The patient's body mass index (BMI) was 37 and she had a past medical history relevant for type 2 diabetes. On physical examination the patient was well appearing, with normal eye, ear, and oral cavity exam. Anterior rhinoscopy demonstrated minimal clear rhinorrhea on the floor of bilateral nasal cavities. Neck exam revealed full range of motion without tenderness to palpation. When asked to flex at the waist with her head down, clear rhinorrhea was noted to drip from the nose. A sample of this fluid was collected and sent for beta-2 transferrin, and a maxillofacial computed tomography (CT) scan without contrast was ordered.

64.2 Differential Diagnosis— Key Points

- Cerebrospinal fluid (CSF) is produced primarily by the choroid plexus in the ventricular system of the brain. The total volume of CSF in an adult is about 150 mL. Normal intracranial pressure (ICP) ranges from 5 to 15 cm H_2O; however, ICP variations occur with changes in position, straining, respiration, and Valsalva maneuvers. Sneezing, for example, can transiently increase ICP to 40 cm H_2O.
- Etiologies for CSF leak include trauma, skull base tumors, and other iatrogenic and idiopathic (spontaneous) causes. The most common cause of CSF rhinorrhea is a spontaneous leak.

Blunt head injury is thought to result in CSF leak in 2 to 4% of cases. Most of these cases will occur within the first 48 hours of injury, however, CSF leaks can occur in a delayed fashion, with presentation years after an injury. Two-thirds of traumatic leaks will close without surgical intervention.

Iatrogenic causes of CSF rhinorrhea include endoscopic sinus surgery (ESS) and neurosurgical procedures. Incidence of CSF leak due to iatrogenic injury during ESS has improved with the use of image guidance systems, with reported rates of 0 to 3%. The most common locations for injury are the lateral lamella of the cribriform plate and the posterior ethmoid roof.

Idiopathic or spontaneous CSF leaks seem to be increasing in incidence. These cases of CSF rhinorrhea occur in the absence of tumor, trauma, or iatrogenic injury. The majority of these patients are middle-aged women with an elevated BMI. The patient may also carry a diagnosis of benign intracranial hypertension (BIH). The pathogenesis of BIH leading to CSF leak is thought to be a result of increased hydrostatic forces causing bony erosion of the thin bony skull base. A recent multicenter study found that the rate of spontaneous CSF leak is twice as high in areas of the United States with a higher average BMI. Surgical repair of a spontaneous CSF leak in an obese patient has a higher rate of failure, likely related to the underlying elevated ICP.

Tumors and encephaloceles can rarely present with CSF rhinorrhea, which results from erosion of the skull base. Basal encephaloceles may present as an intranasal mass causing unilateral obstruction of the nasal passage. Malignant sinonasal neoplasms or pituitary tumors may cause bone erosion due to direct invasion or by tumor growth causing mass effect on the nearby thin bony walls. Surgical intervention is needed for resection of the tumor and CSF leak repair in these cases to avoid the risk of meningitis.

- The risk of meningitis after posttraumatic CSF leak ranges from 10 to 37%, and the risk following transnasal skull base surgery is reported to be 0.3 to 7%. Antibiotics are frequently prophylactically prescribed in the setting of CSF leak to prevent meningitis. However, there is no definitive recommendation regarding the role of prophylactic antibiotics due to conflicting data. While one meta-analysis did show a benefit with the use of antibiotics, three larger meta-analyses have shown no benefit.

64.3 Test Interpretation

- Beta-2 transferrin is a protein found almost exclusively in the CSF as a result of neuraminidase activity in the brain, and as a result, it is a highly sensitive and specific screening test that can be performed on fluid collected from the nose.

- High-resolution CT scan with triplanar views is useful for the evaluation of bone anatomy to identify skull base defects. CT scan obtained for the patient above revealed pneumocephalus with an associated bone defect in the left sphenoid roof with air–fluid levels in the left sphenoid cavity (▶ Fig. 64.1).
- Magnetic resonance imaging (MRI) is useful to define the soft tissue components of a skull base defect. MRI is particularly useful in differentiating between a meningocele and an encephalocele. MRI may also aid in the identification of empty sella syndrome resulting from chronic

elevated ICP. MRI obtained postoperatively in this patient demonstrated fluid signal contained within the left sphenoid (▶ Fig. 64.2).
- CT cisternography may be performed using intrathecal injection of contrast to aid in the identification and location of a CSF leak. This test has a high sensitivity for identifying active leaks (92%). However, the test is not as useful for inactive or intermittent leaks. To improve the accuracy in the setting of an intermittent leak, the test can be performed with pledgets in the nose. These pledgets are removed 6 to 24 hours later, and then radioactive tracer is measured in

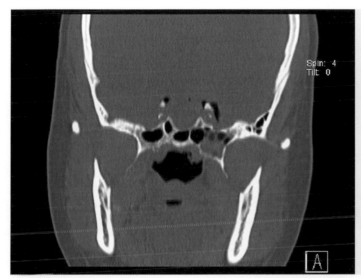

Fig. 64.1 Coronal noncontrast CT scan demonstrating pneumocephalus and air–fluid levels in the left sphenoid.

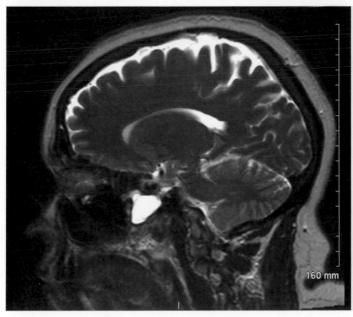

Fig. 64.2 Postoperative sagittal T2 MRI with fluid signal isolated to the left sphenoid.

comparison to serum levels. Ratio of 1.5–3:1 is diagnostic of a leak. While useful for identifying the presence of a CSF leak, this test does not accurately identify the location of the leak.

- Intrathecal fluorescein can be used intraoperatively to identify a leak under direct visualization. Fluorescein injection into the intrathecal space results in fluorescein leakage at the site of defect. Visualization via endoscope, with or without a blue light filter, will aid in determining the presence of an active leak either before or after surgical repair. Intrathecal use of fluorescein is not Food and Drug Administration (FDA) approved, and as a result, care must be taken when using this drug due to the known side effects of seizure, pulmonary edema, and neurologic deficits when given in high doses.

64.4 Diagnosis

Spontaneous CSF rhinorrhea

64.5 Medical Management

Conservative management is often sufficient to stop CSF leaks. Sixty percent to 70% of posttraumatic CSF leaks close because of using CSF precautions, which include bed rest, no nose blowing, no drinking through a straw, stool softeners, and sneezing with the mouth open. Antiemetics, antitussives, and stool softeners may be effective in reducing Valsalva maneuvers, but these medications have not been shown to reduce risk in controlled studies. A lumbar drain can also be inserted to decrease and/or measure the ICP in an attempt to allow the CSF leak to close. Lumbar drains are frequently used as adjuncts to surgical repair; however, there are data to suggest that surgical success rates are independent of lumbar drain use. Acetazolamide, which decreases the ICP by a mean of 10 cm H_2O, is the only medication that is used to indirectly treat CSF leak and is typically only used in patients with chronically elevated ICP, such as those with BIH.

64.6 Surgical Management

Surgical repair for CSF leak should be done in a timely manner to prevent intracranial complications such as meningitis, pneumocephalus, and cerebral or epidural abscess. Surgical management varies depending on the anatomic location of the

CSF leak. Cribriform plate, ethmoid roof, sella, clival, and sphenoid sinus leaks are amenable to endoscopic repair. Frontal sinus CSF leaks have traditionally been treated via extracranial approaches; however, leaks from the frontal recess can be repaired using an endoscopic frontal sinusotomy or Draf IIB approach. Intraoperative CSF leaks are encountered in 20 to 50% of transsphenoidal pituitary surgery and can be closed in a layered fashion using fat, hemostatic material, and cartilage. The mainstays of repair, regardless of the site, are good surgical technique and multilayered closure, unless the leak is in the olfactory cleft, where single-layer closure should be employed. Materials used to close CSF leaks include fat grafts, bone grafts, cartilage, fascia, fibrin glue, and absorbable packing. The nasoseptal pedicled flap based on the posterior septal artery is also an effective source of vascularized tissue to facilitate faster healing of the defect repair. Published success rates following endoscopic repair of CSF leaks range from 70 to 100% after first attempt. For patients who are refractory to repair, ventriculoperitoneal shunt may be necessary to divert the flow of CSF. The patient above underwent repair with a fat graft, septal cartilage, and nasoseptal flap, with resolution of her CSF rhinorrhea.

64.7 Rehabilitation and Follow-up

Postoperatively, patients are typically kept on strict bed rest for 3 to 5 days with the head of the bed at 15 degrees. CSF precautions are employed. If a lumbar drain is placed at the time of surgery, it is typically clamped 24 to 48 hours after surgery and removed after an observation period to ensure no further signs of CSF leak. Pain control and nasal hygiene are also important after surgery. Following discharge, the patient should avoid vigorous activity for 6 to 8 weeks, and they should have frequent follow-up for endoscopic evaluation and débridement as necessary. Additionally, continuous positive airway pressure should be avoided in the immediate postoperative setting.

64.8 Questions

1. What is the rate of spontaneous cerebrospinal fluid (CSF) leak closure in trauma-induced CSF leak?
   a) 10 to 20%.
   b) 60 to 70%.

c) 80 to 90%.

d) 30 to 40%.

2. What is the role of antibiotics in the prevention of meningitis in the setting of CSF leak?

a) Antibiotics should be given only in the acute setting of CSF leak.

b) Prolonged antibiotics are necessary during active CSF leak.

c) The role of antibiotics is not clear at this time.

d) Antibiotics should not be given in the perioperative period.

3. Which of the following should not be used in the postoperative setting to reduce the risk of increased intracranial pressure (ICP) and repair failure?

a) Bed rest.

b) Head elevation to 15 degrees.

c) Lumbar drain.

d) Drinking through a straw.

Answers: 1. b 2. c 3. d

Suggested Readings

Jiang ZI, Mclean C, Perez C, Barnett S, Friedman D, Batra P. Long-term surgical outcomes of spontaneous CSF rhinorrhea. Journal of Neurological Surgery. 2014; 75:91

Johnson J, Rosen CA. Bailey's Head and Neck Surgery: Otolaryngology. Lippincott Williams & Wilkins; 2013: 662–674

Nelson RF, Gantz BJ, Hansen MR. The rising incidence of spontaneous cerebrospinal fluid leaks in the United States and the association with obesity and obstructive sleep apnea. Otol Neurotol. 2015; 36(3):476–480

Oakley GM, Orlandi RR, Woodworth BA, Batra PS, Alt JA. Management of cerebrospinal fluid rhinorrhea: an evidence-based review with recommendations. Int Forum Allergy Rhinol. 2016; 6(1):17–24

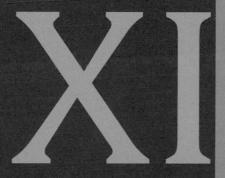

XI

65 Stomatitis

Hayley L. Born and Allen M. Seiden

65.1 History

A 7-year-old girl was brought in by her mother at the suggestion of their primary care provider. The patient had repeated episodes of sore throat, high fevers, cervical lymphadenitis, and painful mouth ulcers. The patient had these symptoms about every 3 to 5 weeks for the past 9 months, and it had required many days away from school and activities. Her mother seemed most concerned with the sudden and frequent high fevers. The patient said that the part that bothered her the most was the "canker sores" in her mouth. She was occasionally unable to eat or drink because of the pain of these ulcerations.

The patient was otherwise healthy and returned to this baseline between episodes. She did not take any medications and she did not chew gum or suck on hard candy. She had never had a "cold sore" or the chicken pox. She was up-to-date on all her vaccines.

On examination the patient looked sick but was in no acute distress. She had bilateral cervical lymphadenitis, which was mildly tender. Examination of her oropharynx revealed widespread posterior pharyngeal erythema. Two half- to 1-cm ulcerations were seen on the lower labial mucosa, consistent with aphthous ulcerations (▶ Fig. 65.1). Her temperature when she arrived was 103.0°F.

65.2 Differential Diagnosis— Key Points

- *Stomatitis* is a general term that refers to inflammation of the mouth and lips. It can involve any part of the oral mucosa and may or may not include discrete ulcerations. Its many causes include infection (viral, fungal, or bacterial), allergic reactions (erythema multiforme), radiation therapy, chemotherapy, and nutritional deficiencies (commonly the B vitamins B_2, B_3, B_6, B_9, and B_{12}). Stomatitis can also be autoimmune as is postulated in aphthous stomatitis and periodic fever adenitis pharyngitis aphthous ulcer (PFAPA) syndrome.

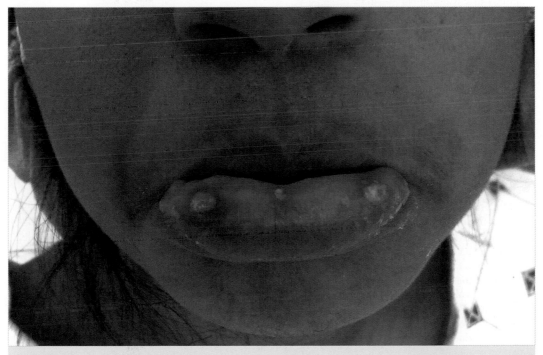

Fig. 65.1 Aphthous stomatitis on lower lip.

- The most common type of stomatitis is aphthous stomatitis or recurrent aphthous ulceration, colloquially referred to as canker sores. The ulcers commonly occur one or two ulcerations at a time in healthy adults and recur periodically (3 to 6 times per year). They are benign and noncontagious and usually last 7 to 10 days. Phenotypically the ulcers consist of a gray-yellow ulceration surrounded by erythema. The initial vesicular stage is rarely observed clinically, as patients present later in the course with painful sores. The underlying cause of aphthous stomatitis is not known, but evidence suggests it is a T cell–mediated autoimmune type of disease. Sores tend to be more common in women and may be related to the menstrual cycle. Treatment is symptomatic.
- Another commonly seen etiology for stomatitis is postirradiation or postchemotherapy stomatitis, or mucositis, as it is sometimes called. Five to 15% of patients undergoing cancer treatment develop mucositis of either the oral cavity or the gastrointestinal (GI) tract. Certain chemotherapeutic agents such as 5-fluorouracil are associated with high rates (40%) of mucositis. Patients who receive a bone marrow transplant have a 75 to 85% chance of developing mucositis. Additionally, radiotherapy is associated with a high degree of mucositis at the site of radiation, often in greater than 50% of patients. Stomatitis in these patients can be compounded by xerostomia, causing irritation to the mucosa and secondary mucosal infection. Unlike the loss of taste that can occur following radiation, xerostomia typically does not improve after radiation and can result in long-term, recurrent stomatitis. In this case, the patient did not have a history of radiation treatment, chemotherapy, or malignancy.
- Viral stomatitis is commonly associated with the herpes simplex virus (HSV), type 1 more commonly than type 2. As with genital HSV infection, oral HSV is often recurrent and associated with a prodrome. It can occur on both keratinized and nonkeratinized mucosa and results in vesicles, which proceed to ulceration. Similarly, herpes zoster can cause vesicular stomatitis, which occurs in a dermatomal pattern.
- Any agent that contacts the mucosa can cause contact and allergic dermatitis. This is seen with inhaled medications, orthodontic devices and glues, and even with food ingestion. Patch testing can be done to determine allergic status, and avoidance testing can be used to rule out contact stomatitis.

- Thought to be a type of allergic or autoimmune reaction, erythema multiforme can also cause stomatitis. While typically confined to a target lesion rash, erythema multiforme major can present with painful mucous membrane erosions. It usually follows a drug exposure or infection, often triggered by a flare of HSV. The condition may be mediated by immune complex deposition that causes epidermal detachment.
- Given this patient's history of concurrent fevers, lymphadenitis, and pharyngitis during stomatitis episodes, the most likely etiology is PFAPA. It is an idiopathic disease most commonly seen in children that may have an autoimmune-like pathogenesis.

65.3 Test Interpretation

History and physical examination are key for determining the etiology of stomatitis. Generally, no further testing is required. Occasionally, cultures of fungal plaques or biopsies of ulcerations can be done for definitive diagnosis.

In this case, diagnostic criteria require at least 6 months of recurrent episodes with negative throat cultures and no other identifiable causes for pharyngitis and adenitis such as mononucleosis.

65.4 Diagnosis

Periodic fever adenitis pharyngitis aphthous ulcer (PFAPA) syndrome

65.5 Medical Management

Medical treatment for PFAPA, like other types of stomatitis, is generally symptomatic. It can include topical numbing agents, analgesia, and occasionally steroids. PFAPA in particular has also been treated using colchicine and other immune-modulating medication.

Correction of other underlying causes for stomatitis may include using secretagogues, topical antibiotics or antifungals, oral antifungals, supplementation of deficient vitamins, or avoidance of offending agents.

65.6 Surgical Management

Generally speaking, there is no role for surgical intervention in stomatitis care. Certain conditions associated with stomatitis may be treated surgically; for example, PFAPA is commonly treated with adenotonsillectomy, though the level of evidence for this treatment modality is only moderate, according to a 2014 Cochrane Review.

65.7 Rehabilitation and Follow-up

Patients with PFAPA usually have resolution of their episodes by adulthood. Surgical intervention may hasten this resolution. It is unknown why tonsillectomy helps in PFAPA syndrome cases, though the prevailing thought is that the lymphoid tissue in the tonsils perpetuates the inflammation brought on during the periodic fever cycles. Follow-up for stomatitis patients is as needed for future symptomatic episodes or postsurgical complications.

65.8 Questions

1. Aphthous stomatitis
   a) Is considered an autoimmune condition.
   b) Is more frequent in women than in men.
   c) May be related to the menstrual cycle.
   d) Is rarely seen clinically with vesicle formation.
   e) All of the above.
2. Radiation therapy causes all of the following conditions. All are reversible except
   a) Dry mouth (xerostomia).
   b) Taste loss (dysgeusia).
   c) Mucositis (stomatitis).
   d) Sore throat (pharyngitis).

3. Deficiencies of the following can cause stomatitis except
   a) Iron.
   b) Vitamin B2 (riboflavin).
   c) Vitamin B3 (niacin).
   d) Vitamin B5 (pantothenic acid).
   e) Vitamin B6 (pyridoxine).
   f) Vitamin B9 (folic acid).
   g) Vitamin B12 (cobalamin).

Answers: 1. e 2. a 3. d

Suggested Readings

Long SS. Syndrome of Periodic Fever, Aphthous stomatitis, Pharyngitis, and Adenitis (PFAPA)–what it isn't. What is it? J Pediatr. 1999; 135(1):1–5

Preeti L, Magesh K, Rajkumar K, Karthik R. Recurrent aphthous stomatitis. J Oral Maxillofac Pathol. 2011; 15(3):252–256

Altenburg A, Zouboulis CC. Current concepts in the treatment of recurrent aphthous stomatitis. Skin Therapy Lett. 2008; 13(7):1–4

Burton MJ, Pollard AJ, Ramsden JD, Chong LY, Venekamp RP. Tonsillectomy for periodic fever, aphthous stomatitis, pharyngitis and cervical adenitis syndrome (PFAPA). Cochrane Database Syst Rev. 2014; 9(9):CD008669

Rubenstein EB, Peterson DE, Schubert M, et al. Mucositis Study Section of the Multinational Association for Supportive Care in Cancer, International Society for Oral Oncology. Clinical practice guidelines for the prevention and treatment of cancer therapy-induced oral and gastrointestinal mucositis. Cancer. 2004; 100(9) Suppl:2026–2046

Hairston BR, Bruce AJ, Rogers RS, III. Viral diseases of the oral mucosa. Dermatol Clin. 2003; 21(1):17–32

Vissink A, Jansma J, Spijkervet FK, Burlage FR, Coppes RP. Oral sequelae of head and neck radiotherapy. Crit Rev Oral Biol Med. 2003; 14(3):199–212

66 Tonsillitis

Andrew J. Redmann and Reena Dhanda Patil

66.1 History

A 51-year-old man presented to the emergency department with a 2-day history of low-grade fever, worsening sore throat, odynophagia, right otalgia, and muffled voice. He denied any difficulty breathing or handling his oral secretions. He had similar symptoms 3 years ago and was diagnosed with a peritonsillar abscess. This was drained in the emergency department. Additionally he reported approximately three episodes of pharyngitis per year for the last 3 years. These had all been treated with antibiotics, which improved his symptoms. His medical history was significant for gastroesophageal reflux disease (GERD) and obstructive sleep apnea, which resolved following an intentional 40-lb weight loss. He was a prior three-pack-per-day smoker but currently only smoked eight cigarettes per day.

Physical exam revealed an adult man in no acute distress. Temperature was 101.1 °F. All other vital signs were within normal limits. Ear and nasal exams were normal. Intraoral examination revealed erythematous oropharyngeal mucosa. Tonsils were 1 + bilaterally, with the right tonsil appearing slightly larger than the left tonsil. There was no uvular deviation or soft palate fullness (▶ Fig. 66.1). Neck examination revealed bilateral shotty lymphadenopathy but full range of motion. There was no trismus. Chest examination was within normal limits.

66.2 Differential Diagnosis— Key Points

• The differential diagnosis of pharyngitis in adults includes infectious etiologies (viral versus bacterial) and inflammatory conditions (laryngopharyngeal reflux, postnasal drip, caustic ingestion, postradiation). In a patient with a history of smoking, a neoplastic process such as squamous cell carcinoma must be considered as a cause of asymmetric tonsillar enlargement. Benign neoplasms are also possible, for example, parapharyngeal tumors such as pleomorphic adenoma. In this patient, the history of peritonsillar abscess, fever, and recurrent pharyngitis made bacterial causes more likely.

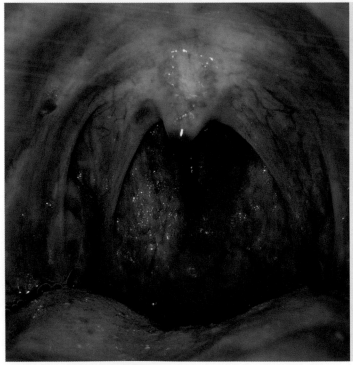

Fig. 66.1 Transoral view demonstrating erythematous pharynx and cryptic tonsils.

- Infectious tonsillitis can be divided into viral and bacterial causes. Bacterial causes of tonsillitis in adults include group A streptococcus (5 to 15% of cases, compared to 30% of cases in children), *Staphylococcus aureus*, anaerobic infection, and less commonly, *Neisseria gonorrhoeae* or syphilis. Viral disease is much more common, with classic pathogens including those traditionally associated with the common cold, such as *Rhinovirus* or *Coronavirus*. Other important viral causes of pharyngitis include Epstein-Barr virus (EBV) and cytomegalovirus (CMV), as these can cause infectious mononucleosis. Characteristic signs of mononucleosis include splenomegaly and hepatomegaly, along with impressive bilateral tonsillar enlargement and bilateral lymphadenopathy. Human immunodeficiency virus (HIV) can also present as pharyngitis, tonsillar hypertophy, and nontender lymphadenopathy, and must be considered in patients with significant risk factors.
- Peritonsillar abscess is the most common complication of tonsillitis and presents with a constellation of symptoms including trismus, odynophagia, inability to tolerate secretions, and a muffled voice. Examination reveals deviation of the soft palate, as the potential space between the capsule of the tonsil and the superior constrictor muscles is filled with purulence. Peritonsillar abscesses are more common in older children and adults than the younger pediatric population.
- Untreated streptococcal pharyngitis may lead to other sequelae, including rheumatic heart disease, poststreptococcal glomerulonephritis, and rheumatic fever. It is estimated that 3% of patients with untreated group A strep infections will develop rheumatic fever, and thus prompt diagnosis is important to allow appropriate antibiotic treatment. Other rare complications include extension of tonsillar infection to the parapharyngeal space or other deep neck spaces.

66.3 Test Interpretation

Initial laboratory testing in this patient included a complete blood count (CBC) and rapid strep antigen testing. In this case, the rapid strep antigen was positive and the CBC showed an elevated leukocyte count of 16,000/μL, with 70% polymorphonuclear leukocytes. Unlike in pediatrics, if the rapid strep test is negative, a throat culture is generally not obtained in an adult.

In teenagers and adults with bilateral tonsillar hypertrophy, malaise, and lymphadenopathy, a monospot test should be obtained. The monospot test evaluates for heterophile antibodies, which are caused by EBV infection and are present in approximately 90% of patients with mononucleosis. If the monospot test is negative but mononucleosis is still highly suspected, specific EBV antibody studies can be obtained.

Imaging studies are not indicated in uncomplicated pharyngitis. Diagnosis of a peritonsillar abscess is primarily clinical, though intraoral ultrasound can be used to evaluate for fluid in the peritonsillar space. Computed tomography (CT) should be avoided unless deep neck space infection is suspected.

66.4 Diagnosis

Chronic tonsillitis

66.5 Medical Management

In this patient with a positive group A strep test, treatment with antibiotics is appropriate, both for treatment of the acute infection and to prevent long-term sequelae such as rheumatic fever. Group A streptococcus is sensitive to penicillin, and either oral penicillin V or amoxicillin is an appropriate first-line treatment. If the group A test is negative, supportive treatment is an appropriate alternative to antibiotics and includes hydration, rest, antipyretics, and analgesics. In patients who have a positive monospot test, supportive treatment is recommended. Amoxicillin should be avoided because it may cause a maculopapular rash. If there is concern for bacterial superinfection in mononucleosis, a first- or second-generation cephalosporin can be used.

In patients with a peritonsillar abscess, primary treatment is surgical as discussed below, but patients should also be started on antibiotics (generally amoxicillin-clavulanate or clindamycin) to cover for anaerobic bacteria after surgical drainage. Steroids may also be administered after abscess drainage. There is some evidence that steroids improve symptoms.

66.6 Surgical Management

The classic Paradise's criteria indicate that surgical treatment is appropriate in patients who experience seven episodes of tonsillitis in 1 year, five episodes in 2 consecutive years, or three episodes in 3 consecutive years. The criteria define tonsillitis as a sore throat plus one of the following:

temperature > 38.3 °C, tonsillar exudate, cervical lymphadenopathy, or positive group A strep culture. In patients with severe symptoms and chronic issues with tonsillitis such as halitosis and tonsilliths, tonsillectomy may improve quality of life. Other factors may also make tonsillectomy appropriate in patients who do not meet the Paradise criteria, including antibiotic allergy, history of rheumatic heart disease, or a history of peritonsillar abscess. In general, after a second peritonsillar abscess, tonsillectomy is indicated. Tonsillectomy can be performed using a variety of techniques, but it commonly involves transoral removal with either electrocautery or a coblation device. Complications of tonsillectomy are well described, but most pertinently include a 2 to 5% risk of posttonsillectomy hemorrhage, about which patients must be counseled.

Surgical intervention is also appropriate in the setting of peritonsillar abscess. In general, incision and drainage (I&D) can be performed under local anesthesia in cooperative adult and adolescent patients. Some advocate needle aspiration of the abscess as the best initial treatment and reserve I&D for treatment failures. Alternatively, in patients who cannot tolerate bedside treatment, or in those who have repeated peritonsillar abscesses, a "quinsy" tonsillectomy can be performed under general anesthesia. However, the risks and benefits of this approach must be carefully considered because surgical planes can be difficult to identify in the acutely inflamed pharynx.

66.7 Rehabilitation and Follow-up

Otherwise healthy patients without indication for tonsillectomy can be discharged with the appropriate treatment (antibiotics and/or supportive measures). In patients with chronic tonsillitis who meet criteria for elective tonsillectomy, the acute infection can be treated with antibiotics and the patient scheduled for surgery at his or her convenience. In peritonsillar abscess, if patients are able to tolerate oral intake after I&D, they can be discharged home with oral antibiotics with or without steroids.

66.8 Questions

1. What is the most sensitive physical exam finding for peritonsillar abscess?
   a) Trismus.
   b) Asymmetric tonsil size.
   c) Dysphagia.
   d) Tonsillar exudate.
2. Which is the appropriate antibiotic choice for uncomplicated pharyngitis in a patient with a positive rapid strep test?
   a) Clindamycin.
   b) Cephalexin.
   c) Penicillin V.
   d) Metronidazole.
3. Which of the following is not a potential sequela of untreated group A strep pharyngitis?
   a) Glomerulonephritis.
   b) Heart disease.
   c) Deep space neck infection.
   d) Vision loss.

Answers: 1. a 2. c 3. d

Suggested Readings

Burton MJ, Glasziou PP, Chong LY, Venekamp RP. Tonsillectomy or adenotonsillectomy versus non-surgical treatment for chronic/recurrent acute tonsillitis. Cochrane Database Syst Rev. 2014(11): CD001802

Bird JH, Biggs TC, King EV. Controversies in the management of acute tonsillitis: an evidence-based review. Clin Otolaryngol. 2014; 39(6):368–374

Paradise JL, Bluestone CD, Bachman RZ, et al. Efficacy of tonsillectomy for recurrent throat infection in severely affected children. Results of parallel randomized and nonrandomized clinical trials. N Engl J Med. 1984; 310(11):674–683

van Driel ML, De Sutter AI, Keber N, Habraken H, Christiaens T. Different antibiotic treatments for group A streptococcal pharyngitis. (Review). Cochrane Database Syst Rev. 2013(4):CD004406

Lee YJ, Jeong YM, Lee HS, Hwang SH. The Efficacy of Corticosteroids in the Treatment of Peritonsillar Abscess: A Meta-Analysis. Clin Exp Otorhinolaryngol. 2016; 9(2):89–97

67 Posttonsillectomy Hemorrhage

Nathan D. Wiebracht and Charles M. Myer III

67.1 History

A 4-year-old girl presented to the emergency department after spitting up blood 7 days following an adenotonsillectomy for obstructive sleep apnea. She had a previously uneventful postoperative course. On the morning of presentation, she awakened and started coughing. Her mother reported that she spit out approximately 2 tablespoons of bright red blood mixed with clots. Since that time, she also had one episode of hematemesis, which was approximately "one cup of blood." At the time of evaluation, she had not had any additional bleeding for 2 hours. Her mother was unaware of any family history of bleeding diathesis. The mother also denied prior abnormal bleeding history for the patient. She had been taking acetaminophen and ibuprofen for pain as needed since surgery but had not required either in the 24 hours preceding the initial bleeding episode. Her last oral intake was 4 oz of apple juice 4 hours prior to presentation.

On physical examination, a large clot was noted in the left superior tonsillar fossa. There was no evidence of active bleeding. The patient was taken to the operating room (OR) where intravenous (IV) access was obtained and she was intubated. The clot was then removed and suction cautery was used to establish hemostasis of the left tonsillar fossa. The right fossa showed no evidence of bleeding. The patient was admitted for observation overnight and discharged home the next day. Laboratory studies were unremarkable for any coagulopathy, and her hematocrit was normal. Follow-up 3 weeks later revealed well-healing tonsillar fossae bilaterally.

67.2 Differential Diagnosis—Key Points

• This patient presented initially with posttonsillectomy bleeding 7 days after adenotonsillectomy. Bleeding in the first 24 hours postoperatively is considered a primary hemorrhage and is usually due to inadequate hemostasis during the initial surgery. Secondary posttonsillectomy hemorrhage occurs more than 24 hours after the procedure. Such bleeding usually occurs between postoperative days 5 and 10.

It is associated with premature separation of the granulation membrane that forms over the tonsillar fossae. The rate of primary hemorrhage generally ranges from 0.2 to 2.2% and that of secondary hemorrhage from 0.1 to 3%. Patients undergoing adenotonsillectomy for obstructive sleep apnea have a lower postoperative hemorrhage incidence than those with recurrent tonsillitis. The risk of hemorrhage increases with age and obesity. Administration of nonsteroidal anti-inflammatory drugs (NSAIDs) in the postoperative period has not been associated with a significant increase in hemorrhage.

• Repeated episodes of postoperative bleeding should raise the possibility of a coagulation disorder. A thorough preoperative medical history regarding the patient and immediate family members should always be obtained. History of easy bruising, epistaxis, oral bleeding, posttraumatic hemorrhage, excessive circumcision bleeding, postoperative or dental hemorrhage, hemarthrosis, perinatal bleeding, and recent use of any anticoagulation medication are all potentially significant. Systemic disorders that may result in excessive bleeding, such as liver disease, renal disease, or hematologic disease, should also be addressed. The preoperative physical examination may also raise suspicion for coagulopathies. The presence of petechiae suggests vascular or platelet disorders. Mucosal and gastrointestinal hemorrhage may be associated with vascular abnormalities such as bleeding into an elbow or knee joint, which is characteristic of hemophilia A (factor VIII deficiency) or factor IX deficiency. The presence of hepatosplenomegaly may indicate a liver disorder or hemolytic neoplasm.

• In cases of recurrent bleeding with normal coagulation studies, vascular abnormalities should be suspected and angiography may be indicated.

67.3 Test Interpretation

Platelet count, activated partial thromboplastin time (PTT), prothrombin time (PT), international normalized ratio (INR), and platelet function assays are useful in the detection of inherited and acquired coagulation disorders. These tests should be obtained preoperatively if the history or physical examination suggests a coagulation disorder. The patient's history and family history are the best screening tools. The conscientious clinician should use discretion because, in the absence of significant history or physical exam findings, routine preoperative testing is low yield and costly. However, if either raises the possibility of a specific coagulation disorder, focused tests should be performed. Discovery of a coagulopathy reduces perioperative complications and may prevent a disastrous surgical outcome.

Coagulation testing should be obtained following a bleeding episode, and if abnormal, hematology consultation is recommended. A complete blood count (CBC) will also help to assess the degree of hemorrhage and as a baseline in case further bleeding occurs.

The combination of multiple bleeding episodes with normal coagulation tests should raise the suspicion of a vascular abnormality, which warrants evaluation with angiography. While angiography is not without risk, in cases of repeated postoperative bleeding, it is essential to detect possible vascular abnormalities that might cause further episodes of hemorrhage.

67.4 Diagnosis

Secondary posttonsillectomy hemorrhage without associated coagulopathy

67.5 Medical Management

Any coagulation disorder detected preoperatively or postoperatively should be addressed and treated as necessary. Two of the most common coagulation abnormalities encountered are platelet dysfunction and von Willebrand's disease (vWD). More than 20 subtypes of vWD have been recognized to date. Some of these subtypes respond to desmopressin acetate (DDAVP) treatment. This should be evaluated by a challenge test 1 or 2 weeks before surgery. If DDAVP is to be used, treatment should be given approximately 1 hour before surgery at a dose of 0.3 mg/kg of body weight during a 30-minute infusion and once daily thereafter until wound healing is complete. Cryoprecipitate or factor VIII concentrate, both of which contain vW multimers, should be available in the event that the DDAVP fails to control hemorrhage. Other subtypes of vWD are treated with exogenous vWD factor replacement in the form of cryoprecipitate or factor VIII concentrate.

Pharmaceuticals are the most common cause of platelet dysfunction, and aspirin is the most commonly used drug known to affect platelet function. When a hemostatically normal patient who is taking aspirin requires a surgical procedure, aspirin should be discontinued for at least 2 weeks. If severe hemorrhage due to deficient platelet function is suspected, either a random donor platelet transfusion or DDAVP would be effective rapidly.

Patients with posttonsillectomy bleeding typically are admitted for observation and coagulopathy testing. If the blood loss is excessive and the patient is symptomatic, blood transfusion should be considered. As a general rule, hemoglobin less than 7 mg/dL is an indication for transfusion in the setting of acute blood loss. In the case of a delayed bleeding episode without signs of clot or active bleeding, the patient can be kept in an observation unit for ~4 hours while being hydrated before discharge.

67.6 Surgical Management

The most important factor in management of postoperative tonsillectomy bleeding is prevention. The actual method of removal of tonsils, either by dissection or electrocautery, is not as important as attention to the detail of staying in the proper plane between the tonsillar capsule and its surrounding fossa. Intracapsular microdebrider tonsillectomy has shown some promise in decreasing the postoperative hemorrhage rate. Other techniques, which include bipolar radiofrequency ablation (Coblation, Smith & Nephew, London, UK) and CO_2 laser, have not proven to decrease the incidence of postoperative bleeding. Hemostasis is generally obtained with electrocautery. Suture should be reserved for persistent bleeding, as it has been shown to increase the risk of pseudoaneurysm. The surgeon must not terminate the procedure until confident of hemostasis. If any bleeding is noted in the mouth during emergence from anesthesia, the surgeon should not be reluctant to have the anesthesiologist deepen the plane of anesthesia in order for the pharynx to be examined again and any bleeding stopped.

Although a small amount of blood-tinged saliva is acceptable in the recovery room and for the first 24 hours, any amount of bright red blood coming from the mouth or nose should alert the surgeon to the possibility of postoperative bleeding. A complete examination of the oropharynx is indicated, and this may need to be done in the OR if the patient is uncooperative.

Frequent swallowing and tachycardia have been reported as indirect evidence of possible postoperative bleeding. If the child has continued emesis with coffee ground material, active pharyngeal bleeding should be suspected and the appropriate investigations and treatment initiated. If a clot is present in the tonsillar fossa during the physical examination, this should be removed because it can prevent normal tissue retraction and subsequent healing. However, because of the risk of brisk arterial bleeding behind a clot, IV access should be obtained prior to clot removal.

The age of the child and his or her ability to cooperate are important in the decision-making process. In the appropriate patient, local or topical anesthesia may be sufficient to allow direct examination and removal of the clot. Hemostasis can be achieved using silver nitrate cautery or electrocautery. If this fails, or if the patient is unable to tolerate care in an awake state, general anesthesia will be required to control the airway and allow the surgeon to work without distraction. The initial step in hemostasis is suctioning off any fresh clot from the tonsillar fossa. Identified bleeding sites are controlled with electrocautery or chemical cautery. If these measures are not successful, suture ligature may be required to stop the bleeding. However, this must be done with extreme care. The tissue in the postoperative tonsillar fossa is fragile. Placement of sutures is often difficult because the suture tends to tear through the tissue and pull out. The surgeon then may attempt to place the suture deeper to hold more securely and may inadvertently lacerate a major vessel deep to the fossa, possibly leading to aneurysm formation. If the measures previously mentioned are not successful in stopping the bleeding, consideration must be given to exploration of the neck and ligation of the external carotid artery or its small distal branches. If possible, preoperative angiography may be helpful and embolization might be considered a surgical alternative or adjunct.

67.7 Rehabilitation and Follow-up

If any coagulation disorder is discovered during the preoperative or postoperative period, this should be addressed and treated properly. The patient and family members should receive a complete hematologic consultation, and the patient should be followed up periodically as necessary.

67.8 Questions

1. Secondary posttonsillectomy hemorrhage most commonly occurs because of which of the following?
   a) Platelet disorder.
   b) Eating food with sharp edges.
   c) An upper respiratory infection.
   d) Premature separation of the granulation membrane.
2. True or false? In a preoperative evaluation, discovery of a relative with a bleeding diathesis is an absolute indication for further evaluation before proceeding with adenotonsillectomy.
3. In a patient noted to have posttonsillectomy hemorrhage, which of the following is considered the last resort for hemostasis?
   a) Ligation of the external carotid artery.
   b) Suction Bovie cautery.
   c) Silver nitrate.
   d) Embolization of tonsillar vascular bed.

Answers: 1. d 2. True 3. a

Suggested Readings

Bolger WF, Parsons DS, Potempa L. Preoperative hemostatic assessment of the adenotonsillectomy patient. Otolaryngol Head Neck Surg. 1990; 103(3):396–405

Burk CD, Miller L, Handler SD, Cohen AR. Preoperative history and coagulation screening in children undergoing tonsillectomy. Pediatrics. 1992; 89(4 Pt 2):691–695

Jeyakumar A, Brickman TM, Williamson ME, et al. Nonsteroidal anti-inflammatory drugs and postoperative bleeding following adenotonsillectomy in pediatric patients. Arch Otolaryngol Head Neck Surg. 2008; 134(1):24–27

Liu JH, Anderson KE, Willging JP, et al. Posttonsillectomy hemorrhage: what is it and what should be recorded? Arch Otolaryngol Head Neck Surg. 2001; 127(10):1271–1275

Lowe D, van der Meulen J, Cromwell D, et al. Key messages from the National Prospective Tonsillectomy Audit. Laryngoscope. 2007; 117(4):717–724

Kshirsagar R, Mahboubi H, Moriyama D, Ajose-Popoola O, Pham NS, Ahuja GS. Increased immediate postoperative hemorrhage in older and obese children after outpatient tonsillectomy. Int J Pediatr Otorhinolaryngol. 2016; 84:119–123

Perkins JN, Liang C, Gao D, Shultz L, Friedman NR. Risk of post-tonsillectomy hemorrhage by clinical diagnosis. Laryngoscope. 2012; 122(10):2311–2315

Schmidt R, Herzog A, Cook S, O'Reilly R, Deutsch E, Reilly J. Complications of tonsillectomy: a comparison of techniques. Arch Otolaryngol Head Neck Surg. 2007; 133(9):925–928

Warad D, Hussain FTN, Rao AN, Cofer SA, Rodriguez V. Haemorrhagic complications with adenotonsillectomy in children and young adults with bleeding disorders. Haemophilia. 2015; 21(3): e151–e155

Windfuhr JP, Chen YS, Remmert S. Unidentified coagulation disorders in post-tonsillectomy hemorrhage. Ear Nose Throat J. 2004; 83 (1):28–39, 30, 32 passim

68 Sialadenitis

Patrick R. Owens and J. Paul Willging

68.1 History

A 71-year-old woman presented to the emergency department (ED) with altered mental status, right-sided facial swelling, and pain. Per reports from the nursing home, she had been complaining of pain on the right side of her face for the past several days, with the onset of swelling the previous afternoon. She had begun showing signs of confusion earlier on the day of presentation. Her past medical history was significant for diabetes mellitus type 2, hypertension, hyperlipidemia, gastroesophageal reflux, and mild dementia.

On physical examination she exhibited confusion and had decreased ability to communicate. She had significant swelling of the right side of her face anterior to the tragus. Her parotid gland was indurated and very tender to palpation. No fluctuance was appreciated. Her cranial nerve exam was intact. Her oral mucous membranes were dry and her dentition was poor. Upon massage of her right parotid, purulent drainage was expressed from the papilla of Stenson's duct and a culture was obtained. There was minimal salivary flow from the left parotid gland. Her white blood cell count was 17 K/µl with a left shift. Her basic metabolic panel showed evidence of dehydration. A computed tomography (CT) scan with contrast demonstrated an enlarged right parotid gland with fat stranding and evidence of inflammation but no abscess or stones.

68.2 Differential Diagnosis—Key Points

- Acute suppurative sialadenitis is the most common cause of acute unilateral swelling of the parotid gland in the setting of infectious symptoms. However, sialolithiasis and chronic sialadenitis should also be considered. A good history from the patient or caregivers can help determine if similar symptoms have occurred before. The differential diagnosis of bilateral parotid gland swelling includes viral etiologies such as mumps, human immunodeficiency virus (HIV), cytomegalovirus (CMV), and Coxsackie A and B. Atypical infections such as tuberculosis and cat-scratch disease are rare but may be considered, especially in the pediatric population. Autoimmune pathologies should also be considered, especially primary or secondary Sjögren's syndrome.

- The primary events leading to acute sialadenitis are salivary stasis, reduced flow, and obstruction. Salivary stasis increases the risk of bacterial overgrowth. Up to 30% of patients over 65 years of age struggle with dry mouth. Common causes of reduced salivary flow are outlined in ▶ Table 68.1. *Staphylococcus aureus* has traditionally been the most common pathogen. More recent studies continue to demonstrate *S. aureus* as the most common pathogen, but there are increasing numbers of other pathogens including *Streptococcus pneumoniae, Escherichia coli,* and *Haemophilus influenzae,* as well as polymicrobial or anaerobic organisms.

- Sjögren's syndrome is an autoimmune disorder that affects exocrine glands leading to xerostomia, dry eyes, and enlargement of the salivary glands. It affects as many as 4 million people in the United States. The male-to-female ratio is 9:1. It can affect all age ranges and can be primary or secondary. Secondary disease results from another systemic autoimmune disease such as rheumatoid arthritis (RA) or systemic lupus erythematosus (SLE). Sjögren's syndrome has well-established diagnostic criteria. Four of the following six criteria must be present: symptoms of dry eyes, sign of dry eyes (abnormal Schirmer's test), symptoms of dry mouth, signs of

Table 68.1 Common causes of reduced salivary flow

Source of Salivary Dysfunction	
Medications—up to 80% of medications cause some degree of xerostomia; diuretics and anticholinergics are very common Postsurgical fluid shifts—gastrointestinal procedures are the most common risk	Diabetes Dehydration Radiation and chemotherapy Alzheimer's disease Systemic autoimmune disease and Sjögren's syndrome

abnormal salivary gland function, minor salivary gland biopsy focus score > 1, and presence of SS-A or SS-B antibodies.

- Sialolithiasis can lead to acute suppurative sialadenitis by impeding salivary flow. Stones are composed of both organic and inorganic substances. The formation of stones is thought to occur around an inorganic nidus, most commonly calcium carbonate or calcium phosphate. Stones most commonly occur in the submandibular gland (80%), followed by the parotid gland (20%). Stones more commonly are located in the submandibular duct due to its length and antigravity flow, while they more commonly occur at the hilum or in the parenchyma of the parotid gland. Despite the chemical composition, sialoliths are radiolucent 90% of the time on standard facial radiographs. Sialography and CT scans are much more accurate. Ultrasonography is an underutilized imaging tool for evaluation for stones and is used more frequently in Europe.
- Chronic sialadenitis is defined as recurrent inflammation and pain of the major salivary glands, most commonly the parotid glands. Recurrent infection leads to permanent damage including acinar destruction and ductal ectasia. These changes eventually lead to xerostomia. Acute exacerbations will mimic acute suppurative sialadenitis.
- In the pediatric population, recurrent parotitis eventually leads to juvenile recurrent parotitis (JRP). JRP is a nonobstructing, nonsuppurative swelling of one or both parotid glands in children. JRP is an idiopathic process that most children grow out of after puberty, but acute episodes require antibiotics, pain management, and often hospital admission.

68.3 Test Interpretation

Diagnosis of sialadenitis is primarily clinical. A good history and physical can help elucidate the acute suppurative sialadenitis from chronic sialadenitis from swelling secondary to sialolithiasis. Chronic sialadenitis is recurrent, with eventual atrophy of the glands. Sialolithiasis can be asymptomatic or have swelling and tenderness that is associated with eating. On physical exam, acute suppurative sialadenitis and an acute exacerbation of chronic sialadenitis will have purulence upon massage of the gland, while an obstructing sialolith will have reduced to no salivary flow. Laboratory tests, such as a complete blood count (CBC) with differential and basic metabolic panel (BMP),

can help determine the degree of infection and dehydration. If there is concern for an underlying autoimmune process such as Sjögren's syndrome (primary or secondary), an autoimmune panel including ANA, rheumatoid factor, and SS-A and SS-B can be obtained. If there is underlying concern for HIV or tuberculosis, a rapid HIV test or PPD can be obtained.

Imaging is important to help determine management of the disease, as well as contributing factors. CT scan with contrast will determine if an abscess is present within the gland. It is also useful in looking for possible sialoliths or underlying parotid mass causing obstruction. Ultrasound is likely underutilized. It can be used to identify obstructing stones. This should especially be considered in the pediatric population to avoid unnecessary radiation exposure.

68.4 Diagnosis

Acute suppurative sialadenitis

68.5 Medical Management

Medical management for sialadenitis primarily consists of warm compresses, glandular massage, sialogogues, and antibiotics. Antibiotics should be directed at penicillinase-resistant *S. aureus* empirically until culture results are available. Aggressive hydration orally and/or parenterally should be pursued as appropriate. The precipitating cause of the infection should be sought and addressed.

68.6 Surgical Management

Surgical management in the setting of acute suppurative sialadenitis is limited to incision and drainage if an abscess is present. This should be performed via a modified Blair's incision to expose the parotid capsule. A hemostat is used to enter the abscess cavity, taking care to spread parallel to the direction of the facial nerve. Ultrasound-guided aspiration can be performed in patients who are poor surgical candidates.

Sialendoscopy is becoming a popular surgical option in the management of sialolithiasis or chronic sialadenitis. It has also been reported to be effective in patients with severe JRP when steroid injection is included. Other surgical options for chronic sialadenitis and sialolithiasis include papillary and ductal dilation or transoral surgical excision of the stone with marsupialization. Rarely, surgical excision of the affected glands is needed in patients with chronic sialadenitis.

68.7 Rehabilitation and Follow-up

Follow-up is necessary to ensure resolution of the infection and to optimize underlying conditions.

68.8 Questions

1. What is the most common pathogen in acute suppurative sialadenitis?
   a) Streptococcus pneumoniae.
   b) Staphylococcus aureus.
   c) Haemophilus influenzae.
   d) Escherichia coli.
   e) Bacteroides melaninogenicus.
2. Which of the following is not part of the diagnostic criteria for Sjögren's syndrome?
   a) Symptoms of eye dryness.
   b) Symptoms of dry mouth.
   c) Positive Schirmer's test.
   d) Positive rheumatoid factor.
3. Which of the following is true of juvenile recurrent parotitis (JRP)?

a) It is nonsuppurative.
b) It is suppurative.
c) It generally leads to chronic sialadenitis.
d) It eventually leads to bilateral superficial parotidectomy.

Answers: 1. b 2. d 3. a

Suggested Readings

Brook I. The bacteriology of salivary gland infections. Oral Maxillofac Surg Clin North Am. 2009; 21(3):269–274

Carlson ER. Diagnosis and management of salivary gland infections. Oral Maxillofac Surg Clin North Am. 2009; 21(3):293–312

Chen S, Paul BC, Myssiorek D. An algorithm approach to diagnosing bilateral parotid enlargement. Otolaryngol Head Neck Surg. 2013; 148(5):732–739

Motamed M, Laugharne D, Bradley PJ. Management of chronic parotitis: a review. J Laryngol Otol. 2003; 117(7):521–526

Bowen MA, Tauzin M, Kluka EA, et al. Diagnostic and interventional sialendoscopy: a preliminary experience. Laryngoscope. 2011; 121 (2):299–303

Katz P, Hartl DM, Guerre A. Treatment of juvenile recurrent parotitis. Otolaryngol Clin North Am. 2009; 42(6):1087–1091

Cornec D, Devauchelle-Pensec V, Tobón GJ, Pers JO, Jousse-Joulin S, Saraux A. B cells in Sjögren's syndrome: from pathophysiology to diagnosis and treatment. J Autoimmun. 2012; 39(3):161–167

69 Angioedema

Jeffery J. Harmon and Alfred M. Sassler

69.1 History

A 73-year-old woman with a past medical history including hypertension and osteoarthritis presented to the emergency department with 4 hours of acute onset upper and lower lip swelling, shortness of breath, dysphagia, and a muffled voice. The patient had been eating dinner at the time of onset of these symptoms. She denied odynophagia, difficulty controlling her secretions, nausea, or diarrhea. She had never developed these symptoms before and had no family history of similar symptoms. Her home medications included metoprolol and ibuprofen.

Physical examination demonstrated moderate upper and lower lip edema and mild anterior tongue edema. There was no swelling of other areas of her face or extremities. There were no rashes present. Flexible nasopharyngoscopy and laryngoscopy demonstrated moderate false vocal fold edema but no edema of the base of tongue, epiglottis, aryepiglottic folds, arytenoids, or posterior oropharynx. The glottis was incompletely visualized due to the edema of the false vocal folds.

The emergency department physician administered intravenous (IV) dexamethasone, IV ranitidine, and IV diphenhydramine prior to evaluation by otolaryngology. Based on her exam findings, the otolaryngology team decided to intubate the patient by means of awake fiberoptic nasotracheal intubation. Treatment with steroids, an H1 blocker, and an H2 blocker was continued for approximately 24 hours. She was successfully extubated approximately 24 hours after intubation.

69.2 Differential Diagnosis— Key Points

- Angioedema is nonpitting edema of the skin and mucous membranes that can occur anywhere in the body. The edema results from a state of hyperpermeability of venules due to vasoactive agents. Angioedema becomes concerning to the otolaryngologist when it involves the head and neck, especially the airway.
- The mechanism of angioedema involves mediators in the kallikrein-kinin system and immunoglobulin E (IgE)–mediated histaminergic

response, both of which result in the release of vasoactive peptides that increase vascular permeability and, therefore, edema.
- Head and neck symptoms of angioedema include shortness of breath, voice changes often described as a muffled or as a "hot potato" voice, hoarseness, stertor, stridor, drooling or difficulty controlling secretions, dysphagia, and odynophagia. Associated signs and symptoms may include extremity edema, edema of gastrointestinal tract manifested by nausea/emesis/diarrhea, edema of the genitourinary system, and urticaria.
- It is important to determine if there is a family or personal history of similar episodes. It is also important to review current medications, exposure to known allergens, and/or recent trauma or surgeries.
- Management of the airway is the most important and immediate focus of management. A decision must be made whether to observe the patient in the emergency department, to observe the patient in an intensive care unit (ICU) setting, or to secure the airway either via intubation or tracheotomy.
- The anatomic locations of swelling include the oral cavity and airway. Sites of oral edema include the lips, tongue, soft palate, uvula, and floor of mouth. Sites of airway edema include the base of tongue, epiglottis, vallecula, pharyngeal wall, aryepiglottic folds, and false vocal cords. The location of swelling and number of sites affected are predictive of the need for intubation.
- Causes of angioedema are allergic or nonallergic. Allergic responses are the result of an IgE-mediated, histaminergic pathway (type 1 hypersensitivity reaction). Allergic etiologies include medications such as antibiotics, food, and insect bites. Nonallergic causes include hereditary angioedema, angioedema secondary to the use of an angiotensin-converting enzyme (ACE) inhibitor, and angioedema secondary to nonsteroidal anti-inflammatory drugs (NSAIDs) that target the cyclooxygenase-1 (COX-1) pathway. The mechanism by which ACE inhibitors can cause angioedema is through reduced degradation of bradykinins. ACE is an enzyme that normally enhances the degradation of bradykinin, a molecule that binds to a receptor on vasculature,

277

resulting in vasodilation and increased vascular permeability. The mechanism by which NSAIDs can cause angioedema is through the production of leukotrienes. Leukotrienes are inflammatory mediators that can lead to increased vascular permeability and, therefore, edema. Leukotrienes are produced as an alternative metabolite of arachidonic acid when NSAIDs block the enzyme COX-1.

- Hereditary angioedema is an autosomal dominant disease that accounts for approximately 2% of angioedema cases. There are two types of hereditary angioedema. The first involves too little C1 esterase inhibitor. The second involves production of a deficient C1 esterase inhibitor. They are clinically indistinguishable. Both result in increased production of bradykinin leading to increased vascular permeability and edema. Clinical presentation is sporadic and unpredictable but can be induced by trauma, dental procedures, and even stress. Unlike an allergic response, hereditary angioedema does not present with urticaria and does not respond to steroids, H1 blockers, or H2 blockers.

69.3 Test Interpretation

Angioedema is a clinical diagnosis. No imaging is required. A work-up for hereditary angioedema can include C4 and C1 esterase inhibitor levels. However, a work-up for hereditary angioedema should be delayed until the patient has been stabilized.

69.4 Diagnosis

Angioedema

69.5 Medical Management

Any potentially causative medications or allergic exposures should be discontinued immediately. Patients taking ACE inhibitors may develop angioedema at any point, even if they have been taking the medication for an extended period of time.

A common initial treatment regimen includes a steroid such as IV dexamethasone, an H1 receptor blocker such as IV diphenhydramine, and an H2 receptor blocker such as IV ranitidine. Treatment with these medications should begin in the emergency department. This management should continue until resolution of symptoms. However, as described above, there are multiple potential causes for angioedema, both allergic and nonallergic. There is a weak theoretical basis for treating nonallergic angioedema with steroids, an H1 receptor blocker, and an H2 receptor blocker. However, as the cause of angioedema is commonly idiopathic and the time frame between what could be multiple potential exposures is often unclear, this remains an appropriate initial intervention.

For hereditary angioedema, medical management is stratified into prophylactic treatment and treatment for acute episodes. Prophylactic treatment for hereditary angioedema targets various points in the kallikrein-kinin pathway. Medications include a C1 esterase inhibitor concentrate, androgens including danazol that increase C1 esterase inhibitor levels, and antifibrinolytics. All of these medications have side effects, making long-term management by an allergist/immunologist important. Acute treatments for hereditary angioedema include C1 esterase inhibitor concentrate, a bradykinin receptor antagonist, and a plasma kallikrein inhibitor. The purpose of each of these treatments is to reduce the release of vasoactive peptides that lead to edema.

69.6 Surgical Management

Management of the airway is of utmost importance when treating an angioedema patient. There are multiple considerations in determining whether a patient requires intubation. One factor is the time to presentation from the onset of symptoms. Presentation within 4 hours of symptom onset has been shown to correlate with need for intubation. The presence of respiratory distress and/or inability to manage oral secretions both indicate the need for intubation. A third factor is the location of swelling. Patients who require intubation most often present with floor of mouth, base of tongue, soft palate, and laryngeal edema. Supraglottic edema with an obstructed view of the glottis is especially concerning. Flexible airway endoscopy is essential in every patient presenting with symptoms suggestive of angioedema. The etiology of the angioedema can be investigated after the airway has been appropriately triaged.

In cases of severe oropharyngeal or laryngeal edema, an awake tracheotomy may be the safest method by which to secure the airway.

69.7 Rehabilitation and Follow-up

The time to resolution of symptoms varies. Those cases of angioedema requiring intubation take longer for resolution of symptoms. The patient is monitored and treated until signs of oral and/or airway edema have resolved.

69.8 Questions

1. Causes of angioedema include all of the following except
   a) Medications, including angiotensin-converting enzyme (ACE) inhibitors and antibiotics.
   b) Insect bites.
   c) Food.
   d) A deficiency in C1 esterase.
   e) All of the above are causes.
   f) None of the above are causes.
2. Which factors are important in determining the risk of airway compromise in a patient and the need to secure an airway?
   a) Location of the edema.
   b) The time course and progression of symptoms.
   c) The associated symptoms, including degree of respiratory distress and ability to control secretions.
   d) All of the above are factors.
   e) None of the above are factors.
3. Consider a patient with known C1 esterase inhibitor deficiency. She has been unable to acquire Cinryze due to its expense and, therefore, has not been taking the appropriate medication for an unknown period of time. She presents to the hospital with facial swelling but no shortness of breath. She is controlling her secretions well. She has had difficulty acquiring Cinryze in the past and has been to the emergency department with airway edema requiring intubation before. Physical exam demonstrates lip swelling. Airway endoscopy demonstrates no oropharyngeal or laryngeal edema. Appropriate management of this patient includes which of the following?
   a) Admission to the intensive care unit (ICU) for monitoring.
   b) Consultation with allergy/immunology for management and administration of C1 esterase inhibitor.
   c) Observation in the emergency department, followed by discharge when patient has received C1 esterase inhibitor.
   d) A + B.
   e) B + C.
   f) None of the above.

Answers: 1. e 2. d 3. d

Suggested Readings

Al-Khudari S, Loochtan MJ, Peterson E, Yaremchuk KL. Management of angiotensin-converting enzyme inhibitor-induced angioedema. Laryngoscope. 2011; 121(11):2327–2334

Bork K. Current management options for hereditary angioedema. Curr Allergy Asthma Rep. 2012; 12(4):273–280

Cicardi M, Aberer W, Banerji A, et al. HAWK under the patronage of EAACI (European Academy of Allergy and Clinical Immunology). Classification, diagnosis, and approach to treatment for angioedema: consensus report from the Hereditary Angioedema International Working Group. Allergy. 2014; 69(5):602–616

Kieu MCQ, Bangiyev JN, Thottam PJ, Levy PD. Predictors of Airway Intervention in Angiotensin-Converting Enzyme Inhibitor-Induced Angioedema. Otolaryngol Head Neck Surg. 2015; 153(4):544–550

Levy JH, Freiberger DJ, Roback J. Hereditary angioedema: current and emerging treatment options. Anesth Analg. 2010; 110 (5):1271–1280

70 Ludwig's Angina

Brittany A. Leader and John F. Barrord

70.1 History

A 50-year-old white man with insulin-dependent diabetes presented to the emergency department (ED) with progressive pain and swelling in the floor of his mouth over a 3-day period.

He underwent a full-mouth dental extraction 7 months earlier, followed by an alveoloplasty 3 months ago. He first noted an infected "blister" under a poorly fitting denture last week, which he squeezed and drained by himself. He sought medical attention when his neck began rapidly swelling over the course of the night and he developed increasing difficulty swallowing and breathing. Despite his dysphagia, he consumed a large breakfast prior to driving himself to the ED.

On physical examination he was found to have significant bilateral submandibular fullness and tenderness. Computed tomography (CT) scan with contrast of the neck demonstrated an abscess along the inside of the mandibular arch (▶ Fig. 70.1). His airway was adequate and his floor of mouth was soft upon arrival in the ED. However, he was felt to be at great risk for rapid progression of the infection. Given the severity of the infection and the potential for rapid airway compromise, a needle aspiration of the abscess was performed in the ED as a temporizing measure to allow time for

his stomach contents to empty. The culture of that aspirate later grew microaerophylic streptococcus. He was taken to the operating room a few hours later for incision and drainage of the abscess with consent for tracheostomy if necessary. Fortunately, he was successfully intubated using a curved GlideScope under mild sedation while he maintained spontaneous respiration. An incision and drainage was performed, and a passive neck drain was left in place for a week to allow all the soft tissue induration to resolve. He was treated with a 2-week course of antibiotics.

70.2 Differential Diagnosis—Key Points

Angioedema may present with symptoms of swelling, drooling, and difficulty swallowing and breathing and tends to involve the tongue, lips, uvula, and/or oropharynx. The edema is typically acute onset. It frequently follows specific triggers including shellfish and is most commonly associated with medications such as angiotensin-converting enzyme inhibitors. The rapid progression of this patient's symptoms, along with leukocytosis, suggested an infectious etiology. Swelling of the floor of mouth is more consistent with

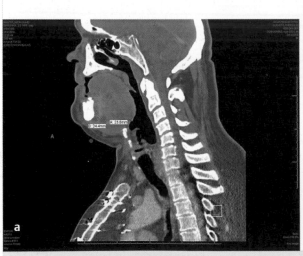
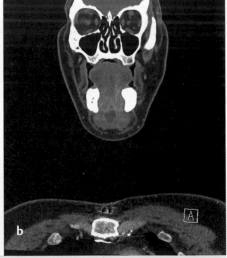

Fig. 70.1 (a) CT of the neck with contrast demonstrating an abscess inside the mandibular arch in the sagittal plane. (b) Abscess as seen in the coronal plane.

Ludwig's angina, as opposed to peritonsillar abscess, epiglottitis, or other pharyngeal and deep neck space infections. Deep neck infections, including masseteric space infections and submandibular space infections, also need to be considered in the differential diagnosis.

Ludwig's angina is named after the German physician Wilhelm Frederick von Ludwig, who first described the condition in 1836. The word *angina* derives from the Greek word *ankhon,* which means "strangling" and describes the feeling patients may have with this condition. Ludwig's angina is a clinical diagnosis, the hallmarks of which include dysphagia, muffled speech, a rapidly progressive cellulitis associated with submandibular and submental neck swelling that is classically hard and tense, and floor of mouth firmness. Pain, fever, neck stiffness, and drooling are common. Trismus is usually not present unless the pharyngeal or masseteric space is also involved. Ludwig's angina is essentially a compartment syndrome of the sublingual and submandibular spaces, as they are enclosed by the rigid superficial layer of the deep cervical fascia. The infection extends superiorly and posteriorly within the compartment elevating the tongue and floor of mouth. Early recognition of the potential for airway compromise can often prevent the need for an emergent tracheostomy. Causes of Ludwig's angina include pharyngitis, tonsillitis, sialadenitis, tongue piercing, and oral trauma, but the most common cause is an odontogenic infection involving the second or third molars. The roots of these two molars are below the attachment of the mylohyoid muscle to the mandible, so they cross the sublingual and submandibular spaces. Predisposing comorbid conditions include poor oral hygiene, diabetes mellitus, malnutrition, alcoholism, neutropenia, lupus erythematous, aplastic anemia, and glomerulonephritis. Ludwig's angina tends to be caused by polymicrobial oral cavity flora. The organisms isolated are often gram-positive cocci, gram-negative rods, and anaerobes most commonly including *Streptococcus* spp., *Staphylococcus aureus*, *Bacteroides* spp., *Fusobacterium* spp., *Actinomyces* spp., and *Haemophylus influenzae.*

70.3 Test Interpretation

CT is the imaging modality of choice for the diagnosis of Ludwig's angina and other deep neck infections. However, it is important to consider that placing patients with airway compromise supine for a CT scan prior to securing the airway can precipitate airway obstruction. Ultrasound can also be used to evaluate for potential abscess. Plain radiographs can help evaluate for gas-producing organisms and mediastinal involvement.

70.4 Diagnosis

Ludwig's angina

70.5 Medical Management

The approach to a patient with Ludwig's angina entails assessment and management of the airway and initiation of broad-spectrum antibiotics. While some cases can be managed with observation and antibiotics, Ludwig's angina needs to be considered an airway emergency. In patients with progressive swelling and dyspnea, it is imperative to establish a safe airway. Flexible fiberoptic nasal intubation should be the initial method of airway management. If the tongue and floor of mouth are not yet firm, a fiberoptic GlideScope with a curved stylet can be used to successfully intubate with only mild sedation. Blind oral and blind nasotracheal intubation are discouraged, given the risk of inducing laryngospasm. In the event intubation is not possible, tracheostomy under local anesthesia is indicated, with the patient spontaneously breathing.

Empiric broad-spectrum antibiotic coverage should be started and can be tailored as cultures and sensitivities arrive later. Activity against beta-lactamase–producing aerobes and anaerobes and against *S. aureus* is important. Common choices include ampicillin-sulbactam, penicillin G with metronidazole, or clindamycin. In patients at increased risk for infection with methicillin-resistant *S. aureus* (MRSA), vancomycin or linezolid are recommended until culture results are available. Intravenous antibiotic coverage should be continued until resolution of the induration begins, after which the patient can be switched to appropriate oral antibiotics. Antibiotics should be continued for 2 to 3 weeks and should not be discontinued until the patient is no longer febrile and shows significant clinical improvement.

70.6 Surgical Management

If the patient is unable to be managed medically, and intubation is either unsuccessful or deemed unsafe, the preferred method for obtaining a surgical airway is an awake tracheostomy. The patient may remain in an upright position, thereby decreasing the risk of airway compromise. Ideally the awake tracheostomy would be performed in an operating room, but if the patient is rapidly deteriorating, it may need to be performed outside the operating room. No sedation should be used if there is concern that it may worsen the patient's respiratory status. A cricothyroidotomy should be considered in particularly urgent situations.

While a frank abscess may not be present, if the cellulitis progresses and does not show signs of resolution within 24 to 48 hours of antibiotic coverage, then drainage may be needed. In this circumstance, several horizontal incisions are made over the submental and submandibular areas. It is important to consider the location of the marginal mandibular branch of the facial nerve when making these incisions. Drainage options then include Penrose's drain, packing, and suction drains. Drains are commonly left in place much longer than routine postsurgical drains, as it may take a long time for the induration to resolve.

70.7 Rehabilitation and Follow-up

After patients demonstrate clinical improvement, they may be discharged on oral antibiotics to follow up as an outpatient with continued clinical exams to monitor for complete resolution. Patients who required a tracheostomy should be decannulated after resolution of their infection. Treatment of the underlying pathology is critical, including addressing dental issues and improving comorbid conditions such as diabetes mellitus.

70.8 Questions

1. Which of the following is not a common presenting symptom for a patient with Ludwig's angina?
   a) Drooling.
   b) Neck stiffness.
   c) Angina.
   d) Fever.
2. Which airway management technique would not be appropriate for a patient with Ludwig's angina?
   a) Fiberoptic nasal intubation.
   b) Awake tracheostomy.
   c) Oral intubation with GlideScope.
   d) Rapid sequence intubation with cricoid pressure.
3. How long do patients with Ludwig's angina typically require antibiotic therapy?
   a) 24 hours.
   b) 72 hours.
   c) 2 to 3 weeks.
   d) 2 to 3 months.

Answers: 1. c 2. d 3. c

Suggested Readings

Bansal A, Miskoff J, Lis RJ. Otolaryngologic critical care. Crit Care Clin. 2003; 19(1):55–72

Botha A, Jacobs F, Postma C. Retrospective analysis of etiology and comorbid diseases associated with Ludwig's Angina. Ann Maxillofac Surg. 2015; 5(2):168–173

Britt JC, Josephson GD, Gross CW. Ludwig's angina in the pediatric population: report of a case and review of the literature. Int J Pediatr Otorhinolaryngol. 2000; 52(1):79–87

Bross-Soriano D, Arrieta-Gómez JR, Prado-Calleros H, Schimelmitz-Idi J, Jorba-Basave S. Management of Ludwig's angina with small neck incisions: 18 years experience. Otolaryngol Head Neck Surg. 2004; 130(6):712–717

Kremer MJ, Blair T. Ludwig angina: forewarned is forearmed. AANA J. 2006; 74(6):445–451

Lawson W, Reino A, Westreich R. Odontogenic infections. In: Bailey B, Johnson J, Newlands S, eds. Head & Neck Surgery—Otolaryngology. Philadelphia, PA: Lippincott Williams & Wilkins; 2006:619

Marple BF. Ludwig angina: a review of current airway management. Arch Otolaryngol Head Neck Surg. 1999; 125(5):596–599

Vieira F, Allen SM, Stocks RM, Thompson JW. Deep neck infection. Otolaryngol Clin North Am. 2008; 41(3):459–483, vii

71 Epiglottitis

Nathan D. Wiebracht and Michael J. Rutter

71.1 History

A 21-year-old woman presented to the emergency department (ED) with acutely worsened respiratory status. She was previously well and had no significant past medical history. Earlier that day she developed a sore throat with rapidly worsening dysphagia, with inability to tolerate her secretions upon presentation to the ED. She reported difficulty breathing that was markedly worse when she tried to lie flat. She denied any recent trauma. She had no prior surgical history. She took no medications but had a penicillin allergy. Her parents reported she had only received some of her childhood vaccines.

On physical examination, she appeared uncomfortable. She was febrile to 102.5 °F. She was leaning forward and occasionally drooling. Her voice was muffled but she had no stridor. Her intraoral exam demonstrated 2 + tonsils with no peritonsillar fullness or uvular deviation or tonsillar exudates. She had some pooling of secretions in the oral cavity. Her hyoid and midline neck demonstrated tenderness on palpation. There was no cervical lymphadenopathy. She had no trismus or limitation to neck range of motion. Flexible fiberoptic examination of the upper airway revealed diffuse supraglottic edema and erythema, with the most profound findings localized at the epiglottis. Both vocal folds were mobile.

71.2 Differential Diagnosis—Key Points

- Odynophagia can result from tonsillitis, pharyngitis, or a deep neck infection or malignancy. In this case, the onset of symptoms was rapid (< 24 hours), decreasing the likelihood of a deep neck space infection, as well as other causes, such as malignancy. The history excluded other causes such as foreign body impaction or other trauma. The combination of fever, progressive odynophagia, sore throat, and fiberoptic findings of erythema and edema should raise the suspicion of epiglottitis. Immediate action should be taken to ensure a safe airway.
- Until the early 1990s, epiglottitis was considered a disease of early childhood, most commonly seen in children aged 2 to 7 years. However, after the introduction of the *Haemophilus influenzae* type B (Hib) vaccine in the 1980s, the incidence in children declined significantly from 5 to 0.5 per 100,000. This disease is now more commonly observed in adults, with an incidence of 1.6 to 3.1 per 100,000 people. Adult mortality rates approach 7%, in many cases owing to a delay in diagnosis or adequate care. Therefore, a high index of suspicion should be maintained.
- Physical examination is diagnostic and requires the use of either indirect mirror or fiberoptic laryngoscopy. Classically, there is concern that performing such an examination in children may precipitate acute airway obstruction, so it is still recommended that a child with suspected epiglottitis be immediately transported to the operative suite to secure the airway. In adults, several studies have demonstrated that indirect laryngoscopy is safe in patients who are not in significant respiratory distress. Alternatively, a lateral airway radiograph could be obtained, which may demonstrate the "thumbprint" sign indicative of severe epiglottic edema (▶ Fig. 71.1). However, the sensitivity and specificity of this imaging study are relatively low (38% and 78%, respectively). Also note that in adults, the inflammation may involve not only the epiglottis, but other supraglottic structures as well, and may even extend toward the pharynx and uvula. In children, the infection tends to classically manifest as a swollen, cherry-red epiglottis.
- This patient was sitting in the "tripod" position, erect and leaning slightly forward, which uses gravity to aid in reduction of the supraglottic obstruction. A muffled or "hot potato" voice and tenderness to direct palpation over the larynx are also characteristic of epiglottitis. However, regardless of age, the three most reliable signs of epiglottitis are fever, respiratory difficulty, and irritability.

71.3 Test Interpretation

A lateral neck (airway) radiograph may be useful in narrowing the differential diagnosis, particularly in children, who are at significant risk of laryngospasm or airway obstruction from indirect or

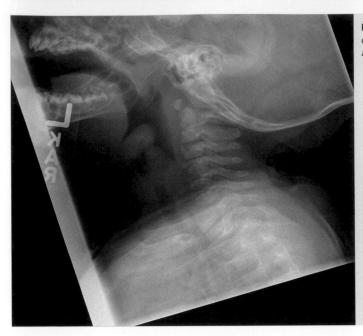

Fig. 71.1 Lateral airway radiograph demonstrating edema of epiglottis and the classic "thumbprint" sign.

fiberoptic laryngoscopy. However, in adults this imaging modality is generally not favored because of its low sensitivity and specificity. Computed tomography (CT) imaging of the neck can rule out the presence of epiglottic or tongue-base abscesses, a complication found almost exclusively in adults, or other deep neck space infection. However, because of the potential for complete airway compromise in epiglottitis, this imaging study should be ordered with extreme caution and only once the patient has been stabilized.

A complete blood count (CBC) will usually reveal leukocytosis. Blood cultures may demonstrate positive results for *H. influenzae*, *Streptococcus* spp., *Staphylococcus aureus*, or other organisms in 8 to 31% of cases. Prior to introduction of the Hib vaccine, *H. influenzae* bacteremia was seen in 90 to 95% of patients. *H. influenzae* and streptococci still constitute most of the bacteriology seen in adult patients with epiglottitis, while anaerobes, fungi, and viral agents are only rarely cited as pathogens. If epiglottitis is suspected, blood cultures should be obtained before initiating antibiotic therapy. Throat swab cultures are of little benefit because the infection is typically limited to submucosal cellulitis in adults. Note that there are numerous noninfectious causes of epiglottitis in adults, such as foreign body trauma, caustic injury, or thermal injury, which may explain the variance in positive blood cultures seen in several studies.

71.4 Diagnosis

Epiglottitis

71.5 Medical Management

Initial medical therapy involves aggressive intravenous fluid resuscitation and broad-spectrum antibiotic coverage for *H. influenzae*, staphylococci, and streptococci, with ampicillin/sulbactam, clindamycin, or a third-generation cephalosporin such as ceftriaxone. Vancomycin may be added if methicillin-resistant *S. aureus* is suspected. Antibiotic therapy should be modified as culture results are obtained. Duration of antibiotic therapy (including oral medications) ranges from 1 to 2 weeks in total, depending on the clinical condition of the patient. Administration of corticosteroids to reduce upper airway edema is controversial but is recommended in most cases.

Morbidity and mortality from epiglottitis in the modern era are typically due to airway obstruction. In children, placing an artificial airway may reduce the incidence of morbidity, but this approach is somewhat more controversial in adults. One study from 1995 recommends automatic airway intervention for patients with obvious signs of airway obstruction; for all patients 5 years of age or younger; for those with respiratory distress when sitting upright; for those with stridor, drooling, or symptom progression over less than 24 hours; or for significant enlargement of the epiglottis on laryngoscopy or radiography.

Several studies indicate that in adults without respiratory distress, close observation with humidified oxygen in an intensive care unit may be all that is required for airway management, with endotracheal intubation and tracheotomy equipment available at the bedside in case the patient develops more significant signs of respiratory distress. It should be noted that delayed respiratory compromise is known to occur in epiglottitis. Emergent intubation and tracheotomy are performed in adults with epiglottitis at a rate of 9 to 16%. Extubation trials may be attempted after a 48-hour period of empiric antibiotics, once an air leak is noted around the endotracheal tube, or if significantly decreased supraglottic edema and erythema are noted on flexible laryngoscopy.

71.6 Surgical Management

Surgical management may be indicated in order to establish a secure airway. Intubation can be quite difficult because of significant edema and distortion of landmarks. If intubation with or without fiberoptic guidance fails, a cricothyrotomy or tracheotomy is required. If an epiglottic abscess is suspected or noted on CT imaging, incision and drainage of the abscess should be performed in the operative suite only after the airway has been secured.

71.7 Rehabilitation and Follow-up

Recurrent epiglottitis is rare and should raise the suspicion of an underlying medical problem such as sarcoidosis, collagen vascular disease, or even malignancy. One complication of epiglottitis that might not be immediately apparent while a patient is sedated and intubated is meningitis. Note that antibiotic regimens suitable for treatment of epiglottitis may not meet the recommended therapeutic dosages for meningitis.

As a result of the Hib vaccine, the incidence of pediatric epiglottitis is on the decline. Even though many adults have never received the Hib vaccine, it has been documented that protection from *H. influenzae* can be transmitted through populations by the herd immunity phenomenon. Nonetheless, a decrease in adult epiglottitis patients has not yet been observed. Medical literature also documents cases in which Hib-vaccinated children were nonetheless diagnosed with *H. influenza*–mediated epiglottitis, with or without bacteremia, because of an inability to produce Hib antibodies or the production of anticapsular antibodies, which provides less protection from *H. influenzae*.

71.8 Questions

1. To which vaccination has the decline in epiglottitis in the pediatric population been attributed?
   a) Tdap.
   b) Flu.
   c) *Haemophilus influenzae* type B.
   d) Chicken pox.
   e) Human papillomavirus.
2. True or false? Visualization of the epiglottis is required for the diagnosis of epiglottitis.
3. Which is the first priority when epiglottitis is suspected?
   a) Ensure a safe airway.
   b) Obtain blood cultures.
   c) Start empiric antibiotics.
   d) Obtain imaging.
   e) Acquire intravenous access.

Answers: 1. c 2. False 3. a

Suggested Readings

Carey MJ. Epiglottitis in adults. Am J Emerg Med. 1996; 14(4):421–424

Mathoera RB, Wever PC, van Dorsten FR, Balter SG, de Jager CP. Epiglottitis in the adult patient. Neth J Med. 2008; 66(9):373–377

Mayo-Smith MF, Spinale JW, Donskey CJ, Yukawa M, Li RH, Schiffman FJ. Acute epiglottitis. An 18-year experience in Rhode Island. Chest. 1995; 108(6):1640–1647

McEwan J, Giridharan W, Clarke RW, Shears P. Paediatric acute epiglottitis: not a disappearing entity. Int J Pediatr Otorhinolaryngol. 2003; 67(4):317–321

Rafei K, Lichenstein R. Airway infectious disease emergencies. Pediatr Clin North Am. 2006; 53(2):215–242

Richards AM. Pediatric respiratory emergencies. Emerg Med Clin North Am. 2016; 34(1):77–96

Rotta AT, Wiryawan B. Respiratory emergencies in children. Respir Care. 2003; 48(3):248–258, discussion 258–260

Shah RK, Roberson DW, Jones DT. Epiglottitis in the Hemophilus influenzae type B vaccine era: changing trends. Laryngoscope. 2004; 114(3):557–560

Sobol SE, Zapata S. Epiglottitis and croup. Otolaryngol Clin North Am. 2008; 41(3):551–566

Wong EY, Berkowitz RG. Acute epiglottitis in adults: the Royal Melbourne Hospital experience. ANZ J Surg. 2001; 71(12):740–743

Zoorob R, Sidani MA, Fremont RD, Kihlberg C. Antibiotic use in acute upper respiratory tract infections. Am Fam Physician. 2012; 86(9):817–822

72 Sjögren's Syndrome

Brian L. Hendricks and John F. Barrord

72.1 History

A 58-year-old Caucasian woman presented for evaluation of dysphagia, which she reported had become an issue over the past 6 months. She also reported chronic dry mouth, hoarseness, and dry throat sensation. She stated that her difficulty swallowing foods was temporarily alleviated if she drank liquids to "wash it down." She denied any history of odynophagia or regurgitation after meals. She did report a history of gastroesophageal reflux disease (GERD), which seemed to be improved after recently being started on a proton pump inhibitor by her primary care physician. She had an esophagram, which was normal. Upon further questioning, the patient also reported that she had the sensation of dry eyes and occasional ocular foreign body sensation. She had been attributing this to allergies, as she had moved to the region within the past year. She had been previously prescribed antihistamine eyedrops, which seemed to make things worse, but she did seem to get some improvement with artificial tears.

Her past medical history was remarkable only for a history of GERD and hypertension. These were managed with omeprazole and hydrochlorothiazide, respectively. She no longer used the antihistamine eyedrops. She reported a family history of hypertension and diabetes. She drank a glass of wine with dinner on weekends, and denied any history of tobacco use. She denied any joint pain or known history of rheumatologic disease.

On physical examination, her conjunctivae were mildly injected but otherwise unremarkable in appearance. Her oral mucosa was moderately dry, and she had dry, chapped-appearing lips. Her nasal examination revealed mild crusting bilaterally and dry mucosa. The remainder of her exam, including flexible laryngoscopy, was unremarkable.

Salivary gland biopsy from the lower lip was performed, and the patient had blood drawn for anti-SSA/Ro, anti-SSB/La, rheumatoid factor (RF), and antinuclear antibody (ANA) testing.

72.2 Differential Diagnosis—Key Points

- While dysphagia is commonly related to xerostomia in patients with Sjögren's syndrome, it is important to consider other possible etiologies. A normal esophagram reduced the likelihood that this patient's dysphagia was related to esophageal diverticuli, mass lesions, stricture, dysmotility disorders, extrinsic compression, or a hiatal hernia. Neurologic disorders and GERD are other important considerations in the differential.

- Xerostomia has a number of possible causes, including granulomatous disease, human immunodeficiency virus (HIV) infection, Sjögren's syndrome, dehydration, prior head and neck irradiation, hypothyroidism, mouth breathing, oxygen use, and a wide variety of medications. A thorough review of the patient's history and medication list is necessary. Minor salivary gland biopsy is helpful to evaluate for disorders of the salivary glands, with the primary concern being Sjögren's syndrome.

- The presence of xerophthalmos (dry eyes) should raise the index of suspicion for Sjögren's syndrome. Tear-deficient dry eye is classified by ophthalmologists into Sjögren's-related and non-Sjögren's tear deficiency, the latter of which is generally associated with systemic medications, graft-versus-host disease, other autoimmune processes, or HIV infection. Schirmer's test measures aqueous tear flow and can be done rapidly in the office. In normal patients, greater than 15 mm of test strip wetting is expected over the course of 5 minutes. Less than 5 mm of wetting is considered a severely decreased volume of tear production. Rose bengal dye, lissamine green, or fluorescein staining of the ocular surface may be able to detect ocular abnormalities such as corneal ulcerations.

- Sjögren's syndrome is an autoimmune disorder characterized by xerostomia and xerophthalmos caused by chronic inflammation of exocrine glands. Its prevalence in the United States is estimated to be between 0.2 and 2%, with a 9:1 female-to-male preponderance. The average age of onset is between 40 and 60 years of age.

- Historically, secondary Sjögren's syndrome has been diagnosed in patients with other underlying autoimmune disorders such as rheumatoid arthritis, systemic lupus erythematosus, and scleroderma, while primary Sjögren's syndrome has been diagnosed in patients without another underlying autoimmune disorder. However, given that primary Sjögren's syndrome is also associated with disorders of other organ systems, some clinicians have begun to move away from distinguishing between the two.

- Sjögren's syndrome affects numerous tissues and organs, including the inner ear, larynx, thyroid, sinonasal passages, lungs, gastrointestinal and hepatobiliary tracts, kidney and bladder, musculoskeletal system, central nervous system, and circulatory system. Chronic oral candidiasis is sometimes seen in Sjögren's syndrome patients. One of the worst associations of Sjögren's syndrome is the increased risk of non-Hodgkin's lymphoma (most commonly mucosal-associated lymphoid tissue type), up to 44 times greater than that of the general population. Non-Hodgkin's lymphoma of the salivary glands may present as a progressively enlarging, painless mass.

72.3 Test Interpretation

Several tests can be helpful in the evaluation of a patient with xerostomia and associated dysphagia. This patient had already had a normal esophagram, but a modified barium swallow could be helpful if any neurologic disorders such as prior stroke or Parkinson's disease were suspected to play a role. A fasting basic metabolic panel could help evaluate for diabetes, dehydration, or diuretic use as potential causes of the patient's symptoms. Thyroid hormone levels may be checked to exclude hypothyroidism.

Several blood tests are helpful in the evaluation of suspected Sjögren's or sicca complex. Serum anti-SSA/Ro, anti-SSB/La, RF, and ANA levels should be ordered.

Sialography may reveal pooling of extravasated contrast material, which would suggest acinar cell inflammation and salivary gland pathology, but does not confirm a specific diagnosis. Minor salivary gland biopsy remains the gold standard for pathologic diagnosis of Sjögren's syndrome. The classic findings are multiple lymphocytic foci or plasma cell infiltrates, as well as acinar and ductal cell destruction (▶ Fig. 72.1). The commonly accepted criteria to establish a diagnosis of Sjögren's syndrome include at least two of the following:

- Positive serum anti-SSA (Ro) and/or anti-SSB (La), or positive RF and ANA ≥ 1:320.
- Ocular staining score ≥ 3 (using lissamine green and fluorescein) to diagnose keratoconjunctivitis sicca.
- Presence of focal lymphocytic sialadenitis in a labial salivary gland biopsy with a focus score ≥ 1 focus/4 mm.

72.4 Diagnosis

Sjögren's syndrome

72.5 Medical Management

The management of Sjögren's syndrome and sicca complex is primarily symptomatic in nature. Given the decreased exocrine gland function, patients benefit from treatment aimed at restoring moisture to the eyes and upper aerodigestive tract.

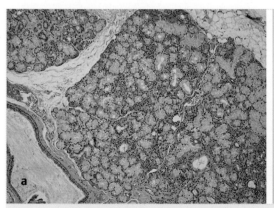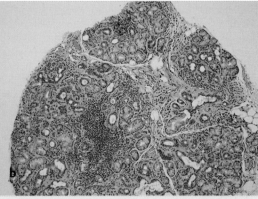

Fig. 72.1 Histopathology of (a) a normal salivary gland, and (b) a salivary gland in a patient with Sjögren's syndrome. Note the lymphocytic infiltrates and disrupted acinar cell architecture. (Acknowledgment to Matthew Hagen in the University of Cincinnati Department of Pathology for this image.)

Artificial tears, salivary stimulants, oral lubricants, and saline nasal sprays are all helpful in reducing complaints related to epithelial dryness. Pilocarpine, cevimeline, and bethanechol are muscarinic agonists used in Sjögren-related xerostomia to stimulate salivary secretions. Sialogogues and mechanical stimulation can also be helpful in increasing saliva production. Medications that cause dry mouth or eyes should be managed judiciously and avoided when possible, including diuretics, antihistamines, decongestants, and antidepressants. Fluoride supplementation may have a role in preventing dental caries.

72.6 Surgical Management

Surgical intervention in routine Sjögren's syndrome is currently limited to salivary gland biopsy for diagnosis. The specimen should preferably provide at least 8 mm² of minor salivary tissue and be sent in formalin. The surgeon should avoid biopsy of grossly inflamed mucosa because this can make it difficult for the pathologist to interpret the lymphocytic response. As these patients are also known to have an increased risk of non-Hodgkin's lymphoma, suspicious gland growth or change should also be biopsied. Though some may advocate superficial parotidectomy as a therapeutic measure for those with chronic sialadenitis, our experience has been that most patients will experience gland involution over time, with a reduction in number of infectious episodes.

72.7 Rehabilitation and Follow-up

Xerostomia is a lifelong problem for patients with Sjögren's syndrome. Because of the possibility of severe dental and periodontal disease associated with xerostomia, close follow-up with a dentist is highly recommended. An ophthalmologist should be consulted for regular eye examinations to monitor for ocular sequelae such as keratitis and corneal ulcerations. If an underlying rheumatologic disorder is diagnosed during work-up, the patient's management should be coordinated with a rheumatologist. Long-term follow-up with a medical provider is also recommended to help monitor for any concerning signs or symptoms of salivary or lymphoproliferative malignancy.

72.8 Questions

1. Sjögren's syndrome is associated with an increased risk of
   a) Glaucoma.
   b) Lymphoma.
   c) Adenoid cystic carcinoma.
   d) Renal failure.
2. What is the most definitive test for diagnosing Sjögren's syndrome?
   a) Schirmer's test.
   b) Anti-SSA/Ro and anti-SSB/La autoantibodies.
   c) Sialography.
   d) Minor salivary gland biopsy.
   e) Antinuclear antibodies.
3. Histopathologic analysis of a salivary gland in a patient with Sjögren's syndrome can be most expected to have which of the following?
   a) Noncaseating granulomas.
   b) Acinar cell dysplasia.
   c) Multiple lymphocytic foci.
   d) Disorganized ductal cells.

Answers: 1. b 2. d 3. c

Suggested Readings

Freeman SR, Sheehan PZ, Thorpe MA, Rutka JA. Ear, nose, and throat manifestations of Sjögren's syndrome: retrospective review of a multidisciplinary clinic. J Otolaryngol. 2005; 34(1):20–24

Mahoney EJ, Spiegel JH. Sjögren's disease. Otolaryngol Clin North Am. 2003; 36(4):733–745

Roh JL, Huh J, Suh C. Primary non-Hodgkin's lymphomas of the major salivary glands. J Surg Oncol. 2008; 97(1):35–39

Shiboski SC, Shiboski CH, Criswell L, et al. Sjögren's International Collaborative Clinical Alliance (SICCA) Research Groups. American College of Rheumatology classification criteria for Sjögren's syndrome: a data-driven, expert consensus approach in the Sjögren's International Collaborative Clinical Alliance cohort. Arthritis Care Res (Hoboken). 2012; 64(4):475–87

Stewart CM, Bhattacharyya I, Berg K, et al. Labial salivary gland biopsies in Sjögren's syndrome: still the gold standard? Oral Surg Oral Med Oral Pathol Oral Radiol Endod. 2008; 106(3):392–402

Zintzaras E, Voulgarelis M, Moutsopoulos HM. The risk of lymphoma development in autoimmune diseases: a meta-analysis. Arch Intern Med. 2005; 165(20):2337–2344

73 Dysphagia

Andrew J. Redmann and Rebecca J. Howell

73.1 History

A 75-year-old man had a long history of acid reflux treated for more than 5 years. Initially he saw a gastroenterologist who started him on a proton pump inhibitor (PPI), but since then had been seeing his primary care physician for all prescribed medications. He had been having progressive worsening of solid food dysphagia for several years. Over the past year, he reported pills and occasional undigested food particles were regurgitated several hours after a meal. At night when he lay down, he immediately started coughing. Most nights, after he coughed up mucus he was able to fall asleep without waking. He denied daytime somnolence. He was a one-half-pack-per-day smoker for 40 years. He was treated for pneumonia once last year and did have known chronic obstructive pulmonary disease (COPD). He denied voice changes, shortness of breath, or weight loss.

The patient was a well-appearing elderly gentleman. Examination of the ears, nose, throat, and neck showed no evidence of tumors or ulceration. Manual compression of the neck did not result in crepitus or a gurgling sensation. The patient had no trismus and could achieve full neck extension. Flexible laryngoscopy revealed no lesions or masses in the larynx, pharynx, or hypopharynx, but there was moderate pooling of secretions in the left pyriform sinus. Mild posterior glottic edema was also present.

73.2 Differential Diagnosis—Key Points

- Differential diagnosis for solid food dysphagia includes neoplastic (squamous cell carcinoma or adenocarcinoma of the esophagus), infectious (esophagitis), mechanical (diverticulum, foreign body, esophageal web, Schatzki's ring, cricopharyngeal dysfunction, achalasia), systemic (eosinophilic esophagitis, inclusion body myositis, dermatomyositis, scleroderma), and neurogenic (oculopharyngeal myodystrophy, Parkinson's, amyotrophic lateral sclerosis) causes. Esophageal diverticulum, and in particular Zenker's diverticulum, is the most common.
- A Zenker's diverticulum is formed at the dehiscence in the oblique muscle fibers of the inferior constrictor and the transverse muscle fibers of the cricopharyngeal muscle, also known as Killian's triangle. Zenker's diverticulum is a pulsion-type diverticulum where the pharyngeal mucosa and submucosa herniate between the muscular layers, also described as a false diverticulum (► Fig. 73.1).
- Dysphagia secondary to dysfunction of the upper esophageal sphincter, also known as cricopharyngeal hypertrophy or spasm, without hypopharyngeal pouch formation is another consideration. This may be an early precursor to development of Zenker's diverticulum. Individuals with dysphagia from cricopharyngeal dysfunction also may have a higher incidence of gastroesophageal reflux, stroke, cranial nerve palsy, and neuromuscular disease.
- Dysphagia to solids with history of tobacco abuse is a warning sign for obstructive lesions of the laryngopharyngeal complex or esophagus where primary lung cancer or mediastinal tumors can cause dysphagia due to compression.

73.3 Test Interpretation

Laryngoscopy is critical in the evaluation of dysphagia to assess for the presence of a laryngopharyngeal neoplasm. Findings specific to Zenker's diverticulum include asymmetric left-sided pooling of pharyngeal secretions in the pyriform sinus. A modified barium swallow or barium esophagram should be obtained to confirm the diagnosis. In this patient, barium coated the lining of a posterior diverticulum superior to the cricopharyngeus, and a contrast-filled pouch was readily seen, confirming the diagnosis of a Zenker's diverticulum (► Fig. 73.2). Modified barium swallow or cineradiography is preferred to evaluate cricopharyngeal dysfunction. A barium esophagram is preferred to evaluate esophageal causes of dysphagia including motility disorders (achalasia), mediastinal or esophageal masses, or other esophageal webs or strictures. Of final note, Killian-Jamieson diverticula are classically anterolateral, and Laimer's diverticula are true diverticula seen posteriorly, but lack a cricopharyngeal bar on esophagram and are found *inferior* to the cricopharyngeus.

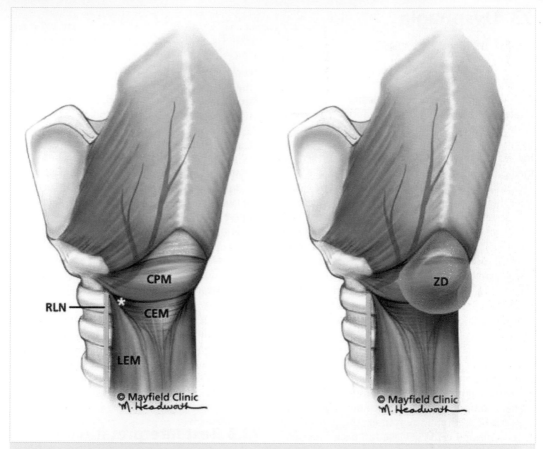

Fig. 73.1 Representation of normal anatomy of Killian's triangle from posterolateral view (CPM=cricopharyngeus, CEM=circular esophageal muscle, LEM=lateral esophageal muscle, RLN=recurrent laryngeal nerve). Note Zenker's diverticulum (ZD) extending out superiorly to the cricopharyngeus muscle. (Printed with permission from Mayfield Clinic.)

73.4 Diagnosis

Zenker's diverticulum

73.5 Medical Management

Zenker's diverticulum is typically diagnosed in patients over the age of 65. In the medically frail, who are not surgical candidates, patients can be monitored for recurrent aspiration pneumonia. A pulmonology consult may be warranted. A speech-language pathologist for dietary modifications and recommendations may be considered. However, there is a paucity of data on long-term follow-up of conservatively managed patients with Zenker's diverticulum; therefore, surgical consultation is recommended.

73.6 Surgical Management

Symptomatic Zenker's diverticula are treated surgically, especially if aspiration pneumonia or severe weight loss has occurred. Zenker's diverticulum can be treated using either an endoscopic or open approach. Regardless of technique, the critical step is performing a cricopharyngeal myotomy, thereby treating the underlying cause. The endoscopic approach has a higher failure rate; however, advantages include lower morbidity and mortality, decreased delay to oral feeding, decreased hospitalization, and decreased operative time compared to the open approach.

Endoscopic diverticulotomy opens the diverticulum into the esophagus and completes a cricopharyngeal myotomy during the resection of the common diverticular wall. A Weerda

symptoms. The advantages of the CO_2 laser include the ability to perform a complete diverticulotomy without a remnant edge at the pouch's base. Disadvantages include (1) a higher risk of perforation and mediastinitis, (2) greater risk of scarring leading to esophageal stenosis, and (3) longer hospital stay. Complications are similar to open diverticulotomy, and include esophageal leak, crepitus, and infection.

For the open transcervical approaches, diverticulectomy, diverticulopexy, or sac inversion with or without myotomy have been described in the literature. Diverticulectomy with myotomy is described here. The procedure begins with rigid esophagoscopy to confirm the surgical site. Next, sterile ribbon gauze is used to pack the diverticulum to allow for easier identification of the pouch, and a small (32Fr) bougie is placed into the esophagus to decrease risk of stenosis, all performed under direct visualization. The neck is prepped and draped in the usual sterile fashion, a cervical incision is made, and dissection is performed lateral to the thyroid gland and laryngotracheal complex to avoid injury to the recurrent laryngeal nerve. A cricopharyngeal myotomy is performed. In smaller diverticula, this is often all that is necessary to resolve symptoms. A surgical stapling device or hand-sewn repair is performed to resect the diverticulum. A passive drain should be considered and the patient is admitted for observation, and discharged on a soft diet after removal of the drain. Potential complications include pharyngocutaneous fistula, esophageal perforation, unilateral vocal cord paralysis, hematoma, and infection.

73.7 Rehabilitation and Follow-up

Repeat imaging is surgeon dependent, but in the senior author's practice is only done for clinical suspicion of esophageal perforation or recurrent symptoms. Patients often describe an immediate cessation of dysphagia and regurgitation. A head and neck examination is performed to rule out neck crepitus and unusual neck pain (abscess formation) during the immediate postoperative period and inpatient hospitalization. If significant neck pain is elicited, computed tomography (CT) of the neck with contrast is warranted to rule out postoperative abscess formation. Otherwise, the patient is discharged on a soft diet for 2 weeks.

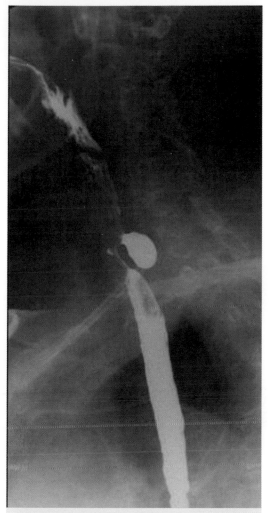

Fig. 73.2 Esophagram showing posteriorly extending Zenker's diverticulum superior to the level of the cricopharyngeus.

diverticuloscope (Karl Stortz) is used to expose both the esophagus and the diverticulum. A diverticulotomy is then performed with either a CO_2 laser, an endoscopic stapler, or a combination of both. The advantages of the stapling technique include (1) simple, efficient diverticulotomy; (2) reliable stapling and sealing of cut mucosal edges; (3) low risk of esophageal perforation or mediastinitis; and (4) outpatient surgical procedure in select patients. The disadvantages of the stapling technique include the inability to perform on small diverticula (<2.5 cm) and a potential 5- to 10-mm mucosal ridge at the base of the pouch. The remnant edge may cause persistent or recurrent

73.8 Questions

1. What should be the first test performed in a patient with solid food dysphagia?
   a) Laryngoscopy.
   b) Barium esophagram.
   c) Computed tomography (CT) of the neck.
   d) Chest X-ray.
2. Which of the following statements concerning open diverticulectomy is false?
   a) Rigid esophagoscopy with placement of packing in Zenker's pouch allows easier identification of the pouch during an open approach.
   b) Sac inversion of the pouch is an effective long-term treatment for Zenker's diverticulum.
   c) Removal of the pouch increases the risk of esophageal stenosis in the postoperative period.
   d) The pexy approach excludes the need for cricopharyngeal myotomy, decreasing the length of time for surgery.
3. The best test to diagnose a Zenker's diverticulum is
   a) Barium esophagram/modified barium swallow.

b) Rigid esophagoscopy.
c) CT of the chest.
d) CT of the neck.

Answers: 1. a 2. d 3. a

Suggested Readings

Anagiotos A, Preuss SF, Koebke J. Morphometric and anthropometric analysis of Killian's triangle. Laryngoscope. 2010; 120(6):1082–1088

Kuhn MA, Belafsky PC. Management of cricopharyngeus muscle dysfunction. Otolaryngol Clin North Am. 2013; 46(6):1087–1099

Ongkasuwan J, Yung KC, Courey MS. Pharyngeal stasis of secretions in patients with Zenker diverticulum. Otolaryngol Head Neck Surg. 2012; 146(3):426–429

Bock JM, Van Daele DJ, Gupta N, Blumin JH. Management of Zenker's diverticulum in the endoscopic age: current practice patterns. Ann Otol Rhinol Laryngol. 2011; 120(12):796–806

Verdonck J, Morton RP. Systematic review on treatment of Zenker's diverticulum. Eur Arch Otorhinolaryngol. 2015; 272(11):3095–3107

Parker NP, Misono S. Carbon dioxide laser versus stapler-assisted endoscopic Zenker's diverticulotomy: a systematic review and meta-analysis. Otolaryngol Head Neck Surg. 2014; 150(5):750–753

74 Thyroglossal Duct Cyst

Brian Ho and Sally R. Shott

74.1 History

A 3-year-old boy was brought to the office by his parents for evaluation of a neck mass first noticed 2 weeks earlier. They initially noticed swelling in the superior midline neck. It arose rapidly in association with an upper respiratory infection (URI). The mass was initially painful to palpation but had no overlying erythema. Antibiotics prescribed by his pediatrician caused the mass to decrease in size slightly, and the tenderness resolved. There was no history of difficulty eating or breathing.

On examination, there was a 11 × 1.5-cm spherical mass located 1 cm below the hyoid bone in the midline of the neck. It was cystic with no tenderness on palpation. It was not freely mobile and was noted to move in a superior/inferior fashion with swallowing and on tongue protrusion. No other cervical lymphadenopathy was present.

74.2 Differential Diagnosis—Key Points

- Thyroglossal duct cyst (TGDC): The thyroid gland originates in the tongue base (foramen cecum) and descends inferiorly through the neck to assume its final position in the pretracheal position. TGDCs are epithelial lined cysts that result if the thyroglossal duct that forms as the gland descends into neck fails to obliterate. This occurs during the development of the thyroid gland in the 8th to 10th week of gestation. Remnants of the descending thyroid tissue may also persist in the anterior compartment of the neck as either extensions of the thyroid (pyramidal lobe) or isolated bits of thyroid. TGDCs may be found anywhere from the base of tongue down to the clavicles. Lingual TGDCs may manifest as a tongue base mass without any visible abnormality in the neck. As the thyroid descends, it passes in close proximity to the hyoid bone, which can often ossify and trap thyroid tissue or the thyroglossal duct in the central portion of the hyoid. Most commonly, TGDCs present just inferior to the hyoid bone. These lesions remain either in the midline, or just adjacent to the midline. With such close association to the hyoid bone, they frequently move with swallowing as the larynx

elevates to protect itself from aspiration, or with tongue protrusion.
- Dermoid cyst: An epithelial inclusion cyst, or a dermoid, is often associated with developmental fusion planes. The dermoid is a benign accumulation of squamous debris. They may become infected and present with pain and swelling, or they may present as a solitary mass. In the neck, they are most commonly found above the level of the hyoid bone. Antibiotics have limited effect beyond management of an acute infection.
- Lymphadenopathy: Cervical adenopathy may occur in any of the nodal chains. Cervical lymph nodes are typically found laterally in the neck. Midline nodes are commonly found in the submental area in level 1A. Nodes can also be located below the level of the thyroid in level 6 or be pretracheal nodes (e.g., node of Delphi). Antibiotics will often lead to resolution of reactive lymphadenopathy.
- Branchial arch anomaly: Failure of branchial apparatus development may cause the persistence of cysts, sinuses, or fistulas in the head and neck region. The location of the anomaly and its relation to the great vessels and cranial nerves are dependent on the arch from which it is derived. Branchial arch anomalies tend to be located along the anterior border of the sternocleidomastoid muscle, not encroaching on the midline.
- Neoplasm: Neoplasms may develop in the neck and must always be considered in the evaluation of a child with a neck mass. In the pediatric population, around 10% of masses will be neoplasms. Examples of pediatric neoplasms would include lymphoma, neuroblastoma, thyroid cancer, and rhabdomyosarcoma.

74.3 Test Interpretation

- Ultrasound: Ultrasound is the primary imaging modality employed in the diagnosis of a midline neck mass. Ultrasound will demonstrate whether the mass is solid or cystic. A TGDC will appear cystic. The most important role of ultrasound is to confirm the presence of the thyroid gland in the normal position in the neck. If the thyroid is not in its normal location, further testing is needed to identify the location of functioning thyroid tissue.

- Computed tomography (CT) imaging: CT imaging is rarely needed when an anterior midline neck mass is encountered, as the location and physical characteristiccharacteristics of an anterior compartment mass often suggest the diagnosis of a TGDC. When there is doubt, a CT provides good visualization of the lesion and its anatomic relationships to other structures. It will show a low-density cystic mass (▶ Fig. 74.1). The associated thyroglossal tract, which traverses the hyoid bone and terminates in the tongue base, is rarely identified. If a CT is obtained, it is important to evaluate the films to confirm that the thyroid gland lies in its proper location at the base of the neck. It is possible that the only functioning thyroid tissue resides within the mass. CT scans are most useful in revision cases.
- Magnetic resonance imaging (MRI): MRI will provide similar anatomic details about the mass and surrounding structures as a CT. It is rarely

necessary in cases of suspected TGDC. Although it avoids ionizing radiation exposure, its higher cost and longer acquisition times decrease its utility.

- Thyroid scan: This radiolabeled iodine study shows concentration of the label within functioning thyroid tissue. This study has been used in the past to determine the presence of a normal thyroid in its normal location. Unless there is a question of normal thyroid tissue presence and function, this test is not required in the evaluation of a patient with a TGDC.
- Needle aspiration: Needle aspiration can be used to evacuate the cyst of its mucinous content and to obtain a specimen for culture and sensitivity. The contents of a noninfected cyst are generally amber colored, thick, and tenacious. It is not necessary to perform this procedure routinely because cytology is not critical to the diagnosis and may hinder palpation when surgery is necessary. If an active infection is present, an incision and drainage procedure may be necessary

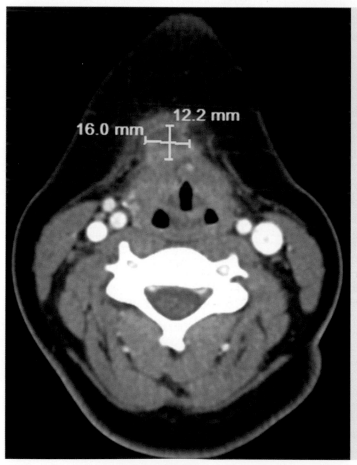

Fig. 74.1 Axial computed tomography scan with contrast demonstrating a cystic lesion closely associated with the hyoid.

to achieve resolution of the infection but may lead to tissue seeding of the skin. Therefore, oral antibiotics are the treatment of choice for acute infections, with planned excision once the infection has resolved.

74.4 Diagnosis

Thyroglossal duct cyst

74.5 Medical Management

Unless an acute infection is present, there is no role for medical management in TGDC. In the setting of infection, antibiotic treatment with coverage of *Staphylococcus* and *Streptococcus* organisms should be initiated.

If a lingual thyroid is identified, hypothyroidism must be ruled out. In this circumstance, thyroid function tests should be obtained. If a lingual thyroid is present, thyroid suppression may be necessary to suppress thyroid growth and minimize the risk of airway obstruction developing secondary to the size of the thyroid tissue within the tongue base.

74.6 Surgical Management

1. The Sistrunk procedure is the surgical approach of choice for management of a TGDC. The cyst is exposed through a horizontal neck incision. Once the cyst is isolated, the tract extending superiorly should be identified. This duct should not be skeletonized to minimize the risk of recurrence. The tissue surrounding the tract should be left attached to the stalk because small extensions or arborizations of the duct lumen are common. The middle section of the hyoid should be transected and removed with the tract. The tract should be followed into the tongue base and a core of lingual tissue should be resected. The tract is ligated and transected, taking care not to violate the tongue base mucosa. A drain should be placed in the operative bed and the incision closed in layers.
2. Care must be exercised to properly identify the hyoid bone and its relationship to the thyroid cartilage. In young children, the larynx remains high in the neck, with the hyoid overlying the thyroid cartilages. It is possible to inadvertently resect portions of the laryngeal framework, resulting in significant airway compromise.

3. The Sistrunk procedure is associated with a 3 to 5% recurrence risk. If a TGDC has been infected on several occasions before excision, the recurrence risk triples. For this reason, the surgical excision should be expedited once a history of infection within the mass has been established.

74.7 Rehabilitation and Follow-up

Wound infections tend to develop between 5 and 7 days after the operation and are associated with surrounding erythema, pain at the incision site, and purulent material below the skin flaps. A recurrent TGDC will generally present within the first few months after surgery and will be associated with a painless swelling at the incision line, with mild surrounding erythema and thick mucoid drainage below the skin flaps.

Most recurrences are located near the incision line, but they may be located anywhere along the previous tract. Initial treatment is preferably antibiotics but could require incision and drainage of the area, with packing placed to allow drainage of the material and induction of fibrosis that may obliterate the residual thyroglossal duct tissue. In most cases, however, reoperation is required.

Excision of a recurrent TGDC requires excision of the original incision line and a broad excision of the material in the anterior compartment of the neck. A defined tract may be seen that directs the excision to a specific area, but often no definable tract can be located. Small pockets of mucoid material may be found in the tissues. All these areas need to be excised.

The initial operation provides the best opportunity for complete excision of the congenital TGDC. Leaving tissue attached to the duct, resecting the central portion of the hyoid bone without extensive skeletonization of the structure, and excision of a cuff of tongue base tissue maximizes the changeschances of complete excision of the mass at the first operation.

74.8 Questions

1. Ultrasound imaging of the neck in a child with a suspected thyroglossal duct cyst (TGDC)
   a) Is necessary to determine the diagnosis of the cervical mass.
   b) Is useful to identify the presence of thyroid tissue in its normal location at the base of the neck.

c) Is less effective in providing needed information regarding the management of the patient than a computed tomography (CT) scan.

d) Should be used only for needle localization during an aspiration procedure.

2. The risk of airway complications following TGDC excisions in young children
   a) Is related to the position of the hyoid bone over the thyroid cartilage of the larynx.
   b) Is secondary to swelling caused by excision of tissue from the tongue base.
   c) Is related to infections in the neck.
   d) Is lower than in older children.

3. Doing the following during TGDC excision minimizes the risk of recurrence:
   a) Skeletonizing the tract that extends to the tongue base.
   b) Removing the entire hyoid bone after isolating it from surrounding structures.
   c) Leaving tissue at the tongue base.

d) Removing the TGDC and its tract along with adherent tissue, the central portion of the hyoid bone, and a core of tissue from the tongue base.

Answers: 1. b 2. a 3. d

Suggested Readings

Ducic Y, Chou S, Drkulec J, Ouellette H, Lamothe A. Recurrent thyroglossal duct cysts: a clinical and pathologic analysis. Int J Pediatr Otorhinolaryngol. 1998; 44(1):47–50

Hewitt K, Pysher T, Park A. Management of thyroglossal duct cysts after failed Sistrunk procedure. Laryngoscope. 2007; 117(4):756–758

Koch BL. Cystic malformations of the neck in children. Pediatr Radiol. 2005; 35(5):463–477

Wootten CT, Goudy SL, Rutter MJ, Willging JP, Cotton RT. Airway injury complicating excision of thyroglossal duct cysts. Int J Pediatr Otorhinolaryngol. 2009; 73(6):797–801

75 Cervical Lymphadenitis in Children

Thomas K. Hamilton and Charles M. Myer III

75.1 History

A 13-month-old former 36-week-premature girl with a past medical history significant for hepatitis C exposure presented with a 10-day history of bilateral posterior cervical lymphadenopathy that acutely worsened, becoming more painful and swollen, despite steroids and three courses of antibiotics. An ultrasound revealed multiple enlarged lymph nodes in the posterior cervical chains, surrounding inflammatory changes, and multiple irregular areas of hypoechogenicity within the lymph nodes bilaterally suggestive of focal suppuration. Computed tomography (CT) with contrast of the neck was then done, confirming the findings of bilateral necrotic/suppurative posterior chain adenopathy (▶ Fig. 75.1). She was admitted to the hospital for incision and drainage (I&D) and started on intravenous clindamycin. Cultures taken at the time of I&D grew methicillin-sensitive *Staphylococcus aureus*. Following the procedure, the patient was kept in the hospital with regular packing changes. Within the next few days, the patient improved clinically and was discharged home in good condition on an oral antibiotic regimen based on the culture sensitivities.

75.2 Differential Diagnosis—Key Points

1. *General considerations:* Cervicofacial lymphoid tissue can be subdivided into three general regions: region 1 tissue is in Waldeyer's ring (palatine tonsils, lingual tonsils, adenoids); region 2 covers lymph nodes in the head/face region (occipital, postauricular, preauricular, parotid, and facial lymph nodes); and region 3 covers lymph nodes in the neck region (submaxillary, submental, and deep cervical/jugular lymph nodes). In general, nodes in regions 1 and 2 all ultimately drain into the nodes of region 3, which is where the majority of cervical lymphadenitis will be detected. This is important to remember, as an enlarged lymph node in the neck may actually be a result of pathology in the oral cavity, pharynx, head, or face. Secondly, the age of the patient can help guide the initial differential diagnosis. For example, while infectious etiologies are the most common reason for lymphadenitis in general, a new onset neck mass in an adult is much more likely to be a malignancy. Certain characteristics of the mass can also help differentiate whether a new

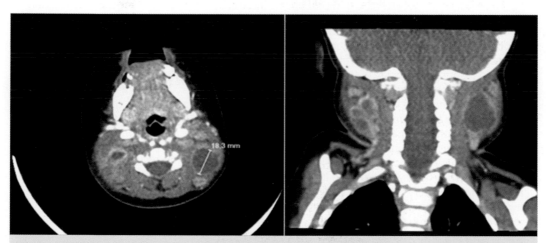

Fig. 75.1 CT with contrast of the head and neck showing bilateral necrotic/suppurative posterior cervical lymphadenopathy.

onset neck mass is likely to be infectious (soft, mobile, tender, overlying erythema, acute time course) versus neoplastic (hard, fixed to the skin, nontender, chronic time course).

2. *Acute lymphadenitis:* As described previously, infectious etiologies are the most common cause of cervical lymphadenitis in both adults and children. The pathogen can be viral, bacterial, or fungal, with self-limited viral infections being the most common overall. When not viral, acute lymphadenitis is most commonly due to *S. aureus* or *Streptococcus pyogenes.* Anaerobic bacteria can be seen in patients with preexisting dental or periodontal disease. Fungal infections are generally only seen in the immunocompromised population and are typically caused by *Candida, Histoplasma,* or *Aspergillus* species.

3. *Chronic lymphadenitis:* The most common causes of chronic lymphadenitis, which develops or persists over weeks to months, include mycobacterial infections, toxoplasmosis, and cat-scratch disease. *Mycobacterium tuberculosis* is the most common cause of chronic lymphadenitis in adults, whereas nontuberculous mycobacterial infections are more common in children. Toxoplasmosis is caused by a protozoan associated with contact with cat litter and most commonly presents in an immunocompetent patient as a discrete, firm, nontender, nonsuppurative cervical mass. Finally, cat-scratch disease, caused by the *Bartonella henselae* bacterium, will present as a single large, tender lymph node, in the setting of a recent cat scratch or cat exposure.

4. *Noninfectious causes:* Four important causes of noninfectious cervical lymphadenopathy are Kawasaki's disease (KD), Rosai-Dorfman disease, sarcoidosis, and neoplastic disease. KD is diagnosed in children with at least 5 days of fever and at least four of the following additional findings: acute, nonpurulent cervical lymphadenopathy; edema or erythema of the extremities; polymorphous exanthema; and bilateral, painless conjunctivitis and oral mucosal infectious changes. Untreated KD can lead to coronary artery disease. KD is the leading cause of acquired heart disease in children in developed countries. Rosai-Dorfman disease, also known as sinus histiocytosis, presents with fever, skin nodules, and massive nontender cervical lymphadenopathy. Sarcoidosis is an autoimmune disease that presents with constitutional symptoms and cervical lymphadenopathy along with a wide variety of other symptoms that vary based on the patient.

Finally, neoplastic disease often can be differentiated from infectious causes of cervicofacial lymphadenitis based on the characteristics of the mass. Neoplastic masses will tend to arise over a longer time period and be rock-hard, fixed in position, and nontender.

75.3 Test Interpretation

Laboratory testing and imaging is not needed for the vast majority of cases of cervical lymphadenitis. However, in certain cases directed tests can be useful. A complete blood count can be useful to help confirm the suspicion of an infectious etiology. Blood cultures and a liver panel may be indicated in severely ill or toxic-appearing patients. If a mycobacterial infection is suspected, a purified protein derivative (PPD) test and chest radiograph can be useful.

If an abscess is suspected, imaging may be useful for localization to help guide biopsy or I&D. Ultrasound is inexpensive and can distinguish between solid and cystic structures. It may be used to guide fine needle aspiration (FNA) of a neck mass for diagnostic purposes. Ultrasound also has the benefit of being noninvasive, relatively easy to perform and free of radiation exposure, which can be especially important in children. A downside of ultrasound is that it is very operator dependent. CT is another option for imaging of the neck. Abscesses are easy to identify on CT, and it is easier to distinguish general head and neck anatomy using this type of scan.

75.4 Diagnosis

Bilateral posterior chain cervical lymphadenitis with abscess formation

75.5 Medical Management

The vast majority of cases of acute cervicofacial lymphadenitis will require no therapy, as they result from self-limited viral illnesses. If a bacterial etiology is suspected, empiric antibiotic coverage should be chosen with the goal of covering *S. pyogenes* and *S. aureus.* Generally, treatment should be initiated with oral antibiotics, such as amoxicillin, amoxicillin-clavulanate or clindamycin. In more severe cases, or in those refractory to oral antibiotics, an intravenous (IV) antibiotic can be used. Commonly used IV antibiotics for this indication include a first-generation cephalosporin (e.g., cefazolin), clindamycin, or ampicillin/sulbactam.

If the patient does not respond to either oral or IV antibiotics or is getting worse, an atypical organism or noninfectious etiology should be considered. Cultures should be obtained with FNA, if possible, to help guide the next step in treatment. *Bartonella* infections often respond to azithromycin or trimethoprim-sulfamethoxazole. Cultures and sensitivities will also help guide therapy in cases of mycobacterial or drug-resistant (e.g., methicillin-resistant *S. aureus* [MRSA]) infections.

Noninfectious causes of cervical lymphadenitis are generally treated conservatively. Specifically, corticosteroids are useful in flares of sarcoidosis, and intravenous immunoglobulin (IVIG) and high-dose aspirin are used for Kawasaki's disease.

75.6 Surgical Management

Surgical management may be necessary to (1) incise and drain an abscess, (2) obtain a biopsy for pathologic analysis, or (3) remove the inflamed lymph node(s). Most cases of cervical lymphadenitis are related to self-limited viral illnesses and will not require surgical intervention. Lymphadenitis related to bacterial infections typically resolves with antibiotics. However, some patients will develop abscesses that will not respond to medical therapy alone. In these cases, a simple I&D coupled with appropriate antibiotic therapy is the gold standard of treatment.

The vast majority (70–95%) of mycobacterial lymphadenitis in the United States is attributable to nontuberculous mycobacterial infections (e.g., *Mycobacterium avium-intracellulare, Mycobacterium scrofulaceum*). The gold standard for treatment in these cases is surgical excision, with some recent evidence suggesting that a postoperative course of macrolide antibiotics may also be of some benefit. Conversely, in tuberculous mycobacterial lymphadenitis, management is primarily medical with a 12- to 18-month course of multiagent antituberculous antibiotic therapy.

75.7 Rehabilitation and Follow-up

The primary goal of follow-up in cervical lymphadenitis is to confirm the resolution of the inciting disease process. Additionally, patients with infection-related cervical lymphadenitis that ultimately require surgical intervention, such as an I&D of an abscess, should be followed to ensure appropriate wound healing. Longer-term follow-up is sometimes needed in cases of chronic lymphadenitis caused by organisms such as mycobacterium that require extended courses of antibiotics. Similarly, patients with certain noninfectious causes of their lymphadenitis may need additional specialized follow-up depending on their particular condition. For example, patients with Kawasaki's disease will need long-term cardiology follow-up to monitor potentially devastating cardiac sequelae.

75.8 Questions

1. The best imaging modality to confirm the presence of a suspected abscess associated with cervical lymphadenitis is
   a) Ultrasound.
   b) Magnetic resonance imaging (MRI).
   c) Computed tomography (CT).
   d) X-ray.
2. Possible causes of noninfectious cervical lymphadenitis include all of the following except
   a) Rosai-Dorfman disease.
   b) Kawasaki's disease.
   c) Sarcoidosis.
   d) Behcet's disease.
3. The next step in an otherwise healthy patient with tender cervical lymphadenitis is
   a) Head and neck CT.
   b) Fine needle aspiration (FNA).
   c) Close follow up with or without empiric antibiotics based on clinical picture.
   d) Complete blood count (CBC) and blood culture.

Answers: 1. c 2. d 3. c

Suggested Readings

Montoya JG, Liesenfeld O. Toxoplasmosis. Lancet. 2004; 363 (9425):1965–1976

Hurley MC, Heran MK. Imaging studies for head and neck infections. Infect Dis Clin North Am. 2007; 21(2):305–353, v–vi

Freeman AF, Shulman ST. Kawasaki disease: summary of the American Heart Association guidelines. Am Fam Physician. 2006; 74 (7):1141–1148

Dulin MF, Kennard TP, Leach L, Williams R. Management of cervical lymphadenitis in children. Am Fam Physician. 2008; 78(9):1097–1098

Dash GI, Kimmelman CP. Head and neck manifestations of sarcoidosis. Laryngoscope. 1988(1);50–53

Al-Dajani N, Wootton Sh. Cervical lymphadenitis, suppurative parotitis, thyroiditis, and infected cysts. Infect Dis Clin North Am. 2007; 21(2):523–541

Brigger MT, Cunningham MJ. Malignant cervical masses in children. Otolaryngol Clin North Am. 2015; 48(1):59–77

Cunningham MJ. The management of congenital neck masses. Am J Otolaryngol. 1992; 13(2):78–92

76 Deep Neck Space Abscess

Colin R. Edwards and Charles M. Myer IV

76.1 History

A 40-year-old woman presented to the emergency department with a 5-day history of progressive right neck pain and swelling, limiting her range of motion. In addition, she noted subjective fevers, chills, and dysphagia to both solids and liquids. There was no history of stridor, shortness of breath, or recent trauma. She was an intravenous (IV) drug user and shared needles with other users. She was unsure of her human immunodeficiency virus (HIV) status.

On exam, the patient was uncomfortable appearing but nontoxic. Her temperature was 102.7 °F. She was tachycardic with a heart rate (HR) of 117 but normotensive. She had an 8-cm area of swelling and induration on her right neck, lateral to the sternocleidomastoid muscle. The skin was warm with blanching erythema, but there was no obvious fluctuance or skin changes. Intra-orally, she had poor dentition but no tender or loose teeth. Her tongue and pharyngeal mucosa were within normal limits. Her tonsils were 2 + and symmetric, and there was no trismus or uvular deviation. She was breathing comfortably without stridor or retractions. Laboratory studies showed a leukocytosis with bandemia. A computed tomography (CT) scan of the neck was performed in the emergency department (▶ Fig. 76.1).

76.2 Differential Diagnosis—Key Points

- The constellation of features in this patient's history and physical examination signifies the high likelihood of a deep neck space infection. Symptoms of cellulitis, warmth, erythema, edema, and induration with associated pain should clue the physician to include abscess on the differential diagnosis. IV drug use and needle sharing can cause bacteremia and are associated with the development of abscesses. Odontogenic infections, from dental carries, are the most common cause of cervical abscess formation in adults. In patients with head and neck cancer or cervical metastases, abscesses can arise in necrotic lymph nodes and may be the first sign of malignancy.
- In contrast, children are more likely to have deep neck space infections following common infections, with tonsillitis and pharyngitis being the two most common causes of deep neck space infection. Retropharyngeal abscesses are typically seen in children less than 6 years of age, as the retropharyngeal lymph nodes tend to involute later in childhood. Other potential causes of pediatric neck abscess include superinfection of a congenital branchial cleft cyst or thyroglossal duct cyst. Some causes of deep neck space infections are not specific to children or adults. Any

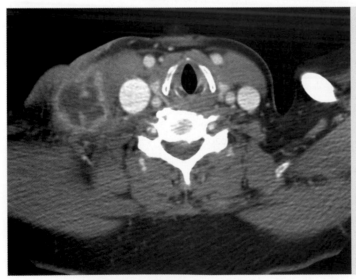

Fig. 76.1 A CT scan of the neck with IV contrast demonstrating a 3-cm ring-enhancing mass posterior to the right sternocleidomastoid muscle with surrounding edema and fat stranding, consistent with an abscess. Note the slight airway deviation to the contralateral side from significant soft tissue edema.

age group may develop an abscess secondary to trauma, surgery, sialadenitis, mastoiditis, or thyroiditis. In approximately 20% of cases a cause of infection is not identified.

- Deep neck space infections can occur at any point along the length of the neck. The deep cervical fascial planes lay medial to the platysma and are divided into the superficial, middle or visceral, and deep layer. Neck spaces are further classified as suprahyoid, infrahyoid, or those that span the entire length of the neck. Suprahyoid spaces include the peritonsillar, masticator, temporal, buccal, parapharyngeal, parotid, and submandibular spaces. Knowledge of the anatomy of the spaces helps to determine the etiology of infection and is useful for surgical planning. The danger space consists of a plane between the visceral and deep layers of cervical fascia that extends up to the skull base and down to the posterior mediastinum. Infections of the danger space can lead to intracranial extension or mediastinitis with grave consequences. Ludwig's angina is a floor of mouth cellulitis, typically from an odontogenic infection. Ludwig's angina involves infection of the bilateral submandibular, sublingual, and submental spaces, causing posterior displacement of the tongue with the potential for the development of airway obstruction.
- Medical comorbidities can contribute to the development of deep neck space infections. Immunodeficiency from HIV, poorly controlled diabetes, chronic steroid use, or chemotherapy may impair the body's ability to fight infection. In some cases, a complete blood count (CBC) may show leukopenia, reflecting the patient's underlying immunodeficiency. Atypical organisms including *Mycobacterium avium* complex (MAC) are often seen in patients with HIV.

76.3 Test Interpretation

Assessment of the patient should begin with a thorough history including associated symptoms and temporal course, previous throat or neck infections, and any medical comorbidities. A set of vitals should be collected, and tachycardia or hypotension may suggest sepsis. IV access should be obtained immediately, and fluid resuscitation should be ordered.

Neck mass or infection can be associated with airway compromise from compression secondary to mass effect or edema. Flexible laryngoscopy can be used to assess the airway and is mandatory in patients who present with dyspnea, stridor, or hypoxemia. Pulse oximetry may provide information regarding respiratory status. Blood gas analysis can provide further information but is often not necessary to make clinical decisions regarding the need for respiratory support.

Laboratory testing should include CBC with differential, renal panel, and blood cultures. A leukocytosis with bandemia is often seen in cases of deep neck space infections. If the patient is immunocompromised, then leukopenia, rather than leukocytosis, may be observed. In the setting of pharyngitis, rapid strep and monospot tests can be useful for identifying the underlying etiology. In patients with sepsis, electrolyte abnormalities may be present and should be corrected to prevent cardiovascular complications in a potentially unstable patient.

Imaging is useful both to diagnose and to localize the infection. Anteroposterior (AP) and lateral airway films may be useful in patients with respiratory distress or if a retropharyngeal abscess is suspected. On lateral plain films prevertebral soft tissue thickening at the C6 vertebrae greater than half of the height of the corresponding vertebral body is indicative of a retropharyngeal process. A computed tomography (CT) scan with IV contrast is the gold standard for diagnosing a deep neck space abscess. The abscess will appear as a ring-enhancing mass with central hypodensity and associated lymphadenopathy, and surrounding edema is often observed. CT can be helpful for differentiating abscess from a neck mass or other acute pathology with similar presentation. In addition, the CT may provide information regarding the underlying nidus of infection, including suppurative lymphadenitis, infected branchial cleft anomaly, or lymphatic malformation. Magnetic resonance imaging (MRI) has the benefit of better definition of soft tissue planes, and no radiation is used. However, CT imaging is faster, easier to obtain, and typically adequate for characterizing the lesion. Ultrasound can also be a valuable tool for identifying drainable fluid collections in deep neck space infection because it is fast and portable and does not subject the patient to ionizing radiation.

76.4 Diagnosis

Deep neck space abscess of the visceral vascular space, involving the posterior triangle of the neck.

76.5 Medical Management

The initial assessment of a patient with a deep neck space infection should focus on determining airway patency and degree of respiratory compromise. Ludwig's angina, as well as retropharyngeal, parapharyngeal, and anterior visceral space infections, may cause airway compression, leading to stridor, increased work of breathing, and oxygen desaturations. Flexible fiberoptic laryngoscopy should be performed to assess for airway patency. Steroids, oxygen, and positive pressure ventilation can temporize a tenuous airway. If there is concern for impending airway collapse, then the airway should be secured with endotracheal intubation. Awake flexible fiberoptic intubation is usually preferable, as direct laryngoscopy may be difficult in the presence of intraoral swelling or trismus. If the airway cannot be secured from above, then an awake tracheostomy can be performed. Sedation and paralytics should be avoided out of concern for further depressing respiratory drive and decreasing muscle tone in a tenuous airway.

Medical therapy should be expedited in patients with deep neck space infections, particularly those who present with hemodynamic instability, suggesting sepsis. IV access should be obtained and fluid resuscitation initiated upon arrival. Hyperglycemia is frequently encountered in poorly controlled diabetics, increasing the risk for infection due to impaired host defences and increased substrate for organism growth. Electrolyte abnormalities may be encountered as well, and electrolytes should be replaced as necessary to restore normal physiologic values. Any carious teeth should be addressed for source control of the infection.

Antibiotic therapy is tailored to the suspected organisms. Oropharyngeal flora are the most common organisms and may include *Streptococcus* spp., *Staphylococcus aureus, Fusobacterium,* and *Bacteroides* spp. Other gram-negative organisms including *Haemophilus influenzae, Escherichia coli,* and *Klebsiella pneumoniae* may occasionally be observed. Hospitalized patients with potential nosocomial infections should raise the suspicion for possible *Pseudomonas aeruginosa* infection. Patients with immune compromise, including those with diabetes or HIV or those affected by chronic steroid use or chemotherapy treatment, are susceptible to additional organisms including *Mycoplasma* spp., *Pneumocystis carinii, Toxoplasma gondii,* and fungal and other atypical infections.

Blood cultures can be collected as part of the initial work-up, and empiric antibiotic therapy should be initiated against oral flora. Ampicillin/sulbactam or ceftriaxone is appropriate antimicrobial therapy for otherwise healthy individuals. In patients with a penicillin allergy, clindamycin is an acceptable treatment alternative. If the patient has a history of previous methicillin-resistant *S. aureus* infection, then vancomycin may be advisable. Piperacillin/tazobactam, ticarcillin/clavulanate, imipenem/cilastin, or ciprofloxacin plus clindamycin can be used if *Pseudomonas* species are suspected or if there is a concern for immunocompromise. If imaging fails to demonstrate a focal abscess, a trial of 24 to 48 hours of medical therapy is undertaken. If there is clinical improvement over this time, then the patient can be transitioned to oral antibiotics. In those patients with symptom persistence or progression, repeat imaging should be performed. An infectious disease consult may be indicated for complex infections or for patients with multiple medical comorbidities complicating treatment.

76.6 Surgical Management

Surgical intervention is indicated when there is a definitive abscess identified on physical exam or imaging or when patients have failed to improve despite appropriate medical therapy. Incision and drainage is the primary treatment for deep neck space infections. Specimens should be collected from the abscess and sent for aerobic and anaerobic culture and Gram stain, as well as any additional cultures, such as acid fast or fungal, that may be indicated based on the clinical picture. Tissue sampling and pathologic examination may be indicated in select cases, such as to rule out malignancy or invasive disease.

The surgical approach is dictated by the location and extent of the abscess. Imaging should be thoroughly reviewed prior to surgical intervention, with particular attention paid to the great vessels and other important structures in the neck. Drainage of retropharyngeal, parapharyngeal, and peritonsillar abscesses is usually performed via an intraoral approach. Peritonsillar abscesses may be drained at bedside under local anesthesia in the teenage and adult population. The majority of deep neck space infections are drained via a transcervical approach, with the specific incision dependent on the site of the abscess. A drain or packing material will often be placed to prevent reaccumulation, to be removed 24 to 72 hours after surgery.

76.7 Rehabilitation and Follow-up

Patients should be observed in the hospital for at least 24 hours after surgery. Cultures should be followed and antibiotics adjusted based on sensitivities. When the patient has shown clinical improvement after source control and IV antibiotics, then they can be transitioned to oral antibiotics and discharged to home. Close follow-up is necessary to ensure resolution. Incomplete drainage or reaccumulation of the abscess is possible and may require prolonged antibiotics and repeat drainage. Underlying sources of infection or anatomic anomalies should be addressed once the acute infection has resolved.

76.8 Questions

1. A 43-year-old man presents to the emergency department with fevers, chills, neck pain, swelling, and shortness of breath. All of the following diagnoses would be high on your differential except
   a) Sialadenitis.
   b) Odontogenic infection.
   c) Retropharyngeal abscess.
   d) Carotid sheath abscess.
   e) Ludwig's angina.
2. In a patient with a deep neck space infection and a tenuous airway, all of the following measures may be appropriate except
   a) Flexible fiberoptic intubation.
   b) Steroids and BiPAP.
   c) Rapid sequence intubation with direct laryngoscopy.
   d) Awake tracheostomy.
3. Ludwig's angina typically arises from what kind of infection?
   a) Peritonsillar.
   b) Masticator space.
   c) Sialadenitis.
   d) Pretracheal.
   e) Odontogenic.

Answers: 1. c 2. c 3. e

Suggested Readings

Baldassari CM, Howell R, Amorn M, Budacki R, Choi S, Pena M. Complications in pediatric deep neck space abscesses. Otolaryngol Head Neck Surg. 2011; 144(4):592–595

Barzan L, Tavio M, Tirelli U, Comoretto R. Head and neck manifestations during HIV infection. J Laryngol Otol. 1993; 107(2):133–136

Daramola OO, Flanagan CE, Maisel RH, Odland RM. Diagnosis and treatment of deep neck space abscesses. Otolaryngol Head Neck Surg. 2009; 141(1):123–130

Reynolds SC, Chow AW. Life-threatening infections of the peripharyngeal and deep fascial spaces of the head and neck. Infect Dis Clin North Am. 2007; 21(2):557–576, viii

Roscoe DL, Hoang L. Microbiologic investigations for head and neck infections. Infect Dis Clin North Am. 2007; 21(2):283–304, v

Tom MB, Rice DH. Presentation and management of neck abscess: a retrospective analysis. Laryngoscope. 1988; 98(8 Pt 1):877–880

Vieira F, Allen SM, Stocks RM, Thompson JW. Deep neck infection. Otolaryngol Clin North Am. 2008; 41(3):459–483, vii

Part XII

Sleep

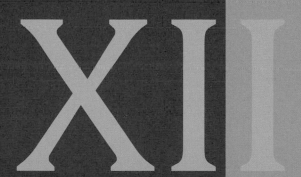

77 Pediatric Obstructive Sleep Apnea

David F. Smith and Stacey L. Ishman

77.1 History

A 10-year-old boy presented with parent-reported snoring, choking, and gasping at night. He also slept with his head extended backward and would routinely wake up with his sheets bunched up or off the bed. His mother was very concerned that he had intermittent periods where he stopped breathing at night. He also began to have bed-wetting after approximately 5 years without nocturnal enuresis. He was doing well in school without behavioral issues. He went to bed at 9 p.m. on weeknights and woke up on his own at 6 a.m. He had no other medical history and took no medications except for a children's multivitamin.

On physical exam, he was a healthy, nonobese boy with a body mass index (BMI) of 24 kg/m². He appeared developmentally appropriate for his age. His oropharyngeal examination revealed a single uvula, 3 + tonsils, normal dentition, and a modified Mallampati's score of 2. He had full neck range of motion with no palpable cervical lymphadenopathy. On nasopharyngoscopy, the inferior turbinates and adenoids were both moderately enlarged.

Based on the history and physical exam findings, the mutual decision was made for him to undergo outpatient adenotonsillectomy for sleep disordered breathing (SDB). His operative and postoperative courses were uncomplicated. He was followed up in the clinic 6 weeks after the procedure. His symptoms had slightly improved; however, his mother reported that he still had loud nightly snoring, choking at night, and episodes of apneas.

77.2 Differential Diagnosis—Key Points

Primary snoring: Snoring without evidence of apneic events, gas exchange abnormalities, or sleep fragmentation is referred to as primary snoring. Snoring is also a frequent presenting symptom of obstructive sleep apnea (OSA). Although primary snoring has traditionally been considered a benign disease, research suggests that snoring can be associated with elevated blood pressures, poor school performance, and an increase in systemic inflammatory markers. Snoring can be diagnosed by clinical history, but a sleep study is frequently used to differentiate between snoring and OSA.

77.2.1 Nocturnal Gastroesophageal Reflux Disease

Patients with nocturnal gastroesophageal reflux disease can present with nighttime coughing and choking and restless sleep. Symptoms will typically include abdominal or chest pain, chronic cough, and sore throat. Children with significant disease can also present with apneas, stridor, or apparent life-threatening events. Diagnosis often includes a diagnostic trial of H_2 blocker medication, manometry, and/or esophagogastroduodenoscopy. A sleep study would commonly be reserved for children with signs or symptoms of OSA after reflux treatment is initiated.

77.2.2 Obstructive Sleep Apnea

This patient presented with signs and symptoms consistent with SDB, a spectrum of disorders that range from primary snoring to OSA. OSA is characterized by partial or complete upper airway obstruction during sleep. When untreated, it results in changes to sleep structure and gas exchange that can lead to a host of clinical sequelae, including poor school performance, metabolic abnormalities, cardiovascular and pulmonary morbidities, and neurocognitive deficits.

OSA occurs in 2 to 4% of children in the United States and is most commonly attributed to adenotonsillar hypertrophy. Adenotonsillectomy (T&A) is first-line treatment for OSA, with resolution rates of 80% in otherwise healthy children. Despite these good results, it is now clear that as many as 40% of children have persistent disease after T&A. For these children, evaluation and further treatment must be individualized.

The patient presented in this clinical vignette had SDB with persistent symptoms after T&A. The following diagnostic testing should be considered to determine if OSA is present.

77.3 Test Interpretation

Polysomnography (PSG) is the gold standard method to diagnosis OSA. It includes the recording of multiple physiologic measures, including airflow, respiratory effort, oxygen saturation, and end-tidal CO_2, which provide objective measurement of disease severity. The severity of OSA is reported using the apnea-hypopnea index (AHI), which is the average number of apneas and hypopneas per hour of sleep. In children, mild OSA is defined as an AHI of 1 to < 5 events/hour, moderate is defined as an AHI of 5 to < 10 events/hour, and severe OSA is defined as an AHI of ≥ 10.

Despite the PSG being the gold standard for diagnosis of OSA, 90% of children undergoing T&A for SDB have not undergone a PSG. The decision to forgo a PSG is often made based upon the fact that the results will not change the clinical decision to perform T&A, as well as the cost and limited availability of this test for children. When utilized, preoperative PSG allows for identification of factors (severe OSA, high carbon dioxide levels) that predict which patients have a higher likelihood of postoperative respiratory complications. As an alternative, screening questionnaires were developed to predict the presence of OSA; the Pediatric Sleep Questionnaire (PSQ) is the most reliable and frequently used screening tool.

Children with OSA will sometimes present with intermittent hemoglobin desaturations. Thus, pulse oximetry studies are used as an inexpensive diagnostic alternative to PSG. A positive oximetry study is very good at predicting the presence of OSA; however, a negative study cannot be used to rule out OSA, as the negative predictive value of this test is less than 20%.

For children that fail to improve after T&A, there are no national treatment guidelines established.

Children typically undergo a physical examination in the clinic that may involve awake flexible laryngoscopy to evaluate for adenoid regrowth, lingual tonsil hypertrophy, or supraglottic collapse. Drug-induced sleep endoscopy (DISE) is also frequently used to determine the site or sites of upper airway obstruction; this is typically performed using flexible nasopharyngoscopes or bronchoscopes during light sedation in an attempt to replicate airway collapse during sleep. This diagnostic technique can be useful for children who cannot tolerate continuous positive airway pressure (CPAP) or who prefer to consider a surgical option.

Similar to DISE, cine magnetic resonance imaging (MRI) is used to evaluate the site of upper airway obstruction for children with persistent OSA. Cine MRI provides a high-resolution image of the dynamic airway, without the radiation risk associated with computed tomography (CT), and allows for complete evaluation of the airway in children who might not otherwise tolerate awake flexible nasopharyngoscopy. It also allows for good visualization of primary and secondary sites of airway obstruction.

The patient presented in this clinical vignette did not have complete resolution of symptoms after the T&A. For this reason, an appropriate next step would be to obtain a PSG as a means to determine the severity of OSA. The PSG demonstrated an AHI of 13 and an oxygen nadir of 78%. DISE performed while in the operating room demonstrated lingual tonsillar hypertrophy (▶ Fig. 77.1), and the cine MRI confirmed circumferential collapse at the tongue base.

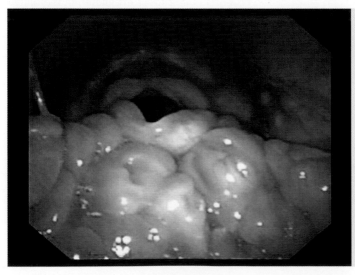

Fig. 77.1 Lingual tonsil hypertrophy in a pediatric patient with persistent OSA.

77.4 Diagnosis

- Severe persistent obstructive sleep apnea
- Lingual tonsillar hypertrophy

77.5 Medical Management

There are limited data regarding the use of medicine for the treatment of pediatric OSA. Intranasal topical steroids can reduce or resolve the severity of disease in children with mild OSA. However, the long-term outcomes with intranasal steroids are unclear. Leukotriene modifiers, like montelukast, have also been shown to decrease the AHI by three to four events/hour when used alone or in combination with intranasal steroids.

Weight loss has also been shown to improve or ameliorate OSA for children with mild to moderate OSA who are overweight or obese. Further, for obese children with severe OSA, weight loss and bariatric surgery have also been shown to reduce CPAP requirements and may lead to resolution of OSA in a subset.

The most common medical therapy recommended for children with persistent OSA in the United States is CPAP. Nasal CPAP has been routinely used in children who fail T&A or have contraindications to surgery since 2006. A CPAP titration is commonly performed in the sleep laboratory in order to determine the appropriate CPAP level at which obstructive events are eliminated. Risks associated with long-term CPAP use include skin breakdown and midfacial growth restriction. While CPAP is effective for the treatment of OSA, the majority of children cannot tolerate this therapy and eventually discontinue use.

Oral appliances are also available as a means to enlarge the upper airway using mandibular or tongue advancement; however, they are typically reserved for older children with secondary dentition. Recent data suggest that mild OSA in children with malocclusion can be safely and effectively treated with the use of oral appliances. Children with high arched palates can be treated with palatal expanders, often between 6 and 12 years of age, which can improve both occlusion and OSA at the same time.

77.6 Surgical Management

T&A is the first-line treatment for OSA in children. For children with persistent OSA, evaluation of adenoid hypertrophy or tonsil regrowth (especially for children who underwent tonsillotomy/

partial tonsillectomy) is part of the initial clinical evaluation. Children with moderate to severe OSA often have obstruction at multiple levels. Recommended surgical management in children should be driven by the anatomic site of upper airway obstruction, including evaluation of the nasal cavity, nasopharynx, oropharynx, hypopharynx, and larynx. The most commonly reported sites of obstruction for children with persistent OSA are the tongue base and the supraglottis (with sleep state–dependent laryngomalacia).

Surgeries of the nasal cavity include, but are not limited to, septoplasty and inferior turbinate reduction. Surgeries to expand the nasopharyngeal space include adenoidectomy and maxillary advancement. Surgeries to improve space in the oropharynx include tonsillectomy and uvulopalatopharyngoplasty. Finally, surgeries that increase space in the hypopharynx include lingual tonsillectomy, partial midline glossectomy, hyoid myotomy and suspension, tongue suspension, and mandibular advancement. Lateral hypopharyngeal collapse may be addressed with expansion pharyngoplasty.

In children with significant disease and other medical comorbidities, such as neurologic impairment or severe cardiopulmonary disease, a tracheostomy may be considered. This therapy may also be recommended for children that need staged surgery for multilevel obstruction. In these children, the goal is to decannulate the children once the surgeries are completed.

77.7 Rehabilitation and Follow-up

This patient underwent T&A as the primary treatment. Despite the initial surgical therapy, he returned to the treating physician with similar untreated symptoms and signs. These patients should be followed with PSG. Also, patients that receive further second-line surgical therapies should be monitored postoperatively with follow-up sleep studies.

77.8 Questions

1. Which of the following tests is the gold standard to diagnose obstructive sleep apnea?
   a) Pulmonary function test.
   b) Polysomnography.
   c) Pulse oximetry.
   d) Chest computed tomography (CT).
   e) Multiple sleep latency test.

2. What is the most common medical therapy recommended for children that have persistent obstructive sleep apnea (OSA) in the United States?
   a) Continuous positive airway pressure (CPAP).
   b) Oral appliance.
   c) Uvulopalatopharyngoplasty.
   d) Distraction osteogenesis.
   e) Septoplasty.
3. Which sign is not typical of nocturnal gastro-esophageal reflux disease?
   a) Stridor.
   b) Chronic cough.
   c) Bedwetting.
   d) Apparent life-threatening events.

Answers: 1. b 2. a 3. c

Suggested Readings

Section on Pediatric Pulmonology, Subcommittee on Obstructive Sleep Apnea Syndrome. American Academy of Pediatrics. Clinical practice guideline: diagnosis and management of childhood obstructive sleep apnea syndrome. Pediatrics. 2002; 109(4):704–712

Baugh RF, Archer SM, Mitchell RB, et al. American Academy of Otolaryngology-Head and Neck Surgery Foundation. Clinical practice guideline: tonsillectomy in children. Otolaryngol Head Neck Surg. 2011; 144(1) Suppl:S1–S30

Bhattacharjee R, Kheirandish-Gozal L, Spruyt K, et al. Adenotonsillectomy outcomes in treatment of obstructive sleep apnea in children: a multicenter retrospective study. Am J Respir Crit Care Med. 2010; 182(5):676–683

Chervin RD, Hedger K, Dillon JE, Pituch KJ. Pediatric sleep questionnaire (PSQ): validity and reliability of scales for sleep-disordered breathing, snoring, sleepiness, and behavioral problems. Sleep Med. 2000; 1(1):21–32

Lumeng JC, Chervin RD. Epidemiology of pediatric obstructive sleep apnea. Proc Am Thorac Soc. 2008; 5(2):242–252

Manickam PV, Shott SR, Boss EF, et al. Systematic review of site of obstruction identification and non-CPAP treatment options for children with persistent pediatric obstructive sleep apnea. Laryngoscope. 2016; 126(2):491–500

Redline S, Tishler PV, Schluchter M, Aylor J, Clark K, Graham G. Risk factors for sleep-disordered breathing in children. Associations with obesity, race, and respiratory problems. Am J Respir Crit Care Med. 1999; 159(5 Pt 1):1527–1532

Roland PS, Rosenfeld RM, Brooks LJ, et al. American Academy of Otolaryngology—Head and Neck Surgery Foundation. Clinical practice guideline: Polysomnography for sleep-disordered breathing prior to tonsillectomy in children. Otolaryngol Head Neck Surg. 2011; 145(1) Suppl:S1–S15

78 Adult Obstructive Sleep Apnea

Christine H. Heubi and Stacey L. Ishman

78.1 History

A 43-year-old man presented with a history of loud snoring and restless sleep that had worsened in the past few years. His wife endorsed gasping and choking at night. He reported extreme tiredness while driving, but denied motor vehicle accidents. He often needed to nap in the evening after coming home from work, slept 8 hours per night, and typically woke up feeling unrefreshed. He often woke with a headache and reported a 20-lb weight gain in the last year. His father had a history of obstructive sleep apnea (OSA) and used a continuous positive airway pressure (CPAP) machine. The patient was seen previously by a pulmonologist, who ordered an overnight polysomnogram (PSG) and started him on auto-PAP for a diagnosis of moderate OSA. He had been unable to tolerate the machine due to nasal obstruction and the sensation of suffocation when he wore his full face mask. His past medical history was significant for hypertension requiring two antihypertensives, and exercise-induced asthma. He was referred to the office to discuss surgical options for the management of his OSA.

Physical examination revealed an obese man (body mass index [BMI] = 38 kg/m^2) with a neck circumference of 18 inches. Oropharyngeal examination revealed a large tongue obscuring the pharynx and soft palate (modified Mallampati III) with lateral tongue grooving. He had a high arched palate, but no evidence of retrognathia, and class I occlusion. Use of a tongue depressor revealed a floppy uvula and soft palate, with small 1 + tonsils. Nasal examination revealed bilateral inferior turbinate hypertrophy with leftward septal deviation and an inferior septal spur on the right. Occlusion of the right nare revealed limitation in leftward nasal flow that was reproduced on the opposite side as well. Mild right external nasal valve collapse was noted, with improvement in breathing with the Cottle's maneuver.

78.2 Differential Diagnosis—Key Points

This patient presented with a diagnosis of OSA based on an in-laboratory PSG, which is the gold standard for diagnosis. He also demonstrated many of the key clinical features of OSA, including daytime somnolence, nonrestorative sleep, loud snoring, frequent nighttime awakenings, choking or gasping during sleep, and witnessed apnea by the bed partner. Additionally, in conjunction with the symptoms above, his past medical history of obesity and refractory hypertension increased his risk for OSA. Additional risk factors include atrial fibrillation, congestive heart failure, cerebral vascular accident, type 2 diabetes, pulmonary hypertension, high-risk driving populations, and patients undergoing evaluation for bariatric surgery.

OSA results from repetitive upper airway collapse during sleep that leads to sleep fragmentation, hypercarbia, hypoxemia, oscillations in intrathoracic pressure, and increased sympathetic activity. If left untreated, this can lead to secondary conditions including hypertension, cor pulmonale, cerebral vascular accidents (CVAs), myocardial infarction, motor vehicle collisions, and decreased daytime alertness.

The severity of disease must be determined before a treatment plan can be established. Objective testing for OSA is performed by two accepted methods: an in-laboratory PSG, or home testing with portable monitoring (PM). PM is only recommended when there is a high pretest probability of moderate to severe OSA. It is not indicated in patients with significant comorbid conditions such as moderate to severe pulmonary disease, neuromuscular disease, or congestive heart failure, or in those patients in whom a comorbid sleep disorder is present. The diagnosis of OSA can be made if any of the above symptoms are present and there are at least five respiratory events (apneas, hypopneas, or respiratory-associated arousals) per hour of sleep. Additionally, in the absence of any of the above symptoms, the diagnosis can be made if there are 15 or more respiratory events per hour of sleep on PSG.

78.3 Test Interpretation

In determining a patient's candidacy for surgical management, the physical exam is of the utmost importance, and special attention should be focused on identification of areas of obstruction. Physical exam findings consistent with OSA in this patient included neck circumference > 17 inches (> 16 in females), obesity (BMI ≥ 30 kg/m^2), high arched palate, modified Mallampati ≥ 3, macroglossia suggested by lateral tongue grooving, enlarged uvula, and nasal abnormalities. He did not have retrognathia or lateral peritonsillar narrowing, which are also associated with OSA.

Awake flexible fiberoptic nasopharyngoscopy in the upright and reclined position is an easily performed office procedure that can be useful to identify nasal obstruction, adenoid hypertrophy, lingual tonsil hypertrophy, and base of tongue obstruction. The Mueller's maneuver, having the patient suck in against a closed nose and mouth, is a traditional method of evaluation that has fallen out of favor. However, evaluation of the airway during end expiration may further reveal lateral pharyngeal wall collapse. Drug-induced sleep endoscopy (DISE) is a commonly utilized diagnostic tool for adults with OSA, as it allows for a dynamic airway evaluation in a sleeplike state in an operating room or endoscopy suite, and is a more accurate estimation of the pattern of collapse. However, it requires sedation and knowledgeable anesthesia staff to administer properly.

The Epworth Sleepiness Scale (ESS) is an eight-question patient-administered questionnaire that can help assess the degree of daytime sleepiness that is present, with a score above 10 (range 0–24) considered suggestive of sleepiness. This can be helpful when counseling patients about avoidance of activities that worsen sleepiness, including drowsy driving.

A PSG is the gold standard test used for the diagnosis of OSA that is reported with the apnea-hypopnea index (AHI) to determine disease severity; an AHI of 5 to 15 events/hour is considered mild, 16 to 30 events/hour is considered moderate, and greater than 30 events/hour is considered severe OSA. Oxygen desaturation is reported as the proportion of time with oxygen levels below 90%, as well as the lowest oxygen saturation; both serve as a measure of OSA disease severity and can suggest underlying pulmonary disease. Coexistent sleep disorders such as periodic limb movement disorder or central sleep apnea syndrome may also be identified on PSG.

This patient's in-laboratory PSG revealed an AHI of 25, with his lowest oxygen saturation of 82% consistent with moderate OSA. His awake fiberoptic examination revealed significant leftward septal deviation with enlarged inferior turbinates, right greater than left, and hypopharyngeal obstruction, primarily at the base of the tongue. His ESS was markedly elevated at 15, consistent with excessive daytime somnolence.

78.4 Diagnosis

Moderate obstructive sleep apnea

78.5 Medical Management

Adult OSA is a chronic disease that necessitates a long-term management plan and a multidisciplinary approach with close follow-up. Ideally, the patient is an active participant in management decisions that may include behavioral, medical, and/or surgical options. Behavioral modification is frequently used in conjunction with other treatment modalities, and should be discussed with all patients with OSA. Specific recommendations include the avoidance of driving while drowsy, the need for significant weight loss (to a BMI < 25 kg/m^2) in obese patients, exercise, positional therapy, and avoidance of sedatives and alcohol before bedtime.

The mainstay of treatment for adults with OSA is PAP therapy, and it should be offered as an option for all patients with moderate or severe disease, as well as those with mild OSA who are symptomatic or have significant comorbidities. The positive pressure functions to maintain airway patency and effectively eliminate pharyngeal collapse and resultant obstruction. PAP therapy can be administered continuously (CPAP), as bilevel, or as auto-PAP (APAP). It is very effective when used consistently; proper mask fitting and elimination of nasal obstruction are essential for successful PAP use. The amount of positive pressure, reported in centimeters of water (cm H$_2$O), is determined during a titration in the sleep laboratory or through auto-titrating devices. The effectiveness of this therapy is dependent on nightly adherence to treatment, with some patients unwilling or unable to comply with PAP use. Because of the high effectiveness of CPAP when tolerated, repeated efforts should be made to optimize therapy for those having difficulty adjusting to the device, particularly in the first few weeks after initiation. Referral to an otolaryngologist is often considered when there is a need for interventions to improve CPAP tolerance such as medical or surgical relief of nasal obstruction. In this regard, an inhaled nasal corticosteroid can be efficacious and aid in mask tolerance. In addition, the pressure from a PAP machine many induce vasomotor rhinitis with resultant obstruction and should be considered; ipratropium spray (0.06%) can be useful for these patients. In addition, nasal valve collapse should be assessed in these patients. CPAP adherence downloads, symptoms, and the ESS can be used to clinically assess the efficacy of CPAP.

For patients who are unable to tolerate CPAP, oral appliances may be a treatment option. These devices are designed to pull the jaw or the tongue forward and have traditionally been recommended for patients with mild to moderate disease. More recently, providers have started to consider these devices for all patients with OSA intolerant to CPAP, even those with severe disease. Custom-made adjustable appliances are preferred to prefabricated devices, as they are more likely to completely ameliorate OSA while minimizing dental malocclusion and temporomandibular joint symptoms. Close follow-up with a dentist is recommended. Once device adjustment is felt to be sufficient, typically when snoring resolves, repeat PSG with the device in place is strongly recommended to confirm improvement in OSA. Oral devices may also be used in conjunction with CPAP, as the device may help with proper mask fitting.

Pharmacologic treatment of OSA is limited but may occasionally include the use of stimulants, such as modafinil, to treat daytime somnolence in patients who are compliant with CPAP.

78.6 Surgical Management

Surgery is most frequently employed as salvage therapy for people who have failed CPAP therapy or for those unwilling to consider long-term CPAP use, with success rates of multilevel surgery typically noted to be in the 50 to 70% range. However, for patients with an obvious source of obstruction, such as tonsillar hypertrophy, surgical cure may be attempted as first-line therapy. Surgical management of adults with OSA requires identification of the level(s) of obstruction in order to appropriately individualize treatment. In order to identify obstructing anatomy, DISE is frequently employed as an adjunct to the clinical exam, particularly in cases where the level of obstruction is not clear. The DISE findings serve as the basis for surgical management, most commonly focused on three areas of obstruction: nasal, retropalatal, and retroglossal.

A careful nasal exam is necessary to determine nasal patency. There is little data to suggest that septoplasty or inferior turbinate reduction alone is curative for OSA, but both have been reported to aid in PAP tolerance. A meta-analysis by Ishii et al showed that overall, nasal surgery for patients with OSA and nasal obstruction improves some sleep parameters, namely ESS and RDI, but does

not significantly change the AHI. However, two prospective studies showed a reduction in AHI of 11 events/hour. For patients who present with CPAP intolerance or who remove their mask unintentionally at night, the presence of nasal obstruction should be identified. Medical therapy with nasal steroids and treatment of comorbid conditions, such as allergic rhinitis, should be initial treatment. Patients should also be screened for vasomotor rhinitis and treated with steroid or iptratropium nasal spray if this screen is positive. If these medical options are unsuccessful, septoplasty and/or inferior turbinate reduction should be considered.

As a curative measure, tonsillectomy is typically reserved for young, nonobese patients with significant tonsil hypertrophy (3–4+). A recent systematic review and meta-analysis looked at evidence for tonsillectomy as an isolated treatment for adult OSA. The authors found a 65.2% reduction in AHI, but carefully noted that all of the patients had significant tonsillar hypertrophy. Furthermore, outcomes were better for patients who were nonobese with mild to moderate disease. There is no evidence to support tonsillectomy as a curative measure for OSA in adults without evidence of tonsillar hypertrophy. Tonsillectomy may, however, be helpful in patients with CPAP intolerance.

Unlike nasal surgery or tonsillectomy, which have both been shown to improve PAP tolerance, palatal procedures are solely utilized as part of salvage surgery for OSA. Uvulopalatopharyngoplasty (UP3) is a common surgical procedure performed for adults with OSA, but it should be approached with caution, as it may worsen mask leak if there is excessive soft palate resection. For this reason, several techniques have been developed that minimize uvular removal and resection of the entire posterior palate. UP3 (which includes tonsil removal) is most effective for adults with minimal palate obstruction (modified Mallampati's position I or II) and tonsillar hypertrophy (3+ to 4+), with a BMI < 40 kg/m^2; the reported resolution rate for this group is 81%. In patients with minimal palatal obstruction and 1+ or 2+ tonsils, as well as those with significant palatal obstruction (modified Mallampati's position III or IV) and tonsillar hypertrophy, the resolution rate is modest at 37%. Lastly, in patients with significant palatal obstruction (Friedman's palate position III or IV) and minimal tonsillar hypertrophy, the resolution rate is very low, at 8%. Given these results, and because many adults with OSA have a BMI > 40 kg/m^2, newer palatal procedures have been introduced, such as relocation pharyngoplasty, lateral pharyngoplasty, and expansion sphincter pharyngoplasty. Preservation of palatal musculature and posterior soft palatal mucosa is advocated to minimize the risk of development of velopharyngeal insufficiency or nasopharyngeal stenosis.

Because of the limited effectiveness of isolated palate surgery for most adults, and the observation that tongue base obstruction is present in up to 80% of OSA patients, multiple procedures to address retroglossal collapse have been developed. The goal of these procedures is to increase the space between the tongue base and the posterior pharyngeal wall by tongue base reduction and/or tongue repositioning; these are typically performed as part of multilevel surgery in order to yield greater success.

Options for tongue base reduction include radiofrequency ablation of the tongue base, posterior midline glossectomy, and lingual tonsillectomy. Radiofrequency ablation to the tongue base can reduce tissue volume with minimal morbidity and can be performed in the office with the patient under local anesthesia, but it requires multiple treatments to be effective. Posterior midline glossectomy more effectively reduces tongue base volume by removing muscle, and studies have shown success rates ranging from 23 to 77% when combined with other procedures. There is minimal data on lingual tonsillectomy in adults, but when found on flexible laryngoscopy, removal is prudent because the tissue crowds the retroglossal space; pediatric studies summarized by Manickam et al note resolution of OSA in 57 to 88% of cases.

Tongue base repositioning procedures include anterior mandibular osteotomy with genioglossus advancement, tongue suspension, hyoid myotomy and suspension (HMS), and hypoglossal nerve stimulator placement. Genioglossus advancement procedures are performed using a limited mandibular osteotomy with advancement and fixation of the mandibular segment and attached genioglossus muscle to the lower anterior mandible. In an attempt to reduce the morbidity of genioglossus muscle advancement with mandibular osteotomy, systems have been developed for tongue suspension with a suture secured to the mandible. HMS can be performed with suspension of the hyoid to the thyroid cartilage or the mandible, and can be quite effective when combined with tongue base reduction or a palatal procedure. The hypoglossal nerve stimulator, approved for use by the Food and Drug Administration in 2014, treats base of tongue obstruction by activating the genioglossus

muscle during inspiration and opening the airway. It has also been shown to increase the retropalatal airway through activation of the palatoglossus muscle and/or anterior displacement of the tongue, allowing the palate to fall forward. The stimulator is implanted as an isolated procedure and is indicated for adults who have moderate to severe OSA, are intolerant to CPAP, and have an AHI > 20 but < 65 events/hour without evidence of circumferential collapse at the level of the palate on DISE. Initial trials with the device included patients with a BMI < 32 kg/m^2 and revealed significant improvements in quality of life measures as well as AHI.

Maxillomandibular advancement (MMA) allows for advancement of both the maxilla and the mandible through bilateral sagittal splits and LeFort's I osteotomies to enlarge the entire posterior pharyngeal airway. MMA has been found to be 80 to 90% effective at ameliorating OSA, and can be considered as first-line therapy in patients with midface and/or mandibular hypoplasia. Its use is limited due to changes in facial profile and dental occlusion.

Bariatric surgery is effective to reduce both the BMI and the AHI in morbidly obese patients (BMI > 35–40 kg/m^2) with OSA who are unable to tolerate CPAP or for whom it is ineffective. The benefits of bariatric surgery obviously include improvement in OSA as well as improvement of other obesity-related comorbidities, and this therapy may be recommended as part of a combination therapy plan. The effectiveness of bariatric surgery for resolution of OSA depends on the weight loss achieved. A 2013 systematic review evaluated this question and found that 75% of patients had improvement or resolution of their OSA, although many patients still had OSA levels (AHI > 15) that would require CPAP after weight reduction.

Tracheotomy can be curative for patients with OSA. A 2014 systematic review of the effect of tracheostomy on OSA reported that the mean AHI resolved after surgery and sleepiness and mortality both improved. Tracheostomy may be necessary in morbidly obese patients (BMI > 40 kg/m^2) with life-threatening OSA who cannot tolerate, or do not benefit from, CPAP and have failed all other surgical options. It may also be selected for patients with significant comorbidities who need timely resolution of their OSA. However, because it is associated with social stigma, significant ongoing care management issues, and inability to participate in water sports, it is not readily accepted as a treatment option by most patients.

78.7 Rehabilitation and Follow-up

This patient was unable to tolerate auto-PAP due to significant nasal congestion. Given the exam findings of significant septal deviation and bilateral inferior turbinate hypertrophy, and after a trial of medical therapy, he was taken to the operating room for DISE, septoplasty, and bilateral turbinate reduction. Tonsillectomy and UP3 were not considered given his 1 + tonsils and Friedman-Friedman's palate position III, as success rates for patients with this clinical exam are very low. His DISE revealed nasal obstruction, as was seen on clinical exam, minimal collapse at the level of the palate, and anterior-posterior collapse at the tongue base with evidence of lingual tonsil hypertrophy and glossoptosis. He recovered well from his septoplasty and bilateral inferior turbinate reduction and underwent a split-night PSG 3 months after the procedure. His residual obstructive AHI was 18 events/hour, and he was started on CPAP of 7 cm H_2O with nasal pillows as his mask device. At his follow-up visit, 1 month after CPAP initiation, his adherence report showed device usage 5 nights per week for 70% of the night. He reported a 5-lb weight loss, and his ESS was 5. His morning headaches had resolved, and he was no longer napping after work. He was encouraged to use his CPAP every night. When he asked about possible additional surgical options, posterior midline glossectomy, lingual tonsillectomy, and tongue suspension were discussed. He plans to continue to work on his CPAP to improve compliance with the help of the providers in the CPAP clinic, and he will consider additional surgery if he is unsuccessful. He will be seen back in clinic in 3 months with a CPAP compliance download.

78.8 Questions

1. Which of the following has not been found to be helpful for improvement in continuous positive airway pressure (CPAP) tolerance?
   a) Septoplasty.
   b) Uvulopalatoplasty (UP3).
   c) Tonsillectomy.
   d) Bilateral inferior turbinate reduction.
   e) Oral appliance.
2. Which of the following clinical exam findings indicates the highest likelihood of success with a UP3?
   a) 1 + tonsils, Friedman's palate position I.
   b) 3 + tonsils, Friedman's palate position IV.
   c) 4 + tonsils, Friedman's palate positon II.
   d) 4 + tonsils, Friedman's palate position III.
   e) 2 + tonsils, Friedman's palate position III.
3. In which patient is a home sleep test with portable monitoring indicated?
   a) A 40-year-old nonobese man, no past medical history, with apneic pauses, snoring, and daytime somnolence.
   b) An 82-year-old woman with congestive heart failure and snoring.
   c) A 35-year-old obese man with frequent nighttime awakenings and chronic obstructive pulmonary disease (COPD).
   d) A 26-year-old man with REM behavioral disorder and gasping and snoring at night.

Answers: 1. b 2. c 3. a

Suggested Readings

Camacho M, Certal V, Brietzke SE, Holty JE, Guilleminault C, Capasso R. Tracheostomy as treatment for adult obstructive sleep apnea: a systematic review and meta-analysis. Laryngoscope. 2014; 124 (3):803–811

Camacho M, Li D, Kawai M, et al. Tonsillectomy for adult obstructive sleep apnea: A systematic review and meta-analysis. Laryngoscope. 2016; 126(9):2176–2186

Epstein LJ, Kristo D, Strollo PJ, Jr, et al. Adult Obstructive Sleep Apnea Task Force of the American Academy of Sleep Medicine. Clinical guideline for the evaluation, management and long-term care of obstructive sleep apnea in adults. J Clin Sleep Med. 2009; 5 (3):263–276

Friedman M, Ibrahim H, Bass L. Clinical staging for sleep-disordered breathing. Otolaryngol Head Neck Surg. 2002; 127(1):13–21

Randerath WJ, Verbraecken J, Andreas S, et al. European Respiratory Society task force on non-CPAP therapies in sleep apnoea. Non-CPAP therapies in obstructive sleep apnoea. Eur Respir J. 2011; 37 (5):1000–1028

Smith DF, Cohen AP, Ishman SL. Surgical management of OSA in adults. Chest. 2015; 147(6):1681–1690

Sarkhosh K, Switzer NJ, El-Hadi M, Birch DW, Shi X, Karmali S. The impact of bariatric surgery on obstructive sleep apnea: a systematic review. Obes Surg. 2013; 23(3):414–423

XIII

79 Choanal Atresia

Michael A. DeMarcantonio and Catherine K. Hart

79.1 History

The neonatal intensive care unit (NICU) requested the evaluation of a 1-day-old full-term male newborn. The pregnancy was otherwise uncomplicated, with an uneventful delivery and normal initial Apgar's scores. After birth, the patient was noted to have progressive respiratory distress, nasal flaring, and suprasternal retractions. There was no report of stridor. The patient was supported initially with nasal cannula with little effect and was subsequently intubated, without difficulty, with an appropriately sized endotracheal tube. Following intubation, NICU staff noted an inability to pass a 6 French nasal cannula through either nostril.

The physical examination revealed an intubated patient. Head and neck examination was normal with the exception of bilaterally small and abnormally shaped pinnae. Flexible nasal endoscopy was performed, revealing thickened secretions and an inability to advance the scope into the nasopharynx.

79.2 Differential Diagnosis—Key Points

- Choanal atresia: Choanal atresia occurs in 1 in 7,000–8,000 births and more commonly presents as unilateral, in females, and on the right side. Bilateral atresia may be associated with CHARGE syndrome. Atresia is described as bony, membranous, or mixed. Historically, 90% of cases were described as bony and 10% membranous. More recent research has described only 30% of atresia as purely bony with the remaining 70% a mix of bony and membranous.
- CHARGE syndrome: CHARGE syndrome is a rare genetic disorder with an incidence ranging from 0.1 to 1.2 in 10,000 live births. The syndrome has six defining features: coloboma, heart defects, atresia of the choanae, retardation, genital anomalies, and ear anomalies. Choanal atresia may result in obstructed breathing in up to 65% of patients. Ear anomalies may include abnormal pinnae and hearing loss.
- Pyriform aperture stenosis: Congenital pyriform aperture stenosis is a rare cause of neonatal respiratory distress. This malformation may occur in isolation, or with other associated midline deformities on the holoprosencephaly spectrum. Other associated head and neck findings include a single maxillary central incisor, absent upper labial frenulum, midface hypoplasia, and cleft palate.
- Major septal deviation: Birth or fetal trauma may lead to significant septal deviation. However, this finding is usually unilateral, and typically presents with mild symptoms.
- Nasal cavity mass: Nasal cavity masses such as teratoma and congenital dacryocystocele should be considered in all neonates with obvious nasal obstruction.

79.3 Test Interpretation

In cases of suspected choanal atresia, computed tomography (CT) scan should be performed to rule out nasal masses, evaluate for pyriform stenosis, and assist with surgical planning. CT scan in this child demonstrated evidence of a bilateral, mixed, but predominately bony choanal atresia (▶ Fig. 79.1). Additional imaging showed cochlear hypoplasia, underdeveloped semicircular canals, an aberrant facial nerve course, and evidence of ocular colobomas.

Given the likelihood of CHARGE syndrome, additional testing is warranted. Genetics should be consulted for a complete evaluation and possible testing. The CHD7 gene represents the most common mutation and typically occurs as a new autosomal dominant mutation with no family history.

CHARGE syndrome is associated with both sensorineural and conductive hearing loss. An auditory brainstem response (ABR) test should be performed. In cases of profound sensorineural hearing loss, magnetic resonance imaging (MRI) is required to confirm normal cochlear nerve anatomy prior to considering a cochlear implant. All children with suspected CHARGE syndrome should also be evaluated by cardiology and have an echocardiogram performed prior to surgical intervention.

The patient was scheduled for a microlaryngoscopy, bronchoscopy, and nasal endoscopy. A rigid 4-mm Hopkins rod telescopic unit was used for evaluation of the airway. The supraglottis, glottis, sublgottis, and trachea were all normal. The airway

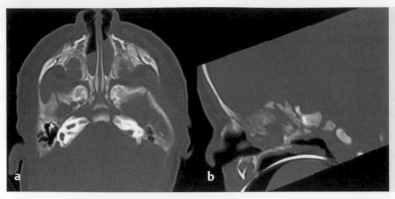

Fig. 79.1 CT scan from a patient with bilateral choanal atresia and CHARGE malformation. (a) Axial and (b) sagittal CT images demonstrating a mixed bony/membranous atresia. Note the postobstructive fluid levels in the nasal cavity anterior to the atresia site.

was sized with an age-appropriate endotracheal tube.

The nasal cavities were then decongested with oxymetazoline-soaked pledgets and evaluated using a rigid nasal endoscope. Bilateral choanal atresia was noted. The decision was made to proceed with the endoscopic repair of bilateral choanal atresia.

79.4 Diagnosis

Bilateral choanal atresia with associated CHARGE syndrome

79.5 Medical Management

Patients with bilateral choanal atresia and CHARGE syndrome must be treated in a multidisciplinary fashion. Patients will likely require evaluation and treatment by genetics, speech pathology, cardiology, ophthalmology, urology, and endocrinology.

79.6 Surgical Management

In patients with significant comorbidities or cardiopulmonary instability, a tracheostomy may be required prior to definitive surgical repair. Once stable, the patient should proceed to operative repair of the atresia. Surgical options include transpalatal repair, transnasal puncture, and transnasal endoscopic repair.

79.6.1 Transpalatal Repair

The transpalatal technique involves the elevation of a palatal flap and drilling of the atresia plates, posterior vomer and medial pterygoid plates. This approach has been associated with a high rate of primary success but has also been linked to palatal

deformities, cross-bite, and velopalatal insufficiency. Due to these associated morbidities, the transpalatal technique is not recommended in children < 6 years of age and is rarely performed.

79.6.2 Transnasal Puncture

This procedure utilizes a 120-degree scope or laryngeal mirror to visualize the atretic plate from the nasopharynx. The area of atresia is then dilated with progressively larger urethral sound dilators. This technique can be considered in small infants where endoscopic visualization may be difficult. Transnasal puncture alone should be avoided in children with CHARGE syndrome due to unacceptably high rates of restenosis. This technique is often performed in combination with an endoscopic repair.

79.6.3 Transnasal Endoscopic Repair

The endoscopic transnasal technique has emerged as the procedure of choice with pediatric otolaryngologists. In this technique a 2.9- or 4.0-mm endoscope is used to visualize the atretic plate. A laterally based mucosal flap is first raised to expose the atretic plate. Using powered instruments or pediatric sinus instruments, the thinnest portion of the plate is then removed, followed by removal of the posterior bony septum. Transnasal puncture can also be used to create the initial opening prior to performing the posterior septectomy. Only one-third of the bony septum may be removed to prevent abnormal nasal growth; however, an adequate posterior septectomy is essential for success. The mean success rate using transnasal endoscopic repair was 85.3% in a large review.

The rarity of congenital choanal atresia has led to the publication of a large number of single-institution case series with small sample sizes. To date there have been no randomized controlled trials evaluating the treatment of congenital choanal atresia. As a result, there is currently no consensus on recommended surgical technique. There also remains no consensus on the use of postoperative stents or stent duration. Given this patient's presumed CHARGE diagnosis, a combined transnasal puncture with endoscopic technique was used.

79.7 Rehabilitation and Follow-up

Following surgery, children must be followed closely for evidence of restenosis with serial endoscopic evaluations. Frequent nasal irrigations and repeat endoscopy with removal of nasal crusting should be performed during the postoperative period. These interventions are particularly important in cases were stenting is not used. Symptoms such as increased work of breathing, nasal flaring, and unexplained desaturations should raise concern for possible restenosis and prompt repeat endoscopy and revision as required.

79.8 Questions

1. Choanal atresia
   a) Occurs commonly in 1 in 100 births.
   b) Is more frequently bilateral.
   c) Most frequently presents as a mix of bony and membranous atresia.
   d) Occurs more commonly in males.
2. The transnasal puncture technique
   a) Is associated with high rates of restenosis in children with CHARGE syndrome.
   b) Should not be used in young children.
   c) Utilizes a 0-degree endoscope to visualize the atretic plate.
   d) Involves performing a wide posterior septectomy.
3. All of the following are true in regard to CHARGE syndrome except
   a) CHARGE is commonly associated with single midline central incisor.
   b) CHARGE is associated with a new autosomal dominant mutation of the CHD7 gene.
   c) Ear anomalies may include abnormal pinnae and hearing loss.
   d) Auditory brainstem response (ABR) should be performed in children with suspected CHARGE syndrome.

Answers: 1. c 2. a 3. a

Suggested Readings

Durmaz A, Tosun F, Yldrm N, Sahan M, Kvrakdal C, Gerek M. Transnasal endoscopic repair of choanal atresia: results of 13 cases and meta-analysis. J Craniofac Surg. 2008; 19(5):1270–1274

Hsu P, Ma A, Wilson M, et al. CHARGE syndrome: a review. J Paediatr Child Health. 2014; 50(7):504–511

Kwong KM. Current Updates on Choanal Atresia. Front Pediatr. 2015; 3:52

80 Juvenile Nasopharyngeal Angiofibroma

Andre M. Wineland and Alessandro de Alarcon

80.1 History

A 16-year-old boy was referred by his pediatrician to evaluate nasal obstruction and recurrent epistaxis. His nasal obstruction had been refractory to antihistamines and nasal steroids for the past 4 months. His epistaxis was predominately on the left side, but it can be bilateral. In the past 3 weeks, his epistaxis had become a daily event. He presented to the local emergency room for further evaluation. He denied any history of facial trauma. He denied headache, facial pain or numbness, or change in his vision.

His medical history was notable for seasonal allergies, for which he took over-the-counter antihistamines and nasal steroids. He had no drug allergies. He had no surgical history. On physical examination, he had a deviated nasal septum and pooling of thick mucoid secretions within the left nasal cavity. He had no cranial nerve deficiencies. His vision was normal and he had full range of extraocular motion. The oral cavity and oropharynx were unremarkable. Nasopharyngoscopy demonstrated a fleshy red mass filling the left nasal cavity (▶ Fig. 80.1).

80.2 Differential Diagnosis—Key Points

The differential diagnosis of a child with a nasal mass is extensive: encephalocele, glioma, nasal dermoid, hemangioma, teratoma, hamartoma, nasolacrimal duct cyst, nasalveolar cyst, nasal polyps, antrochoanal polyp, nasopharyngeal angiofibroma, hemangiopericytoma, squamous papilloma, inverted papilloma, sinus mucocele, lymphoma, esthesioneuroblastoma, lymphoid hyperplasia, rhabdomyosarcoma, or carcinoma.

Juvenile nasopharyngeal angiofibroma (JNA) is the most common type of benign nasopharyngeal tumor, accounting for 0.05% of all head and neck tumors. It is the most common vascular mass in the nose. JNA has a frequency of 1 in 5,000 to 60,000 otolaryngology patients. Onset is most commonly in the second decade and rare in patients older than 25 years. JNA occurs exclusively in males; females diagnosed with JNA should undergo genetic testing.

JNAs arise near the posterior attachment of middle turbinate close to the superior aspect of the sphenopalatine foramen. There are multiple theories about JNA etiology. When compared to normal nasal mucosa, JNAs are associated with increased hormonal receptors and elevated vascular endothelial growth factor (VEGF). Nonchromaffin paraganglionic cells have been found on the terminal branches of the maxillary artery. Alterations of p53 and Her-2/neu on chromosome 17 have also been associated with JNA. Desmoplastic response of the nasopharyngeal periosteum or embryonic fibrocartilage during the development of the cranial bones between the basiocciput and

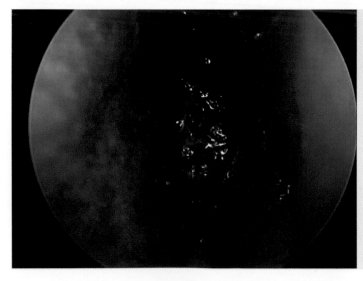

Fig. 80.1 Nasal endoscopic image of a vascular lesion obstructing the left nasal cavity.

basisphenoid has also been proposed as a possible causative factor. Because this tumor arises near the sphenopalatine foramen and is slow growing, it is not uncommon to have extension from the nasal cavity into the pterygopalatine fossa. Additional patterns of spread include into the nasopharynx, paranasal sinuses, infratemporal fossa, orbital cavity, intracranial, cavernous sinus, and intradural. The most frequent symptom associated with JNA is nasal obstruction (80–90%); less common findings include epistaxis (45–60%), headache (25%), and facial swelling (10–18%). On physical examination, the nasal mass typically appears as a red, smooth, mucosa-covered mass in the nasal cavity and nasopharynx. JNA is an aggressive benign neoplasm with a recurrence rate that can be as high as 50%.

80.3 Test Interpretation

Although not routinely ordered, plain-film findings include displacement of the nasal septum and erosion of the sphenoid, hard palate, or medial maxillary sinus. Computed tomography (CT) with contrast and/or magnetic resonance imaging (MRI) are often included in the initial work-up of nasal mass. A slow-growing nasal mass can produce subtle bowing of the posterior wall of the maxillary antrum. However, bony erosion is pathognomonic for JNA. This particular finding is often called the antral sign or Holman-Miller sign.

MRI provides additional anatomic details to define the extent of tumor extension in relation to the dura, which impacts staging. With proper imaging, a biopsy is rarely indicated. Common histologic findings include "staghorn-shaped" vessels

that lack smooth muscle (▶ Fig. 80.2). VEGF and vimentin are typically positive. Adjuvant therapy may be applicable in tumors that express testosterone and estrogen receptors.

Several staging systems for JNA have been published based on the extent and location of the tumor. The majority of these staging systems were developed before the widespread use of endoscopic approaches. The University of Pittsburgh Medical Center (UPMC) published a new endoscopic staging system for JNA. Unique to this staging system, tumor size and extent of sinus disease are less important than the tumor vascularity and the route of skull base involvement, which often limits complete tumor resection (▶ Table 80.1).

In this case, the CT revealed an enhancing polypoid nasopharyngeal mass that was centered in the posterior nasopharynx near the sphenopalatine foramen with extension along the posterior nasopharyngeal mucosa obliterating the nasopharyngeal airway (▶ Fig. 80.3). The posterior wall of the left maxillary sinus was bowed anteriorly and thinned. Within the left greater wing of the sphenoid, there was destruction and bony remodeling. Tumor extended into the left sphenoid sinus without erosion of the skull base. The bony nasal septum was eroded with deviation into the right nasal cavity. There was no intracranial involvement and no extension into the oropharynx, oral cavity, or orbit.

80.4 Diagnosis

Juvenile nasopharyngeal angiofibroma, UPMC stage II

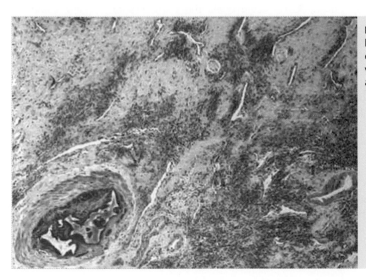

Fig. 80.2 Fixed hematoxylin and eosin histologic slide with multiple vascular clefts without muscular walls. A large vessel with a normal muscular wall is also seen.

Table 80.1 University of Pittsburgh Medical Center (UPMC) staging of JNA

Stage	UPMC staging system
I	Nasal cavity, medial pterygopalatine fossa
II	Paranasal sinuses, lateral pterygopalatine fossa; no residual vascularity
III	Skull base erosion, orbit, infratemporal fossa; no residual vascularity
IV	Skull base erosion, orbit, infratemporal fossa; residual vascularity
V	Intracranial extension, residual vascularity; medial/lateral extension

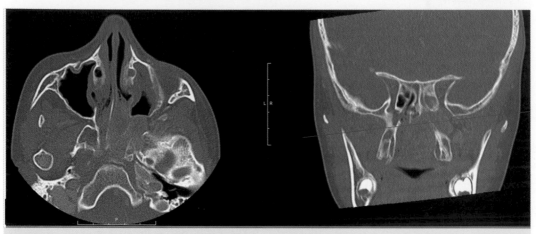

Fig. 80.3 Axial CT revealing expansion of the pterygopalatine fossa and anterior bowing of the posterior wall of the left maxillary sinus.

80.5 Medical Management

JNA is a surgically managed disease. However in families who refuse surgery or when the morbidity of surgery outweighs the risk, nonsurgical options must be explored.

Since one of the predominant theories of JNA etiology is hormonally based, antiandrogen medications have been a focus of research in the management of JNA. Flutamide is a drug used in treating prostate cancer. It is an antagonist of the androgen receptor. Although there are only a small number of patients reported in the literature, preoperative treatment with flutamide appears well tolerated and better suited for postpubertal patients in providing presurgical partial regression.

Both external beam radiation and CyberKnife treatments have been reported in the literature in the management of JNA. A multidisciplinary approach is often warranted in the management of higher-stage tumors.

80.6 Surgical Management

The preferred management for JNA is complete surgical removal. Prior to advanced endoscopic techniques, the morbidity of surgery could be quite significant with the incorporation of lateral rhinotomy and craniotomy approaches. Currently, even advanced skull based tumors can often be approached completely endoscopically.

Given that these tumors are vascular in origin, angiography is often incorporated for further evaluation and preoperative embolization. Residual vascularity after embolization is a prognostic variable in the UPMC angiofibroma staging system. The main blood supply generally comes from the internal maxillary artery or the ascending pharyngeal artery (▶ Fig. 80.4).

Tumors with intracranial extension with incomplete embolization have the highest rates of residual tumor, as they are usually firmly attached to the ICA, and are often managed via staged procedures because of excessive blood loss. The UPMC

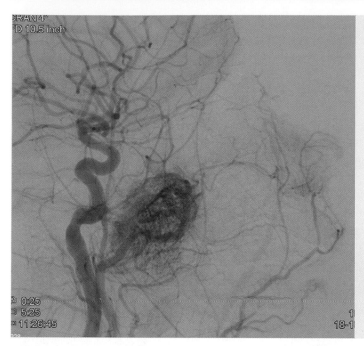

Fig. 80.4 Angiogram revealing the blush of the nasopharyngeal angiofibroma.

staging system divides these stage V tumors based on the relationships to the paraclival and cavernous segments of the ICA. The tumors that spread laterally often require combined endonasal and infratemporal approaches.

This case illustrates management of a stage II JNA. Preoperative embolization was performed 24 hours prior to surgery to reduce intraoperative blood loss. By decreasing intraoperative bleeding, embolization also improves endoscopic visualization. Complete tumor removal was performed using an endoscopic approach. The patient remained in the intensive care unit for overnight monitoring and was discharged home on postoperative day (POD) 1.

80.7 Rehabilitation and Follow-up

Given the lower tolerance for in-office nasal endoscopy with débridement in pediatric patients, he returned to the operating room on POD 10. At 6 months a repeat MRI was obtained, and no evidence of recurrence was seen. Surveillance may be performed with in-office endoscopy to visualize the resection site and postoperative MRI imaging on a yearly basis if there is suspicion for regrowth or residual tumor.

80.8 Questions

1. Which of following have been used as medical treatments in management of juvenile nasopharyngeal angiofibroma (JNA)?
   a) Adriamycin.
   b) Decarbazine
   c) External beam radiation.
   d) Gamma Knife.
   e) Flutamide.
   f) All of the above.
2. Girls with JNA should undergo what testing?
   a) Sex hormone levels for possible hirsutism.
   b) Attention-deficit hyperactivity disorder levels.
   c) Karyotype and sex chromosome analysis for testicular feminization.
   d) Complete coagulation studies.
   e) Pregnancy test.
3. What is the most appropriate preoperative imaging work-up for an obstructing nasal mass?
   a) Computed tomography (CT).
   b) Magnetic resonance imaging (MRI).
   c) Angiography.
   d) CT, embolization.
   e) A and B.

Answers: 1. e 2. c 3. e

Suggested Readings

Beham A, Kainz J, Stammberger H, Auböck L, Beham-Schmid C. Immunohistochemical and electron microscopical characterization of stromal cells in nasopharyngeal angiofibromas. Eur Arch Otorhinolaryngol. 1997; 254(4):196–199

Bremer JW, Neel HB, III, DeSanto LW, Jones GC. Angiofibroma: treatment trends in 150 patients during 40 years. Laryngoscope. 1986; 96(12):1321–1329

Fagan JJ, Snyderman CH, Carrau RL, Janecka IP. Nasopharyngeal angiofibromas: selecting a surgical approach. Head Neck. 1997; 19 (5):391–399

Herman P, Lot G, Chapot R, Salvan D, Huy PT. Long-term follow-up of juvenile nasopharyngeal angiofibromas: analysis of recurrences. Laryngoscope. 1999; 109(1):140–147

Sessions RB, Bryan RN, Naclerio RM, Alford BR. Radiographic staging of juvenile angiofibroma. Head Neck Surg. 1981; 3(4):279–283

Snyderman CH, Pant H, Carrau RL, Gardner P. A new endoscopic staging system for angiofibromas. Arch Otolaryngol Head Neck Surg. 2010; 136(6):588–594

Thakar A, Gupta G, Bhalla AS, et al. Adjuvant therapy with flutamide for presurgical volume reduction in juvenile nasopharyngeal angiofibroma. Head Neck. 2011; 33(12):1747–1753

Wiatrak BJ, Koopmann CF, Turrisi AT. Radiation therapy as an alternative to surgery in the management of intracranial juvenile nasopharyngeal angiofibroma. Int J Pediatr Otorhinolaryngol. 1993; 28 (1):51–61

81 Cleft Palate

Nathan D. Wiebracht and J. Paul Willging

81.1 History

A female infant was delivered at 39 weeks' gestation to a healthy mother. Apgar scores were 7 and 10. Initial physical examination in the newborn nursery demonstrated abnormal facies with downward-slanting palpebral fissures and micrognathia. Intraoral exam revealed a cleft of the secondary palate. Additionally, the auricles were abnormally small.

The infant experienced no respiratory distress in the postnatal period, but she experienced feeding difficulty with frequent choking episodes. After transitioning to a special cleft palate bottle and nipple, feedings improved significantly. A genetics consultation was obtained, and the infant was diagnosed with Treacher Collins syndrome. The child returned to her birth weight by the end of the first week of life, and the family was discharged home with close follow-up.

At 10 months of age, the palate was repaired and tympanostomy tubes were inserted for chronic middle ear effusions. By 36 months of age, she had achieved normal speech and resonance.

81.2 Differential Diagnosis—Key Points

- The embryologic sequence necessary for normal closure of the palate includes (1) an intrinsic force that enables the palatal shelves to change from a vertical to a horizontal orientation, (2) migration of the tongue in an anteroinferior direction away from the shelves, and (3) palatal fusion. The configuration of the skull base and the size and migration of the tongue and mandible may be responsible for the development of an isolated cleft of the palate.
- When the aforementioned process is disrupted, Pierre Robin's sequence may occur. This sequence consists of (1) mandibular hypoplasia, (2) glossoptosis, and (3) midline cleft of the palate. The sequence usually occurs as an isolated triad of abnormalities but occasionally constitutes part of more complex entities such as trisomy 18 or Stickler syndrome. The cause of cleft palate in Pierre Robin's sequence is thought to be from retropositioning or underdevelopment of the mandible, leading to upward displacement of the tongue, which then blocks the palatal shelves from fusing medially. The resultant gap between the palatal shelves is the cleft in the palate.
- A cleft palate should alert the clinician to the possibility of other anomalies or associated syndromes. A genetic consultation is advisable. Other anomalies, such as 22q11 deletion syndrome, can occur in up to 50% of patients with cleft palate. The most common anatomic systems that present with abnormalities associated with a cleft palate involve the nervous, musculoskeletal, and cardiovascular systems.
- Palatal clefts represent one of the most frequently occurring congenital deformities. The frequency is higher in whites (1.34 per 1,000 births) than in blacks (0.41 per 1,000 births). The chances for a future offspring to have an isolated cleft palate are (1) one sibling has a cleft with no parent with a cleft, 2%; (2) one sibling has a cleft with one parent with a cleft, 17%; and (3) no sibling with a cleft with one parent with a cleft, 7%.
- Children with a cleft palate are best managed by a team approach to ensure coordinated care. Timing of surgical interventions is often dependent on the achievement of particular milestones: tooth eruption, craniofacial skeletal development, and language development.
- Feeding difficulties exist in nearly all infants with cleft palate. The cleft defect prevents sealing of the oral cavity from the nasopharynx, resulting in an inability of the infant to develop adequate negative pressure required for sucking. Unless specific intervention through the use of adaptive feeding devices is done, these infants fail to gain weight appropriately. It is also recommended that feedings be done while the infant is sitting upright, thereby allowing gravity to help with swallowing.
- Over 80% of patients with cleft palate will develop otitis media with middle ear effusion before cleft repair. Eustachian tube dysfunction is the cause of middle ear effusions in this patient population. The eustachian tube cartilage is abnormally formed, and the attachment of the tensor tympani muscle to the eustachian tube cartilage is abnormal. Cleft repair usually leads to improvement in eustachian tube function and resolution of the effusion.

81.3 Test Interpretation

Apart from a complete physical examination, no specific laboratory or other diagnostic study is needed to make the diagnosis of cleft palate. Genetic consultation should be obtained in all children with a cleft palate. Genetic testing may be obtained if other findings on physical examination warrant suspicion of a syndrome, as in the above case.

81.4 Diagnosis

Treacher Collins's syndrome with cleft palate

81.5 Medical Management

Airway issues are a major concern in this patient population. Patients tend to stratify into three distinct groups: (1) no problem with airway or feeding ability, (2) intermittent airway and feeding problems, and (3) severe airway issues. Severe airway problems require immediate intervention. Endotracheal intubation can temporize the problem, but is often difficult because of retrognathia. A laryngeal mask airway may mitigate the situation until definitive treatment is achieved. Patients with intermittent problems should undergo a sleep study to define the severity of the problem.

Feeding difficulties are often exaggerated by airway problems. Supplemental oxygen during feedings, or when sleeping, may allow time for growth and development of the mandible, which may lead to spontaneous resolution of the airway issues. This management option requires close monitoring to ensure ongoing improvement. Children with no airway or feeding issues are followed expectantly.

Feeding is an immediate concern following the birth of an infant with a cleft deformity. It is essential that the parents be taught how to properly feed the infant. It is necessary to deliver the milk or formula to the posterior surface of the tongue in order for the infant to swallow effectively. Many commercially available nipples of various shapes and sizes can be used to accomplish this goal. Special bottles are available that allow the caregiver to actively express the formula into the oropharynx to improve feeding efficiency. Breastfeeding is difficult without the use of prosthetic feeding devices. The primary caregiver is taught to feed the child slowly and allow for frequent burping throughout the feeding.

Genetic evaluation is important to ensure the cleft is not secondary to an underlying syndrome. Patients with retrognathia associated with a syndrome tend to have more symptoms of airway obstruction than those without a syndrome. Positioning of the infant, supplemental oxygen, high-flow nasal cannula support, mandibular distraction, and tracheotomy are options for management of the airway in neonates with retrognathia depending upon the severity of the airway obstruction.

Hearing and middle ear function must be evaluated in patients with a cleft because of the high incidence of middle ear disease. Acute otitis and chronic middle ear effusions are common. Ventilation tube insertion is associated with a high incidence of otorrhea when performed before the palate is repaired. Hearing screens are helpful in determining if intervention is required.

Velopharyngeal insufficiency (VPI) occurs when the soft palate is unable to seal the nasopharynx from the oropharynx during connected speech. Children with a history of a cleft palate are at higher risk for developing VPI. An adequate evaluation of resonance cannot be reliably performed until the child has developed connected speech. This is generally around 3 years of age. If VPI is present, early intervention is associated with the best results. Compensatory speech patterns are best prevented by early intervention.

Dental hygiene is important in children with a cleft palate. The potential for future orthodontic intervention warrants developing good dental hygiene habits in childhood to optimize the ability to correct any maxillary crowding or malocclusion.

Regular follow-up with a craniofacial anomalies team ensures coordinated management of the medical, surgical, and psychosocial problems that commonly develop in children with a cleft.

81.6 Surgical Management

The ideal method for management of airway obstruction secondary to retrognathia or glossoptosis is controversial. Conservative measures need to be considered before moving to surgical interventions. Tracheotomy is the most definitive method of bypassing the area of obstruction. In select patients, mandibular distraction may be appropriate to avoid tracheotomy. Distraction may also be used as a means of achieving earlier decannulation compared with waiting for natural growth and development to occur.

Surgical closure of the palate should occur when the tissue on the palatal shelves is sufficient to close the defect in the palate easily. Generally, waiting until the child is between 9 and 12 months of age permits transposition of reliable flaps. Early repair (before the development of speech patterns) aids in overall speech-language development.

Management of chronic otitis media with ventilation tube insertion should be considered to ensure normal hearing and maximize speech-language development. Tube otorrhea rates decrease once the palate has been repaired because the repair also improves eustachian tube function.

81.7 Rehabilitation and Follow-up

Long-term follow-up of children with cleft palate is required to ensure adequate midface development, occlusion, and speech-language development. Regular evaluations by the craniofacial anomalies team ensure timely interventions to stem problems developing over time. Speech pathologists can identify resonance problems and recommend interventions before the child develops speech strategies to compensate for the difficulty with abnormal resonance occurring because of the cleft palate.

81.8 Questions

1. Which of the following describes the order of Pierre Robin's sequence?
   a) Mandibular hypoplasia, glossoptosis, cleft palate.
   b) Glossoptosis, mandibular hypoplasia, cleft palate.
   c) Cleft palate, glossoptosis, mandibular hypoplasia.
   d) Cleft palate, mandibular hypoplasia, glossoptosis.
2. In an infant with cleft palate, which of the following takes the greatest priority?
   a) Evaluation of feeding.
   b) Ensuring a safe airway.
   c) Genetic evaluation.
   d) Involvement of multidisciplinary craniofacial team.
3. Timing for surgical repair of cleft palate depends on which of the following?
   a) Tooth eruption.
   b) Palatal expansion.
   c) Language development.
   d) All of the above.

Answers: 1. a 2. b 3. d

Suggested Readings

Bassett AS, McDonald-McGinn DM, Devriendt K, et al. International 22q11.2 Deletion Syndrome Consortium. Practical guidelines for managing patients with 22q11.2 deletion syndrome. J Pediatr. 2011; 159(2):332–9.e1

Kummer AW. Cleft Palate and Craniofacial Anomalies: Effects on Speech and Resonance. Florence, KY: Cengage Learning; 2007

Losee JE, Kirschner RE. Comprehensive Cleft Care. New York, NY: McGraw-Hill; 2008

Meyer AC, Lidsky ME, Sampson DE, Lander TA, Liu M, Sidman JD. Airway interventions in children with Pierre Robin Sequence. Otolaryngol Head Neck Surg. 2008; 138(6):782–787

Milerad J, Larson O, Hagberg C, Ideberg M. Associated malformations in infants with cleft lip and palate: a prospective, population-based study. Pediatrics. 1997; 100(2 Pt 1):180–186

Posnick JC. Treacher Collins syndrome: perspectives in evaluation and treatment. J Oral Maxillofac Surg. 1997; 55(10):1120–1133

Valtonen H, Dietz A, Qvarnberg Y. Long-term clinical, audiologic, and radiologic outcomes in palate cleft children treated with early tympanostomy for otitis media with effusion: a controlled prospective study. Laryngoscope. 2005; 115(8):1512–1516

82 Stridulous Child

Amy M. Manning and Charles M. Myer IV

82.1 History

A previously healthy, former full-term 2-month-old infant was transferred to a tertiary pediatric hospital for management of a small hemangioma noted on her lower left lip. Her parents first noticed the lesion approximately 5 days after birth, and since that time it had grown slightly and had ulcerated. Additionally, the patient's mother noted "noisy breathing" since about 1 week of age, which had progressed recently. The infant had been gaining weight appropriately, but her mother noted she was difficult to feed and frequently spit up. She noted retractions and stridor that worsened with agitation and feeding. The patient had no apnea or cyanotic spells. She had an older sibling with a history of laryngomalacia that resolved without operative intervention. The patient had no history of intubation or surgery. There was no known history of the patient swallowing anything other than milk. There were no reported sick contacts.

Physical examination revealed an afebrile, well-developed infant with mild suprasternal and intracostal retractions and soft inspiratory stridor at rest. With agitation the stridor became louder and the patient was noted to have head bobbing and intermittent nasal flaring. Her respiratory rate was normal for her age and she was saturating well on room air. Her cry was not hoarse, breathy, or high pitched. Inspection of the head and neck revealed a hemangioma of the left lower lip approximately 4 mm in diameter, completely contained within the mucosa with resolving ulceration. The remainder of the oral cavity exam was normal. The neck exam was normal without palpated masses. Chest auscultation revealed equal breath sounds bilaterally with transmitted upper airway noise. Flexible nasolaryngoscopy revealed bilaterally patent nasal cavities and choanae. The supraglottis had shortened aryepiglottic folds bilaterally and redundant arytenoid mucosa with dynamic prolapse of the arytenoids into the glottic inlet during inspiration. Bilateral vocal cords were mobile. An anteroposterior neck film was normal without tracheal or subglottic narrowing, and chest radiographs showed no hyperinflation or mediastinal shift. Microlaryngoscopy and rigid bronchoscopy along with supraglottoplasty were planned.

82.2 Differential Diagnosis— Key Points

- Airway complaints, especially those in young children, are frequently challenging consultations for otolaryngologists. The urgency of evaluation and intervention are dictated by the degree of respiratory distress (indicated by dyspnea, retractions, grunting, cyanosis, and apnea), along with the degree of feeding difficulty. Within moments, it was possible to place this patient into the "not acutely ill" category. For a stidulous child who presents in respiratory distress, urgent airway stabilization may be necessary.

- The quality of sound observed in a child with noisy breathing may provide information as to the etiology of the airway obstruction. Stridor is an abnormal sound due to turbulent airflow through an airway with partial obstruction. Stertor is a fluttering sound caused by soft tissue structures in the pharynx or nasopharynx. Wheezing is a musical or whistling sound produced by turbulent airflow through constricted small airways.

- The differential diagnosis for stridor is extensive, as the obstructed area can be located anywhere along the length of the airway. The quality of the stridor may help the clinician ascertain the level of obstruction. Supraglottic obstruction tends to produce inspiratory stridor, while intrathoracic tracheal obstruction generally presents with expiratory stridor. Biphasic stridor is most commonly seen with a fixed obstruction at the level of the glottis or subglottis.

- The time of onset of stridor may also aid in determining its etiology. This patient's symptoms of stable inspiratory stridor starting the week after birth are consistent with laryngomalacia. Although physical exam revealed a moderate to severe degree of laryngomalacia, the clinician must maintain suspicion for a synchronous airway lesion, as this has been reported in a significant proportion of patients with severe laryngomalacia. Additionally, the presence of a cutaneous hemangioma in the so-called beard distribution increases the likelihood of a subglottic hemangioma. Subglottic hemangiomas often present slightly later, several months after birth, due to the natural history of infantile hemangioma and the onset of the proliferative phase.

- There were no signs or symptoms of acute inflammation, such as fever, to support the diagnosis of croup, supraglottitis, or bacterial tracheitis. The patient's breathing was normal after birth, and nasopharyngoscopy had revealed bilateral cord motion, ruling out vocal cord paralysis. The patient had no intubations, thus ruling out acquired subglottic stenosis, subglottic cyst, or arytenoid dislocation. Congenital subglottic stenosis remained a possibility, as did tracheomalacia.
- Foreign body aspiration must always be considered in a young child with respiratory complaints. A witnessed choking spell accompanied by immediate onset of stridor is suggestive of foreign body aspiration; however, this history may not always be reported because the event may be unwitnessed and index of suspicion must be high.

82.3 Test Interpretation

Anteroposterior and lateral high-kilovolt neck films to evaluate the airway can demonstrate subglottic and tracheal narrowing. Symmetric subglottic narrowing, rising to a superior point ("steeple sign") is commonly found in croup, although the presence of subglottic narrowing on radiographs can also be seen in subglottic stenosis. Asymmetric narrowing may indicate a subglottic hemangioma. The presence of irregularities along the tracheal wall or in the subglottis points to an exudative tracheitis.

Chest radiographs complement airway films and evaluate for extrinsic tracheal compression such as that caused by neck or mediastinal masses. Mediastinal shift or air trapping, often better demonstrated on lateral decubitis series, may indicate the presence of a foreign body or a more distal obstructive lesion.

Barium esophograma is useful in select cases, such as those infants who have symptoms concerning for tracheoesophageal fistula or vascular compression. A computed tomography (CT) scan with contrast may also be used to evaluate for aberrant vasculature as well as to better delineate masses of the neck or chest. In cases of vascular anomalies, magnetic resonance imaging (MRI) can provide a more complete evaluation.

Awake flexible nasolaryngoscopy should be included in the complete physical examination of the stridulous infant, provided impending airway obstruction has been ruled out clinically. The examination should include both nasal cavities and choanae. Examination should note presence of obstructing lesions or dynamic collapse. It is essential to document vocal fold mobility. Any pooling of secretions should be noted. Attention should be paid to sequelae of reflux disease, including postcricoid and laryngeal edema as well as cobblestoning of the pharynx.

Microlaryngoscopy and bronchoscopy (MLB) allows for complete evaluation of the airway and is the gold standard for children who present with significant stridor. This is performed in the operating room under a general anesthetic, and therapeutic intervention may also be performed in the same setting in select patients. In this patient, operative endoscopy confirmed very short aryepiglottic folds, as well as dynamic prolapse of the bilateral arytenoids (▶ Fig. 82.1a,b), and the absence of any other contributory lesions.

The use of laboratory testing in the patient who presents with stridor is not routine although pulse oximetry and blood gas analysis may be useful. Polysomnography may also provide information regarding severity of obstruction and the need for intervention in select cases.

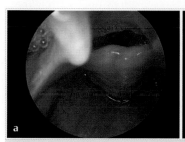 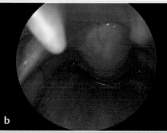 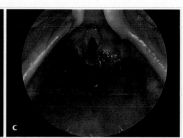

Fig. 82.1 Intraoperative view of the larynx. (a) Preoperative view demonstrating short aryepiglottic folds. (b) Preoperative view demonstrating bilateral arytenoid prolapse. (c) Postoperative view.

82.4 Diagnosis

Laryngomalacia

82.5 Medical Management

Management of the stridulous child depends on the underlying etiology and degree of respiratory distress. Immediate stabilization and resuscitation may be necessary in those children who present in acute distress. The use of oxygen or heliox, which improves laminar flow past an obstructive lesion, may help resolve hypoxemia and avert intubation. Racemic epinephrine is a rapidly acting treatment of airway edema and can be helpful in cases of acute inflammation of the airway. Concomitant treatment with steroids provides a long-acting treatment of airway edema.

Most children with laryngomalacia do not present as seen in this case with concomitant risk factors for a secondary airway lesion. Laryngomalacia is the most common etiology of neonatal stridor. The stridor is classically inspiratory, and frequently aggravated by feeding, sleep, agitation, and supine positioning. It is thought to be due to immaturity of neuromuscular tone and weak, immature cartilages of the supraglottis. The natural history of laryngomalacia is resolution over the first 1 to 2 years of life, and infants without feeding difficulties, failure to thrive, cyanosis, hypoxia, apnea, or pulmonary hypertension can be managed expectantly. Gastroesophageal reflux disease (GERD) is frequently associated with laryngomalacia, and up to 80% of infants with laryngomalacia have symptoms including regurgitation, recurrent emesis, dysphagia, coughing or choking with feeds, feeding intolerance, or weight loss. Treatment with antireflux medication and feeding in an upright position are recommended if there are feeding-related symptoms.

Subglottic hemangiomas are usually asymptomatic at birth. Once the hemangioma enters the proliferative phase (usually at 2 to 3 months of age), biphasic stridor is noted. MLB confirms the presence of a subglottic hemangioma. The proliferative phase lasts approximately 1 year. The natural history of a hemangioma is typically to involute slowly, over years. Until recently, corticosteroids were considered first-line treatment for subglottic hemangiomas. Propranolol has now become the mainstay of medical management for infantile hemangioma, and the mechanism by which it treats infantile hemangioma is unknown. Treatment is typically initiated in an inpatient setting, with the dose titrated up to 2 mg/kg/day and continued for approximately 15 months before weaning. Studies indicate that responders typically experience resolution of their airway symptoms within 24 to 48 hours after initiation of propranolol. Recommended duration of therapy is based upon studies of use of propranolol in treatment of cutaneous infantile hemangioma.

82.6 Surgical Management

Up to 10 to 20% of infants with laryngomalacia have severe enough symptoms to warrant surgical intervention. Indications for surgical intervention include apnea, failure to thrive, recurrent cyanosis, hypoxia, and pulmonary hypertension. The first-line surgical procedure for laryngomalacia is a supraglottoplasty, with microlaryngeal instrumentation or, less frequently, the CO_2 laser (▶ Fig. 82.1c). Supraglottoplasty is successful in the great majority of patients and has a low complication rate. Tracheostomy to bypass the obstruction is rarely performed for laryngomalacia, but may be required in surgical failures or children with multiple medical comorbidities.

82.7 Rehabilitation and Follow-up

Because the natural history of laryngomalacia is resolution in the first 12 to 24 months of life, the majority of infants can be managed expectantly, with the addition of acid-suppressive medication if feeding difficulties or reflux is present. Infants being managed medically or expectantly should be followed up in clinic regularly for symptom evaluation, weight checks, and repeat flexible laryngoscopy until resolution occurs. If aspiration is suspected, a video swallow study (VSS) or fiberoptic endoscopic evaluation of swallowing (FEES) study can be helpful. For those with significant nocturnal symptoms, a polysomnogram may be indicated. Acid-suppressive medication is continued for an average of 9 months and can be weaned when symptoms begin to resolve.

82.8 Questions

1. Inspiratory stridor with onset within the first few weeks of life and that worsens with feeding, sleep, or agitation likely represents obstruction at which level of the airway?

a) Supraglottis.

b) Glottis.

c) Subglottis.

d) Trachea.

e) Distal airways.

2. Laryngomalacia management may include all but which of the following?

a) Observation.

b) Tracheotomy.

c) Systemic steroids.

d) Supraglottoplasty.

e) Acid supression.

3. A stable 2-year-old child with up-to-date vaccinations and respiratory compromise of acute onset without viral prodrome likely has which of the following?

a) Croup.

b) Epiglottitis.

c) Bacterial tracheitis.

d) Laryngomalacia.

e) Airway foreign body.

Answers: 1. a 2. c 3. e

Suggested Readings

Dohar JE, Anne S. Stridor, aspiration and cough. In: Johnson JT, Rosen CA, et al, eds. Bailey's Head and Neck Surgery—Otolaryngology 5th.th ed. Philadelphia, PA: Lippencotti Williams & Wilkins; 2014

Stern Y, Cotton RT. Evaluation of the noisy infant. In: Cotton RT, Myer CM, et al, eds. Practical Pediatric Otolaryngology. Philadelphia, PA; Lippencotti-Raven; 1999

Ida JB, Thompson DM. Pediatric stridor. Otolaryngol Clin North Am. 2014; 47(5):795–819

Landry AM, Thompson DM. Laryngomalacia: disease presentation, spectrum, and management. Int J Pediatr. 2012; 2012:753526

Richter GT, Thompson DM. The surgical management of laryngomalacia. Otolaryngol Clin North Am. 2008; 41(5):837–864, vii

Elluru RG, Friess MR, Richter GT, et al. Multicenter Evaluation of the Effectiveness of Systemic Propranolol in the Treatment of Airway Hemangiomas. Otolaryngol Head Neck Surg. 2015; 153(3):452–460

83 Recurrent Respiratory Papillomatosis

David F. Smith and Alessandro de Alarcon

83.1 History

A 2-year-old Caucasian boy presented to his pediatrician with a history of worsening hoarseness over the last several months. His parents also described a high-pitched sound on inspiration when he was physically active. Besides the voice complaints and slight increased work of breathing while playing outside, he had no other complaints. His history was negative for weight loss, choking or snoring at night, apneic spells or cyanotic events, or any problems with eating or drinking. Further questioning revealed that he had no history of abnormal vocal abuse or overuse. He had met all of his developmental milestones and was up-to-date on his vaccinations. His past medical history was negative except for several viral upper respiratory infections over the winter that resolved without any antibiotic therapy. His birth history was normal, and he was the first child of a young family in a nonsmoking household with no pets. His review of systems was negative except for the vocal and respiratory complaints.

Physical examination revealed a well-appearing child in no acute distress. He was appropriately active for his age. His voice was moderately hoarse with a small amount of inspiratory stridor when the patient was breathing deeply. A full head and neck examination was otherwise normal, and he had no retractions. Flexible nasopharyngoscopy in the office revealed an exophytic mass on the left true vocal fold and with asymmetry that extended to the anterior commissure. No other supraglottic masses or lesions could be appreciated.

Based on the history and physical examination, the patient was taken to the operating room for a microlaryngoscopy and bronchoscopy with a biopsy.

83.2 Differential Diagnosis—Key Points

83.2.1 Key Symptoms

The patient in this clinical vignette was presenting with two major symptoms: hoarseness and inspiratory stridor. Hoarseness typically indicates that the opposing vocal fold surfaces have been altered from the baseline. It is a common complaint, even among the pediatric population. The differential diagnosis of hoarseness is lengthy, ranging from inflammation secondary to common viral upper respiratory infections, vocal fold lesions, and laryngopharyngeal reflux to more complex disorders, including nerve deficits and neoplastic processes. A thorough history and physical examination can help to narrow the list of possible diagnoses. Further tests should be used to definitely diagnose the appropriate pathology. Stridor is another symptom seen with multiple disease processes and conditions. The presence of stridor implies that the supraglottic, glottic, subglottic, and/or tracheal passage is narrowed.

83.2.2 Allergic or Irritant Inflammation

Hoarseness caused by allergic or irritant inflammation will be temporally related to exposure and may be accompanied by other symptoms as well.

83.2.3 Gastroesophageal Reflux Disease

Gastroesophageal reflux disease (GERD) results in laryngeal inflammation, which can cause hoarseness as a symptom. This type of hoarseness may be chronic and recurrent, occurring more consistently in the morning. A course of antireflux therapy may be tried and the patient's presumed diagnosis confirmed by his or her response to therapy. Additional pH probe, impedance study, and/or esophagogastroduodenoscopy may be warranted.

83.2.4 Recurrent Respiratory Papillomatosis (RRP)

Characterized by papillomas of the aerodigestive tract, RRP is caused by the double stranded DNA human papillomavirus (HPV) in the Papovaviridae family, most commonly types 6 and 11. As the most common neoplasm of the larynx in children, it has an incidence among children in the United States of 4.3 per 100,000. Airway obstruction and voice changes are common due to papillomas in the airway. In more aggressive cases, papillomas can extend below the larynx and into the trachea and main stem bronchi. RRP involves the lung parenchyma in less than 1% of cases. The course of

RRP is variable and difficult to predict. The course may consist of spontaneous resolution, stable disease with occasional fluctuations in severity, and aggressive disease requiring frequent surgical intervention and adjuvant therapy.

83.2.5 Viral Upper Respiratory Infections

Viral upper respiratory infections can routinely cause hoarseness in the pediatric and adult populations, but they are usually accompanied by other complaints consistent with the disease process. These infections are self-limited.

83.2.6 Vocal Abuse

Vocal abuse is any behavior that strains the vocal folds. This can include excessive talking, yelling, coughing, and throat clearing. Although hoarseness can be seen with vocal abuse, stridor and other signs seen with papillomatosis are uncommon.

83.2.7 Vocal Fold Lesions

Different vocal fold lesions can be seen in pediatric patients, including vocal fold nodules, vocal fold cysts, and malignant lesions. Constant or progressive hoarseness is commonly due to a vocal fold lesion. The differential diagnosis of a vocal fold lesion differs from that in the adult population. The most common lesions are vocal fold nodules. In some cases, these lesions may be related to vocal abuse. Other lesions include neoplastic processes, of which laryngeal papilloma is the most common. Less common lesions include hemangiomas, benign and malignant mesenchymal tumors, and squamous cell carcinoma. Biopsy is required for diagnostic confirmation in cases of neoplasia.

83.2.8 Vocal Fold Paresis or Paralysis

Impaired vocal fold mobility may cause hoarseness. This will likely be recognized on flexible nasopharyngoscopy. If impaired vocal fold mobility is a congenital problem or one acquired as an infant (e.g., after cardiac surgery), it is likely to have been identified earlier than 2 years of age, as in our clinical vignette. Acquired recurrent laryngeal nerve dysfunction may also be caused by metabolic disorders, nutritional deficiency, or heavy metal poisoning, or as part of a postinfectious polyneuropathy. Recurrent laryngeal nerve injuries may result from an overinflated or high-riding endotracheal tube cuff. Vocal fold mobility problems may also cause trauma to the cricoarytenoid joint. Arytenoid dislocation can occur during traumatic intubation or blunt trauma to the external neck.

83.3 Test Intepretation

Flexible nasopharyngoscopy, including an examination of the nasal cavity, nasopharynx, oropharynx, hypopharynx, and glottic inlet, can be performed in the office setting. Although flexible endoscopy does not offer a detailed view of the subglottis or trachea, it is well tolerated and provides an excellent diagnostic evaluation of the supraglottis and true vocal folds for children presenting with hoarseness and/or stridor.

Microlaryngoscopy and bronchoscopy can be performed in the operative suite for a thorough examination of the airway, including the trachea and main bronchi. Further, biopsy and surgical debulking with or without intralesional injections of adjuvant therapy can be performed at the same time. Microlaryngoscopy in this patient revealed a discrete focus of exophytic tissue emanating from the surface of the left true vocal fold, extending from midcord region to the anterior commissure (▶ Fig. 83.1). The surgeon performed an excisional biopsy with a cup forceps followed by removal of all gross disease using the microdebrider and/or the potassium titanyl phosphate (KTP) laser. Removal of the disease at the anterior commissure was limited to prevent potential webbing. Histopathologic evaluation revealed polypoid frondlike projections of connective tissue covered by stratified squamous epithelium without evidence of dysplasia. Viral typing of the lesion revealed HPV type 6.

83.4 Diagnosis

Recurrent respiratory papillomatosis (RRP)

83.5 Medical Management

RRP can be a persistent disease, often requiring multiple surgical excisions. Indications for adjuvant medical therapy include the presence of papillomas outside of the larynx or the need for surgical excision more than four times in a 1-year

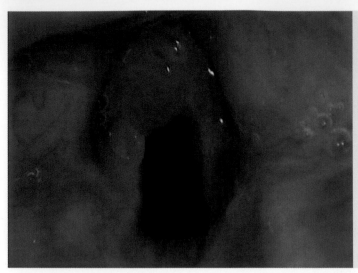

Fig. 83.1 Recurrent respiratory papillomatosis: exophytic lesion on left true vocal fold.

period. Adjuvant therapy is required in as many as 20% of children with RRP. However, despite the use of a variety of adjuvant therapies in children, no single agent has been effective at eliminating RRP in all of the pediatric patients. Adjuvant therapies include Interferon-α, Cidofovir, Ribavirin, Acycloviricra, indole-3-carbinol (a dietary supplement), and retinoids, all with variable success. The most commonly used adjuvant therapies are discussed below.

The monoclonal antibody bevacizumab (Avastin, Genentech, San Francisco, CA), is designed to bind vascular endothelial growth factor (VEGF) and block interaction with the VEGF-receptor. It has shown promise when used as an adjuvant therapy when used with angiolytic laser therapy. Avastin was most often used systemically to inhibit neovascularization seen with certain metastatic carcinomas. For RRP, it is typically used as an intralesional therapy to reduce angiogenesis. In severe cases with pulmonary spread, intravenous (IV) therapy has shown some promising early results in several case studies. Common side effects with IV therapy include dry mouth, cough, voice changes, diarrhea, nausea, vomiting, and cold symptoms. These side effects are rarely seen with intralesional injection.

Cidofovir, an antiviral, is the most frequently used adjuvant therapy in pediatric RRP. Originally designed and approved by the Food and Drug Administration as an agent for cytomegalovirus retinitis, evidence supporting the use of cidofovir in RRP is limited to reports of case series. Studies with similar levels of evidence have failed to show significant benefit. Animal studies have demonstrated carcinogenic potential, an aspect of therapy that must be reviewed in informed consent. Other reported side effects of cidofovir include rash, headache, nephrotoxicity, and neutropenia (more commonly in doses used for cytomegalovirus retinitis), although it should be noted that no systemic side effects have been reported when cidofovir is given intralesionally.

Interferon-α therapy usually consists of daily treatment for 6 months followed by thrice weekly treatment. There is conflicting evidence regarding success rates with this therapy. Certain patients experience a relapse when therapy is stopped. Common side effects include acute reactions such as fever and flulike symptoms. Chronic reactions include a decrease in growth rate, elevation of liver enzymes, leukopenia, seizures, and spastic diplegia. Interferon-α may be more effective on HPV type 6 than on type 11.

Multiple other agents have been investigated, but none of these has shown convincing benefit. Emerging therapy is focused on HPV vaccines and prevention of disease, including the quadrivalent HPV vaccine. Targeting HPV types 6, 11, 16, and 18, this vaccine may prevent the maternal infection and the subsequent vertical transmission.

83.6 Surgical Management

Surgical therapy is the mainstay for treatment of RRP. Surgical management begins with microlaryngoscopy and bronchoscopy with biopsy. After histopathologic confirmation of disease, surgical management consists of papilloma removal for unacceptable voice or airway compromise. In the setting of disease that requires surgical intervention, yearly biopsy is recommended to evaluate for dysplastic change. Malignant transformation is a rare occurrence.

There are multiple methods of surgical treatment for RRP, including cold steel techniques, CO_2 laser, KTP laser, and powered microdebrider. Recent literature supports the use of the microdebrider as a safe and cost-effective alternative to the CO_2 laser therapy. Each technique has its own advantages and disadvantages. Surgeon preference and comfort often dictate the choice of method. Any surgical procedure should have as its goal the removal of gross disease with preservation of normal structures, because latent viral infection exists in surrounding tissue and eradication of this infection is not surgically possible.

83.7 Rehabilitation and Follow-up

Yearly biopsy of recurrent lesions is recommended. Aggressive lesions that are rapidly growing or spreading should be biopsied more frequently. The physician may consider an immunodeficiency work-up. In addition, controlling laryngopharyngeal reflux is recommended.

83.8 Questions

1. In a child with newly diagnosed recurrent respiratory papillomatosis (RRP), what is the primary therapy?
   a) Interferon.
   b) Surgical excision.
   c) Viral vaccine.
   d) Surgical excision with cidofovir.
   e) Topical steroid.

2. A 4-year-old boy with progressive hoarseness is most likely to have which of the following?
   a) Vocal cord paralysis.
   b) Laryngopharyngeal reflux.
   c) Vocal cord nodules.
   d) RRP.
   e) Arytenoid dislocation.

3. Avastin is an antibody that controls the growth of RRP by
   a) Inhibiting DNA polymerase.
   b) Decreasing the number of circulating immune cells.
   c) Decreasing the number of circulating cytokines.
   d) Blocking vascular endothelial growth factor from binding the receptor.

Answers: 1. b 2. c 3. d

Suggested Readings

Derkay CS, Wiatrak B. Recurrent respiratory papillomatosis: a review. Laryngoscope. 2008; 118(7):1236–1247

Goon P, Sonnex C, Jani P, Stanley M, Sudhoff H. Recurrent respiratory papillomatosis: an overview of current thinking and treatment. Eur Arch Otorhinolaryngol. 2008; 265(2):147–151

Schraff S, Derkay CS, Burke B, Lawson L. American Society of Pediatric Otolaryngology members' experience with recurrent respiratory papillomatosis and the use of adjuvant therapy. Arch Otolaryngol Head Neck Surg. 2004; 130(9):1039–1042

Block SL, Nolan T, Sattler C, et al. Protocol 016 Study Group. Comparison of the immunogenicity and reactogenicity of a prophylactic quadrivalent human papillomavirus (types 6, 11, 16, and 18) L1 virus-like particle vaccine in male and female adolescents and young adult women. Pediatrics. 2006; 118(5):2135–2145

Sidell DR, Nassar M, Cotton RT, Zeitels SM, de Alarcon A. High-dose sublesional bevacizumab (avastin) for pediatric recurrent respiratory papillomatosis. Ann Otol Rhinol Laryngol. 2014; 123(3):214–221

Best SR, Friedman AD, Landau-Zemer T, et al. Safety and dosing of bevacizumab (avastin) for the treatment of recurrent respiratory papillomatosis. Ann Otol Rhinol Laryngol. 2012; 121(9):587–593

84 Airway Foreign Body

Brian Ho and Michael J. Rutter

84.1 History

A 15-month-old boy presented to the emergency department from an outside hospital after undergoing an "aspiration event." The child was not with the parents during this episode, but was under supervision by a caretaker. He was noted to have an acute change in respiratory status, but no choking episode was witnessed. There was no history of recent infections, or any other relevant medical history. He was evaluated at an outside hospital and was noted to have oxygen saturations in the upper 80 s on room air and to be in mild respiratory distress. He was therefore urgently transferred for evaluation and management.

On initial examination, the patient was on oxygen at 15 L/min with oxygen saturations in the mid-90 s. He had no stridor or retractions and his skin and lips were pink. His respirations were regular with decreased breath sounds on the left. He did not tolerate being placed supine.

84.2 Differential Diagnosis—Key Points

- Foreign bodies must always be considered in the pediatric population, particularly in children between 10 and 24 months of age. The majority of foreign body aspirations occur in children under the age of 5 years and are frequently unwitnessed events.
- The most common aerodigestive foreign body in a child is an esophageal foreign body, typically a penny at the cricopharyngeus. An esophageal foreign body may present with airway symptoms if the foreign body is very large, or if it is chronic and causing edema of the anterior wall of the esophagus with resultant posterior compression of the trachea. The most concerning esophageal foreign body is a button battery, which may cause severe damage to the esophagus and surrounding structures.
- The most common airway foreign body in Western society is the peanut. Foreign bodies most commonly lodge in the right mainstem bronchus, which is straighter and shorter than the left mainstem bronchus. Acutely, a bronchial

foreign body typically presents with wheezing and respiratory distress after an episode of coughing and/or choking. Far rarer, but much more concerning, are tracheal or laryngeal foreign bodies. These present with stridor or acute airway compromise, and may be lethal.

- In a child with a history suggestive of a foreign body, a normal physical examination and negative radiographs do not rule out the presence of a foreign body.
- Infectious and inflammatory processes frequently affect the pediatric airway and can present with symptoms that mimic a foreign body. These patients will often have a prodromic upper respiratory illness that leads to stridor or wheezing.
- The possibility of a foreign body should be considered in patients with a history of recalcitrant asthma, chronic cough, or recurrent pneumonia.

84.3 Test Interpretation

In a stable patient, the initial evaluation of the airway consists of lateral neck and chest radiographs. The structural elements of the airway are outlined and radiopaque foreign bodies may be identified. The lung fields can also be evaluated for signs of postobstructive emphysema. If a foreign body is ball-valving into a bronchus, there could be air trapping and hyperinflation of the lung field on that side, and mediastinal structures will shift away from the obstruction. Conversely, a completely obstructed bronchus may lead to absorption of the air trapped distally with widespread atelectasis. In these cases, the mediastinum will shift toward the obstruction. Normal radiographs do not exclude the possibility of an airway foreign body.

When doubt arises as to the presence of a radiolucent foreign body in the distal airway, decubitus films and, rarely, airway fluoroscopy can be of assistance in determining the presence of an object in the airway. In the left lateral decubitus view, a normal examination will demonstrate the left lung volume to be compressed. If the lung remains inflated, this suggests a foreign body within the left mainstem bronchus, which is obstructing extravasation of airflow.

The diagnostic gold standard for aerodigestive tract foreign bodies is endoscopy. Evaluation with rigid telescopes allows proper visualization of the entire upper aerodigestive system and provides the means for removal of any foreign body that might be present. Endoscopy also allows the physician to assess inflammation related to the foreign body and provide a prognosis for the recovery of normal airflow dynamics once the foreign body is removed. There is no substitute for evaluation of the airway with the patient under general anesthesia anytime the question of a foreign body has been raised. The onus is on the physician to rule out the presence of a foreign body in the airway. It is accepted that it is better to have a percentage of negative bronchoscopies rather than to miss a foreign body by not performing a bronchoscopy. Most suspected airway foreign bodies should be evaluated by bronchoscopy urgently, if not necessarily emergently.

84.4 Diagnosis

Bronchial foreign body, identified as edamame

84.5 Medical Management

In the emergency room, the child required oxygen to maintain his oxygen saturations above 90%. The child was stable enough to permit radiologic evaluation prior to transfer to the operating room. If the child is unstable with complete airway obstruction, a Heimlich maneuver may be attempted. If complete glottic or supraglottic obstruction is present, immediate steps must be taken to remove the foreign body and secure the airway. This can often be accomplished using a laryngoscope and Magill forceps. In a stable patient, endoscopy and foreign body removal should be performed in the operating room. Once a decision has been made to transfer to the operating room, the appropriate equipment to manage the airway and retrieve the foreign body should be assembled, and double-checked. This includes verifying that the appropriate-size telescopes are in the bronchoscopes and foreign body forceps, and ensuring that the suction catheters are of appropriate length and diameter and that the telescopes are all functional. The anesthesia and nursing teams should ideally be briefed about the case and the risks and expectations of management in a "prebrief huddle" before the child enters the operating room. Great care must be exercised to prevent undue agitation

of the child, which may lead to airway compromise. When general anesthesia is induced, the airway may be unstable and the surgeon should be prepared to secure the airway with a ventilating bronchoscope if necessary.

84.6 Surgical Management

This child underwent mask induction of general anesthesia and spontaneous ventilation was maintained. Endoscopic evaluation of the larynx and trachea demonstrated normal anatomy without any foreign object. Distally, the left mainstem bronchus was normal and the right mainstem was noted to have secretions present. This was gently suctioned and a foreign body was seen occluding the right mainstem bronchus (▶ Fig. 84.1). The optical peanut-grasping forceps were used to safely extract the foreign body. Repeat bronchoscopy demonstrated no additional foreign bodies in the tracheobronchial tree. Mild edema and mucosal laceration were noted at the site of the foreign body impaction in the right mainstem bronchus. The patient tolerated the procedure well and had no postoperative complications.

All equipment to secure the airway was present but not needed in this case. A ventilating bronchoscope must be assembled and ready for use before induction, and a tracheotomy tray should be readily available. Foreign bodies may be impacted at the level of the larynx, trachea, or bronchus. Complete airway obstruction is possible in all of these areas.

Extraction techniques often vary according to the site of obstruction. Deploying optical extraction forceps through a rigid ventilating bronchoscope is the current standard of care for removing foreign bodies from the airway. A variety of graspers are available, and practicing on a copy of the suspected foreign body with different forceps before induction is helpful.

In some cases, due to either the size or shape, a foreign body may not fit through the bronchoscope. These items should be removed in continuity with the bronchoscope. When this occurs, care must be taken not to lose the foreign body in the subglottis or at the glottis. These levels may completely occlude the airway. If this situation arises, the foreign body should be pushed back down one of the mainstem bronchi to allow for ventilation. Once the oxygen saturation improves, additional attempts at removal can be made.

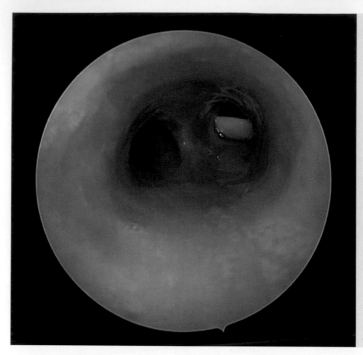

Fig. 84.1 Endoscopic examination demonstrating a foreign body in the right mainstem bronchus.

In rare situations, the foreign body can be firmly grasped, but due to geometry, can still not be removed through an endoscopic approach. In such situations one must not hesitate to perform a tracheotomy to gain adequate access to the airway for removal of the foreign body transtracheally. Impacted distal foreign bodies or chronic foreign bodies that have caused extensive granulation tissue may require a thoracotomy for removal.

The key to successful management of airway foreign bodies is a high index of suspicion. The benefits associated with prompt diagnosis and removal of an airway foreign body outweigh the risks of endoscopy. The difficulty of extraction and the complication rates associated with airway foreign bodies increase dramatically when their duration extends beyond 72 hours. Early diagnosis and timely removal are essential to satisfactory resolution of these life-threatening events.

84.7 Rehabilitation and Follow-up

When the airway problem has been adequately addressed and successfully managed, no long-term follow-up is necessary. Chronic foreign bodies may induce granulation tissue and scarring, occasionally requiring surveillance endoscopy to ensure appropriate healing. Parent education is an important component of preventing recurrent episodes of airway aspiration.

84.8 Questions

1. A partially obstructing, ball-valving foreign body in the left mainstem bronchus would show which of the following on radiography?
   a) Atelectatic left lung with mediastinal shift to the right.
   b) Hyperinflated left lung with mediastinal shift to the right.
   c) Compressed left lung on left lateral decubitus positioning.
   d) Hyperinflated left lung with mediastinal shift to the left.
2. What is the diagnostic gold standard for airway foreign bodies?
   a) Endoscopy.
   b) High-kilovolt radiography of the neck.
   c) History and physical examination.
   d) Computed tomography (CT).
3. True or false? A large or chronic esophageal foreign body can result in symptoms mimicking an airway foreign body.

Answers: 1. b 2. a 3. True

Suggested Readings

Bloom DC, Christenson TE, Manning SC, et al. Plastic laryngeal foreign bodies in children: a diagnostic challenge. Int J Pediatr Otorhinolaryngol. 2005; 69(5):657–662

Holinger LD. Management of sharp and penetrating foreign bodies of the upper aerodigestive tract. Ann Otol Rhinol Laryngol. 1990; 99(9 Pt 1):684–688

Hong SJ, Goo HW, Roh JL. Utility of spiral and cine CT scans in pediatric patients suspected of aspirating radiolucent foreign bodies. Otolaryngol Head Neck Surg. 2008; 138(5):576–580

Kadmon G, Stern Y, Bron-Harlev E, Nahum E, Battat E, Schonfeld T. Computerized scoring system for the diagnosis of foreign body aspiration in children. Ann Otol Rhinol Laryngol. 2008; 117 (11):839–843

Reilly JS. Prevention of aspiration in infants and young children: federal regulations. Ann Otol Rhinol Laryngol. 1990; 99(4 Pt 1):273–276

Swanson KL. Airway foreign bodies: what's new? Semin Respir Crit Care Med. 2004; 25(4):405–411

Walner DL, Ouanounou S, Donnelly LF, Cotton RT. Utility of radiographs in the evaluation of pediatric upper airway obstruction. Ann Otol Rhinol Laryngol. 1999; 108(4):378–383

Zerella JT, Dimler M, McGill LC, Pippus KJ. Foreign body aspiration in children: value of radiography and complications of bronchoscopy. J Pediatr Surg. 1998; 33(11):1651–1654

85 Subglottic Stenosis

Niall D. Jefferson and Catherine K. Hart

85.1 History

A 2-year-old boy with a history of former 28-week prematurity, tracheostomy, and ventilator dependence presented for evaluation. He was intubated for his first 6 weeks of life prior to undergoing tracheostomy. He was no longer ventilator dependent. He had a weak cry and did not tolerate capping of his tracheostomy tube. He was otherwise well with a history of a persistent ductus arteriosis that closed spontaneously soon after birth. He was fed entirely by mouth and was not taking any medications.

On physical examination, he was a well-appearing toddler with a 4.0 pediatric tracheostomy tube in place. He did not vocalize. When his tracheostomy tube was capped, he developed significant retractions and audible biphasic stridor with increased work of breathing. Flexible nasopharyngoscopy demonstrated a normal supraglottis with mobile vocal cords bilaterally. The subglottis was not well visualized.

85.2 Differential Diagnosis—Key Points

- The history of prematurity and prolonged intubation prior to tracheostomy suggest that subglottic stenosis (SGS) is the most likely diagnosis, although other levels of airway obstruction are also possible.
- SGS can be congenital or acquired. Congenital SGS is the third most common laryngeal disorder, following laryngomalacia and vocal fold paralysis. The incidence of congenital SGS is difficult to determine, as many neonates with congenital SGS require intubation shortly after birth, making it difficult to determine if the SGS is congenital or acquired. Congenital SGS may be due to incomplete recanalization during embryogenesis, a small-diameter cricoid (an elliptical cricoid), or a trapped first tracheal ring. It commonly presents in the first few months of life with respiratory distress and/or stridor. SGS should be considered in any infant that presents with recurrent croup symptoms.
- Acquired SGS is most commonly caused by injury from intubation but may be caused by

blunt external trauma, infection, or caustic ingestion. Endotracheal intubation may result in edema, ulceration, infection, and chondronecrosis. As the injured mucosa heals, granulation tissue forms, followed by fibrosis that eventually leads to stenosis.

- The weak cry may be due to cricoarytenoid joint fixation or scarring of the vocal cords due to the intubation. However, the presence of bilateral vocal cord mobility on flexible laryngoscopy does not support this diagnosis.
- Upper airway obstruction such as adenotonsillar hypertrophy, glossoptosis, or laryngomalacia may also cause or contribute to increased work of breathing with tracheostomy tube capping.
- SGS is a condition that can be compounded by gastroesophageal reflux and eosinophilic esophagitis. A reflux-specific history as well as impedance probe testing and esophagogastroduodenoscopy (EGD) with biopsies should be considered, especially if airway reconstruction is anticipated.
- Any case of stridor should raise the possibility of an airway foreign body or mass lesion; therefore, the examination must include microlaryngoscopy and bronchoscopy (MLB) to formally evaluate the airway.

85.3 Test Interpretation

A detailed history including birth history, previous intubation, and other congenital anomalies is essential. Other nonlaryngeal causes of airway obstruction need to be considered, including nasal, nasopharyngeal, palatal, oropharyngeal, hypopharyngeal, and tracheobronchial etiologies. If there is a history of intubation, the size of the endotracheal tube and the duration of intubation are important facts to obtain.

An MLB must be performed to examine the anatomy of the supraglottis, glottis, subglottis, and trachea. This will define the anatomy, levels of airway obstruction, and degree of stenosis.

There is a limited role for imaging in the evaluation of SGS. Chest radiographs may demonstrate steepling of the subglottis and indicate the length of the stenosis. They may also identify concurrent pulmonary pathology.

Table 85.1 Myer-Cotton grading scale for subglottic stenosis

Grade	% narrowing
I	0–50%
II	51–70%
III	71–99%
IV	No detectable lumen

Computed tomography (CT) scans can be useful in selected cases to aid in evaluation of the lung parenchyma or to determine if vascular anomalies are present that may be contributing to airway stenosis.

This patient had a formal airway evaluation in the operating room. Flexible bronchoscopy was performed to assess the dynamics of both the upper and lower airways. A bronchoalveolar lavage was performed, which did not demonstrate inflammation or signs of chronic aspiration. An MLB was performed. The supraglottis was normal, with no cricoarytenoid joint fixation. The subglottis demonstrated circumferential SGS and suprastomal collapse. The airway was sized according to the Myer-Cotton scale (▶ Table 85.1) and a 2.5 uncuffed endotracheal tube had a leak at 25 cm of water pressure, corresponding to a grade III stenosis. Esophagoscopy with biopsies and overnight impedance probe testing were performed and were normal.

85.4 Diagnosis

Subglottic stenosis secondary to prolonged neonatal intubation

85.5 Medical Management

Children with grade I or II SGS who are asymptomatic or have mild symptoms may be managed expectantly, as the symptoms will likely resolve as the child grows. In this case, the tracheostomy tube could be left in place. This would allow the child to have a safe airway and to continue to feed orally without aspiration, but he would continue to have a significantly compromised voice. Given the degree of SGS, he is at high risk for significant morbidity or mortality in the event of accidental decannulation.

Prior to airway reconstruction, concurrent medical conditions should be optimized. Patients with gastroesophageal reflux should be treated with antireflux medications. Patients with eosinophilic esophagitis must have their esophageal disease controlled prior to reconstruction. If methicillin-resistant *Staphylococcus aureus* (MRSA) is present, preoperative antibiotics are administered.

85.6 Surgical Management

SGS may be managed using both endoscopic and open techniques. Grade I and II stenosis can often be managed endoscopically. High-grade stenosis (grade III or IV) usually requires an open reconstruction. Patients with high-grade stenosis may require a tracheotomy to establish a safe airway prior to reconstruction. Due to the high grade of this stenosis, open airway reconstruction with anterior and posterior costal cartilage grafts was indicated.

The other consideration in this case was whether surgery should be performed as a single- or double-stage procedure. Factors that would favor a double stage include a history of difficult intubation, poor pulmonary function, a previous history of reconstruction failures, or sedation issues. In this case a double-stage laryngotracheal reconstruction with stent placement was performed due to the patient's history of prematurity and chronic lung disease.

85.7 Rehabilitation and Follow-up

The patient was admitted for 5 days following the reconstruction until the tracheostomy stoma was mature. The patient returned 6 weeks following the reconstruction for MLB and removal of the suprastomal stent. The patient returned 1 week later for repeat airway evaluation. The airway continued to be evaluated at regular intervals until healing was complete and a stable lumen size had been achieved.

After a period of observation, airway patency was confirmed by MLB and the tracheostomy tube was downsized and capped. The patient tolerated capping and returned a few months later to have the tracheostomy tube removed in an inpatient setting. Periodic MLBs were performed to ensure ongoing growth of the airway.

85.8 Questions

1. Indications for double-stage laryngotracheal reconstruction include all of the following except
   a) Difficult exposure.
   b) Previous failed reconstruction.
   c) Known airway inflammation.
   d) Anterior grafting only.
2. Appropriate work-up prior to open airway reconstruction includes all of the following except
   a) Thorough history and physical examination.
   b) Microlaryngoscopy and bronchoscopy.
   c) Computed tomography (CT) scan with fine cuts through the subglottis.
   d) Evaluation of vocal cord mobility.
3. True or false? Subglottic stenosis is the most common cause of stridor in infants.

Answers: 1. d 2. c 3. False

Suggested Readings

de Alarcon A, Cotton RT, Rutter MJ. Laryngeal and tracheal airway disorders, in.I: Wilmott RW, Boat TF, et al, eds. Kendig and Chernick's Disorders of the Respiratory Tract in Children. 8th ed. Philadelphia, PA: Elsevier; 2012:969–975

Hart CK, Yang CJ, Rutter MJ. Reconstruction of the airway, in.I: Thompson JW, Vieira FO, Rutter MJ, eds. Managing the Difficult Airway: A Handbook for Surgeons. London, UK: JP Medical Publishers; 2015:115–124

Maresh A, Preciado DA, O'Connell AP, Zalzal GH. A comparative analysis of open surgery vs endoscopic balloon dilation for pediatric subglottic stenosis. JAMA Otolaryngol Head Neck Surg. 2014; 140(10):901–905

86 Branchial Arch Anomaly

Andrew J. Redmann and J. Paul Willging

86.1 History

A 1-year-old boy presented to clinic with a right ear lesion obstructing the external auditory canal and intermittent drainage from a pit in the right cheek just inferior to the ear lobule. He had no history of hearing loss, renal disease, or other systemic illness. Facial nerve function was intact and symmetric. The ipsilateral tympanic membrane and remainder of the head and neck examination were normal. Computed tomography (CT) imaging demonstrated a well-defined, low-attenuating mass anterior to the floor of the right cartilaginous external auditory canal. The mass measured 15 × 9 mm and was partially surrounded by parotid tissue.

86.2 Differential Diagnosis—Key Points

- The differential diagnosis of a pediatric neck mass can be divided into congenital and acquired lesions. Congenital masses can further be divided into midline and lateral anomalies.
  ▸ Table 86.1 illustrates the differential diagnosis of pediatric neck masses.
- Knowledge of the embryology of branchial development is essential for understanding the pathway that an anomaly will follow (▸ Table 86.2). There are six branchial arches. Between these arches are clefts externally that are lined with ectoderm and pouches internally that are lined with endoderm. The fifth branchial arch degenerates. Each arch has an associated nerve, artery, cartilaginous structure, and muscle. Of note, the sternocleidomastoid (SCM) muscle derives from the cervical somites posterior and inferior to the branchial arches.
- Branchial anomalies related to arch development include cysts, sinuses, and fistulas. Cysts are lined by mucosa or epithelium, have no external opening, and arise from embryonic rests trapped inside developing tissue. Sinuses result from the incomplete closure of branchial pouches and clefts, and they communicate with a single body surface, either the skin or pharynx. Fistulas also result from the incomplete closure of pouches or clefts; however, they communicate with two body surfaces. Fistulas often present at an earlier age than cysts or sinuses.

- Traditional teaching holds that the path of a branchial anomaly can be predicted based on knowledge of branchial arch embryology. Cysts, sinuses, and fistula tracts course posterior-medial-deep to other derivatives of their own branchial arch, and anterolateral and superficial to the derivatives of the arch behind them.

Table 86.1 Differential diagnosis of pediatric neck masses

Congenital	
Midline	**Lateral**
Thyroglossal duct cyst	Branchial cleft cyst
Dermoid/epidermoid cyst	External laryngocele
Teratoma	Pseudotumor of infancy (fibromatosis coli)
Plunging ranula	Thymic cyst
Lymphatic/vascular malformation	Lymphatic/vascular malformation
Hemangioma	Hemangioma
Normal thyroid gland	
Acquired	
Benign	
Infectious or inflammatory: reactive lymphadenopathy	
Sialadenitis	
Granulomatous (atypical mycobacteria, cat-scratch, sarcoidosis)	
Neoplastic (lipoma, neurofibroma, pilomatrixoma, mixed tumor)	
Malignant	
Lymphoma (Hodgkin's, non-Hodgkin's)	
Rhabdomyosarcoma	
Thyroid carcinoma	
Salivary tumors	
Neuroblastoma	
Langerhans histiocytosis	

Table 86.2 Branchial arch derivatives

Arch	Cranial nerve	Artery	Cartilage	Muscle	Pouch
First (mandibular)	V (trigeminal)	Maxillary (degenerates)	Meckel's cartilage Malleus head/neck Anterior malleolar ligament Incus body/short process Mandible Sphenomandibular ligament	Tensor tympani Tensor veli palatini Muscles of mastication Digastric anterior belly Mylohyoid	Middle ear
Second (hyoid)	VII (facial)	External carotid Stapedial (degenerates)	Reichert's cartilage Malleus manubrium Incus long process Stapes Pyramidal eminence Styloid process Hyoid lesser cornu	Stapedius tendon Muscles of facial expression Digastric posterior belly Stylohyoid	Tonsillar fossa Palatine tonsils
Third	IX (glossopharyngeal)	Internal carotid Common carotid	Hyoid greater cornu	Stylopharyngeus	Inferior parathyroids Thymus
Fourth	X (superior laryngeal)	Right subclavian Aortic arch	Thyroid cartilage Cuneiform	Cricothryoid membrane Inferior pharyngeal constrictors	Superior parathyroids
Sixth	X (recurrent laryngeal)	Right pulmonary Ductus arteriosis	Cricoid Arytenoid Corniculate	Intrinsic laryngeal muscles	Parafollicular C cells

First arch anomalies account for less than 15% of all branchial arch anomalies. Work divided first branchial anomalies into types I and II based on their histology and location. Type I first branchial anomalies are ectoderm-derived duplications of the membranous external auditory canal that are lined by squamous epithelium. They are usually located anterior and medial to the external auditory canal and course lateral to the facial nerve. Type II first branchial anomalies are more common than type I first branchial anomalies. They derive from ectoderm and mesoderm, are lined by squamous epithelium, and contain cartilage. They usually open into the concha or external auditory canal as well as the anterior border of the SCM at the angle of the mandible. Retrospective case series indicate that first arch anomalies have a variable relationship to the facial nerve, and can pass superficial to, deep to, or between branches of the nerve. Tracts passing deep to the facial nerve are more common in women, children presenting at a young age, children with fistulas as compared with

sinuses, and tracts that did not open into the external auditory canal.

Second branchial anomalies are the most common of the branchial anomalies (~ 90%). Their path begins along the anterior border of the SCM, courses deep to the platysma and facial nerve, deep to the external carotid artery, superficial to the internal carotid artery, deep to the posterior belly of the digastric, and superficial to the glossopharyngeal and hypoglossal nerves, and enters the pharynx in the region of the tonsillar fossa. A second branchial anomaly is three times more likely to be a cyst than a sinus or fistula, and it can be located anywhere along this path. Branchio-oto-renal syndrome most commonly presents with second branchial arch anomalies, bilateral preauricular pits, cup-shaped pinnae, deafness, and renal anomalies. Other findings may include facial asymmetry and palate anomalies.

Third branchial anomalies are rare. Theoretically, their path should begin along the anterior border of the SCM, course deep to the platysma and facial nerve, deep to both carotid arteries, deep and posterior to the glossopharyngeal nerve, superficial to the hypoglossal nerve, and deep to the stylopharyngeus muscle, and enter the pharynx medial to the greater cornu of the hyoid bone at the base of the pyriform sinus.

Theoretically, the path of a fourth branchial anomaly would begin low in the neck along the anterior border of the SCM, course deep to the platysma and facial nerve, deep to the common carotid artery, loop around the aortic arch on the left or the subclavian artery on the right, deep to the superior laryngeal nerve, superficial to the recurrent laryngeal nerve, and deep to the inferior pharyngeal constrictor muscles, and enter the pharynx at the apex of the pyriform sinus.

Most cases of third and fourth branchial anomalies present as left-sided cystic infections that became fistulas only after drainage, are closely associated with the ipsilateral thyroid lobe, and pass directly from the posteromedial surface of the thyroid through the inferior constrictor into the pyriform fossa, traveling lateral and posterior to the recurrent laryngeal nerve. Some authors suggest that third and fourth branchial anomalies may derive from the thymopharyngeal duct, which forms during descent of the thymus into the mediastinum during the eighth week of embryogenesis. It remains to be determined whether these branchial anomalies and thymopharyngeal remnants are three discrete entities or are in fact simply one entity derived from the thymopharyngeal duct.

86.3 Test Interpretation

Radiographic evaluation of a lateral neck mass can help to confirm the diagnosis and assist with management. Ultrasound will show a low attenuation mass in the lateral neck. On a CT scan with contrast, a branchial cleft cyst will be homogeneous with low attenuation centrally and a smoothly enhancing rim. Magnetic resonance imaging (MRI) will demonstrate a low to intermediate T1- and high T2-weighted signal. Third and fourth branchial anomalies often have a hypodensity within the ipsilateral (usually left) thyroid lobe. Gas bubbles in the cyst or along the tract are diagnostic.

86.4 Diagnosis

First branchial arch anomaly

86.5 Medical Management

Acutely infected branchial cleft anomalies should be treated medically with antimicrobial coverage against *Staphylococcus aureus*. Clindamycin is a lincosamide that covers *S. aureus*, methicillin-resistant *S. aureus*, and respiratory tract anaerobes. Trimethoprim-sulfamethoxazole (Bactrim) is an effective alternative, but it should not be used in infants younger than 2 months of age. In patients who do not improve on antibiotics, ultrasound-guided needle aspiration to obtain cultures should be considered. Incision and drainage should be avoided if possible. Surgical excision should be delayed until the infection resolves and should proceed shortly after resolution to avoid increased scarring and fibrosis.

86.6 Surgical Management

First branchial arch anomalies that swell, become infected, or drain require surgical excision. First arch anomalies are located close to the facial nerve and therefore require identification of the facial nerve trunk at an early stage of dissection, as in parotid surgery. In older children and adults, the facial nerve is protected by the mastoid tip, and landmarks such as the digastric muscle, external auditory canal cartilaginous pointer, and tympanomastoid suture can be used to identify and preserve the nerve. In infants and young children, the mastoid tip is less developed because the pull of the SCM has not yet caused it to lengthen. The extratemporal facial nerve is therefore more superficial in young children and has a greater risk of being damaged. To decrease the risk of facial nerve injury, a curvilinear incision is made 2 cm below the mandible extending in a skin crease over the mastoid and ending 1 to 2 cm behind the postauricular crease. A subplatysmal flap is elevated up to the ramus of the mandible. The facial nerve is identified in the triangular space formed by the posterior belly of the digastric muscle, the anterior border of the SCM, and the cartilaginous external auditory canal. If the mass is in this area, consideration should be given to identifying the facial nerve in the mastoid and following it out the stylomastoid foramen.

Controversy exists regarding the optimal age for excision of first branchial arch anomalies because of the inherent risk to the facial nerve. Waiting until the child is older to excise the anomaly makes identification and preservation of the facial nerve easier. However, observation over a long period increases the risk of infection and fibrosis, rendering surgical dissection more difficult. In general, it is prudent to wait until the child is ~2 years of age, at which time the mastoid tip and facial nerve are larger.

When the tract involves the cartilaginous external auditory canal, the cartilage and overlying skin must be excised with the tract. Tracts entering the middle ear or temporal bone may be amputated with curettage of the bone if necessary. Tracts with extensive involvement of the external auditory canal may require the canal to be packed for 3 to 4 weeks to prevent subsequent stenosis.

Second branchial arch anomalies that swell, become infected, or drain also require surgical excision. The resection should include a rim of skin around the fistulous tract if present, careful dissection of the tract with a cuff of normal tissue, and removal of any cystic structures and the tract up to the tonsillar fossa mucosa, where the tract is amputated. Care must be made not to injure the numerous vessels and nerves in close proximity to the tract. Fistulas or sinuses with an external skin opening may be cannulated using a lacrimal probe to facilitate dissection.

Controversy exists surrounding the management of third and fourth branchial anomalies. When clinical suspicion is high for a third or fourth anomaly, microlaryngoscopy is recommended to evaluate the pyriform sinuses. Tracts ending at the pyriform sinus can be treated with endoscopic electrocauterization of the opening with resolution of symptoms in greater than 75% of patients. Cystic anomalies and those failing endoscopic treatment require open resection, including hemi-thyroidectomy and meticulous dissection of the tract to the pyriform sinus apex. Great care must be taken to preserve the recurrent laryngeal nerve.

86.7 Rehabilitation and Follow-up

The rate of recurrence following resection of branchial anomalies is less than 5% when there is no history of prior infection or surgery. This rate increases to 20% when these risks are present. Permanent injury to the facial nerve is rare when first branchial anomalies are approached in a systematic fashion.

86.8 Questions

1. The differential diagnosis of congenital midline neck mass includes all of the following except
   a) Thyroglossal duct cyst.
   b) Dermoid/epidermoid cyst.
   c) Plunging ranula.
   d) Branchial cleft cyst.
   e) Hemangioma.
2. Concerning the embryology of branchial arches, the first branchial arch gives rise to what?
   a) Head and neck of the malleus.
   b) Upper half of hyoid bone.
   c) Stylopharyngeus.
   d) Sphenomandibular ligament.
   e) Stapedius tendon.
3. Which of the following statements regarding branchial cleft cysts is true?
   a) First branchial arch cysts often present as thyroid abscesses.
   b) Acutely infected cysts should receive incision and drainage prior to antibiosis.
   c) Cysts, sinuses, and fistulas course superior to other derivatives of their own arch.
   d) Second branchial arch anomalies are the most common.
   e) First branchial arch cysts are always superficial to the facial nerve.

Answers: 1. d 2. a 3. d

Suggested Readings

Adams A, Mankad K, Offiah C, Childs L. Branchial cleft anomalies: a pictorial review of embryological development and spectrum of imaging findings. Insights Imaging. 2016; 7(1):69–76

Prosser JD, Myer CM, III. Branchial cleft anomalies and thymic cysts. Otolaryngol Clin North Am. 2015; 48(1):1–14

Work WP. Newer concepts of first branchial cleft defects. Laryngoscope. 1972; 82(9):1581–1593

D'Souza AR, Uppal HS, De R, Zeitoun H. Updating concepts of first branchial cleft defects: a literature review. Int J Pediatr Otorhinolaryngol. 2002; 62(2):103–109

Shinn JR, Purcell PL, Horn DL, Sie KC, Manning SC. First branchial cleft anomalies: otologic manifestations and treatment outcomes. Otolaryngol Head Neck Surg. 2015; 152(3):506–512

James A, Stewart C, Warrick P, Tzifa C, Forte V. Branchial sinus of the piriform fossa: reappraisal of third and fourth branchial anomalies. Laryngoscope. 2007; 117(11):1920–1924

Josephson GD, Black K. A Review Over the Past 15 Years of the Management of the Internal Piriform Apex Sinus Tract of a Branchial Pouch Anomaly and Case Description. Ann Otol Rhinol Laryngol. 2015; 124(12):947–952

87 Vascular and Lymphatic Malformations

Kareem O. Tawfik and Charles M. Myer IV

87.1 History

The otolaryngology team was consulted by the obstetric service regarding a 35-year-old G1P0A0 woman in her 35th week of pregnancy. Routine screening ultrasound revealed a right-sided fetal cervicofacial mass. Magnetic resonance imaging (MRI) confirmed the presence of a complex predominantly T2-hyperintense infiltrative lesion centered in the right cheek soft tissues and parotid space, extending superiorly toward the scalp and medially into the parapharyngeal space, surrounding the carotid sheath, and extending into the right posterior cervical space. The mass also extended inferiorly into the floor of mouth and bilateral submandibular/sublingual soft tissues as it crossed the midline. The parapharyngeal component mildly impinged upon the airway (▶ Fig. 87.1). Plans were made for an elective cesarean section delivery with the otolaryngology team present in the delivery room to assist with management of the neonate's airway.

Cesarean section proceeded uneventfully. The neonate cried upon delivery but shortly thereafter became bradycardic with heart rate < 60.

87.2 Differential Diagnosis—Key Points

Several key points in this history point to potential problems in the care of this child:

- Airway obstruction at birth is a life-threatening condition associated with a high mortality rate, especially if there is delay in securing an airway or if there is inability to ventilate the neonate. Hypoxia, acidosis, and ischemic brain injury will result in significant morbidity, even death. When fetal airway obstruction is diagnosed antenatally, a planned multidisciplinary approach to delivery is advocated to maximize the outcome for both the mother and child. An ex utero intrapartum treatment (EXIT) procedure allows the fetus to be delivered while maintaining the uteroplacental circulation until secure fetal airway has been established. The obstetric team, two anesthesiology teams, otolaryngology, neonatology, pediatric surgery, maternal-fetal medicine specialists, an echocardiographer, and two full surgical scrub teams should be briefed and prepared for every contingency. Reliable maternal-fetal circulation can be maintained for longer than 1 hour.

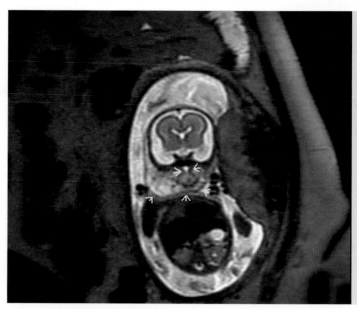

Fig. 87.1 A prenatal magnetic resonance imaging scan depicting T2-hyperintense complex infiltrative lesion centered in the right cheek soft tissues/parotid space, extending medially into the parapharyngeal space and inferiorly into the floor of mouth and bilateral submandibular/sublingual soft tissues as it crosses the midline. The parapharyngeal component abuts the airway wall but does not appear to cause significant compression.

If an experienced team of clinicians and surgeons is not available, a child might be delivered by cesarean section, maintaining the child at the level of the maternal heart, on placental support (operation on placental support [OOPS]). Reliable maternal-fetal circulation can be maintained for only 5 minutes using this approach.

- The mother and neonate have specific individual needs that must be met, and a separate team dedicated to the management of each is important. Planning for the delivery should occur as soon as the lesion is identified by imaging. The largest operating room available needs to be set up to accommodate the two teams so that each will have access to equipment without interference from the other. For the neonate, a range of appropriately sized laryngoscopes with light sources, endotracheal tubes, introducers, laryngeal mask airways, ventilating bronchoscopes, and tracheotomy instruments are essential. If a tracheotomy is required, a second surgical nurse should be available to assist with that procedure. A pediatric surgeon should also be available if there is concern that access to the mediastinal trachea may be necessary. A pediatric anesthesiologist should be in attendance to provide for the anesthetic needs of the child.

- The EXIT procedure differs from a routine cesarean section in that the goal is to achieve a state of uterine hypotonia with preservation of uterine volume to maintain the uteroplacental circulation. A level of fetal anesthesia without cardiac depression is also desired. In contrast, during a cesarean section, the goal is to maximize uterine tone to prevent postpartum hemorrhage and to avoid fetal anesthesia and potential respiratory depression.

- The differential diagnosis of a congenital cystic cervicofacial mass causing extrinsic airway obstruction such as described in this case includes teratoma, lymphatic malformation, and arteriovenous malformation. Less common lesions causing extrinsic obstruction of the airway include branchial cleft cyst, fetal goiter, sarcoma, and neuroblastoma. The term CHAOS (congenital high airway obstruction syndrome) has been used to describe intrinsic fetal upper airway obstruction. Intrinsic airway lesions include laryngeal atresia, stenosis, or web and tracheal atresia or stenosis. If there is no tracheoesophageal connection, the secretions produced by the fetal lungs cannot be excreted, causing the lungs to expand and the diaphragm to flatten or invert. If the esophagus is compressed or obstructed, fetal swallowing is impaired and polyhydramnios may occur. Regardless of the precise diagnosis of the obstructing lesion, the initial approach to the airway will be the same.

- The approach to the compromised newborn airway must be orderly. If a neonate is spontaneously breathing, the degree of airway obstruction must be assessed to determine the need for elective intubation in the delivery room. If the airway is compromised, endotracheal intubation with a reinforced endotracheal tube should be attempted. If the endotracheal tube cannot be passed because of a mass compressing the lumen of the trachea (most of these can be overcome with gentle pressure on the endotracheal tube), a rigid bronchoscope can be passed into the airway. In some situations, traction on the mass by an assistant may help to elevate it off of the airway structures, allowing for intubation. With a bronchoscope in place, a tracheotomy can then be performed in a controlled fashion.

- If a bronchoscope cannot be passed, a tracheotomy must be performed immediately. This may require reflection or partial resection of a neck mass. If the cervical component of the mass precludes access to the anterior base of the neck, a thoracotomy should be performed to access the mediastinal trachea. Proper positioning of the tracheotomy between the second and third tracheal rings is important because the fetal trachea may be pulled out of the chest owing to hyperextension of the neck.

- In an EXIT procedure, depending on the length of the umbilical cord, procedures on the fetus may need to be performed on the partially delivered child (head, neck, and one arm delivered through the hysterotomy), with the child across the legs of the mother or occasionally on a sterile instrument tray on a movable stand positioned at right angles to the mother. In the case described, the patient did not require a formal EXIT procedure. Rather, she was promptly intubated after a controlled cesarean section. After stablilization, microlaryngoscopy and bronchoscopy were performed, revealing grade 1 laryngeal exposure despite the presence of soft tissue fullness of the right lateral pharyngeal wall and right supraglottis. The glottic, subglottic, and tracheal airway appeared normal. The patient was transferred to the intensive care unit. Five days later, after being weaned to minimal ventilator support, the patient was extubated successfully in the operating room.

87.3 Test Interpretation

- Prenatal ultrasound: Because of the widespread use of prenatal ultrasound, there has been an increase in the diagnosis of fetal airway malformations. Polyhydramnios is seen in up to 40% of cases due to concomitant fetal esophageal obstruction that is often seen in association with large tumors. The two most common cervical fetal masses are lymphatic malformations and teratomas. Lymphatic malformations, formerly known as *lymphangiomas*, are a type of vascular malformation. Vascular malformations, in contrast to vascular tumors, are present at birth and grow commensurately with the child. Histologically, they display no evidence of proliferation but progressive dilation of their channels. They are classified according to the predominant channel type present: capillary, venous, lymphatic, arterial, or combined. Whereas arterial malformations exhibit fast flow, capillary, venous, and lymphatic malformations are slow-flow anomalies. Lymphatic malformations may be classified as *macrocystic*, *microcystic*, or *mixed* according to the size of the cysts that constitute the lesions. In the head and neck, macrocystic lesions are often located below the mylohyoid muscle, whereas microcystic lesions often lie above the mylohyoid. On ultrasound, lymphatic malformations typically appear as multiloculated cystic masses with poorly defined, infiltrating borders. They have a proclivity for forming in the head and neck and do not have malignant potential. Fifty percent of lesions are apparent in the neonatal period, and 75% present within the first year of life. Those diagnosed early in gestation tend to be associated with chromosomal abnormality. Teratomas, in contrast, are germ cell tumors composed of tissues foreign to their anatomic site (such as neural elements, cartilage, and respiratory epithelium). All three germ cell layers are represented. They may involve the floor of the mouth or the tongue and can extend into the mediastinum. On ultrasound they tend to be cystic appearing with well-defined margins, although the two lesions may be difficult to distinguish. The availability, portability, and ease of obtaining an ultrasound are the main benefits of ultrasonography for vascular anomalies of the head and neck.
- Magnetic resonance imaging (MRI): Visualization of the mass allows for precise surgical planning and helps to predict the need for airway intervention at birth. Fetal MRI can provide information about the physical characteristics, extent, and vascularity of the lesion and about its relationship to surrounding structures. Radiation is avoided and there are no deleterious effects on the developing fetus. Postnatal MRI for evaluation of a vascular malformation should include T1- and T2-weighted spin-echo imaging, fat-saturated T1-weighted imaging with the intravenous administration of a gadolinium-based contrast agent, and gradient-recalled echo (GRE) imaging. Imaging should be reviewed by a radiologist familiar with the diagnosis and classification of vascular malformations. Biopsy is rarely required to differentiate tumors that arise in the neck. The child in this case had a lymphatic malformation diagnosed prenatally. Once the neonate's airway was stable, MRI was repeated to assist in planning for therapy (► Fig. 87.2).
- Computed tomography (CT): This modality may provide further information about osseous involvement and skeletal abnormality, but it generally plays a limited role given the inherent lack of soft tissue detail and significant exposure to unnecessary ionizing radiation.
- Plain radiographs: Radiographic films may assist assessment of dental development in later years because cervicofacial lymphatic malformations can cause skeletal distortion, malocclusion, mandibular overgrowth, and anterior open bite.

87.4 Diagnosis

Cervicofacial lymphatic malformation causing fetal airway obstruction

87.5 Medical Management

The neonate must be stabilized after the airway is secured and thoroughly evaluated for associated anomalies. Only after the child is considered stable should surgical excision of the mass be planned. Pulmonary function must be maximized preoperatively or the resection must be delayed until the neonate's pulmonary function has been optimized. Nutritional support may be required by means of a nasogastric or orogastric tube. If long-term support is required because of impaired swallowing ability, gastrostomy tube placement may be prudent.

Most lymphatic malformations of the head and neck are not diagnosed prenatally and do not present emergently. An asymptomatic neck mass

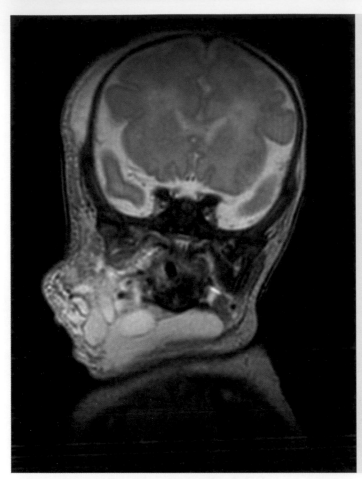

Fig. 87.2 A postnatal magnetic resonance imaging scan depicting a mixed microcystic and macrocystic mass. Macrocystic components resolved with sclerosing therapy. Microcystic components continue to be treated with systemic rapamycin therapy.

is the most common presentation. While lymphatic malformations do not regress, expansion and contraction of these lesions can occur depending on the amount of lymphatic flow. The most significant complications of lymphatic malformations are intralesional bleeding and infection, which often result in rapid expansion of the mass. Pain, concerns regarding cosmesis, and ulceration may also drive patients to seek therapy. Intravenous antibiotics are prescribed if there is an acute infection but are generally not given prophylactically. Some children with limited disease are successfully managed expectantly. Aspiration of the cysts has been described for the treatment of macrocystic lymphatic malformations but often results in recurrence. Sclerotherapy has emerged as an acceptable alternative to surgery in select vascular anomalies. Under ultrasound guidance, the cysts are aspirated and then injected with a sclerosant such as hypertonic saline, sodium tetradecyl sulfate, absolute ethanol, doxycycline, bleomycin, or

Streptococcus pyogenes–derived OK-432, which causes inflammation and subsequent fibrosis of the vascular channels. Admission to hospital for overnight observation is recommended if there is a risk of airway compromise secondary to the manipulation of the lesion. Microcystic lymphatic malformations are not generally suitable for sclerosant therapy, although it has been described as beneficial in limited reports.

For large complex or complicated vascular anomalies, the use of sirolimus has been shown to be beneficial. Sirolimus acts on the phosphatidylinositol 3-kinase (PI3K)/AKT signaling pathway, which regulates normal angiogenesis and vascular development. Case reports and a larger prospective trial have shown improvement in pain, quality of life, and stabilization and regression of these complicated lesions. The potential for adverse effects and need for close monitoring limit its applicability to those patients with significant disease burden and limited therapeutic options.

This particular patient was successfully intubated at birth due to respiratory distress. She was stabilized in the neonatal intensive care unit and was successfully extubated in the operating room several days later. Since that time, she has not exhibited symptoms of airway obstruction and is growing appropriately. The macrocystic components of her malformation have been treated successfully with sclerotherapy. Her microcystic disease is being treated with rapamycin. Surgical therapy to address residual malformation will be pursued as she grows.

87.6 Surgical Management

The indications for surgical treatment of vascular anomalies include functional limitations, intolerable symptoms, and disfigurement. The benefit of surgery must be weighed against the risk of potential morbidity from operating in a small and distorted surgical field, especially given the benign nature of these lesions. Due to the complex nature and varied presentation of vascular anomalies, treatment must be individualized for each patient, and evaluation by a multidisciplinary team well versed in the management of these lesions is beneficial. Surgery may need to be staged over months to years depending on the symptoms and site of the disease.

The goal of surgery is complete resection, although this is seldom possible because malformations are often closely related to essential structures that must be preserved. The approach to the large cervicofacial lymphatic malformation is dictated by the extent of the lesion. Macrocystic and unilocular masses can be easily dissected. Microcystic and infiltrative lesions are resected with the goal of maintaining function. The recurrence rate of these lesions is high.

Anomalies involving the tongue base, pharyngeal walls, and supraglottic or glottic structures have the potential to cause airway obstruction or difficulty with deglutition. The airway should always be evaluated to determine the extent of involvement. A tracheotomy may be required for long-term management of the patient. However, a combination of medical and surgical therapy, such as tongue base reduction or radiofrequency ablation, may allow for decannulation.

Tongue reduction surgery may be helpful if bulky infiltrating disease prevents oral closure. Laser resurfacing of the oral mucosa may be beneficial for those patients with leakage or bleeding.

Orthodontics and orthognathic procedures may be required for facial skeletal deformities in later years.

87.7 Rehabilitation and Follow-up

Long-term follow-up of these patients is required. The need for further resection is based on the location of persistent disease, the degree to which the recurrent mass becomes symptomatic for the patient, and the degree to which function is impaired. The mere presence of persistent lymphatic malformation does not necessitate resection. Multidisciplinary input from otolaryngology, plastic surgery, dentistry, nutritionists, and speech-language therapy is essential in the long-term management of these children.

87.8 Questions

1. Maternal-fetal circulation is best maintained via which of the following?
   a) EXIT (ex utero intrapartum treatment) procedure.
   b) OOPS (operation on placental support) procedure.
   c) Cesarean section with umbilical cord left intact.
   d) Spontaneous vaginal delivery.
2. Polyhydramnios is a predictor of which of the following?
   a) Teratoma.
   b) Lymphatic malformation.
   c) Gastric obstruction.
   d) Esophageal obstruction.
3. Regarding the nature of vascular malformations, which of the following statements is false?
   a) Lesions grow commensurately with the child.
   b) Lesions display no evidence of cellular proliferation on histologic analysis.
   c) Lesions are often absent at birth.
   d) Lesions may be classified as capillary, arterial, venous, lymphatic, or combined.

Answers: 1. a 2. d 3. c

Suggested Readings

Adams DM, Trenor CC, III, Hammill AM, et al. Efficacy and Safety of Sirolimus in the Treatment of Complicated Vascular Anomalies. Pediatrics. 2016; 137(2):e20153257

Arneja JS, Gosain AK. Vascular malformations. Plast Reconstr Surg. 2008; 121(4):195e–206e

Dasgupta R, Adams D, Elluru R, Wentzel MS, Azizkhan RG. Noninterventional treatment of selected head and neck lymphatic malformations. J Pediatr Surg. 2008; 43(5):869–873

Elluru R. Congenital Vascular Lesions.vl In: Bailey BJ, Johnson JT, et al, eds. Head & Neck Surgery—Otolaryngology.Vol 1. 5th ed. Philadelphia, PA: Lippincott Williams & Wilkins; 2014:1574––1588

Farrell PT. Prenatal diagnosis and intrapartum management of neck masses causing airway obstruction. Paediatr Anaesth. 2004; 14 (1):48–52

Hartnick CJ, Rutter M, Lang F, Willging JP, Cotton RT. Congenital high airway obstruction syndrome and airway reconstruction: an evolving paradigm. Arch Otolaryngol Head Neck Surg. 2002; 128 (5):567–570

Lim FY, Crombleholme TM, Hedrick HL, et al. Congenital high airway obstruction syndrome: natural history and management. J Pediatr Surg. 2003; 38(6):940–945

Marwan A, Crombleholme TM. The EXIT procedure: principles, pitfalls, and progress. Semin Pediatr Surg. 2006; 15(2):107–115

Ogamo M, Sugiyama T, Maeda Y, et al. The ex utero intrapartum treatment (EXIT) procedure in giant fetal neck masses. Fetal Diagn Ther. 2005; 20(3):214–218

Wassef M, Blei F, Adams D, et al. ISSVA Board and Scientific Committee. Vascular Anomalies Classification: Recommendations From the International Society for the Study of Vascular Anomalies. Pediatrics. 2015; 136(1):e203–e214

88 Down Syndrome

Christine H. Heubi and Sally R. Shott

88.1 History

A 7-year-old girl with Down syndrome presented to the otolaryngology clinic with a 2-month history of draining ears. She had been on multiple oral antibiotics prescribed by her pediatrician, but her ears continued to drain. Her father reported that the pediatrician had difficulty visualizing the patient's tympanic membrane, but treated with oral antibiotics whenever there was drainage. He had also been applying the ear drops that were prescribed when her third sets of pressure equalizing tubes (PE tubes) were placed for her repeated ear infections. The father also reported nasal obstruction and rhinorrhea for many months, and that he often found his daughter breathing with her mouth open. He denied any snoring or apneic pauses at night, but on further questioning about her sleep, he reported that she slept in unusual positions, including in a sitting up position or with hyperextension of her neck and sometimes folded over forward at the waist; she often fell asleep with passive activities, particularly when riding in the car.

On review of her past medical history, the father reported that his daughter was full term and did not require supplemental oxygen or intubation at birth. She did have a ventriculoseptal defect (VSD) that was repaired shortly after birth. She also had multiple episodes of croup as an infant requiring emergency room visits, but had not had any symptoms of this for many years. She underwent an adenotonsillectomy at age 4 years. Her sleep improved after the surgery, but her father reported that she was back to waking up several times each night once again. She had been developing well, with mild delay in regard to her milestones. She was in an integrated classroom with an aide, currently in the first grade. Recently, the father had noted bed-wetting at night after being dry for at least 2 years. Her father also questioned a possible balance problem because his daughter had several recent falls.

Physical examination revealed a mildly obese 7-year-old girl with the epicanthal folds and midface hypoplasia commonly seen in Down syndrome and an open-mouth breathing posture at rest. Her external auditory canals were stenotic and filled with yellow mucoid discharge, making it difficult to visualize the tympanic membranes. She had poor nasal airflow, her inferior turbinates were slightly congested, and yellow rhinorrhea was evident. The oral cavity showed macroglossia, a small oropharynx, and tonsillar fossae that were well healed from her previous surgery. There was no cervical lymphadenopathy. She would not cooperate for a flexible nasoendoscopy, and a lateral neck X-ray was ordered. The ears were examined under the microscope and suctioned, revealing bilateral external otitis and bilateral otorrhea with patent PE tubes.

88.2 Differential Diagnosis—Key Points

Several key points in this history pointed to potential problems in the care of this child:

The patient had a history of chronic ear disease and eustachian tube dysfunction requiring multiple sets of PE tubes. Children with Down syndrome are more predisposed to this condition because of midface hypoplasia with nasopharyngeal abnormalities and the effects of generalized hypotonia, including poor function of the muscles of the palate, immaturity of the immune system, and adenoid hypertrophy. Otoscopic exam by an otolaryngologist every 3 to 6 months is recommended by the American Academy of Pediatrics (AAP) until the external auditory canal is of an adequate size for the pediatrician to reliably examine the tympanic membranes. Chronic tympanic membrane retraction and potential for acquired cholesteatoma should also be considered in this population of patients. They also have a higher incidence of hearing loss than other children, which may have a significant impact on their speech-language development.

The child had symptoms of nasal obstruction for many months. Anatomic abnormalities of the midface in children with Down syndrome can cause crowding of the nasal cavities and nasopharynx and contribute to chronic rhinorrhea and sinusitis. Immature immunologic development might also have been a factor here. Although she had a previous adenoidectomy, it was important to consider adenoid regrowth as a potential cause, which is more common in children with Down syndrome.

This child's symptoms of sleep-disordered breathing improved initially after her adenotonsillectomy, but symptoms of sleep-disordered breathing had returned. Unfortunately, because a large percentage of children with Down syndrome have airway obstruction during sleep and the onset of obstructive sleep apnea at a very young age, many parents frequently assume that this is "normal" for their child and do not seek treatment. Airway obstruction in children with Down syndrome can be due to multiple levels of pathology: medially displaced tonsils in the face of midface hypoplasia and a contracted oropharynx and nasopharynx, hypotonia with oropharyngeal and hypopharyngeal collapse during sleep, and macroglossia with associated base of tongue collapse and resultant airway obstruction. In addition, central sleep apnea can be seen. Although removal of the tonsils and adenoids usually cures airway obstruction in typical children, studies have shown persistent obstructive sleep apnea (OSA) in 50 to 70% of children with Down syndrome after adenotonsillectomy, and this can be difficult to treat. The long-term effects of OSA disorders include failure to thrive, pulmonary hypertension, and behavioral issues, as well as decreased school performance.

This child presented with a history of recurrent croup. Children with Down syndrome are known to have smaller subglottic airways than the typical population and are prone to recurrent episodes of croup. This is important if surgery with anesthesia and intubation is being considered. Studies have shown that a child with Down syndrome will need a smaller endotracheal tube than what is usually used in typical children for intubation.

The patient's history of recently noted balance problems, particularly after active play and rolling on the ground, may be due to some coordination problems but could also be due to atlantoaxial instability and resultant compression of the spinal cord. This is of particular importance if contemplating a surgical procedure where the patient's neck will be manipulated.

88.3 Test Interpretation

Before any surgical procedure in which manipulation of the neck is required, parents should be questioned on symptoms that may be related to cervical spine abnormalities in children with Down syndrome including atlantoaxial instability, abnormal congenital fusion of the vertebral bodies, degenerative changes in the C2–C3 and C3–C4 cervical interspaces, and spinal cord compression. This is particularly important since hyperextension

and hyperflexion, in the presence of atlantoaxial instability, can cause compression of the spinal cord. Because it has been shown that plain radiographs are a poor predictor of the development of spine problems, it is no longer recommended to obtain neck radiographs in asymptomatic children with Down syndrome. Instead, universal positioning precautions should be carried out during any anesthetic or surgical procedure. However, patients with symptoms of significant neck pain, weakness, change in tone, gait abnormalities, change in bowel or bladder function, or signs of myelopathy should undergo imaging. Given the patient's history of recent falls, and onset of secondary enuresis, a plain cervical spine film in the neutral position, as well as flexion and extension views, should be performed. Any radiographic abnormality or concern for cervical spine anomalies merits prompt referral to a pediatric neurosurgeon or orthopaedic surgeon. The cervical spine films of the patient described in this case were normal. Regardless, the plan for positioning precautions at the time of the operative procedure was discussed with the family.

With this patient's history of recurrent croup, airway films may suggest some subglottic narrowing. Special precautions, particularly in terms of the size of endotracheal tubes used and documentation of an air leak around the endotracheal tube, should be taken at the time of any surgery. The nasopharynx can also be assessed with these radiographs, especially when the patient will not tolerate a flexible endoscopic examination. In this case, the subglottic airway appeared narrow, and review of her previous surgical records showed that she required an endotracheal tube two sizes smaller than usual for her age. Significant adenoid regrowth obstructing the nasopharynx was also identified on the lateral neck film.

With this patient's long history of upper airway obstruction, a chest radiograph can be helpful to rule out signs of cor pulmonale secondary to the chronic upper airway obstruction. In patients with known OSA that is untreated, it is necessary to obtain an echocardiogram. Her radiograph was normal.

Patients with Down syndrome have a higher incidence of hypothyroidism. Again, this would be important to know if general anesthesia were being considered and may be contributing to the history of fatigue. Current AAP recommendations include yearly thyroid function tests. Thyroid studies were within normal limits for this child.

The current guidelines for audiologic testing in children with Down syndrome is for screening at birth followed by behavioral audiograms every 6 months until normal hearing is seen bilaterally with ear-specific testing, which most patients are unable to perform until after 4 years of age. After normal hearing has been established in both ears, annual testing can be performed. Conductive hearing loss, which is more common in children with Down syndrome secondary to chronic otitis media with effusion, has been shown to improve after placement of PE tubes. Therefore, as stated previously, a careful otoscopic exam is essential to determine the presence of middle ear pathology. In this patient, a baseline audiogram was performed at the initial visit and showed a 45 dB conductive hearing loss bilaterally. Treatment of the ear drainage included suctioning of the ears under the office microscope, with cultures sent of each ear to confirm appropriate medication choices. Cultures were positive for Candida albicans and a mixture of three bacteria in each ear. She was treated with clotrimazole drops twice daily and Ciprodex drops twice daily, alternating the drops. Follow-up exam 2 weeks later showed resolution of the otorrhea and external otitis with patent, dry PE tubes in place. Repeat audio showed borderline mild conductive hearing loss bilaterally.

A formal polysomnogram (PSG) was indicated at this point for this patient's treatment course to evaluate objectively for OSA and determine the severity of disease. It has been well established that in children with Down syndrome there is poor correlation between parental report of sleep symptoms and the degree of OSA on PSG. It is the recommendation of the AAP that all children with Down syndrome should undergo PSG by the age of 4 years. Because children with Down syndrome have multiple potential sources of airway obstruction, persistent OSA after adenotonsillectomy is not uncommon. Additionally, obesity is a risk factor for OSA, and this should be discussed with families. Other findings on the PSG that may merit referral to a pediatric sleep specialist include nonapneic hypoxemia and central sleep apnea. The need for airway support, such as continuous positive airway pressure (CPAP) therapy, can then be determined. In this patient, moderate OSA was found on PSG with an obstructive apnea–hypopnea index of 9 events per hour associated with mild hypoxemia, mild hypercarbia, and an elevated arousal index. A trial of CPAP was not tolerated.

In patients with Down syndrome and persistent OSA after adenotonsillectomy, it is often helpful to obtain a cine sleep magnetic resonance imaging to identify the level, or levels, of obstruction. It provides a high-resolution dynamic assessment of the airway without subjecting the child to ionizing radiation. Performed under light anesthesia, consecutive fast gradient echo sequence images are taken to capture periods of snoring, obstruction, or oxygen desaturation and are then displayed in a cine format. Multiple levels of the airway can be assessed at the same time. Drug-induced sleep endoscopy is another method to evaluate the airway for sites of obstruction during sleep. Treatment can be tailored for the individual, directed toward the sites of the obstruction. In this patient, adenoid regrowth was confirmed, and relative macroglossia with lingual tonsillar hypertrophy was also found to be contributing to ongoing upper airway obstruction (▶ Fig. 88.1).

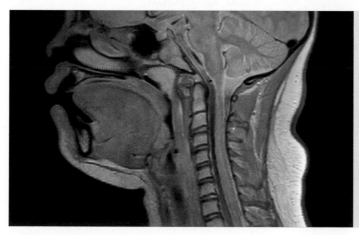

Fig. 88.1 Sagittal magnetic resonance imaging scan showing prominent adenoid regrowth and lingual tonsillar hypertrophy.

88.4 Diagnosis

Chronic otitis media with chronic otorrhea, external otitis, chronic rhinitis, and persistent OSA attributable to lingual tonsillar hypertrophy and adenoid regrowth in a girl with Down syndrome

88.5 Medical Management

The patient had multiple concurrent problems. The external auditory canals needed to be cleaned under the office microscope to allow examination of the tympanic membranes and a swab collected for microbiologic analysis, due to repeated previous treatment courses that were not successful. Topical antibiotics were warranted, but she might have required repeated débridements of the ear canals. If a child is systemically unwell and has other symptoms of an upper respiratory tract infection and/or chronic purulent rhinitis, oral antibiotics may be necessary. In some cases, a biofilm may have developed on the tympanostomy tube, and replacement of the tubes should be considered.

Adenoid regrowth has been identified as a cause for nasal obstruction and chronic rhinorrhea as well as contributing to airway obstruction. In cases of chronic rhinitis that is not purulent, nonsedative antihistamines and nasal steroids can be helpful. Topical nasal saline spray may provide symptomatic relief. Oral antibiotics should be considered when the rhinitis becomes purulent and lasts over 2 weeks.

88.6 Surgical Management

In the described case, surgical management was likely to be required to provide ear toilet and otologic microscopy, to treat the adenoid regrowth (revision adenoidectomy), and to address the lingual tonsillar hypertrophy (lingual tonsillectomy). Given that the child had Down syndrome, special precautions needed to be taken during the surgical procedure to avoid hyperextension/hyperflexion of the neck. The surgery was performed with the patient's neck in the neutral position and no shoulder rolls were used.

With this patient's history of recurrent croup, at the time of intubation, a smaller tube than would be expected for the patient's age and size needed to be used. The appropriateness of the tube chosen had to be confirmed with the presence of an air leak around the endotracheal tube.

Lingual tonsillectomy has been described using cautery, microdebrider, and coblation techniques. For this child, a handheld Lindholm laryngoscope was used to provide exposure of the base of tongue and the lingual tonsils were removed with a coblation wand.

Postoperatively, patients with Down syndrome may have a higher rate of complications than other children because of multiple sources of airway obstruction combined with hypotonia and central apnea. There is a higher incidence of postoperative airway obstruction that will need to be monitored closely in the inpatient setting.

88.7 Rehabilitation and Follow-up

The patient was treated with ototopical antibiotics and antifungals after débridement of the bilateral ears in the clinic. Follow-up examination revealed patent PE tubes with no evidence of retraction or cholesteatoma. Repeat audiogram showed improvement in hearing thresholds. The nasal discharge improved after revision adenoidectomy, and the number of episodes of otorrhea greatly reduced.

The patient's stay in the hospital was uneventful, and she was discharged on the first postoperative day tolerating adequate oral intake. She was seen in the clinic, and a follow-up polysomnogram was arranged 3 months later. This showed improvement in all parameters. The patient will continue to be followed in the future to monitor for the development of recurrent problems.

88.8 Questions

1. True or false? Parental report of sleep symptoms in children with Down syndrome correlates well with findings on polysomnography.
2. Based on the most recent recommendations by the American Academy of Pediatrics (AAP), children with Down syndrome should have audiograms at which interval?
   a) Every year until normal bilaterally on behavioral audiogram, then yearly.
   b) Every 3 months until normal bilaterally on behavioral audiogram, then yearly.
   c) Every month until normal bilaterally on behavioral audiogram, then yearly.
   d) Every 6 months until normal bilaterally on behavioral audiogram, then yearly.

3. Important considerations when intubating a child with Down syndrome include which of the following?
   a) Using an endotracheal tube that is larger than expected.
   b) Using an endotracheal tube that is smaller than expected.
   c) Using an endotracheal tube that is appropriate for the child's age.
   d) Gentle hyperextension of the neck to improve airway visualization.

Answers: 1. False 2. d 3. b

Suggested Readings

Bull MJ, Committee on Genetics. Health supervision for children with Down syndrome. Pediatrics. 2011; 128(2):393–406

Jacobs IN, Gray RF, Todd NW. Upper airway obstruction in children with Down syndrome. Arch Otolaryngol Head Neck Surg. 1996; 122(9):945–950

Kanamori G, Witter M, Brown J, Williams-Smith L. Otolaryngologic manifestations of Down syndrome. Otolaryngol Clin North Am. 2000; 33(6):1285–1292

Mitchell RB, Call E, Kelly J. Ear, nose and throat disorders in children with Down syndrome. Laryngoscope. 2003; 113(2):259–263

Shott SR. Down syndrome: analysis of airway size and a guide for appropriate intubation. Laryngoscope. 2000; 110(4):585–592

Shott SR. Down syndrome: common otolaryngologic manifestations. Am J Med Genet C Semin Med Genet. 2006; 142C(3):131–140

Shott SR, Amin R, Chini B, Heubi C, Hotze S, Akers R. Obstructive sleep apnea: Shoulds all children with Down syndrome be tested? Arch Otolaryngol Head Neck Surg. 2006; 132(4):432–436

Part XIV

Trauma

XIV

89 Frontal Sinus Fracture

Ryan A. Crane and David B. Hom

89.1 History

A 22-year-old man was involved in a motorcycle collision in which his vehicle struck a deer. The patient was unconscious with no gross focal neurologic deficits, and his hemodynamic status was stable. No clear rhinorrhea was evident. Neurosurgical consultation and head computed tomography (CT) scan evaluation showed anterior and posterior table commuted fractures with pneumocephalus. No evidence of intracranial parenchymal injuries or of intracranial bleeding was seen. The lateral cervical spine film was clear. Additional imaging revealed the presence of multiple comminuted midface fractures. The patient was admitted to the surgical intensive care unit for stabilization, and was then taken to the operating room by the neurosurgical and otolaryngology services for repair of his frontal sinus fractures, in addition to repair of his midface fractures.

89.2 Differential Diagnosis—Key Points

- In a patient with multiple trauma, the overall status must be emergently evaluated and be the top priority (airway, breathing, circulation, cervical status, intracranial status). Only after these steps are stabilized can facial injuries be addressed. In some instances, facial fractures may need to be addressed in a later setting, depending on the medical status. In this instance, the major goal of the neurosurgical team was to evaluate for intracranial injuries and to address his comminuted frontal sinus fractures with the assistance of otolaryngology.
- It is optimal to obtain a CT of the face (axial and coronal views) in patients with significant head trauma. In some instances, due to the patient's injuries, the otolaryngology service may be contacted while the patient is being expeditiously transported to the operating suite by the trauma or neurosurgical services.
- In a patient who has multiple major body traumas, it is imperative to have clear communication with all the involved surgical teams to approach the patient in a staged, coordinated manner to prevent lengthy procedures by multiple services at one sitting if the patient's status is precarious.

- For any head trauma, the possibility of cervical spine injury must be ruled out with cervical spine radiographs and clinical examination. However, if the patient is unconscious, the clinical assessment of a cervical spine cannot be performed, and frequently the patient is left in a cervical collar because an occult cervical injury may still be present. Even in the emergent setting when the clinical situation dictates against complete cervical spine radiographs, the neck must be immobilized and protected from any out-of-axis movements until appropriate cervical injury is ruled out. In some instances low cervical spine injury can be missed despite performance of full cervical radiographic series owing to the difficulty of radiographically imaging this area.
- In depressed anterior frontal sinus wall fractures, soft tissue edema can mask a contour deformity in the acute phase. Thus, a CT scan is required. High-resolution CT scan (axial and coronal images using 1.5-mm cuts) is very helpful in delineating the extent of bony displacement. Associated findings with frontal sinus fractures are central nervous system (CNS) injuries and cerebrospinal fluid (CSF) leaks. As in this case, injury to the posterior frontal sinus wall significantly increases the risk of dural tears (70% of displaced posterior walls have CSF leaks). Other possible CNS injures includes brain contusion, subdural hematoma, pneumocephalus, and frontal lobe laceration.

89.3 Test Interpretation

The CT image (▶ Fig. 89.1) shows anterior and posterior frontal sinus fractures, which are comminuted and depressed with pneumocephalus and a right orbital roof fracture. The lateral cervical spine radiographs did not have any evidence of cervical injury.

89.4 Diagnosis

1. Multiple facial lacerations
2. Depressed commuted frontal sinus fractures involving the anterior and posterior table
3. Orbital roof fracture
4. Pneumocephalus
5. Comminuted midface fractures

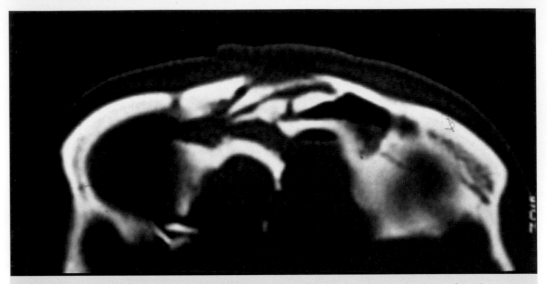

Fig. 89.1 Computed tomography image showing comminuted and displaced anterior and posterior frontal sinus fractures with associated pneumocephalus.

89.5 Medical Management

Prophylactic antibiotics (broad-spectrum) needed to be considered preoperatively because this was a clean contaminated wound. Given the nature of the displaced posterior table fracture, a dural tear with subsequent CSF leak was highly likely. This possibility had to be kept in mind during the initial management of the patient and surgical exploration of the frontal sinus.

Because the patient was young and healthy with no other bodily injury, no other medical issues besides stabilization and monitoring for the intracranial injury appeared to affect the medical management immediately. In the operating room, his eye status was evaluated and cleared by the ophthalmology team in light of the orbital roof fracture.

89.6 Surgical Management

After the life-threatening factors from multiple injuries had been stabilized, a plan for surgical treatment of the frontal sinus injury could be performed. Many times, a CT scan of the head might not give appropriate image resolution, and thus a finer-cut facial CT scan (1.5-mm axial and coronal views) may be helpful. If the patient is in a cervical collar, the coronal CT views will need to be reconstructed to prevent manipulation of the cervical spine.

The surgical treatment of frontal sinus fractures is based on whether the anterior or posterior table fracture is involved. If only the anterior table is fractured, with the nasofrontal duct uninjured, the surgical repair is done primarily to restore the contour of the forehead. In these cases, the depressed bony segment can be raised with bony fixation by several approaches (coronal, pretrichial, prior open laceration, transverse forehead incision, or endoscopically). At times bony fixation might not be needed if the reduced bone segment can maintain its correct anatomic position. If severe comminution is present, titanium mesh can be used to stabilize the bone pieces. If there is significant missing bone, an outer calvarial bone graft can be placed to restore contour of the bony gap. If neurosurgery performs a frontal craniotomy, an inner table calvarial bone graft can be obtained from the bicortical bone window on the table ex vivo before it is placed back to its original site.

For posterior table fractures, which are not comminuted or significantly displaced, many surgeons remove all the intrasinus mucosa, plug the nasofrontal ducts with fascia, and obliterate the sinus with abdominal fat. This procedure is performed to reduce the risk of mucocele formation from trapped mucosa between the bony fracture edges. Frontal sinus mucoceles may take many years to grow. In the setting of an intact anterior table with a posterior table fracture, an osteoplastic flap can be done for surgical exploration and exposure of the frontal sinus.

Only one patent nasal frontal duct is required for the frontal sinus to function. This patency can be tested by placing water dyed with methylene blue into the frontal sinus and by placing dry pledgets intranasally. One can then examine for blue dye on the intranasal pledgets, which would confirm nasofrontal duct patency. If needed, the midline frontal sinus septa may need to be burred down to ensure full communication of the bilateral frontal sinus cavities to the remaining nasofrontal duct. In instances when the nasofrontal duct has been disrupted by a transverse fracture, frontal sinus obliteration should be considered.

For a comminuted posterior table fracture, a cranialization procedure with neurosurgery should be considered. This procedure involves removing the posterior table of the frontal sinus with complete removal of all the frontal sinus mucosa and plugging the nasofrontal duct. In this case, a cranialization procedure with neurosurgery was performed and no dural tears were found.

89.7 Rehabilitation and Follow-up

This patient may need care at a rehabilitation facility for his closed head injury.

In regard to frontal sinus injury, subsequent mucocele formation can still develop over years. Thus, if a patient should have signs of future chronic sinus discomfort or infection, follow-up CT scans would be indicated. If a persistent air–fluid level in the frontal sinus is evident, it may suggest a CSF leak at the posterior frontal sinus wall or decreased function of the nasofrontal duct.

89.8 Questions

1. A 34-year-old man involved in an altercation has multiple comminuted posterior table frontal sinus fractures. What is the best treatment?
a) Cranialization.
b) Obliteration with abdominal fat.
c) Open reduction and internal fixation of comminuted pieces.
d) Placement of titanium mesh.
e) Performing a Reidel's procedure.
2. A 24-year-old woman involved in a motor vehicle accident has an isolated depressed anterior table frontal sinus fracture. What is the best treatment?
a) Cranialization.
b) Obliteration with abdominal fat.
c) Open reduction and internal fixation of depressed bone.
d) Placement of titanium mesh.
e) Performing a Reidel's procedure.
3. A 35-year-old man involved in a motor vehicle accident has transverse fracture through both of his frontal nasal ducts. What is the best treatment?
a) Cranialization.
b) Obliteration with abdominal fat.
c) Open reduction and internal fixation of depressed bone.
d) Placement of titanium mesh.
e) Performing a Reidel's procedure.

Answers: 1. a 2. c 3. b

Suggested Readings

Davidson JS, Birdsell DC. Cervical spine injury in patients with facial skeletal trauma. J Trauma. 1989; 29(9):1276–1278

Donald PJ. Frontal sinus ablation by cranialization. Report of 21 cases. Arch Otolaryngol. 1982; 108(3):142–146

Ducic Y, Hom DB. Reconstruction of frontal sinus fractures. In: Rengachary S, Benzel E, eds. Calvarial and Dural Reconstruction. Park Ridge, IL: American Association of Neurological Surgeons; 1998:102–116

Stanley RB, Jr. Management of frontal sinus fractures. Facial Plast Surg. 1988; 5(3):231–235

Wilson BC, Davidson B, Corey JP, Haydon RC, III. Comparison of complications following frontal sinus fractures managed with exploration with or without obliteration over 10 years. Laryngoscope. 1988; 98(5):516–520

90 Orbital Blowout Fracture

Ryan A. Crane and David B. Hom

90.1 History

The patient was a 67-year-old woman who presented to the emergency department after a fall at home. The patient stated that she slipped on her hardwood floor in the kitchen and struck her face on the counter and a stool. She reported that she was struck in the right periorbital area. She denied loss of consciousness. Subjectively, she reported blurred vision in her right eye and noted no cheek numbness. She was otherwise healthy, with no medical or ocular history.

Physical examination showed a healthy-appearing woman with periorbital ecchymosis. Pupil and visual examination demonstrated subconjunctival hemorrhage and a small corneal abrasion. Significant diplopia was present in upgaze, and she complained of mild pain with eye movements. She had decreased right ocular mobility on upward gaze with no enophthalmos. A step-off deformity was noted at the right lateral orbital rim. Her vision was 20/30 by the handheld Snellen's vision chart. A computed tomography (CT) scan of the maxillofacial region was done (▶ Fig. 90.1).

90.2 Differential Diagnosis—Key Points

- When evaluating patients with orbital and facial trauma, the more serious injuries need to be ruled out first, such as airway, breathing, circulation, intracranial injury, and vision-threatening problems. The patient had no loss of consciousness with the injury and had a normal neurologic examination. The other major concern would be ruling out an injury to the globe.
- The entire injury appeared to be localized to the periorbital area, and the extent of the injury could not be fully determined on external appearance alone. The motility examination indicated that extraocular muscles may be impinged or paretic, possibly from an orbital fracture. It is important to consider the surrounding facial structures for injury when an orbital fracture is present, namely, a zygomatic complex fracture or other facial fractures. The orbital rims should be palpated for tenderness and step-offs, as should the malar eminence. Any malposition or depressions in comparison to

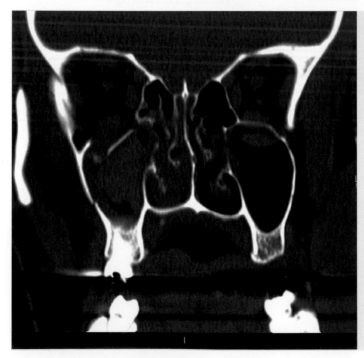

Fig. 90.1 Coronal computed tomography scan showing a right orbital floor fracture and prolapse of orbital soft tissue.

the normal side by the supra vertex and sub-mental clinical views should be noted.

- Cheek and lip numbness can also indicate that an orbital floor fracture is present, given that the infraorbital nerve runs along the floor. It is often involved and may be the only sign of a fracture on the examination. These should be evaluated and documented in trauma patients.
- A significant eye injury occurs in one-third of patients with orbital fractures, and thus a dilated fundoscopic examination by an ophthalmologist is recommended to rule out asymptomatic globe injuries.

90.3 Test Interpretation

A vital diagnostic test is a thorough ophthalmic evaluation to rule out globe injury. Corneal abrasions, hyphema, lens dislocation, retinal detachment, and rupture of the globe are among the injuries that should be ruled out with dilated examination. Delay in diagnosing severe eye problems may result in loss of vision; thus, ophthalmologic consultation in a timely fashion is recommended.

High-resolution CT imaging (axial and coronal views) provides the best information for evaluating orbital bones in relation to the soft tissues and orbital fat. When fractures are identified, herniation of orbital contents into the surrounding sinuses can lead to extraocular muscle entrapment within or below the bony fragments. In this case, there was an orbital floor blowout fracture and herniation of the inferior rectus with associated zygomaticomaxillary complex fracture.

An important part of the examination in patients with orbital fractures is forced duction testing. If it is unclear whether the muscle is entrapped, the insertion of the muscle can be grasped with a fine forceps with the aid of a topical anesthetic, and the globe is rotated. Severe restriction indicates that the muscle is entrapped and needs to be released surgically. This patient had limited upgaze and decreased mobility on forced duction, indicating extraocular muscle entrapment.

Hertel's exophthalmometry is another important examination that can be attempted, but may be difficult in the traumatic setting since this measures the outward protrusion of both eyeballs relative to each other and with respect to the bony orbital rim. The Hertel's measurements determine whether relative enophthalmos or exophthalmos

is present. The instrument is placed on the lateral orbital rims, so if they are not intact from a large tripod fracture or there is too much discomfort, the test is not useful. An easy alternative is to have the patient tilt his or her chin up so the globes can be viewed from below, giving a gross assessment of the eye positions. This patient had no enophthalmos at presentation.

The findings of periorbital ecchymosis, edema, restricted eye motility, cheek numbness, and radiographic evidence of an orbital floor fracture are all diagnostic of a blowout fracture. The compressive forces of the blow to the inferior orbital rim are transmitted posteriorly and the weakest portion of the orbit, the floor, or the medial orbital wall is fractured.

A distinct form of blowout fracture is the medial orbital wall blowout. Medial rectus incarceration can rarely occur in these cases, and the diagnosis is made based on physical exam and radiographically. When there is entrapment, horizontal motility is limited in both directions to some degree, depending on where the muscle is incarcerated.

90.4 Diagnosis

Right orbital floor blowout fracture with entrapment

90.5 Medical Management

Most orbital floor and medial wall fractures do not require surgical intervention, and if surgery is needed, it is rarely on an urgent basis in the adult. One exception is the "trapdoor fracture" that is seen in the pediatric population. The bones of children are thick and elastic and tend to snap back into position after being fractured. Thus, the orbital contents are compressed into the maxillary sinus when a fracture occurs and the bone transiently bends downward but can return to its normal position, leaving orbital contents trapped below the bone. When the inferior rectus is incarcerated in such a fracture, this is an emergent situation. Delay in releasing the muscle from the fracture will lead to ischemia and fibrosis of the muscle, resulting in permanent problems with motility. Early repair of these fractures is indicated to provide the best chance of preserving the function of the inferior rectus.

Other cases of blowout fractures (with the exception of large fractures, muscle entrapment, or enophthalmos > 3 mm) can be observed for resolution of the edema and motility problems. Ophthalmic consultation is required to rule out injury to the globe because 33% of orbital fractures are associated with a significant eye injury. The patient should be instructed not to blow his or her nose to prevent orbital emphysema and should not take medications containing blood thinners in case surgery will be required. If double vision and pain are present, a 1-week course of oral prednisolone (1 mg/kg/day) can be considered to hasten resolution of the edema and abnormal eye movement. Patients should be monitored closely to ensure that the motility is improving and that they are not developing enophthalmos.

Patients with smaller fractures, no enophthalmos evident, and normal forced duction testing can usually be observed without surgery. However, late enophthalmos from fat atrophy and fibrosis can still develop over the first month as the edema from the trauma resolves and may require surgery. Most authorities believe a delayed repair can achieve acceptable results with regard to eye position.

90.6 Surgical Management

Surgery is indicated if enophthalmos or muscle entrapment is present. The orbital floor is explored (through either a transconjunctival or an external approach), and the orbital soft tissues are carefully elevated away from the fracture. Forced duction testing should be done before and after surgery to ensure that release of the tissues has been accomplished. Once the entire fracture is exposed, the orbital floor needs to be resurfaced. Alloplastic sheeting materials are commonly used and readily available; these include nylon, porous polytetrafluoroethylene, and titanium sheets, which can be tailored to the proper size to cover the bone gap and rest on the surrounding bone edges. Care should be taken not to entrap orbital tissues between the posterior part of the implant and the bone, and forced ductions should be rechecked after the implant is placed.

Following surgery, the patient is usually admitted for 23 hours of observation with frequent vision checks, head elevation, and cold compress dressings. Orbital hemorrhage is the most worrisome complication that may occur in this period. It manifests by pain, proptosis, decreasing vision, and inability to move the eye. The hematoma develops in a closed space (the orbit) and can compress the optic nerve and blood supply to the eyeball. This is a surgical emergency that may require opening of the wounds, canthotomy and inferior cantholysis of the lateral canthal tendon, drainage of any hematomas, and control of any active bleeding.

Long-term complications include undercorrection of the enophthalmos. If more surgery needs to be done, one should wait 6 months for adequate resolution of the edema and healing before considering augmenting the floor with additional implants or repositioning of the implant. Persistent muscle entrapment may also occur and can be confirmed with forced duction testing and CT. If entrapment is present, exploration of the floor with release is indicated. If the muscle is only paretic or scarred from the trauma, one should wait at least 6 months before considering muscle surgery to allow for spontaneous improvement.

90.7 Rehabilitation and Follow-up

Patients should be monitored closely for the first 2 weeks following surgery. Eye motility and eye position should be measured until most of the edema has resolved and the patient has an adequate result. No Valsalva activities or nose blowing should be done by the patient for several months.

90.8 Questions

1. Which is not a surgical indication for orbital floor fracture repair?
   a) Entrapment of an extraocular muscle.
   b) Fracture of greater than 50% of the floor.
   c) Enophthalmos of 4 mm.
   d) Double vision from orbital hemorrhage adjacent to the fracture.
   e) Gross inferior placement of the globe into the maxillary sinus.
2. What is the best way to confirm that extraocular muscle entrapment is present?
   a) A dilated examination of the eye.
   b) Computed tomography (CT) imaging alone.
   c) Magnetic resonance imaging alone.
   d) Restriction on forced ductions combined with imaging.
3. What is the goal of orbital floor fracture repair?
   a) Release entrapped contents, improve globe position, and resurface the floor.
   b) Resolve double vision.

c) Release the infraorbital nerve to improve cheek and lip sensation.
d) Improve visual acuity.
e) Precise repositioning of the bones without using implants.

Answers: 1. d 2. d 3. a

Suggested Readings

Brannan PA, Kersten RC, Kulwin DR. Isolated medial orbital wall fractures with medial rectus muscle incarceration. Ophthal Plast Reconstr Surg. 2006; 22(3):178–183

Cole P, Boyd V, Banerji S, Hollier LH, Jr. Comprehensive management of orbital fractures. Plast Reconstr Surg. 2007; 120(7) Suppl 2:57S–63S

Nam SB, Bae YC, Moon JS, Kang YS. Analysis of the postoperative outcome in 405 cases of orbital fracture using 2 synthetic orbital implants. Ann Plast Surg. 2006; 56(3):263–267

Parbhu KC, Galler KE, Li C, Mawn LA. Underestimation of soft tissue entrapment by computed tomography in orbital floor fractures in the pediatric population. Ophthalmology. 2008; 115(9):1620–1625

Rinna C, Ungari C, Saltarel A, Cassoni A, Reale G. Orbital floor restoration. J Craniofac Surg. 2005; 16(6):968–972

91 Nasal Fracture

Adam D. Goodale and David B. Hom

91.1 History

A 24-year-old baseball player presented after being struck in the nose with a baseball during a game. He reported being struck along the left side of his nose with immediate onset of epistaxis but denied loss of consciousness. He was brought to the emergency room for evaluation. Upon evaluation, he reported pain over his nasal bridge and nasal obstruction but denied additional complaints. He reported intact vision and no change in teeth occlusion. On physical examination he had left inward depression of his nasal sidewall with an obvious asymmetry (▶ Fig. 91.1). There was moderate swelling over this area, with pain on palpation. Nasal endoscopy showed significant obstruction of the right nasal cavity with a mucosal tear along the maxillary crest. There was no septal hematoma.

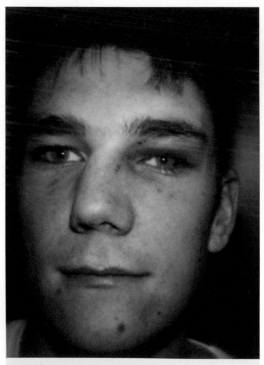

Fig. 91.1 Patient on initial presentation after injury.

91.2 Differential Diagnosis— Key Points

- The patient's history and physical presentation were suggestive of a nasal fracture. Depression of the nasal bones is often apparent on examination, which permits a clinical diagnosis in the majority of cases.
- Fracture of the nasal bones is the most common facial fracture, accounting for 40% of all facial fractures. Approximately 20% of patients with nasal fractures will have multiple fractures, and thus a thorough examination is important.
- The nasal septum should be closely evaluated in patients with nasal fractures. In 47% of patients with nasal fractures, the nasal septum will also be fractured, which can lead to significant airway obstruction.
- Patients with nasal fractures may have additional injuries and should have a comprehensive examination. With any significant impact to the nose, a maxillofacial computed tomography (CT) scan may be warranted to evaluate for nasal orbital ethnocide fractures.
- All patients with nasal trauma should be evaluated for a septal hematoma. A septal hematoma will present with septal mucosa bulging along the septal cartilage; these can be either unilateral or bilateral in presentation. If left untreated, a septal hematoma can develop into a septal abscess, cartilage necrosis with subsequent nasal deformity, or even cavernous sinus thrombophlebitis.
- The goal of treating nasal fractures is twofold: (1) reestablish the nasal airway and (2) restore nasal contour back to its pretrauma status as much as possible.
- Oftentimes it is difficult to determine if a nasal deformity is present, or the degree of deformity, soon after the injury due to overlying soft tissue swelling. Reevaluation several days after the injury allows for more accurate assessment once the swelling has resolved. If the patient has available facial photos from before the nasal injury, it is helpful to assess the baseline pretrauma nasal contour.

91.3 Test Interpretation

A nasal fracture can often be diagnosed on physical exam. The utility of nasal radiographs in the treatment of nasal injuries remains controversial. Plain X-rays have a high degree of false positives and negatives from old fractures, suture lines, and overlapping bone shadows. In addition, cartilage disruption cannot be detected by plain X-rays. CT scans are recommended when more extensive trauma is suspected, but are of limited utility for straightforward nasal fractures. Treatment goals of nasal fractures are to improve nasal breathing and nasal alignment. At times, nasal endoscopy is helpful to evaluate the nasal passage, especially with a prior history of nasal trauma or nasal surgeries.

91.4 Diagnosis

Displaced nasal bone and nasal septal fractures

91.5 Medical Management

Disruption of the nasal mucosa is often associated with nasal fractures, resulting in epistaxis. Control of the epistaxis is commonly the initial focus of treatment. Compression of the lateral cartilages and topical nasal decongestants, such as oxymetazoline, can be used initially. When unsuccessful, intranasal packing can be used. All patients with nasal packing should be treated with antistaphylococcal antibiotics. The patient's pain should be adequately treated.

91.6 Surgical Management

Surgical treatment of nasal fractures focuses on improving nasal airflow and overall nasal contour. In order to accurately assess the nasal contour, swelling should be minimal. Thus, closed reduction is optimally performed either 2 to 3 hours after injury when swelling is limited, or 3 to 5 days after the swelling has subsided. Ideally, closed reduction of nasal fractures should be performed within 5 to 7 days in children and 7 to 14 days in adults. After this time, bony malunion can occur, necessitating later bone osteotomy repair.

Closed reduction of nasal fractures is the most commonly used technique for treating nasal fractures. The majority of patients with uncomplicated nasal fractures are good candidates for closed reduction technique to obtain a satisfactory result. The failure rate increases significantly with the presence of increased severity of the nasal injury, a nasal dorsal septal fracture, and previous history of nasal trauma. Open reduction techniques have the benefit of realigning the displaced bones after bony union has occurred. Typically, open reduction is reserved for cases when patients fail to respond to closed reduction or if a significant nasal injury deformity exists.

For closed reduction, blunt elevator instruments are used endonasally to reduce the fracture site. This technique can be done under local anesthesia, intravenous sedation, or general anesthesia. The choice of clinical setting and anesthesia depends on several factors including the degree of injury, patient cooperation, and surgeon preference. The benefit of general anesthesia or monitored intravenous sedation is that additional procedures can be performed, such as a septal fracture repair, to improve overall outcome. The choice of surgical treatment should be based on the nature and degree of the nasal fracture.

The septum should be closely examined in all patients undergoing nasal fracture repair. Previous reports showed that as many as 80% of patients with nasal fractures have a concomitant septal fracture, with at least 60% of these being classified as severe. Failure to reduce septal fractures at the time of nasal fracture repair leads to higher rates of postreduction nasal deformities. When the septum remains misaligned, the nasal bones will migrate in the direction of the septal deformity with time. Septal fractures can be seen on nasal endoscopy as tears in the septal mucosa, shifted septal cartilage, or new onset nasal obstruction. The presence of a displaced septal fracture may require a closed or open septal fracture repair. However, when septal fractures are repaired, only conservative removal of cartilage and bone should be done to ensure adequate nasal dorsal support by leaving at least a 2-cm dorsal and caudal strut.

If a closed nasal and septal fracture repair is done, the patient should be informed before the procedure that a later open nasal septal fracture repair may still need to be done 6 to 12 months later.

The patient in this case was taken to the operating room for a closed reduction of his nasal bone fracture and an open acute septal repair of his severely deviated nasal septal fracture 7 days after his injury. Intranasal splints were placed to support the septal repair, as well as an external nasal splint. Both splints were removed 1 week after surgery. The patient had improved nasal symmetry and airflow after swelling resolved (▶ Fig. 91.2).

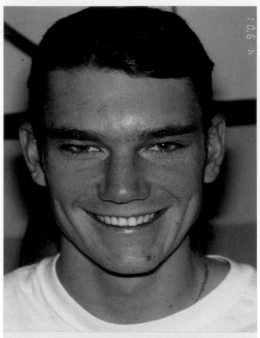

Fig. 91.2 Patient after closed reduction of nasal bone fracture and nasal septal fracture repair 2 months later.

91.7 Rehabilitation and Follow-up

Patients should be evaluated optimally for at least 2 to 3 months postoperatively to ensure adequate reduction and healing. Patients should be counseled to avoid additional nasal trauma for at least 6 weeks postoperatively and to wear nasal protection whenever it is possible that facial trauma may occur as the nasal bones heal. As stated previously, it is best to instruct the patient before any procedure is done that a possible later open nasal septal fracture repair may still need to be done 6 to 12 months later, depending on the severity of the nasal fracture.

91.8 Questions

1. In children, what is the most common type of injury from trauma?
   a) Nasal fractures.
   b) Midface fractures.
   c) Dentoalveolar injury.
   d) Mandible fractures.
2. Following nasal trauma, at what location along the septum are septal fractures most commonly seen?
   a) At the bony–cartilaginous junction.
   b) Along the perpendicular plate of the ethmoid.
   c) Along the dorsal septal cartilage.
   d) Along the quadrangular cartilage, above the maxillary crest.
3. Nasal fractures account for what percent of all facial fractures?
   a) 15%.
   b) 30%.
   c) 40%.
   d) 55%.

Answers: 1. c 2. d 3. c

Suggested Readings

Hom DB. Acute Nasalnasal ractures. In: Maisel R, ed. Maxillofacial Trauma. Rochester, MN: American Academy of Otolaryngology–Head and Neck Surgery Foundation, Inc.; 2001:25--34

Fernandes SV. Nasal fractures: the taming of the shrewd. Laryngoscope. 2004; 114(3):587–592

Rhee SC, Kim YK, Cha JH, Kang SR, Park HS. Septal fracture in simple nasal bone fracture. Plast Reconstr Surg. 2004; 113(1):45–52

Ducic Y, Hilger PA. Surgical correction of the deviated septum. Fac Plast Surg Clin North Am. 1999:7:319-331

92 Midface Fractures

Adam D. Goodale and David B. Hom

92.1 History

A 28-year-old woman presented to the emergency department after being involved in a motor vehicle collision, sustaining facial injuries and an extremity fracture. She was the driver in a two-car collision and was reportedly unrestrained, but was not ejected from the vehicle. Per the report from emergency medical services (EMS), she did not lose consciousness. She was transported by ambulance to the emergency department for evaluation.

On physical exam, she was alert and oriented with stable vital signs. She had a cervical collar (C-collar) in place, as well as a lower extremity stabilizing device. There was a 4-cm stellate laceration over her left brow and there were several abrasions over her left cheek. She had significant periorbital edema with an intercanthal distance of 38 mm. There was palpable crepitus and pain and swelling over her left cheek and midface region. Her nasal cavities were filled with dried blood, but there was no evidence of a septal hematoma or cerebrospinal fluid (CSF) leak. Her vision was grossly intact to finger counting and to reading fine print with no diplopia. She denied malocclusion or trismus.

The remainder of her exam was significant for a left tibia fracture. Her C-spine was clinically cleared. A maxillofacial computed tomography (CT) scan was performed (▶ Fig. 92.1).

92.2 Differential Diagnosis— Key Points

- As with any trauma patient, a thorough history and physical examination should be performed on initial evaluation. The overall status of the patient must be evaluated, and the critical body systems take the top priority (airway, breathing, circulation, cervical status, intracranial status). Only after the patient's status has been stabilized, then the obvious facial injuries can be addressed. In some instances, the facial fractures may need to be addressed at a later setting, The mechanism of the facial injury is also important, since it helps determine the degree of severity and diagnostic work-up.
- Patients with midface trauma should have a thorough neurologic evaluation with particular attention to orbital mobility, pupillary function, and visual acuity. Occult globe injury may be

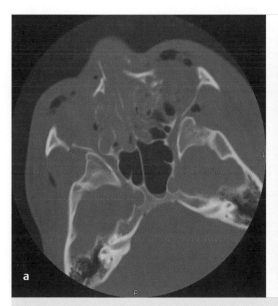
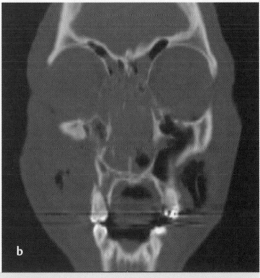

Fig. 92.1 (a,b) Maxillofacial computed tomography scan (axial and coronal cuts) of the face shows bilateral splaying of the lacrimal crests consistent with naso-orbito-ethmoid (NOE) fractures, bilateral orbital fractures involving the lateral and orbital floors, and a left zygoma fracture.

present even when the patient is asymptomatic (i.e., retinal detachment, lens injury).

- Fractures of the midface include fractures of the nose, maxilla, zygoma, orbit, and frontal sinus. Blunt trauma, including motor vehicle accidents, falls, and altercations, is the most common cause of these fractures. Penetrating trauma is less common in this area.

- The structural support of the midface is composed of horizontal and vertical bony buttresses. The main focus of repairing midface fractures is to restore these buttresses to reestablish facial height, width, and projection, as well as preinjury occlusion. Also, special attention should be given to ensuring that traumatic telecanthus has not occurred at the naso-orbito-ethmoid (NOE) complex.

- Midface fractures can be categorized by Le Fort's type. While most fractures do not exactly match this classification, it gives a general idea of the fracture lines. Le Fort I fractures extend across both maxillae and extend posteriorly to involve the inferior pterygoid plates. Le Fort II fractures involve both maxillae laterally, then extend superiorly to involve the anterior, inferior, and medial orbits, as well as the nasal bones. Le Fort III fractures involve complete separation of the facial bones from the skull base. The fracture line traverses laterally from the zygomatic arch to the lateral orbital wall, then to the medial orbital wall and nasofrontal suture line. Le Fort III fractures consist of complete craniofacial separation. By their definition, all Le Fort fractures have pterygoid plate involvement.

- Zygomaticomaxillary complex fractures (ZMC fractures) are the second most common facial fracture after nasal fractures. (Nasal fracture treatment is covered in chapter 91.) ZMC fractures involve trauma to the malar eminence with disruption of the articulations of the zygoma to the maxillary, temporal, sphenoid, and frontal bones. Approximately 90% of patients with ZMC fractures will have associated facial numbness and paresthesia in the infraorbital nerve distribution.

- The orbit should be carefully evaluated in all midface fractures. Fractures of the orbital wall commonly occur with midface fractures, with the orbital floor most commonly involved. Ocular mobility and function should be carefully evaluated, with a low threshold for ophthalmology consultation. Approximately 10% of patients with ZMC fractures will have ocular injuries that require repair.

92.3 Test Interpretation

High-resolution maxillofacial (axial and coronal) CT scans are essential to diagnose midface fractures. The bony horizontal and vertical buttresses should be closely evaluated. Open reduction is considered when there is comminution, displacement, instability, or mobility of these buttresses. The orbital walls should be closely evaluated with particular attention to the orbital floor, which is best evaluated on coronal or sagittal cuts. In the absence of entrapment, orbital floor fractures are typically repaired when more than 50% of the floor is fractured.

Classic clinical findings supporting NOE injury include the following: (1) an intercanthal distance greater than one-half the interpupillary distance and (2) an intercanthal distance greater than 35 mm. The clinical diagnosis of NOE fractures might not be obvious because of significant soft tissue swelling masking the underlying skeletal injury of the central midface. Classic nasal findings include a loss of height of the nasal dorsum with superior rotation of the nasal tip (the pig-nose deformity). At times, NOE fractures will be detected only by imaging studies. Bimanual examination by placing a mosquito clamp in the nose and digitally palpating the medial canthus on the same side can help determine whether free mobility is present at the NOE area. In the past, the eyelid traction test (pulling the lower eyelid laterally away from the nose) has been described as the classic sign for traumatic telecanthus; however, this finding may be evident only in severe cases. New three-dimensional reconstruction can be performed to assist with surgical planning.

92.4 Diagnosis

Naso-orbito-ethmoid (NOE) fracture, bilateral orbital fractures involving the lateral and orbital floors, and a left zygoma fracture

92.5 Medical Management

Displaced midface fractures are typically managed with open reduction and internal fixation. When orbital fractures are present, patients should be advised to avoid nose blowing to prevent orbital emphysema and subsequent pressure on the orbital nerve for at least 2 months.

Ocular trauma management is dependent on the nature of injury. With any evidence of orbital wall or floor fractures, ophthalmology consultation evaluation is recommended to rule out ocular injury. Nondisplaced orbital fractures without entrapment or significant orbital floor involvement can be managed conservatively. Retrobulbar hemorrhage is an orbital emergency and should be treated with mannitol, acetazolamide, steroids, and possible lateral canthotomy and inferior cantholysis. Ophthalmologic consultation should be obtained emergently to evaluate and follow the ocular status.

92.6 Surgical Management

The goal of surgical reduction of midface fractures is to reestablish facial height, facial projection, and preinjury occlusion. Early surgical intervention is favorable to limit soft tissue contracture and bony malunion (especially with NOE fractures). However, surgical repair should be deferred until the patient is clinically stable and more critical injuries, such as intracranial injuries, have been addressed.

Radiographic images should be thoroughly reviewed prior to surgery to assist with surgical planning. There are numerous surgical approaches to repair midface fractures, and the type of approach is dependent upon the location and severity of fractures, as well as surgeon preference. Cosmetically favorable incisions, such as sublabial, transconjunctival, or using preexisting lacerations, should be considered to improve the overall cosmetic result. More severe fractures may involve using multiple approaches to address all fractures.

To treat the bilateral NOE fractures, the displaced bony fragments need to be adequately reduced to restore the normal medial canthal distance (<30mm). The preferred vector pull of the medial canthi should be applied in the medial, posterior, and superior direction. Approaches to NOE fracture are through (1) the traumatic laceration (if present), (2) lateral nasal (Lynch's) incisions, (3) an H incision (transverse nasion with bilateral Lynch's incisions), or (4) a bicoronal approach.

When exposing the medial orbital rims, an attempt should be made to locate the medial canthal tendon attachment and not to strip the bony insertions of the medial canthal tendon off the lacrimal crest. The most important surgical step in treating NOE fractures is correcting the traumatic telecanthus. This step involves proper reduction and internal fixation of the medial orbital bone bearing the medial canthal tendon. Depending on the degree of the NOE fracture, optimal stabilization requires one or more of the following:

• Junctional fixation.
• Interfragmentary fixation.
• Transnasal wiring.

Junctional fixation involves attaching the central medial orbital bony fragment (a single piece or reconstructed bone from multiple pieces). Interfragmentary fixation can be used to fuse comminuted medial orbital bone pieces together using wires or miniplates. Transnasal wiring is used to reduce and secure laterally displaced central fragments near the medial canthal attachment. For splayed NOE fractures, transnasal wiring (30 gauge) is required to bring the medial canthi together to best correct the traumatic telecanthus. Transnasal wiring is often the most challenging surgical step. In most cases the medial canthi are still attached to the lacrimal bone. However, if the medical canthus is avulsed off the bone or if the medial canthal–bearing bone fragment is too small to work with for fixation, medial canthal reconstruction is required. One favored technique identifies the medial canthus and secures it with braided wire (32-gauge stainless steel), which is then passed transnasally through a point slightly posterior and superior to the upper end of the lacrimal fossa. The wire is then secured to a screw on the contralateral frontal bone at the supraorbital rim. If the medial canthi are detached bilaterally, a separate wire is passed for each medial canthus and secured with a small bone graft to secure the medial canthal tendon to the bone. In this case, the secured medial canthal tendon–bone graft unit is positioned using the transnasal wiring technique. Other surgical options are transnasal intercanthal wiring over plates to maintain canthal position and support of the comminuted nasal bones. Primary repair of traumatic telecanthus is much easier to perform early (<5 days) than secondary correction of residual telecanthus because of soft tissue scarring and retraction of the displaced bone fragments over time. If a laceration or tear of the lacrimal drainage system is noted, then the lacrimal duct can be probed and cannulated with cannulicular stents.

Maxillomandibular fixation (MMF) may play a role in the repair of midface fractures if midface instability is present. The relationship between the maxilla and upper midface can be altered during these fractures. MMF creates a rigid guide to reestablish facial contour. Oftentimes, patients are placed into MMF at the outset of surgical repair to guide realignment, and then released at the conclusion of surgical repair. Although rigid fixation is used to repair midface fractures, patients should be continued on a soft diet postoperatively. In cases of severe panfacial fracture, patients may be left in MMF for several weeks postoperatively.

Open reduction with placement of rigid fixation is the mainstay of treating midface fractures of the central facial buttresses of the maxilla. Direct visualization of the fracture site is important to ensure adequate reduction as well as facilitate plating of the fracture line. In this patient case, the left lateral buttress of the zygoma fracture also required open reduction and internal fixation.

92.7 Rehabilitation and Follow-up

Patients should be closely evaluated postoperatively to ensure adequate fracture reduction and healing of incision sites. When orbital fractures are present, the patient's ocular status should be monitored to ensure intact visual acuity and function. With orbital fractures, patients should be advised to avoid nose blowing to prevent orbital emphysema for at least 2 months.

92.8 Questions

1. Ectropion is most common after utilizing which surgical lower eyelid approach?
   a) Transconjunctival.
   b) Subciliary.
   c) Subtarsal.
   d) Lateral canthotomy.
   e) Infraorbital.

2. On physical exam, a helpful way to determine if an unstable naso-orbito-ethmoid (NOE) fracture is present acutely is to
   a) Place a mosquito clamp in the nose and digitally manipulate the medial canthal area.
   b) Manually push the nasal bones medially to determine stability.
   c) Have the patient in the Valsalva position to check for evidence of proptosis.
   d) Measure the intercanthal distance to see if it is greater than 35 mm.
   e) Perform rigid in-nasal endoscopy looking for bone disruption at the lamina papyracea.

3. What is the average intercanthal distance in an adult?
   a) 15 mm.
   b) 30 mm.
   c) 35 mm.
   d) 40 mm.
   e) 45 mm.

Answers: 1. b 2. a 3. b

Suggested Readings

Ochs MW. Fractures of the upper facial and bifacial skeleton. In: Myers EN, ed. Operative Otolaryngology. Philadelphia, PA: Saunders; 2008:pp 905-933

Shumrick KA, Kersten RC, Kulwin DR, Smith CP. Criteria for selective management of the orbital rim and floor in zygomatic complex and midface fractures. Arch Otolaryngol Head Neck Surg. 1997; 123(4):378-384

Jamal BT, Pfahler SM, Lane KA, et al. Ophthalmic injuries in patients with zygomaticomaxillary complex fractures requiring surgical repair. J Oral Maxillofac Surg. 2009; 67(5):986-989

Markowitz BL, Manson PN, Sargent L, et al. Management of the medial canthal tendon in nasoethmoid orbital fractures: the importance of the central fragment in classification and treatment. Plast Reconstr Surg. 1991; 87(5):843-853

93 Mandibular Fracture

Colin R. Edwards and David B. Hom

93.1 History

A 34-year-old man was assaulted in a barroom altercation. He was struck several times in the face and briefly lost consciousness. He presented to the emergency department (ED) complaining of neck pain, jaw pain, and malocclusion. He spoke in full sentences and did not have any stridor or dysphonia. On exam he had tenderness, ecchymosis, and edema over the right anterior mandible. Intraorally he had anterolateral mandibular mobility and premature contact of his right first mandibular molar (teeth no. 3 and no. 30).

He had no numbness of his anterior chin. He had tenderness to palpation of his C5 and C6 vertebrae but denied upper extremity numbness or weakness. He had full range of motion of his neck.

93.2 Differential Diagnosis—Key Points

- The initial management of all trauma patients begins with the ABCs. A for airway and cervical spine stabilization, B for breathing and ventilation, and C for circulation. All patients presenting with neck pain or depressed neurologic status should have their cervical spine stabilized with a cervical spine collar in order to prevent any neck movement that could exacerbate an undetected spine injury. Cervical spine plain film or computed tomography (CT) radiographs should be obtained to evaluate for vertebral fracture or malalignment. Plain film X-rays are often taken as part of the trauma triage process, whereas CT imaging should be deferred until the initial assessment and resuscitation has been performed. Lateral plain film cervical X-rays may be inadequate for evaluating inferior cervical spine injuries due to the shoulder and chest sometimes obscuring the C7 vertebral body. If the radiologist is unable to clear the cervical spine, the neck collar should be left in place until a spinal injury has been ruled out.
- Evaluation of the airway is an essential part of the initial trauma assessment. Hoarseness, stridor, crepitance, dysphonia, and tenderness to palpation over the anterior neck suggest possible laryngotracheal injury. Subcutaneous emphysema, or crepitus, may be palpated on physical exam and results from free air escaping from a laryngotracheal injury to the subcutaneous tissues. Flexible laryngoscopy using a nasopharyngoscope is a valuable tool for assessing laryngeal injuries and any impending airway collapse. Fractures of the thyroid and cricoid cartilages are possible and may be reflected in soft tissue edema, ecchymosis, or distortion of the supraglottis and glottis on flexible nasopharygeal laryngoscopy. Laryngotracheal separation is rare but may be suspected in the setting of subcutaneous emphysema. The patient may still maintain an airway but will eventually deteriorate. In such instances, an awake tracheotomy should be performed because intubation from above may cause complete laryngotracheal separation.
- Blunt cervical trauma can cause vascular injury to the carotid artery or other major vessels of the neck. Trauma can cause intimal disruption, pseudoaneurysm, or rupture of the vessel. Occult vascular injury can be detected on CT angiogram of the neck. Patients with a ruptured vessel may present with expanding hematoma or active bleeding causing hemorrhagic shock. Surgical exploration of the neck may be necessary to control bleeding.
- In the awake patient, complaints of malocclusion should raise the index of suspicion for a mandible fracture. Subtle alterations less than 1 mm can be detected by patients with normal dentition. Malocclusion may also be caused by maxillary fractures, dental or alveolar ridge fractures, and soft tissue edema impairing occlusion. Other physical exam findings may include mobile segments of mandible on palpation and chin numbness from inferior alveolar or mental nerve injury. In instances of fractured or missing teeth, a chest X-ray should be performed to evaluate for aspiration of the tooth.
- Mandible fractures frequently occur in pairs. Bilateral subcondylar fractures may present with posterior displacement of the mobile mandibular segment by the muscles of mastication. Posterior displacement of the mandible, coupled with destabilization of the suprahyoid musculature, may cause airway narrowing and obstruction. In addition, secretion management may be impaired in the facial trauma patient. These signs should clue the physician to the potential for

airway collapse, and an airway plan should be formulated quickly.

93.3 Test Interpretation

The initial assessment should include focus on any respiratory difficulty, and an airway should be established if necessary. Any patients with direct or indirect cervical trauma should be assessed for cervical spine injury. Complaints of neck pain or depressed neurologic status with inability to participate in the exam should prompt cervical spine collar placement, and plain film radiographs of the cervical spine should be obtained. If plain films are inadequate or subcutaneous air is present, then an axial CT should be obtained.

Once the primary survey is completed and life-threatening hemodynamic, vascular, spinal, and laryngotracheal injuries are ruled out, then the facial injuries can be evaluated. A thorough head and neck history and physical exam should be performed. The patient may complain of focal pain, malocclusion, loose or missing teeth, numbness, or inability to close the mouth. By placing firm manual posterior pressure on the chin, the region of the fracture can usually be ascertained. On bimanual exam, the physician may observe mobile mandible segments. If facial fractures are suspected, then a maxillofacial CT or panoramic x-ray should be obtained (▶ Fig. 93.1). If these imaging modalities

are unavailable, then plain film X-rays of the mandible using posterior–anterior, right and left lateral oblique, and reverse Towne's views can be done.

93.4 Diagnosis

Right mandibular parasymphyseal fracture

93.5 Medical Management

The initial medical management should be focused on maintenance of an adequate airway. In cases of bilateral subcondylar fractures, close attention should be paid to the airway and intubation may be necessary. Pain control is also a significant issue for mandibular fractures. Multimodal pain therapy, including acetaminophen and narcotic pain medications, can be used. Adequate analgesia with narcotics should be balanced against the possibility of depressing respiratory drive, especially in the setting of a tenuous airway. Patients should be considered to be placed on continuous pulse oximetry to monitor their respiratory status. Mandibular fractures may be associated with intraoral or skin lacerations, exposing the underlying bone to potential infectious sources. Antibiotic prophylaxis against oral flora and chlorhexidine mouthwash should be used to help prevent infection. Oral intake is often decreased in patients with mandible fractures and intravenous (IV) fluids may be required to maintain adequate

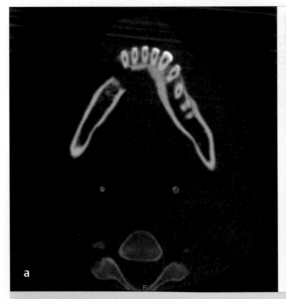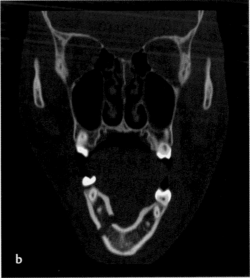

Fig. 93.1 (a,b) CT scan of the mandible (axial and coronal) showing a right displaced mandibular parasymphyseal fracture.

hydration. Many patients are able to tolerate a mechanical soft diet. For those patients unable to chew, protein shake supplements can provide a good source of nutrition.

93.6 Surgical Management

Surgical management of mandibular fractures involves establishing the patient into their best premorbid occlusion. In addition to occlusion, examining the dental cusps may reveal articular facets that represent areas of dental wear. Dental occlusion is usually established with arch bars and intermaxillary fixation (IMF). Next the fractures are exposed through either intraoral or external incisions and the bony segments are reduced and rigidly fixated with mandibular plates and screws. Open reduction and internal fixation with reapproximation of the fracture segments for bony union and reestablishing premorbid occlusion is the goal of surgery. The specific repair will be dictated based on the fracture sites, presence of comminution or bony displacement, dentition, and presence of other associated facial fractures. The patient should be nasally intubated to facilitate the assessment of occlusion and placement of arch bars. If there is any concern for the stability of the airway postoperatively, a tracheostomy can be performed at the beginning of the case. Occlusion can be assessed in the anteroposterior, vertical, and medial-lateral planes, and condylar repositioning may be required to restore anatomic positioning.

Attention should then be turned to the fractures, which can be exposed via intraoral or external incisions. The mandibular fragments should be reduced to their anatomic position and fixated using a 2.0-mm mandibular plating system with multiple screws on either side of the fracture plane. Plates can be placed along the lines of osteosynthesis. In this case, IMF can be removed at the end of the case or maintained for 2 weeks postoperatively if additional stability is required. If the patient is at increased risk for aspiration as an outpatient, from either alcohol abuse or seizure disorder, then IMF should be avoided. All patients in IMF should be provided wire cutters to clip their IMF wires in the event of an episode of emesis.

93.7 Rehabilitation and Follow-up

Adequate nutrition is paramount for wound healing. Patients in IMF will be limited to a liquid diet, while those without IMF should eat a mechanical soft diet in order to minimize stress along fracture planes. Suboptimal occlusion can be modified at postoperative appointments using elastic bands to adjust the bite. Radiographs can be obtained to verify reduction of fractures and document occlusion. Once arch bars are removed, jaw rehabilitation exercises should be performed 4 to 6 times daily. Specifically, for jaw exercises, physicians should instruct patients to touch the distal tip of their tongue to the roof of the mouth when opening their mouth, shift the jaw from side to side, and practice jaw opening range of motion exercises. Most bone plates are left in permanently; however, if the patient requests, they can be removed after 6 months. In addition, loose or infected hardware is a latent complication from surgery and usually requires hardware removal.

93.8 Questions

1. Which of the following patterns of mandibular fracture are especially prone to airway compromise?
   a) Parasymphyseal fracture.
   b) Bilateral subcondylar fracture.
   c) Angle and contralateral body fracture.
   d) Coronoid process fracture.
   e) Dental alveolar fracture.
2. A 45-year-old man presents after a motor vehicle crash with blunt trauma to the right face and neck. On exam he has dyspnea, hoarseness, and diffuse crepitus along his neck, chest, and bilateral shoulders. All of the following should be part of this patient's immediate management except
   a) Airway X-ray.
   b) Obtain two peripheral intravenous (IV) lines.
   c) Nasopharyngoscopy.
   d) Sedation and intubation via direct laryngoscopy.
   e) Maxillofacial and neck computed tomography (CT).
3. A 56-year-old alcoholic man falls down a flight of stairs, causing mandibular angle and parasymphyseal fractures, which are subsequently repaired. His postoperative management should include all of the following except
   a) Oral hygiene.
   b) 4 weeks of maxillomandibular fixation.
   c) Pain control.
   d) Mechanical soft diet.
   e) Range of motion exercises.

Answers: 1. a 2. d 3. b

Suggested Readings

Ellis E. J Oral Maxillofac Surg. 1996; 54(7):864–871, discussion 871–872

Jewett BS, Shockley WW, Rutledge R. External laryngeal trauma analysis of 392 patients. Arch Otolaryngol Head Neck Surg. 1999; 125(8):877–880

Kellman R. The cervical spine in maxillofacial trauma. Assessment and airway management. Otolaryngol Clin North Am. 1991; 24 (1):1–13

Levy FE, Smith RW, Odland RM, Marentette LJ. Monocortical miniplate fixation of mandibular angle fractures. Arch Otolaryngol Head Neck Surg. 1991; 117(2):149–154

Morrow BT, Samson TD, Schubert W, Mackay DR. Evidence-based medicine: Mandible fractures. Plast Reconstr Surg. 2014; 134 (6):1381–1390

O'Connor RC, Shakib K, Brennan PA. Recent advances in the management of oral and maxillofacial trauma. Br J Oral Maxillofac Surg. 2015; 53(10):913–921

Valentino J, Marentette LJ. Supplemental maxillomandibular fixation with miniplate osteosynthesis. Otolaryngol Head Neck Surg. 1995; 112(2):215–220

94 Auricular Avulsion

Hayley L. Born and Ryan M. Collar

94.1 History

A 24-year-old woman was involved in an ATV accident while intoxicated. Her only injury was a completely avulsed ear. She arrived at the emergency department approximately 40 minutes following the accident with her ear in a plastic bag (▶ Fig. 94.1). The patient was alert and oriented, but mildly intoxicated. She had a negative trauma assessment including complete skeletal survey and cervical spine clearance.

94.2 Differential Diagnosis—Key Points

- Initial survey of traumatic auricular avulsion must include a preliminary trauma survey and evaluation for occult head injury. Advanced Trauma Life Support (ATLS) principles should be upheld, and providers should have a low threshold for obtaining a computed tomography (CT) scan of the head. Stabilization of the cervical spine should be established and maintained until injury can be excluded.
- Evaluation of auricular injury should qualify presence of cartilaginous injury and any missing tissue defects. The surgeon should thoroughly examine the external auditory canal and middle ear space when possible. Facial nerve function should be tested and documented.
- Amputated tissue and remaining defect should be examined closely, irrigated, and cleared of any foreign bodies. Care should be taken to avoid excessive cautery, clamping, or vessel ligation to maximize revascularization potential. Any pedicled tissues should not be amputated because even a small tissue bridge can supply adequate vascularization due to the dense and redundant blood supply to the auricle.

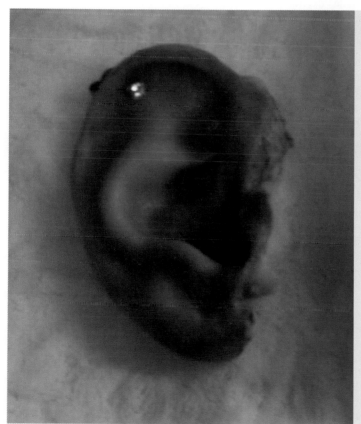

Fig. 94.1 Completely avulsed auricle, 40 minutes after injury, lateral view.

94.3 Test Interpretation

Diagnosis is based on physical exam. Imaging studies and hemoglobin measurement should be considered when there is suspicion for associated injuries or excessive bleeding.

94.4 Diagnosis

Traumatic complete auricular avulsion with intact external auditory canal

94.5 Medical Management

Prior to surgical repair, completely avulsed tissue should be stored in gauze soaked in normal saline solution and placed on ice until repair is possible. This is thought to decrease metabolic demand of the tissue to minimize ischemic injury.

Adjunct use of anticoagulation (when microvascular repair techniques are used), leech therapy, hyperbaric oxygen, and steroids may aid in healing, but use varies among surgeons. Vigorous data evaluating these therapies are not available. Possible anticoagulation therapies include dextran, heparin, or aspirin. Leeches (*Hirudo medicinalis*) have the multilevel benefit of decongesting flaps used in reconstruction and introducing hirudin, a natural anticoagulant leeches produce, into the tissue. Antibiotic prophylaxis to *Aeromonas hydrophila,* bacteria transmitted by leeches, using trimethoprim-sulfamethoxazole or ciprofloxacin and blockage of external auditory canal using cotton should be employed when using leeches.

94.6 Surgical Management

Several surgical methods are used, with varying success, when reconstructing a partially or completely avulsed auricle. As previously mentioned, if a pedicle remains connecting avulsed tissue and remaining intact tissue (partial avulsion), a combination of primary closure and, if necessary, one of the following techniques should be used to maintain this vascular connection.

Use the following techniques when there is complete avulsion of an auricular segment and the avulsed tissue is not lost.

1. Primary repair: This is used when avulsion is limited to skin, the defect is less than 15 mm, and/or when cosmesis is not a priority. This technique may also be used if reconstruction is planned at a later date in order to preserve the maximum amount of remaining tissue and minimize prerepair scarring at that time. This technique typically results in partial or complete necrosis of the reapproximated tissue if cartilaginous tissue is involved.

2. Delayed stage reconstruction: Used in this case, this is a two-step technique that involves deepithelialization of the amputated tissue, reattachment of the amputated cartilage to the remaining stump on the patient, and burying of the cartilage in a pocket created by raising the postauricular skin. The surviving cartilage, along with the overlying postauricular skin, is raised with a pedicle several months later and a skin graft and/or locoregional flaps are used to cover the defect on the posterior aspect of the auricular cartilage and the postauricular space to re-create the retroauricular sulcus (▶ Fig. 94.2).

3. Baudet technique: This is a variation of the delayed stage reconstruction that involves deepithelialization of only the posterior side of the avulsed auricle and creation of fenestrations in the cartilage to increase exposure of the anterior skin to underlying vascularized bed. The anterior skin is reattached in its original anatomic position to the residual skin. The posterior epithelial defect is attached to the postauricular pocket. Several months later the remaining cartilage is lifted off the postauricular surface and a skin graft and/or locoregional

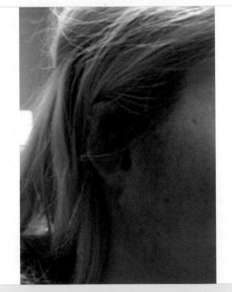

Fig. 94.2 Second stage of a delayed stage recontruction.

grafts are used to cover the defect and re-create the retroauricular sulcus.

4. Microvascular reattachment: The most successful repair technique, when possible, is microvascular reattachment. This requires presence of an adequate artery and vein on the amputated segment and the recipient site. Standard microsurgical techniques are used with possible adjunct therapies as discussed above in the Medical Management section.

All techniques may be combined with concomitant or subsequent reconstruction using rib or contralateral conchal grafts. Additionally, for total avulsions, osseointegrated implants for mounting of prostheses may be used, especially in cases where amputated tissue is lost.

If the external auditory canal is transected, a stent should be placed to maintain patency and avoid stenosis of the canal.

94.7 Rehabilitation and Follow-up

This patient underwent stage 1 at the time of injury that included deepithelialization of the framework and advancement flaps for coverage, given the associated posterior skin defect. Concurrently she underwent split-thickness skin grafting and wick placement to restore and stent the involved lateral external auditory canal. No external auditory canal stenosis ensued with careful cleaning and regular exams. At the time of initial surgery, meticulous wound examination did not reveal vessels available to support a microvascular repair. Approximately 8 weeks postoperatively the patient underwent elevation of the framework and placement of a costal cartilage graft in a postauricular pocket to sustain auricle projection. Due to a pregnancy, we deferred the final stage of reconstruction that included tragal restitution and lobule creation.

Discussion with the patient regarding difficulty in perfectly matching contralateral ear appearance should precede all reconstruction techniques. Clearly, multistage procedures and those requiring later reconstruction using grafts will require the patient to follow up. The patient should participate in decision making regarding which reconstruction technique will be used given this information. All patients should be followed in clinic for several weeks/months to reassess viability of reconstruction.

94.8 Questions

1. A 30-year-old woman sustained a traumatic complete auricular avulsion injury from a knife wound 2 hours ago involving the entirety of the auricle. There is profuse bleeding with large vessels present. What is the best method for treatment when possible?
   a) Microvascular anastomosis.
   b) Osseointegrated alloplastic reconstruction.
   c) Delayed auricular reconstruction discarding the avulsed piece.
   d) Burying and fenestrating the avulsed cartilage.
   e) Placing a rib graft to the auricle.

2. A 60-year-old man arrives via ambulance after a motorcycle accident. He is disoriented and has a nearly avulsed auricle on the right side. His vital signs are stable. What is the first step?
   a) Primary closure of the auricular avulsion in multiple layers.
   b) Stabilization of the cervical spine.
   c) Computed tomography (CT) of the head without contrast.
   d) Hearing exam.
   e) Detachment of the auricular tissue and immediate transfer to operating room for cleaning and reconstruction.

3. An 8-year-old child who is 2 hours away sustains an avulsion injury involving the upper fourth of his left auricle. To maximize salvage of this avulsed piece, what should the patient be instructed to do with the piece during transport?
   a) Wrap it in isotonic saline–soaked gauze and place it in a cooler surrounded with ice.
   b) Wrap it in hypertonic saline–soaked gauze and place it in a cooler surrounded with ice.
   c) Wrap it in isotonic saline–soaked gauze and place it in a thermos with warm water.
   d) Immerse it in dry ice.
   e) Wrap it in a dry gauze covered with antibiotic ointment.

Answers: 1. a 2. b 3. a

Suggested Readings

Bai H, Tollefson TT. Treatment strategies for auricular avulsions: best practice. JAMA Facial Plast Surg. 2014; 16(1):7–8

de Chalain. Replantation of the avulsed pinna: 100 percent survival with a single arterial anastomosis and substitution of leeches for a venous anastomosis. Plast Reconstr SurgSurg.; 95(7):1275–1279

Destro MW, Speranzini MB. Total reconstruction of the auricle after traumatic amputation. Plast Reconstr Surg. 1994; 94(6):859–864

Frodel JL, Jr, Barth P, Wagner J. Salvage of partial facial soft tissue avulsions with medicinal leeches. Otolaryngol Head Neck Surg. 2004; 131(6):934–939

Magritz R, Siegert R. Reconstruction of the avulsed auricle after trauma. Otolaryngol Clin North Am. 2013; 46(5):841–855

Norman ZI, Cracchiolo JR, Allen SH, Soliman AM. Auricular reconstruction after human bite amputation using the Baudet technique. Ann Otol Rhinol Laryngol. 2015; 124(1):45–48

Steffen A, Katzbach R, Klaiber S. A comparison of ear reattachment methods: a review of 25 years since Pennington. Plast Reconstr Surg. 2006; 118(6):1358–1364

95 Penetrating Neck Trauma

Hayley L. Born and Ryan M. Collar

95.1 History

A 17-year-old boy was brought into the emergency department by emergency medical services (EMS) after sustaining a gunshot wound to the neck. Upon arrival, the patient was awake and alert. He was not actively bleeding but was in severe respiratory distress. Intubation had been attempted in the field, but direct visualization of the vocal cords was not possible and the patient was not oxygenating or ventilating adequately. Respiratory rate was 35 and the patient had severe stridor. The oxygen saturation level was 86% and the patient was unable to speak. Pulses were intact and no expanding swelling was present in the neck. An entrance wound on the anterior right side and exit wound on the posterior side of the neck were present. Air bubbles were seen at the anterior wound. No neurologic deficits were found on exam. Paradoxical chest movement was seen during breaths, and some crepitus was felt in the neck tissue.

95.2 Differential Diagnosis—Key Points

- Initial survey of penetrating neck trauma must include a preliminary trauma survey. Advanced Trauma Life Support (ATLS) principles should be upheld.
- Airway management is the primary concern in these patients, in addition to prompt hemostasis. Emergent awake surgical airway may be necessary, especially in cases of laryngotracheal injury. Use of occlusive balloons such as Foley catheters may be required to tamponade large vessel hemorrhage. Resuscitation using two large-bore intravenous (IV) lines should be utilized according to trauma management protocol. Life-threatening injuries that cannot be controlled with related techniques should prompt immediate surgical exploration. Such injuries include massive hematoma, hemorrhage, shock, airway injury, and thoracic injuries.
- Evaluation of penetrating neck trauma has classically been divided into regions. The posterior triangle is the space between the posterior border of the sternocleidomastoid and the anterior border of the trapezius. It contains the vertebral arteries and brachial plexus. The anterior triangle is the area of the neck anterior to the posterior border of the sternocleidomastoid bilaterally. The anterior triangle is further divided into zones, and the management of penetrating neck wounds traditionally varies based on the zone of injury. Other considerations are depth of injury and mechanism of injury.
- Zone I extends from the clavicle to the cricoid and contains the aortic arch, innominate artery, brachiocephalic vein, subclavian artery and vein, common carotid artery, esophagus, trachea, thyroid, brachial plexus, lung apices, and thoracic duct. Injuries to this region are the most life threatening.
- Zone II includes the space between the cricoid and the angle of the mandible. It contains such structures as the common, internal, and external carotid arteries, jugular vein, pharynx, larynx, and esophagus. This is the most common zone of injury.
- Zone III is the space between the angle of the mandible and the skull base. Structures at risk in this area include the internal carotid artery, external carotid artery branches, internal jugular vein, pharynx, and trunk of the facial nerve. This space is very difficult to evaluate due to physical constraints.
- Techniques used to determine extent of injuries in non–life-threatening cases include computed tomography (CT); angiography; CT angiography (CTA); rigid and flexible endoscopy, both esophageal and laryngotracheal; esophagram; selective surgical exploration; and physical exam. Testing should be based primarily on presentation and can be limited to observation if the platysma is not violated. Suggested testing for deeper trauma based on area of injury are as follows: posterior triangle—angiogram; zone I—angiogram/CTA, EGD/esophagram, bronchoscopy; zone II—same as zone I; zone III—angiogram, direct evaluation of oropharynx.

95.3 Test Interpretation

Direct laryngoscopy to establish a definitive airway revealed blood in the oropharynx without direct visualization of the vocal folds. Placement of endotracheal tube was unsuccessful and an emergent tracheostomy was attempted. A large defect in the trachea was found upon entering the deep neck space. The defect was under tension and the distal tracheal segment was pulling into the lower neck/chest. An endotracheal tube was inserted in the distal tracheal segment, and bilateral chest rise and drop in end tidal CO_2 was observed. Auscultation revealed bilateral coarse breath sounds, and saturations improved to 96%. The patient was emergently transferred to the operating room. During neck exploration, an obvious tracheal injury was noted (▶ Fig. 95.1). After repair of the tracheal injuries, CTA, CT of the neck and cervical spine, and esophagram were completed without discovery of further injuries.

95.4 Diagnosis

Acute tracheal separation due to gunshot wound without concomitant injuries

95.5 Medical Management

Management should adhere to ATLS tenets such as prioritization of airway, breathing, circulation, and disability. Early placement of definitive airway and necessary chest tubes and establishment of bilateral large-bore access should accompany control of any active bleeding. This may require controlling bleeding with balloon devices, interventional radiology occlusion, direct packing, or ligation. All patients with penetrating neck wounds should be placed into rigid cervical spine splinting with a cervical collar. Stabilization of the thoracic spine should be considered depending on the mechanism of injury. Wounds should not be probed

because further injury or clot dislodgement may occur.

95.6 Surgical Management

In this case, direct observation of tracheal injury warranted emergent operative management following stabilization. A tracheoplasty and tracheotomy was completed, and the patient was transferred to the intensive care unit (ICU) for further care. The patient was decannulated at a later date.

Surgical management is based on diagnosis and repair of injuries. It may involve repair of vascular, laryngotracheal, and/or esophageal structures.

95.6.1 Vascular Injuries

Most vascular injuries manifest within 48 hours. Zone I vascular perforation requires thoracic surgery, for which a mediastinotomy extension or a formal lateral thoracotomy may be needed. Zone III injuries at the skull base may be temporarily controlled with pressure; however, access to the injury may require a mandibulotomy for accessibility.

All veins in the neck can be safely ligated to control hemorrhage; if both internal jugular veins are interrupted by the injury, an attempt to repair can be done. External carotid artery injuries are easily managed by suture ligation because collateral circulation is good. Common carotid or internal carotid injury in zone II is explored once the diagnosis is made, with attempts for vascular repair. End-to-end anastomosis or autogenous grafting is recommended when stenosis is evident by arteriography.

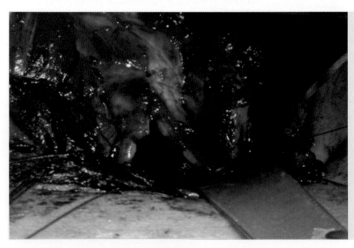

Fig. 95.1 Intraoperative view of transected trachea. An endotracheal tube was placed in the distal tracheal segment.

Ligation of the common or internal carotid injuries is generally reserved for irreparable injuries and in patients who are in a profound coma state with bilateral fixed and dilated pupils. Delayed complications from unrepaired vascular injuries include aneurysm formation, dissecting aneurysm, and arteriovenous fistulas.

Interventional radiologists have used angiographic techniques to treat vascular injury. In many instances, embolization procedures can help control arterial disruption. For arterial injuries in zone III, transcatheter arterial embolization can be an effective modality to obtain hemostasis. Penetrating injuries in zone III can have multiple vascular injuries involving the internal carotid artery, internal maxillary artery, and external carotid artery. In areas of difficult vascular access at the skull base, detachable balloons or steel coils can be placed for carotid occlusion.

Control of hemorrhage from vertebral artery penetration can be very difficult, owing to its location in the bony canal within the cervical spine. Because vertebral artery injuries often result in both neurologic and hemodynamic sequelae, they are frequently associated with higher morbidity and mortality rates. Surgical vascular repair in zone III can be complex, so endovascular treatment approaches are very helpful.

95.6.2 Laryngotracheal Injuries

Laryngeal mucosal lacerations from penetrating injury ideally should be repaired early (within 24 hours) because the time elapsed before repair can affect airway, scarring, and voice quality.

Significant glottic and supraglottic lacerations and displaced cartilage fractures need surgical approximation. Endoscopy and CT will differentiate between the patients that need only observation (small laceration, shallow laceration, nondisplaced fracture) and those that require a thyrotomy or open fracture reduction and mucosal approximation. A soft laryngeal stent may be needed for badly macerated mucosa.

In severe cases, a low tracheotomy with the patient under local anesthesia is advocated. Tracheal injuries may be repaired primarily using 3–0 monofilament sutures that go through the cartilage rings but do not pass into the tracheal lumen. For minor, incomplete lacerations, tracheotomy might not be required. Suprahyoid-releasing incisions may be required for additional length.

Simple tracheal lacerations that do not detach a tracheal ring or encroach on the airway can be repaired without a tracheotomy. More severe disruptions (gunshot wound directly to the trachea) imply more soft tissue injury, and a 6-week tracheotomy either below or through the tracheal injury is the safest procedure. Later, the stenosis may require sleeve resection but, if the stenosis is soft, a T-tube tracheotomy tube can often manage it.

95.6.3 Digestive Tract Injuries

To rule out possible esophageal perforation, most radiologists recommend a water-soluble iodinated radiopaque contrasted swallow study initially, because barium extravasation can radiographically distort soft tissue planes and is more toxic. A barium swallow should follow a negative Gastrografin study if suspicion remains high.

Missed esophageal tears represent most of the delayed injuries and can progress to mediastinitis and increased mortality. Some centers claim that flexible esophagoscopy can be used to circumvent the need for general anesthesia during rigid endoscopy; however, flexible endoscopy can miss perforations near the cricopharyngeus and hypopharynx.

Some trauma centers recommend neck exploration for patients who have air in the soft tissues of the neck despite yielding normal endoscopy results. To rule out pharyngeal and esophageal injuries during the surgical exploration, a nasogastric tube can be gently pulled up to the level of the neck and methylene blue infused through the nasogastric tube to help localize the injury site.

By using the combination of flexible endoscopy and rigid esophagoscopy to examine the entire cervical and upper thoracic esophagus, reportedly no perforations are missed.

If a pharyngeal perforation is still strongly suspected but unconfirmed, the patient is given no food and is observed for several days. Fever, tachycardia, or widening of the mediastinum on serial chest radiographs requires a repeat endoscopy, or a neck exploration should be considered.

When an esophageal injury is found early, management involves a two-layer closure with wound irrigation, débridement, and adequate drainage. After repair of the mucosa perforation, a muscle flap may be interposed over the esophageal suture line for further protection. If an extensive esophageal injury is present, it may necessitate a lateral cervical esophagostomy and later definitive repair.

Many surgeons perform direct laryngoscopy, bronchoscopy, and rigid esophagoscopy with the patient under anesthesia for penetrating injuries of the neck when air is seen in the soft tissues or if hemoptysis, hematemesis, or other suspicious clinical findings are present. Direct laryngoscopy and rigid bronchoscopy can be combined with flexible airway examination to recognize and stent a lacerated trachea temporarily. In the setting of a cervical spine fracture, rigid esophagoscopy might need to be omitted.

Even if the clinical examination is benign, follow-up examination at least three times every 24-hour shift for several days is needed to monitor vital signs, and the neck examination change is needed. Odynophagia, subcutaneous emphysema, hematemesis (or blood from the nasogastric aspirate), and fever are the most common findings for esophageal injury. A patient with negative physical examinations, normal radiographs, and normal endoscopies will most likely have a negative neck exploration, and no significant injury will be discovered.

95.7 Rehabilitation and Follow-up

The patient in this case completed a 1-week hospital stay and was subsequently followed in an outpatient setting. Several months later a revision tracheoplasty with closure of tracheostomy was completed. No significant stenosis resulted. The patient recovered to baseline mental and respiratory status. No neurologic deficits resulted from the hypoxic episode.

Patients with more extensive injuries may require long-term neurologic rehabilitation or repeated esophageal or tracheal ligations. Extensive revision surgeries are occasionally required.

Morbidity and mortality depends on area of injury, with zone I being the most life threatening. Up to 66% of common carotid injuries are fatal. Those that require ligation of common or internal carotid arteries have a 30% rate of stroke. Undiagnosed esophageal injuries may result in up to 20% mortality. Iatrogenic fistula formation may help control resulting infection and salivary flow.

Follow-up appointments depend on management, but sutures should be removed after 7 to 10 days. Reevaluation at 1, 3, and 6 months is recommended to evaluate for any evolving vascular/neurologic injury.

95.8 Questions

1. A 35-year-old man is stabbed in the neck in the midline 3 cm above the sternal notch. What zone is the injury in?
   a) Posterior triangle.
   b) Zone I.
   c) Zone II.
   d) Zone III.
   e) Zone IV.
   f) Zone V.
2. A patient is dropped off at the door of the emergency department with a penetrating trauma to the left neck. The patient is bleeding profusely. What is the first step in management?
   a) Tamponade the bleeding with direct pressure.
   b) Explore the wound for debris.
   c) Write down the license plate of the car that dropped off the patient.
   d) Establish a definitive airway.
   e) Call time of death.
3. If not grossly obvious, what is the best way to evaluate for an esophageal injury during a penetrating neck trauma?
   a) Rigid esophagoscopy.
   b) Barium swallow esophagram.
   c) Gastrografin esophagram.
   d) Surgical exploration.

Answers: 1. b 2. d 3. c

Suggested Readings

Brywczynski JJ, Barrett TW, Lyon JA, Cotton BA. Management of penetrating neck injury in the emergency department: a structured literature review. Emerg Med J. 2008; 25(11):711–715

Hom DB. Penetrating Neck Trauma. Otolaryngology Cases: The University of Cincinnati Clinical Portfolio (2011): 81

Maisel RH, Hom DB. Blunt and penetrating trauma to the neck. Cummings Otolaryngology Head and Neck Surgery. 2005; 3:2525–2539

Rickard J. Penetrating neck trauma. In Common Surgical Diseases: An Algorithmic Approach to Problem Solving, Third Edition. Springer New York; 2015:37–39. Available from DOI: 10.1007/978–1-4939–1565–1_9

Sclafani AP, Sclafani SJ. Angiography and transcatheter arterial embolization of vascular injuries of the face and neck. Laryngoscope. 1996; 106(2 Pt 1):168–173

Stassen NA, Hoth JJ, Scott MJ, et al. Laryngotracheal injuries: does injury mechanism matter? Am Surg. 2004; 70(6):522–525

Stiernberg CM, Jahrsdoerfer RA, Gillenwater A, Joe SA, Alcalen SV. Gunshot wounds to the head and neck. Arch Otolaryngol Head Neck Surg. 1992; 118(6):592–597

Part XV

Facial Plastic and Reconstructive Surgery

XV

96 Otoplasty

Colin R. Edwards and Ryan M. Collar

96.1 History

A 13-year-old otherwise healthy girl presented to clinic with complaints of large, protruding ears. She was previously evaluated for her prominent ears, but the family elected to observe her condition. In recent years, children at school had started to tease her about her appearance. She was approaching high school and becoming increasingly anxious about her ears. Her family was concerned about her confidence and was interested in pursuing surgical correction. On physical exam her bilateral pinnae demonstrated hypoplastic antihelical folds, causing lateral protrusion of the helices. She had deep conchal bowls, which also contributed to her ear projection. Her auriculocephalic angles were increased at 45 degrees bilaterally (▶ Fig. 96.1).

96.2 Differential Diagnosis—Key Points

Prominauris affects nearly 5% of the population to some degree. It is often present at birth and may be corrected with molding in the first 2 months of life. Growth of the external ear occurs early in childhood, reaching approximately 90% of the adult size by age 3. Surgical repair should be deferred until age 5 or 6 when the ear has completed development. In addition, this age cohort corresponds with school matriculation and self-awareness of the child and may benefit from surgical repair from a psychosocial standpoint.

The work-up of prominauris should begin with the patient's history, including birth history and any associated syndromic or genetic disorders, as well as social and emotional development in older children. The diagnosis of prominauris is made on physical exam, paying special attention to specific anatomic relationships. The auriculocephalic angle is the angle between the mastoid and the posterior helical rim and is typically 20 to 35 degrees. The conchal bowl depth is the distance between the tragus and the medial depth of the conchal bowl and is approximately 15 mm. The conchomastoid and conchoscaphal angles are typically 90 degrees and perpendicular to each other, giving the antihelix its characteristic appearance.

In patients with prominauris there is abnormal projection of the ear from the mastoid portion of the temporal bone, most often from underdevelopment of the antihelical fold. In these cases, the auriculocephalic, conchomastoid, and conchoscaphal angles are all increased. This causes

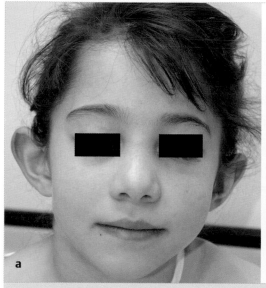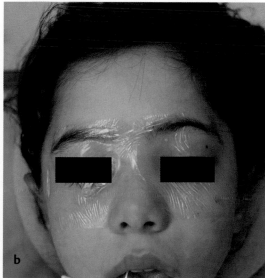

Fig. 96.1 (a,b) Preoperative and postoperative photos of a patient with prominauris.

protrusion of the ear, which can be measured in the distance from the mastoid cortex to the edge of the helix. An increased conchal bowl depth may also contribute to ear protrusion. While prominauris is often bilateral, it is important to examine each ear individually because there may be differences in the irregularities of each ear.

There are several terms to describe various types of prominauris. The *protruding ear* features a hypoplastic antihelix and superior crus, causing protrusion of the helix. The ear is otherwise normal in individuals with a protruding ear. In contrast, a *lop ear* arises due to a soft, weak cartilaginous framework of the ear, causing the ear to hang or tilt forward. In the lop ear the weak cartilage may be limited to the helix or may involve the entire framework in severe cases. The *cup ear* refers to the combination of both a protruding and lop ear and features a deep conchal bowl, coupled with a hypoplastic antihelix and superior pole.

The degree of deviation in the deformed ear, when compared to population norms, can be helpful when trying to decide when to intervene. As previously discussed, the auriculocephalic angle typically ranges between 20 and 35 degrees, with angles greater than 40 degrees considered abnormal. In the adult ear, the vertical height of the ear, from the lobule to the dome, is approximately 55 mm. The horizontal axis is measured from the tragus to the helix and typically measures approximately 34 mm. The distance from the helix to the mastoid cortex varies depending on what level of the ear one measures from. At the level of the external auditory canal, the helix to mastoid distance ranges from 15 to 18 mm. In prominauris, these distances are increased. Other deformities may include a hypoplastic antihelical fold or superior and inferior crus, a distorted scapha, and an overdeveloped or prominent conchal bowl. Assessment of the physical characteristics of the deformed ear, as well as the deviations in measurements, will help the surgeon develop an operative plan for repair.

96.3 Test Interpretation

Patients with isolated prominauris do not require any additional testing beyond a thorough physical exam. If the patient has evidence of external auditory canal stenosis or atresia, then a temporal bone computed tomography (CT) scan and audiogram are warranted to assess for malformation of the middle ear structures arising from the first and second branchial arches. If surgical intervention is being considered, then thorough photographic documentation of the ear is necessary. Photographs should be taken from multiple angles including anterior and posterior views, a lateral view, and a close-up of the deformed ear. Coagulation studies may be warranted if a family history of bleeding disorder exists, as postoperative hematoma is the most common complication of surgery and can cause significant wound healing issues.

96.4 Diagnosis

Prominauris, or prominent ears

96.5 Medical Management

In newborns with prominauris, ear molding may be beneficial but can only be used in the first 1 to 2 months of life. Beyond this point, the patient should be observed until approximately 5 to 6 years of age, when surgical correction may be considered. It is important to consider the social and emotional development of the child with prominent ears and provide support if any teasing or self-esteem issues arise.

96.6 Surgical Management

The definitive treatment for prominauris is otoplasty with the aim of providing the patient with a more natural sized, shaped, and contoured ear that is of normal proportion and symmetric with the contralateral side. The surgical technique used will be dependent on the specific deformity and training of the surgeon. Goals of surgery should include repositioning of the ear to a normal auriculocephalic angle, decrease in the size of an enlarged conchal bowl, and creation of natural-appearing helical and antihelical folds when indicated. One key to creating a natural-appearing ear is maintaining a gentle, natural contour to the helix. This is often achieved using a combination of cartilage scoring, trimming, and carefully placed sutures. If bilateral deformities are present, they can be addressed at the same surgery with care taken to create symmetry between the two sides.

96.6.1 Perioperative Preparation

In the pediatric population, otoplasty should be performed under general anesthesia. Some teenagers and adults may be able to tolerate surgery with MAC anesthesia and local anesthesia using an auricular ring block. Thorough photo-documentation of both ears should be obtained prior to any surgical intervention. Both ears should be assessed and any specific deformities identified and documented for surgical planning.

The most common approach to treating prominauris is the Mustarde suture technique. The Mustarde technique involves placement of three or four horizontal mattress sutures to bring the scapha closer to the fossa triangularis and the concha. A 25-gauge needle can be used to reapproximate the antihelix prior to suturing. Typically, a permanent suture, such as a 4–0 Prolene (Ethicon Inc.) or nylon, is used with good long-term results. In adult patients, the helical cartilage may calcify, leading to delayed reprotrusion of the ear. In these patients, scoring of the cartilage at the time of the initial surgery may soften the helix and prevent reprotrusion. When performed correctly, the Mustarde technique creates a new, natural-appearing antihelix while displacing the helical rim slightly posteriorly, in a normal anatomic position. If the central one-third of the ear is overcorrected relative to the superior and inferior poles, then a telephone ear deformity results.

In some patients, an enlarged conchal bowl is a cause of prominauris. In these patients the posterior conchal cavum can be shaved down and the cartilage can be sutured to the mastoid periosteum to decrease auricular projection. The specific surgical techniques used are dependent on the deformity present, and one ear may require a combination of techniques to create a natural appearance.

96.7 Rehabilitation and Follow-up

At the end of the surgery, petroleum ointment-soaked cotton balls are placed in the concha cavum, fossa triangularis, and scaphoid fossa to provide moisture and support. A mastoid dressing is then applied and kept in place for 12 to 24 hours postoperatively. After removal of the mastoid dressing, a soft elastic head wrap is then applied around the head, including the superior pole of the helix in order to maintain the new position of the ear as it heals.

Early complications following otoplasty include hematoma, cellulitis, chondritis, and cartilage or skin necrosis. Hematomas should be drained to prevent devascularization of the helix or abscess formation. Cellulitis and chondritis can be particularly problematic, as infection can create a secondary deformity that may be difficult to later correct. Any evidence of infection should be treated with a fluoroquinolone due to good *Pseudomonas* coverage and cartilage penetration.

Late complications following otoplasty may include hypertrophic scar or keloid formation, suture exposure, telephone deformity, overcorrection of the antihelix, narrowing of the external auditory canal meatus, and over- or underprojection of the helix. Additional surgery may be necessary to correct any persistent deformity. Revision surgery should be deferred until at least 1 year after the original surgery in order to allow for complete wound healing and stabilization of the shape of the auricle following the initial procedure.

96.8 Questions

1. The auricular helix is approximately 90% of its adult size by what age?
   a) 2 years old.
   b) 3 years old.
   c) 5 years old.
   d) 7 years old.
   e) 10 years old.
2. All of the following may be characteristic of a cup-ear deformity except what?
   a) Deep concha cavum.
   b) Hypoplastic helix.
   c) Decreased auriculocephalic angle.
   d) Weak cartilaginous framework.
   e) Drooping of the superior helical pole.
3. Overcorrection of the middle one-third of the helix is referred to as what?
   a) Lop ear.
   b) Cup ear.
   c) Protruding ear.
   d) Vertical post deformity.
   e) Telephone ear.

Answers: 1. b 2. c 3. e

Suggested Readings

Adamson PA, Litner JA. Otoplasty technique. Facial Plast Surg Clin North Am. 2006; 14(2):79–87, v

Becker DG, Lai SS, Wise JB, Steiger JD. Analysis in otoplasty. Facial Plast Surg Clin North Am. 2006; 14(2):63–71, v

Converse JM, Nigro A, Wilson FA, Johnson N. A technique for surgical correction of lop ears. Plast Reconstr Surg (1946). 1955; 15 (5):411–418

Furnas DW. Complications of surgery of the external ear. Clin Plast Surg. 1990; 17(2):305–318

Handler EB, Song T, Shih C. Complications of otoplasty. Facial Plast Surg Clin North Am. 2013; 21(4):653–662

Mustarde JC. The correction of prominent ears using simple mattress sutures. Br J Plast Surg. 1963; 16:170–178

Pawar SS, Koch CA, Murakami C. Treatment of Prominent Ears and Otoplasty: A Contemporary Review. JAMA Facial Plast Surg. 2015; 17(6):449–454

97 Blepharoplasty

Colin R. Edwards and Ryan M. Collar

97.1 History

A 75-year-old woman presented with sagging eyelids and a visual field deficit. The patient complained of several years of progressive eyelid droop, which now limited her superior visual fields. In addition, she noted visual fatigue and headaches when reading or looking at a computer screen for an extended period of time. She denied previous trauma, ocular surgery, or botulinum toxin use. She denied a history of dry eye, tearing, and thyroid disease. She was unhappy with her appearance because her family said she constantly looked sleepy.

On physical exam, her extraocular muscles were intact, and vision was grossly normal. Pupils were equally round and reactive to light. She had upper lid dermatochalasis with minimal pseudoherniation of fat (▸ Fig. 97.1a). The marginal reflex

distance-1 was 4 mm with palpebral distance of 11 m bilaterally. Distraction and snap testing were within normal limits.

97.2 Differential Diagnosis—Key Points

Eyelid droop can be due to a number of causes, both intrinsic and extrinsic. A thorough history and physical should be elicited as part of any eyelid complaints. The patient should be assessed for systemic conditions that affect eyelid position prior to any planned intervention.

Proper nomenclature is essential for accurately describing eyelid pathology. A common finding in the elderly population is *dermatochalasis,* which describes age-related skin laxity and upper eyelid skin redundancy. *Blepharoptosis* refers to the

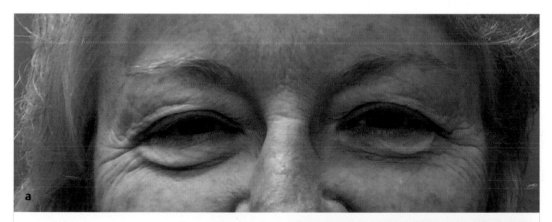
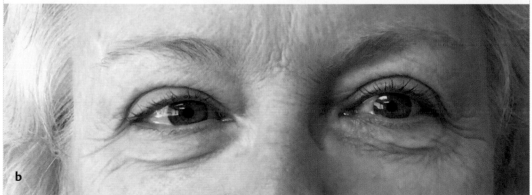

Fig. 97.1 (a) Preoperative photo of the patient. (b) Postoperative photo of the patient.

downward position of the upper eyelid, often partially obscuring the upper pupil, causing a superior visual field deficit. *Pseudoptosis* is a catchall term for conditions that mimic blepharoptosis but may be a result of levator muscle weakness, eyebrow or forehead ptosis, or enophthalmos with decreased eyelid support from the globe. *Blepharochalasis* refers to a specific condition usually seen in females featuring episodic, recurrent upper eyelid edema, which can lead to thinning of the eyelid skin. *Lagophthalmos* is seen when lid retraction or globe proptosis prevents complete closure of the eyelid over the eye, often resulting in exposure keratopathy and corneal abrasion.

Systemic causes of eyelid pathology range from common to rare. Allergies often cause waxing and waning periorbital edema and itchy or watery eyes. Graves disease may be associated with ophthalmopathy featuring proptosis of the globes with upper and lower lid retraction. Horner's syndrome features unilateral ptosis and may be the result of a an ischemic stroke or mass interrupting sympathetic input to the superior tarsal (Mueller's) muscle. Myasthenia gravis is an autoimmune-mediated process that features autoantibodies against nicotinic acetylcholine receptors at the neuromuscular junction. Often ocular findings, including ptosis from levator palpabrae superior muscle weakness and extraocular muscle weakness, are the first signs of myasthenia gravis.

The most common cause of ptosis in the aging population is aponeurotic blepharoptosis, in which the levator tendon involutes or dehisces from the tarsal plate slowly over time, leading to progressive eyelid droop. Patients with aponeurotic blepharoptosis will often have a high or absent upper eyelid crease and thinning of the eyelid above the tarsal plate. Another potential cause of decreased visual acuity and eyelid droop is brow ptosis, where increased skin laxity causes the brow tissues to sag downward. Brow ptosis can cause pseudoptosis of the eyelid, where the loss of eyelid support causes the appearance of redundant eyelid tissue. It is important to identify the underlying structural issues and rule out any systemic or neuromuscular causes of blepharoptosis prior to considering surgical intervention.

97.3 Test Interpretation

Careful examination of the eye, eyelids, brow, and orbital rims should be performed in order to determine the cause of the patient's eyelid heaviness. Measurement of the anatomic relationships of the

eyelids to the surrounding structures can be helpful in guiding the surgeon toward a treatment plan. Measurements may include the *palpebral fissure,* which is the vertical distance between the upper and lower eyelid at the center of the pupil. The *marginal reflex distance* may be assessed by shining a light on the cornea and measuring the distance from the upper eyelid to the pupillary light reflex.

The eyelid should be assessed with the brow relaxed, in a neutral position. The position of the brow in relationship to the orbital rim will allow one to assess for brow ptosis. Close attention should be paid to the eyelid skin and any degree of overhang into the visual field. An ophthalmology consult may be useful for documenting visual field deficits. The levator function can be assessed by manually fixing the brow and having the patient look up and down. The distance of excursion between upgaze and downgaze is an approximation of the levator function and is normally between 12 and 16 mm.

If the history suggests it, the patient should be assessed for dry eyes prior to any planned surgical intervention. Schirmer's strips can be placed in each fornix and are used to wick out tears. A failure to wick 10 mm of moisture on the strip in 5 minutes is abnormal. Dry eye symptoms may worsen after blepharoplasty due to increased corneal surface area exposure. However, these symptoms can be managed with artificial tears and lubricants.

97.4 Diagnosis

Dermatochalasis with minimal pseudoherniation of fat

97.5 Medical Management

Dermatochalasis is an anatomic issue. There are no medical therapies to treat the diminished visual fields associated with dermatochalasis. Dry eye symptoms can be treated with artificial tears and lubricants.

97.6 Surgical Management

The patient's bilateral dermatochalasis can be treated with blepharoplasty with the aim of rejuvenating the periorbita through precise excision of redundant eyelid soft tissue. Surgery can be performed in the clinic with light sedation and local, or in the operating room with conscious sedation anesthesia and local. Skin incisions are designed preoperatively to assure appropriate excision dimensions through pinching upper lid skin with blepharoplasty forceps with the patient in an upright position. After excision of the skin layer alone, a strip of muscle may be excised to expose the orbital septum. Current philosophy is to limit orbital fat excision to avoid a hollowed and skeletonized appearance. If heavy lids with excess adipose are present, the orbital septum may be transgressed to allow excision of fat from the medial and central fat pads. More recently surgeons have utilized a medial fat pad transposition approach in which the medial pad is transposed as a soft tissue pedicle into the central upper lid to avoid A-frame deformity. Other complications from blepharoplasty include cellulitis, chemosis, eyelid malposition, ptosis, and lagophthalmos causing dry eye, keratitis, and corneal abrasions.

Brow ptosis can be addressed via a number of different procedures and approaches. The direct browplasty and midforehead approaches involve masking the incision in an existing rhytid, but can lead to visible scarring. The pretrichial approach attempts to mask the scar in the hairline but causes forehead numbness due to transection of the neurovascular bundles of the forehead. The endoscopic browlift is a highly effective means to elevate the forehead soft tissues while also minimizing scarring but requires additional equipment. Myriad implantable devices are available to anchor the bone to the deep subcutaneous tissues of the brow so that the periosteum heals in an elevated position, raising brow height. Complications from browlifts include hematoma, infection, scarring, numbness, and forehead weakness from injury to the frontalis branch of the facial nerve.

97.7 Rehabilitation and Follow-up

Postoperative care for blepharoplasty and browlift surgery should include antibiotic ointment to all incisions. If lagophthalmos is anticipated, artificial tears and ointments should be provided for eye moisture, to prevent keratitis. Cold compresses can be used for bruising and edema. Patients should be seen in clinic 1 to 2 weeks after surgery.

97.8 Questions

1. A 54-year-old woman presents with complaints of bilateral ptosis and diplopia that wax and wane throughout the day. On exam she has bilateral ptosis with left greater than right eyelid droop. She has limited lateral gaze in her left eye. What is the most likely diagnosis?
   a) Graves disease.
   b) Dermatochalasis.
   c) Myasthenia gravis.
   d) Horner's syndrome.
   e) Seasonal allergies.
2. Lagophthalmos may be observed in which clinical scenarios?
   a) Complication following blepharoplasty.
   b) Graves disease.
   c) Blepharochalasis.
   d) a and b.
   e) a and c.
3. The most common cause of eyelid ptosis in the aging population is what?
   a) Brow ptosis causing pseudoptosis.
   b) Blepharochalasis.
   c) Ischemic stroke.
   d) Seasonal allergies.
   e) Levator aponeurosis involution.

Answers: 1. c 2. d 3. e

Suggested Readings

Ahmad SM, Della Rocca RC. Blepharoptosis: evaluation, techniques, and complications. Facial Plast Surg. 2007; 23(3):203–215
Drolet BC, Sullivan PK. Evidence-based medicine: Blepharoplasty. Plast Reconstr Surg. 2014; 133(5):1195–1205
Graf RM, Tolazzi AR, Mansur AE, Teixeira V. Endoscopic periosteal brow lift: evaluation and follow-up of eyebrow height. Plast Reconstr Surg. 2008; 121(2):609–616, discussion 617–619
Moskowitz BK, Patel AD, Pearson JM. Aesthetic and functional management of eyelid and orbital reconstruction. Facial Plast Surg. 2008; 24(1):69–77
Pereira LS, Hwang TN, Kersten RC, Ray K, McCulley TJ. Levator superioris muscle function in involutional blepharoptosis. Am J Ophthalmol. 2008; 145(6):1095–1098
Rohrich RJ, Coberly DM, Fagien S, Stuzin JM. Current concepts in aesthetic upper blepharoplasty. Plast Reconstr Surg. 2004; 113 (3):32e–42e
Tabatabai N, Spinelli HM. Limited incision nonendoscopic brow lift. Plast Reconstr Surg. 2007; 119(5):1563–1570
Viana GA, Sant'Anna AE, Righetti F, Osaki M. Floppy eyelid syndrome. Plast Reconstr Surg. 2008; 121(5):333e–334e
Zoumalan CI, Roostaeian J. Simplifying Blepharoplasty. Plast Reconstr Surg. 2016; 137(1):196e–213e

98 Septoplasty

Thomas K. Hamilton and David B. Hom

98.1 History

A 30-year-old man presented to clinic complaining of a 10-year history of nasal obstruction and occasional nosebleeds, worse on the left side. He had a past history of blunt trauma to the nose 5 years ago. He denied intranasal drug use and had never had nasal surgery in the past.

He denied nasal allergies and was a nonsmoker. He worked as a chef in a restaurant and sang in his church choir. He was not using over-the-counter steroid nasal sprays currently since they had not helped him in the past when he had tried them for 2 months.

On exam, the external nose appeared normal with patent nares. On anterior rhinoscopy, severe caudal septal deviation to the left was present, with compensatory right inferior turbinate hypertrophy. The mucosa was pink and healthy throughout both nasal cavities, and there were no polyps or masses seen. After administering decongestant nasal spray, his inferior turbinates shrunk significantly. In lifting his external and internal nasal valves with a cotton swab, it did not improve his nasal breathing.

Fiberoptic nasal endoscopy confirmed the above findings.

98.2 Differential Diagnosis—Key Points

- Common anatomic causes of nasal obstruction include a deviated septum, turbinate hypertrophy, static or dynamic narrowing of the external and/or internal nasal valves, and adenoid hypertrophy.
- Constant unilateral nasal obstruction from the nasal septum deviation was the probable etiology for his nasal obstruction. The fact that the nasal obstructive symptoms were minimally responsive to topical therapy made the case that isolated turbinate hypertrophy was not the major component of his nasal obstruction.
- The patient was a nonsmoker whose symptoms were constant, rather than seasonal or situational, and there was no history of atopy, which would make allergic or irritation-related etiology more likely.

- There was no history of prior nasal surgery. This is important to establish as it may factor into surgical planning due to the presence of scar tissue, synechia, or previous cartilage harvest.
- As with any nasal surgery, the patient's goals and expectations must be carefully established. In this case, the patient had realistic goals for the surgery. He was aware that his smell, taste, and singing voice resonance might change after nasal septal surgery.

98.3 Test Interpretation

Anatomic nasal obstruction due to septal deviation is a diagnosis based on physical exam and sometimes on imaging when other anatomic etiologies are suspected. Laboratory imaging is not useful in these scenarios.

98.4 Diagnosis

Nasal obstruction due to a deviated nasal septum

98.5 Medical Management

Due to the severe degree of anatomic septal deviation in this patient, medical therapies were unlikely to be useful. In other cases, medications such as nasal steroid sprays, mast cell inhibitors, antihistamines, commercial nasal support devices, and environmental allergy immunotherapy may be of some benefit, depending on whether other anatomic components are contributing (such as turbinate hypertrophy, static or dynamic narrowing of the external and/or internal nasal valve, adenoid hypertrophy).

98.6 Surgical Management

Nasal surgery is generally divided into two categories: (1) surgery done to correct a nasal obstruction and (2) surgery done to improve a perceived cosmetic defect. Oftentimes, these two goals can be accomplished simultaneously during the same procedure. In this case, the patient was primarily interested in just improving his nasal breathing which was limited due to his caudal septal deviation.

The most appropriate operation for this patient is septoplasty and possible turbinate reduction. A full transfixion incision is initially made on the side of the septum most convenient to the surgeon. A mucoperichondrial flap is elevated to provide access to the septal cartilage. If the exposed side is the concave side, partial-thickness scoring can be used to decrease the memory of the septal bend. To release the memory of the caudal septal deflection, a contralateral septal mucoperichondrial flap is lifted from the cartilage. A horizontal 2- to 3-mm inferior strip of septal cartilage is then removed ventrally over the nasal spine using iris scissors to create a swinging door. At least 1-cm dorsal and caudal struts are left on the septal cartilage to minimize nasal dorsal and nasal tip collapse. Removal of spurs or other abnormalities of the septal cartilage contributing to the nasal obstruction should also be performed. A 3–0 Chromic is placed through the caudal septum and through the mucosa over the nasal spine to keep the caudal septum anchored to the midline (Suture of Wright). At times, an elongated caudally deviated septum after straightening can be placed between the medial crura and act as a medial crura strut to give additional nasal tip support, which is then secured with 5–0 Vicryl mattress sutures. The mucosa can then be closed with a 4–0 Chromic gut suture with an SC-1 needle in a running quilting fashion to eliminate dead space where the septal cartilage was removed. This helps to minimize the occurrence of postoperative septal hematoma. Internal nasal splints are then placed and secured with 3–0 nylon to reduce synechia. Packing of the nasal cavities after septoplasty is rarely required and is used only for persistent epistaxis not controlled with more conservative measures (i.e., oxymetazoline nasal spray, cautery, or thrombin hemostatic nasal products).

Certain procedures are often done concomitantly with septoplasty in order to further improve function of the nose. If there is internal nasal valve narrowing, spreader grafts can be placed to widen the internal valve angle. Additionally, there is often contralateral compensatory inferior turbinate hypertrophy for which turbinate reduction can be performed to improve nasal breathing function. External nasal valve function can be improved with techniques such as suture suspension, medial collumella struts, lateral crura struts, and alar batten grafts. Complications include epistaxis, infection, septal hematoma, and septal perforation. Some patients may develop a change in taste and smell, as well as a change in resonance of the voice.

98.7 Rehabilitation and Follow-up

The external and internal nasal splints can be removed in 1 week. Bruising and swelling can be expected to persist for up to a year. Daily saline spray four puffs each nostril four times a day for 3 to 4 months should be used to minimize crusting and enhance mucosa healing. Any additional crusting can be removed with 3% hydrogen peroxide–soaked cotton swabs.

98.8 Questions

1. Components of the internal nasal valve include all of the following except
   a) Inferior turbinate.
   b) Middle turbinate.
   c) Caudal septum.
   d) Pyriform aperture.
   e) Distal end of the upper lateral cartilage.
2. The most important portion of the nose from an airflow perspective in a leptorrhine nose is
   a) External nasal valve.
   b) Internal nasal valve.
   c) Choanae.
   d) Pyriform aperture.
3. What finding often accompanies chronic septal deviation?
   a) Nasal valve collapse.
   b) Pyriform aperture stenosis.
   c) Contralateral inferior turbinate hypertrophy.
   d) Eustachian tube dysfunction.

Answers: 1. b 2. b 3. c

Suggested Readings

Arden RL, Coleman GB. Nasal obstruction. In: Mathog RH, Arden RL, Marks SC, eds. Trauma of the Nose and Paranasal Sinuses. New York, NY: Thieme; 1995:171–203

Ballert JA, Park SS. Functional rhinoplasty: treatment of the dysfunctional nasal sidewall. Facial Plast Surg. 2006; 22(1):49–54

Ducic Y, Hilger P. Surgical correction of the deviated septum. In: Murakami C, ed. Functional Reconstructive Rhinoplasty. Facial Plast Surg Clin North Am. 1999;7:319–331

Kridel RW, Scott BA, Foda HM. The tongue-in-groove technique in septorhinoplasty. A 10-year experience. Arch Facial Plast Surg. 1999; 1(4):246–256, discussion 257–258

99 Rhinoplasty

Jamie L. Welshhans and David B. Hom

99.1 History

A 35-year-old man presented to the clinic seeking improvement of his appearance on lateral profile (▶ Fig. 99.1). He stated that he had nasal surgery 4 years ago by another physician that improved his nasal breathing. However, he felt his nose was now beaklike on side profile. He could breathe through both sides without difficulty. He was in good health and did not smoke. He was married and worked as a contractor. He was pleasant and realistic and sought improvement of his lateral nasal profile. He had been considering a second nasal surgery for over the last 3 years. His motivation for the nasal surgery was for self-improvement. He had had no nasal trauma since his previous surgery.

On physical examination he was a Fitzpatrick's type 2 skin type. The facial skin appeared thick with many sebaceous units. His face was fairly symmetric. On frontal view (▶ Fig. 99.2), the upper and middle thirds of the nose were widened and slightly deviated to the right. His nasal tip lobule was amorphous, widened, and bulbous (▶ Fig. 99.2). On lateral view, his chin appeared to have some anterior projection for a male. His nasal tip projection and nasal tip rotation (approximately 95°) were adequate and his nose was not ptotic. The lower dorsum of his nose did reveal a convexity of the cartilaginous dorsum and supratip region. With palpation of his nasal tip, the tip recoiled nicely upon removal of fingertip pressure, but was less projected than the supratip region. Intranasal examination revealed pink mucosa with

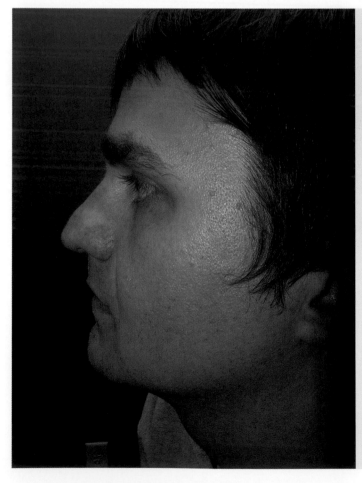

Fig. 99.1 Right lateral view of this patient.

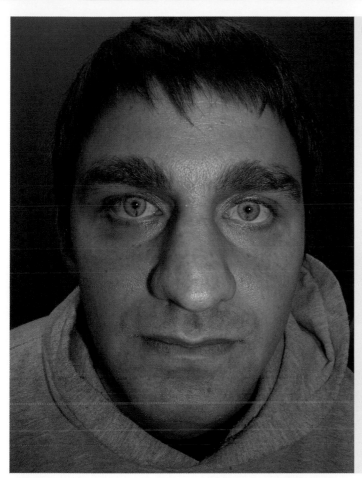

Fig. 99.2 Frontal view of this patient.

normal-size inferior turbinates. A well-healed previous marginal incision scar was present. The septum was midline. Opening the internal and external nasal valve with cotton-tipped applicators offered no changes in nasal breathing.

99.2 Differential Diagnosis—Key Points

This patient had several concerns about the external appearance of his nose, and he was presenting for revision rhinoplasty. He was realistic about his goals and expected finite changes to address specific issues. His anatomic lower dorsal elevation and supratip fullness were most likely secondary to his previous surgery. The abnormal tip-supratip relationship in this patient is referred to as a polly-beak deformity. This deformity usually results from a rhinoplasty complication leading to postoperative fullness of the supratip region and disruption of the tip-supratip relationship. The patient also had thick nasal skin; a widened upper, middle, and lower nose; a deviated upper and middle third of his nose; and an amorphous and bulbous nasal tip.

It is essential to be able to pick out important aspects of the history and physical exam that greatly impact the patient's surgical plan and postoperative outcome. The good recoil of the nasal tip showed adequate strength of underlying support structures. The patient's thick sebaceous skin would make the revision rhinoplasty more challenging and the outcome less predictable.

It is important to inspect the face in its entirety and not just the nose. This will allow you to determine overall symmetry and the relationship of the chin, cheeks, eyes, and forehead to the nose. The chin is especially important in the way the nose is perceived. In a prognathic patient, the nose will seem smaller in comparison, and in a retrognathic patient or a patient with microgenia, the nose will seem larger in comparison. In addition, skin thickness, pigmentation, and the degree of sebaceous units should be noted. All of these can influence surgical outcome.

99.3 Test Interpretation

The diagnosis and surgical plan is made exclusively on the basis of the history and physical exam. Laboratory or radiologic testing is of little benefit. However, standard rhinoplasty view photography can be helpful for the patient and surgeon. Standard oblique views include right and left lateral, frontal, and submental.

99.4 Diagnosis

Pollybeak deformity refers to the fullness of the supratip causing a convexity of the nasal dorsum with a low lying tip. This gives the appearance of a parrot's beak. There are several causes for pollybeak deformity, including loss of tip support, overresection of the bony dorsum, under-resection of the cartilaginous hump, excessive supratip soft tissue, and supratip scar formation. Soft tissue scar formation can occur when thicker skin in supratip regions is present, which causes slower contraction allowing for scar formation in the potential supratip dead space. A soft tissue pollybeak is even more likely to occur in a patient with thick sebaceous skin such as this patient. On physical exam, this patient had an excessive cartilaginous dorsum and soft tissue fullness at the supratip region.

99.5 Medical Management

Medical therapy offers some benefit in the early postoperative period. Small quantities (less than 0.1 mL) of dilute steroid (triamcinolone 10 mg/mL) injected in the subcutaneous plane (not intradermal) can help reduce early supratip edema and scar formation. Nightly paper taping over the supratip region for up to 6 weeks may also help in redraping the nasal skin.

In this case, it would be too late to institute steroid injections from the first nasal surgery. However, 1 month after the revision nasal surgery, if supratip edema persists, dilute steroid injection can be considered.

99.6 Surgical Management

Nasal surgery can be divided into three components depending on the cause of the pollybeak.

The best approach, regardless of cause, is an open approach to provide maximum exposure to all of the nasal components. This is performed by first performing bilateral marginal incisions and then incising the columella with an inverted V incision and then connecting the two incisions. Iris scissors are then used to separate the columellar skin off of the medial crura of the lower lateral cartilages. The elevation is then continued along the nasal tip and dorsum until the nasal bones are visualized. The cartilaginous framework of the nose is delivered into the field and the skin retracted superiorly.

If the pollybeak is from soft tissue only, conservative resection of this scar and subcutaneous tissue is performed and the skin is then redraped. The underlying skin should not be cauterized. A high trans-septal mucosal transfixion suture can also be placed to help reduce this dead space. If the pollybeak is from under-resected cartilage, then the extra cartilage is resected. A columellar strut can be placed concurrently to help maintain tip support. If the pollybeak deformity is overresection on the bony dorsum, then onlay grafting can be implemented. This is especially helpful for a low lying nasion.

If additional nasal tip projection is required, a tip graft (Peck's graft, 9 mm x 4 mm x 1.5 mm thick cartilage) can be placed on top of the superior aspect of the domes to increase nasal tip projection to minimize the supratip fullness. A columellar baton can be placed at the anterior columella to increase the columellar show at the columella–labial junction in this patient. Also, a medial crura strut can be placed to increase and maintain nasal tip projection. The nasal skin is then reapproximated using interrupted sutures, cleaned, and then taped. Taping and an external nasal splint are then applied.

To address his widened deviated nose of the upper and middle third, medial and lateral osteotomies can be performed. His bulbous tip can be addressed by multiple tip defining methods including cephalic trim and dome-binding sutures and dome division.

The following materials can be used for augmentation during rhinoplasty with some key points regarding their use:

- Septal—can be harvested directly in surgical field for rhinoplasty; low rate of infection.
- Conchal—easily available but is more difficult to sculpt and cannot be morselized.
- Split calvarium—very rigid and higher morbidity.
- Rib—much material is available, but surgery is more prolonged with more postoperative discomfort.
- Allograft—shorter surgical time; however, increased risk of infection and extrusion, especially in revision cases.

99.7 Rehabilitation and Follow-up

The patient returned to the clinic in 1 week for removal of the dressing. Edema are expected for up to 1 year following open rhinoplasty techniques. Intranasal crusting is removed with half-strength peroxide. Antibiotic ointment is applied for less than 1 week. Nightly paper taping over the supratip region up to 6 weeks may help the redraping of the nasal skin and reduce the empty space. The patient was instructed on proper incision care and was scheduled to return in 1 week. After one month, one can consider giving a dilute steroid (triamcinolone) injection (less than 0.1 mL, 10 mg/mL) in the subcutaneous space if needed.

99.8 Questions

1. Assessment of a patient prior to rhinoplasty should include which of the following?
   a) Assessment of facial skin type and thickness.
   b) Assessment of facial symmetry.
   c) Assessment of chin placement and size including occlusion.
   d) All of the above.
2. A 21-year-old woman comes to your office following rhinoplasty that was done when she was 18. She has an indentation in the middle third of the nose that is bothersome to her. She mentions that she previously had a large dorsal hump and that is why she pursued rhinoplasty in the first place. What is the best treatment of this deformity?
   a) Medial osteotomies only.
   b) Bilateral spreader grafts.
   c) Cephalic trim to draw the eye away from the middle third that is deformed.
   d) Columellar strut to increase tip support.
3. When using a conchal cartilage graft for rhinoplasty, what is the most important factor to consider?
   a) Extend the cartilage into the external auditory canal when harvesting.
   b) Ear cartilage is more likely to warp than rib.
   c) Excising conchal cartilage should not distort auricular contour.
   d) The patient's preoperative audiogram.

Answer: 1. d 2. b 3. c

Suggested Readings

Johnson CM, Toriumi DM. Open Structure Rhinoplasty. Philadelphia, PA: WB Saunders; 1990

Papel ID, Frodel J, Holt GR, et al. Facial Plastic and Reconstructive Surgery. 2 ed. New York, NY: Thieme; 2002

Sheen JH, Sheen AP. Problems in secondary rhinoplasty. In: Sheen JH, ed. Aesthetic Rhinoplasty. 2nd ed. St. Louis, MO: Mosby-Year Book; 1987; pp 1136 - 1365

Tardy ME, Jr, Kron TK, Younger R, Key M. The cartilaginous pollybeak: etiology, prevention, and treatment. Facial Plast Surg. 1989; 6(2):113–120

Hanasono MM, Kridel RW, Pastorek NJ, Glasgold MJ, Koch RJ. Correction of the soft tissue pollybeak using triamcinolone injection. Arch Facial Plast Surg. 2002; 4(1):26–30, discussion 31

Tosun F, Arslan HH, Hidir Y, Karslioglu Y, Durmaz A, Gerek M. Subcutaneous approximation suture for preventing soft tissue pollybeak deformity. Am J Rhinol Allergy. 2012; 26(4):e111–e114

100 Rhytidectomy (Facelift)

Douglas C. von Allmen and Ryan M. Collar

100.1 History

A 52-year-old woman presented to the office due to concerns about redundant tissue under her chin. Her friend had recently had a procedure performed to address a similar concern and she was wondering what cosmetic options were available. After further inquiry the patient stated that she felt like her skin tension was not what it used to be and she would like more definition along her jawline. She had a past medical history relevant for hypertension and her body mass index (BMI) was 30. She denied prior cosmetic surgery. She was a nonsmoker and drank alcohol socially on occasion. Physical exam revealed a well-appearing woman with normal head and neck exam including normal facial nerve function. She had fair skin with laxity in the submental region, prominent nasolabial folds, and obtuse cervicomental angle. Additionally, she had prominent wrinkles in the perioral and glabellar region.

100.2 Differential Diagnosis—Key Points

- When discussing the options for facial rejuvenation surgery it is important to identify the areas of concern from the patient's point of view. Defining expectations, goals of the procedure, number of procedures necessary, and risks of the procedure are especially important in the setting of elective surgery.
- When assessing a patient for candidacy for rhytidectomy, it is important to distinguish true laxity from intrinsic changes in the skin. Skin laxity can be improved with rhytidectomy; however, deep and fine lines can be better addressed by resurfacing techniques such as chemical peel and laser exfoliation. Favorable characteristics for surgery to address laxity include a high posterior hyoid bone and appropriate chin projection to allow for maximal elevation of the submental contour. Rhytidectomy does not address the upper third of the face and may need to be combined with additional procedures to complete the desired cohesive cosmetic result. Additionally, existing asymmetries, scars, or lesions should be documented prior to proceeding with surgery.

- Contraindications to surgery include American Society of Anesthesiologists (ASA) class IV/V, uncontrolled diabetes, steroid therapy, and connective tissue abnormalities. Smoking's known effects on vasoconstriction can affect wound healing in the postoperative phase of care. Smokers are at higher risk of skin sloughing. Similarly, excessive alcohol consumption may contribute to poor nutrition and wound healing.

100.3 Test Interpretation

Photographs should be obtained preoperatively to review with the patient, including frontal, profile, and oblique views.

100.4 Diagnosis

Submental skin ptosis resulting in rhytids and cosmetic deformity

100.5 Medical Management

Medical management is limited to medical optimization prior to surgery. Smoking cessation, optimization of nutrition, and stabilization of any medical comorbidities is important to establish prior to surgery. In addition, if the patient intends to pursue significant weight loss, surgery should be delayed until the patient reaches a stable weight to avoid further skin laxity following the loss of subcutaneous fat. Patients seeking cosmetic surgery who are unhappy with their appearance are at an inherent risk of depression and should be screened prior to surgery. Those who have undergone multiple procedures without enhanced satisfaction in their appearance may be exhibiting symptoms of body dysmorphic disorder.

100.6 Surgical Management

Rhytidectomy to address the lower face and upper neck can be performed using various approaches including the subcutaneous, sub-SMAS, deep plane, and subperiosteal techniques (▶ Fig. 100.1).

The superficial muscular aponeurotic system (SMAS) is the critical anatomic structure and plane distinguishing these approaches. The SMAS is a layer of musculature and fascia that extends from

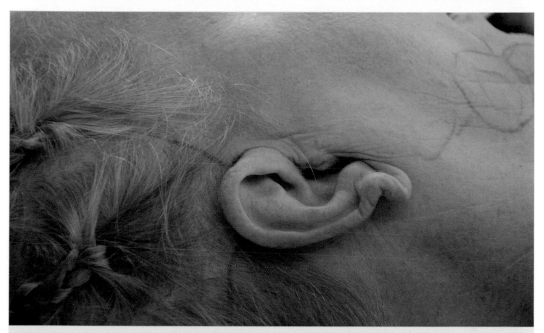

Fig. 100.1 Example of a hytidectomy incision design in a female. Vector of pull is posterior-superior.

the galea aponeurotica and temporoparietal fascia to the platysma and contains the superficial temporal artery, frontal branch of the facial nerve, and muscles of facial expression. The SMAS in the lower face is immediately superficial to the parotidomasseteric fascia and hence superficial to the facial nerve, which innervates the facial mimetic muscles from the undersurface except for the levator anguli oris, the buccinator, and mentalis muscle.

The subcutaneous approach carries the lowest risk to inadvertent facial nerve complications but results in shorter-term improvement of the jowl and does not allow for correction of the midface. In addition, the thin skin flap raised is not ideal in smokers due to potential for skin necrosis. This approach is not commonly employed for these reasons.

Sub-SMAS lifts provide longer-term improvement of the jowl and a study performed in 2015 demonstrated no significant increase in complication rate compared to subcutaneous facelift. This dissection is performed below the SMAS and superficial to the parotidomasseteric fascia and the lift can be executed as a plication or imbrication to suspend ptotic lower third facial soft tissue (▶ Fig. 100.2).

The deep plane lifting aims to correct jowling and neck ptosis, but also midface ptosis and to some degree deep melolabial folds. The approach includes additional supra-SMAS dissection in the midface to separate the malar fat pad and skin complex to allow suspension.

Subperiosteal rhytidectomy is performed by carrying dissection over the maxilla and zygoma and may be combined with endoscopic browlift. The principle difference in this technique allows for vertical elevation of the soft tissue of the midface and the orbicularis oculi may be included. While this has a potentially more dramatic effect on the entire midface and neck, there is added risk to the facial nerve, particularly the temporal and buccal branches.

100.7 Rehabilitation and Follow-up

Postoperative wound care is important both to minimize scarring and to monitor for possible complications. The most common perioperative complication is hematoma, which may occur in up to 8% of patients. Development of a hematoma may lead to skin necrosis, which will result in scarring and a poor cosmetic outcome that will overshadow the improvement in skin laxity. Best practice guidelines after extensive review of the literature in a recent study for hematoma

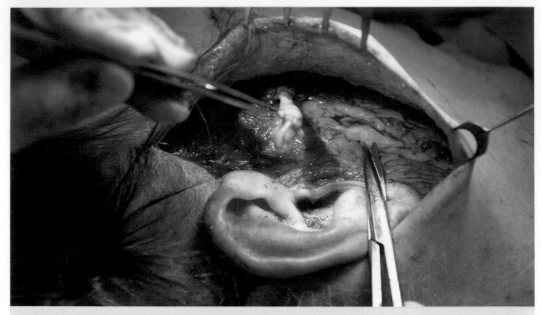

Fig. 100.2 Intraoperative facelift image demonstrating elevation of skin flap with SMAS strip excision prior to sub-SMAS dissection and plication.

prevention include the control of risk factors such as elevated blood pressure, control of pain and nausea, intraoperative hemostasis, and a pressure dressing for the first 24 hours.

100.8 Questions

1. What is the most commonly injured nerve during rhytidectomy?
   a) Temporal branch of facial nerve.
   b) Buccal branch of facial nerve.
   c) Great auricular nerve.
   d) Zygomatic branch of facial nerve.
2. Which of the following muscles is not innervated from its undersurface by the facial nerve?
   a) Buccinator.
   b) Risorius.
   c) Zygomaticus major.
   d) Orbicularis oris.
3. The orbicularis oculi muscle may be included in rhytidectomy performed with which approach?
   a) Subcutaneous.
   b) Supra–superficial muscular aponeurotic system (SMAS).
   c) Sub-SMAS.
   d) Subperiosteal.

Answers: 1. c 2. a 3. d

Suggested Readings

Flint PW, Haughey BH, Lund VJ, et al. Cummings otolaryngology-head and neck surgery. Elsevier Health Sciences, 2014

Johnson JT, Rosen CA. Bailey's Head and Neck Surgery: Otolaryngology. Lippincott Williams & Wilkins, 2013. 3103–3130

Rammos CK, Mohan AT, Maricevich MA, Maricevich RL, Adair MJ, Jacobson SR. Is the SMAS Flap Facelift Safe? A Comparison of Complications Between the Sub-SMAS Approach Versus the Subcutaneous Approach With or Without SMAS Plication in Aesthetic Rhytidectomy at an Academic Institution. Aesthetic Plast Surg. 2015; 39(6):870–876

Index